The Science
of Photomedicine

PHOTOBIOLOGY

Series Editor: Kendric C. Smith
Stanford University School of Medicine
Stanford, California

THE SCIENCE OF PHOTOMEDICINE
Edited by James D. Regan and John A. Parrish

The Science
of Photomedicine

Edited by
James D. Regan
Oak Ridge National Laboratory
Oak Ridge, Tennessee

and
John A. Parrish
Harvard Medical School
Massachusetts General Hospital
Boston, Massachusetts

Plenum Press • *New York and London*

Library of Congress Cataloging in Publication Data

Main entry under title:

The Science of photomedicine.

(Photobiology)
Bibliography: p.
Includes index.
1. Light – Physiological effect. 2. Light – Therapeutic use. 3. Photobiology. I.
Regan, James D. II. Parrish, John Albert, 1939-   . III. Series.
QP82.2.L5S35 1982   615.8′31   82-9072
ISBN 0-306-40924-0   AACR2

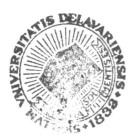

© 1982 Plenum Press, New York
A Division of Plenum Publishing Corporation
233 Spring Street, New York, N.Y. 10013

Printed in the United States of America

TO THE MEMORY OF DR. NIELS RYBERG FINSEN,

NOBEL LAUREATE, THE FATHER OF PHOTOMEDICINE

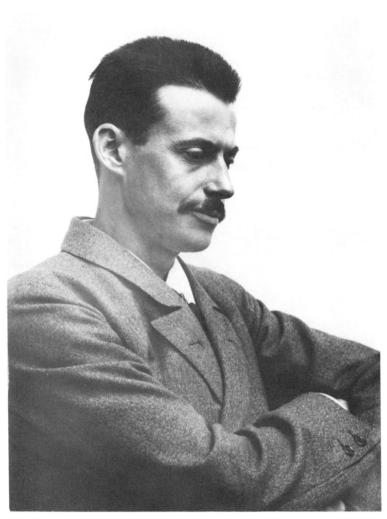

DR. NIELS RYBERG FINSEN

Contributors

R. R. Anderson • Department of Dermatology, Harvard Medical School, Massachusetts General Hospital, Boston, Massachusetts 02114

D. G. Boyle • Division of Radiation Biology, Roswell Park Memorial Institute, Buffalo, New York 14263

W. L. Carrier • Biology Division, Oak Ridge National Laboratory, Oak Ridge, Tennessee 37830

T. J. Dougherty • Division of Radiation Biology, Roswell Park Memorial Institute, Buffalo, New York 14263

T. B. Fitzpatrick • Department of Dermatology, Harvard Medical School, Massachusetts General Hospital, Boston, Massachusetts 02114

L. C. Harber • Department of Dermatology, Columbia University College of Physicians and Surgeons, New York, New York 10032

J. L. M. Hawk • Department of Photobiology, Institute of Dermatology, St. John's Hospital for Diseases of Skin, London, England

M. F. Holick • Department of Medicine, Harvard Medical School, Vitamin D Laboratory and Endocrine Unit, Massachusetts General Hospital, Boston, Massachusetts 02114; and Department of Nutrition and Food Sciences, Massachusetts Institute of Technology, Cambridge, Massachusetts 02139

W. Hubler, Jr. • Department of Dermatology, Baylor College of Medicine, Houston, Texas 77030

H. Ippen • Hautklinik und Poliklinik, Kliniken der Universität Göttingen, Göttingen, West Germany

M. Jarratt • Department of Dermatology, Baylor College of Medicine, Houston, Texas 77030

I. E. Kochevar • Department of Dermatology, Columbia University

College of Physicians and Surgeons, New York, New York 10032 Present address: Department of Dermatology, Harvard Medical School, Massachusetts General Hospital, Boston, Massachusetts 02114

N. I. Krinsky • Department of Biochemistry and Pharmacology, Tufts University School of Medicine, Boston, Massachusetts 02111

J.-L. H. Li • Department of Microbiology, University of Texas School of Medicine, Galveston, Texas 77050

J. W. Longworth • Biology Division, Oak Ridge National Laboratory, Oak Ridge, Tennessee 37830

J. A. MacLaughlin • Department of Medicine, Harvard Medical School, Vitamin D Laboratory and Endocrine Unit, Massachusetts General Hospital, Boston, Massachusetts 02114; and the Department of Nutrition and Food Sciences, Massachusetts Institute of Technology, Cambridge, Massachusetts 02139

M. M. Mathews-Roth • Channing Laboratory and Department of Medicine, Harvard Medical School, Boston, Massachusetts 02114; and Brigham and Women's Hospital, Boston, Massachusetts 02115

J. L. Melnick • Department of Virology and Epidemiology, Baylor College of Medicine, Houston, Texas 77030

W. L. Morison • National Cancer Institute, Frederick Cancer Research Facility, Frederick, Maryland 21701

W. Panek • Department of Dermatology, Baylor College of Medicine, Houston, Texas 77030

J. A. Parrish • Department of Dermatology, Harvard Medical School, Massachusetts General Hospital, Boston, Massachusetts 02114

M. A. Pathak • Department of Dermatology, Harvard Medical School, Massachusetts General Hospital, Boston, Massachusetts 02114

F. Rapp • Department of Microbiology, The Milton S. Hershey Medical Center, The Pennsylvania State University, College of Medicine, Hershey, Pennsylvania 17033

J. D. Regan • Biology Division, Oak Ridge National Laboratory, Oak Ridge, Tennessee 37830

D. E. Rounds • Pasadena Foundation for Medical Research, Pasadena, California 99101

A. R. Shalita • Division of Dermatology, Department of Medicine, State University of New York, Downstate Medical Center, Brooklyn, New York 11203

T. R. C. Sisson • Department of Pediatrics, Rutgers University School of Medicine, Perth Amboy, New Jersey 08861

R. D. Snyder • Biology Division, Oak Ridge National Laboratory, Oak Ridge, Tennessee 37830

J. D. Spikes • Department of Biology, University of Utah, Salt Lake City, Utah 84112

R. S. Stern • Department of Dermatology, Harvard Medical School, Beth Israel Hospital, Boston, Massachusetts 02215

F. Urbach • Department of Dermatology, Skin and Cancer Hospital, Temple University School of Medicine, Philadelphia, Pennsylvania 19140

T. P. Vogl • Departments of Radiology and Pediatrics, Columbia University College of Physicians and Surgeons, New York, New York 10027 Present address: Nutrition Coordinating Committee, Office of the Director, National Institutes of Health, Bethesda, Maryland 20205

C. Wallis • Department of Virology and Epidemiology, Baylor College of Medicine, Houston, Texas 77030

K. R. Weishaupt • Division of Radiation Biology, Roswell Park Memorial Institute, Buffalo, New York 14263

S. S. West • Division of Engineering Biophysics, School of Public Health, University of Alabama in Birmingham, Birmingham, Alabama 35294

Preface to the Series

Photobiology became an officially organized discipline at the national level in the United States in 1972, with the establishment of the American Society for Photobiology. The Society divided photobiology into 14 sub-specialty research areas, namely: bioluminescence, chronobiology, environmental photobiology, medicine, photochemistry, photomorphogenesis, photomovement, photoreception, photosensitization, photosynthesis, phototechnology, spectroscopy, ultraviolet radiation effects, and vision. People working in these diverse areas of photobiology could finally meet under one roof to exchange ideas and data. This intellectual exchange has provided an important stimulus to the field of photobiology.

To meet the need for a comprehensive textbook on photobiology, *The Science of Photobiology** was published in 1977. It contains chapters on each of the 14 subspecialties, written as lectures for advanced undergraduate and graduate students. For a more thorough coverage of subtopics within these 14 subspecialties, the series *Photochemical and Photobiological Reviews** was initiated in 1976.

Photomedicine is one of the subspecialities of photobiology that has shown phenomenal growth in the last few years. This has been both due to the fact that society is currently looking to science for what it can do to benefit mankind, and also because the introduction of new phototherapies by clinicians has stimulated many basic scientists to study the molecular basis of these therapies and to attempt to develop new tools for phototherapy.

When new people enter a field they usually need to do a great deal of "catching up" on the literature. The recognition of this need has led to the introduction of this treatise series on photobiology. It is most appropriate that the first treatise in this series is on *Photomedicine*.

Kendric C. Smith

*K. C. Smith (ed.), Plenum Press, New York.

Foreword

Although the history of photomedicine dates back thousands of years, with even preliterate cultures appreciating the healing properties of sunlight, for many workers in the discipline photomedicine is associated with the observation about 100 years ago of Niels Finsen, a Danish physician. Finsen recognized that people with tuberculosis who lived in Norway and who had very little exposure to sunlight often developed facial lesions (lupus vulgaris) which would decrease and sometimes disappear during the summer months. This very observant physician reasoned that artificial light ought to produce the same effect as sunlight and began utilizing the radiation from the newly available carbon arc. At first, he used a glass lens to concentrate the radiation, but since this produced considerable burning, he replaced this with a hollow glass lens filled with water. However, while this reduced the heat burns, it did not actually duplicate the effect of direct sunlight. Finally, using a hollow lens filled with water but equipped with quartz windows, Finsen was able to imitate, even improve upon, the effect of sunlight. As a result, lupus vulgaris was practically eliminated from the Scandinavian countries.

Finsen sought to understand the mechanism of how this occurred, and so he conducted some very interesting quantitative photobiology studies, using the intense artificial source with a great deal of success. The Scandinavian people were so grateful for the beneficial results of Finsen's research that they set up an institute in Copenhagen, naming it "The Finsen Institute." At that time, when no journals in this area of interest were available, the Finsen Institute published its own journal, *The Proceedings of the Finsen Institute*, offering several papers in photomedicine which, even for today, contain several important observations. Niels Finsen was highly honored and was awarded one of the first Nobel Prizes. Though he died as a young man, I had an opportunity to discuss his work with his widow at the Copenhagen Photobiology Congress in celebration of his 100th birthday, a few years ago.

It was at this occasion that I gained an even broader perspective of Dr. Finsen's accomplishments for the Scandinavian countries.

It is most appropriate to dedicate this volume to Niels Finsen, since his research truly initiated modern photomedicine. Finsen's reports were very carefully documented, always attempting to measure and provide quantitative data, which, at that time, had not become the usual practice. The Finsen Institute has developed over the years and has become one of the most important centers for photomedicine, photobiology, and radiobiology and is also developing as a center for the study of chemical mutagenesis. It is remarkable that the excellent group of investigators at the Finsen Institute conducted outstanding pioneering work during the 1930s, many years before photomedicine got its start in other countries.

Alexander Hollaender

Preface

The roots of photomedicine are ancient. Belief in the health-giving properties of sunlight stems from sun worship reinforced by an awareness that all life on earth ultimately owes its existence to the sun. In the late 19th century the health image of the sun was endowed with scientific rationale in the discovery that microorganisms were killed by invisible ultraviolet radiation. Photomedicine was further enriched when sunlight and artificial ultraviolet sources were used in the prevention and treatment of vitamin D-deficient rickets as well as the treatment of some forms of cutaneous tuberculosis. Solar and artificial sources of ultraviolet radiation could kill germs, make strong bones, and treat disease, and thus rosy cheeks or cutaneous evidence of sun exposure came to signify glowing health. But by the middle of the 20th century specific chemotherapy for tuberculosis and other infections replaced ultraviolet phototherapy or heliotherapy, and vitamin D was added to food. Except for the use of ultraviolet lamps to prevent rickets in Siberian school children and phototherapy of certain skin diseases, photomedicine began to drift back into history and folk medicine.

In the past two decades, however, there has emerged a new science of photomedicine based on molecular photobiology, scientific method, and creative use of physics and sophisticated electrooptical capabilities. Ultraviolet radiation and visible light can now be used to prevent brain damage in newborn infants, successfully treat chronic common skin disease, prevent certain forms of blindness, and perform bloodless surgery. The optical properties of human skin and other tissues are being defined and quantified. Techniques are available to selectively modify these properties by both increasing and decreasing transmission of specific wavelength regions. The details of photobiochemistry are being delineated. Synthetic photoactivated organic molecules are being designed as probes or therapeutic agents. As a result it is possible to selectively initiate specific photochemical reactions in vivo. The in vivo effects of ultraviolet radiation on normal and abnormal cells of skin, blood, and immune system are being studied and manipulated. Photochemical changes in circulating proteins, metabolites, and mediators are being described and the information applied to diagnose and explain a variety of illnesses.

This book describes the paradigms, experimental data, technical procedures, and science which form the basis of photobiology in medicine. Observations range from atomic to epidemiologic. Section I paints a broad, introductory picture of the scope of photomedicine, defines the electromagnetic radiation spectral regions of interest, and introduces a language, context, and perspective in which to place the science to follow. While the interaction of interest is that of the photon with the biomolecule, the frame of reference is the intact living human. Most of the reactions of interest take place in skin and blood, and these are the human organs most often studied by photobiologists. Visual and nonvisual photobiology of the eye is not considered in this book except in the context of potential ophthalmologic hazards of phototherapy.

Section II of this book describes the photophysics, luminescence, and photochemistry which initiate and compete with biologic responses to nonionizing electromagnetic radiation. The principles are provided in a historical perspective but in a way that instructs and reinforces the belief that understanding these laws must form the basis of practical applications of photobiology to medicine. One example is the successful use of fluorescence as a diagnostic probe. In biologic systems applicable to photomedicine, the most studied photoproducts are those derived from DNA. This is in part because of the importance of this molecule in cell regulation and replication, but also because some of the photoproducts are stable enough to study extensively. Other photochemistry occurs affecting proteins, RNA, and membrane function. Photodynamic reactions applicable to understanding human photobiology are categorized and explained.

Section III describes the interaction of normal human skin with nonionizing electromagnetic radiation and the immediate, subsequent, and long-term biologic consequences of that interaction. The optical properties of the skin and the photochemistry and photobiology of vitamin D in human skin are described and quantified. The short-term responses of normal skin to ultraviolet radiation include sunburn, suntan, and thickening. One long-term response of major importance is the malignant transformation of skin cells; skin cancer is the most common malignancy of humans. Skin is not the only organ system that reacts to ultraviolet and visible radiation. Components of blood and the immune system are also affected, with both harmful and potentially beneficial results. Section IV describes abnormal responses to ultraviolet and visible radiation which result from the presence of exogeneous chemicals or abnormal skin, immune systems, or inflammatory response. The photodermatoses are described only in a very general way. The reader interested in these disorders should use this textbook for a scientific framework and overview and study dermatology textbooks to further understand the diseases caused by or made worse by radiation. Section V gives examples of natural and synthetic agents used to protect skin from normal and abnormal reactions to sun.

The final portion of the book (Section VI) describes the scientific basis of the therapeutic applications of photobiology in medicine. Because many of the treatments began from chance observations that sun improved certain diseases, and developed by trial and error, the molecular mechanisms are not always certain. However, the laws of photophysics must still apply. This section summarizes what is known about several forms of phototherapy and photochemotherapy in the hope that an organized presentation of the molecular, cellular, and clinical facts will provide help and stimulus to those able to correct our immense ignorance in this area.

Contents

Photobiology in Medicine

The Scope of Photomedicine

J. A. Parrish

Photomedicine is the application of the principles of photobiology to the diagnosis, treatment, and understanding of health and disease. Photobiology is the study of the interactions of nonionizing electromagnetic radiation with biomolecules, and the ensuing biologic responses. Electromagnetic radiation affects living tissue in various ways. Only radiation that is absorbed can result in photochemistry. The energy of photons in the ultraviolet (UV; 200–400 nm) and visible wavelengths is sufficient to cause electronic excitation of specific chromophore molecules, leading to specific chemical reactions. Thus, use of UV and visible radiation offers the possibility of selecting among a wide variety of specific target molecules and causing specific photochemical reactions. Human color vision is an excellent example of how specific and biologically significant such processes may be. Photobiology is concerned predominantly with radiation of wavelengths 200–800 nm and with photochemical alterations in biomolecules that eventually affect the viability or function of living matter.

In contrast to the relatively specific effects of the UV and visible wavebands of electromagnetic radiation, longer and shorter wavelengths are less specific in their actions. The low quantum energy of infrared photons and microwaves excites specific vibrational or rotational modes, and therefore affects certain target molecules. However, the most significant biologic effects of these wavebands is the heating caused by such kinetic excitation. A high intensity of the radiations is usually required to be effective and the resultant effects on biologic systems is often not specific. X-rays, γ-rays, and other very high-energy, short-wavelength photons affect the highly organized and

J. A. Parrish • Department of Dermatology, Harvard Medical School, Massachusetts General Hospital, Boston, Massachusetts 02114.

complex human tissues and any other matter by relatively indiscriminate ionization of molecules. The ionized molecules are highly reactive, and bonds may be broken or formed, but since the absorption is relatively nonspecific, the ability to select "target" molecules is limited.

The general scope of modern photomedicine is broad. It includes the manipulation of exposure dose parameters and the alteration of the host with exogenous agents to maximize the beneficial and/or minimize the adverse effects of nonionizing electromagnetic radiation. This necessitates identification and quantification of the effects of that radiation on normal and abnormal human tissue. Photomedicine also includes the study of molecular and cellular mechanisms of pharmacology, chemistry, physiology, and pathology as they apply to photobiology. The study, diagnosis, treatment, and prevention of photodermatoses, skin cancer, and chronic actinic changes of skin are also important tasks within photomedicine. One specific aspect of photomedicine is the use of nonionizing electromagnetic radiation, with and without the addition of photoactive drugs, to treat disease. This represents the use of in vivo photochemistry to change the properties of metabolites and to alter the viability and function of normal and abnormal cells.

THE SKIN

Electromagnetic radiation in the range of 200–800 nm passes into the skin and peripheral circulation. The skin is the organ most often injured by UV radiation, and the organ of access for most forms of phototherapy. The skin accounts for about 15% of the total body weight and can be considered the largest organ of the body. In an adult, it is a living tissue system almost 6 ft long and 3 ft wide (approximately $2 m^2$). The skin contains cells and structures usually thought to be part of other organ systems, for example, blood cells and nerves.

Compared to most other land mammals, human beings are relatively naked. Because of a lack of insulating fur, they have developed a unique combination of features: a thick outer layer of skin with a well-developed dead horny layer, a widespread system of thermal-sensitive sweat glands and vascular overperfusion, and an extensive layer of thermally insulating fatty tissue at the undersurface of the skin (Figure 1-1). This complex arrangement allows humans to survive in a wide range of temperatures and humidities. The purpose of the skin is to protect the host from a noxious environment and to maintain a homeostatic internal milieu. The skin absorbs much of the mechanical stresses of our world and also shields us from chemicals, sunlight, and bacteria. Acting as an insulator and a selective membrane, the skin keeps the environment within the body at a relatively constant temperature and saltwater content. The skin has a vast network of nerve endings which mediate the sensations of touch, heat, and cold to provide an environmental testing

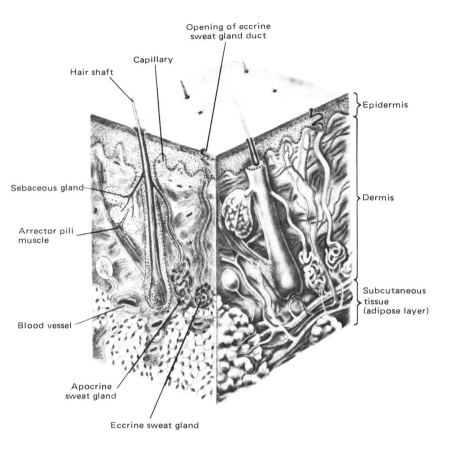

Fig. 1-1. Diagrammatic cross section of normal skin.

facility. When the skin performs these life-supporting functions normally, we notice it only for its aesthetic qualities. But if any of the protective mechanisms malfunction or become overwhelmed, we suffer embarrassment, discomfort, disfigurement, and possibly death.

The thin, outermost epidermis is composed of tightly packed sheets of cells called keratinocytes beneath a very thin but tough outer layer called the stratum corneum (Figure 1-2). The stratum corneum provides protection against water loss and surface abrasion and attenuates UV radiation before it reaches living cells. The epidermal cells are called keratinocytes because they produce keratin, which are heterogeneous fibrous protective proteins of the skin. Keratinocytes stem from a single layer of germinative cells (basal cells). After these cells divide, the daughter cells are pushed toward the surface. They no longer divide, but differentiate to form the precursors of keratin. As differentiation and outward migration continue, the keratinocytes lose their

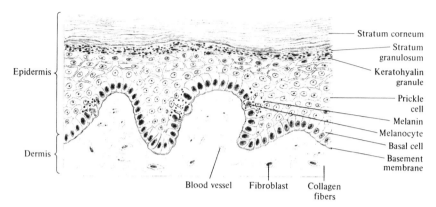

Fig. 1-2. Diagrammatic cross section of epidermis. This drawing is a magnification of part of Fig. 1-1.

nuclei, dehydrate, extrude lipids, and flatten out into dead, polygonal cells with a surface area about 25 times that of the basal cells. This closely packed, cemented, flat, dead cell layer laden with keratin and lipids forms a tough, protective stratum corneum.

Specialized cells called melanocytes reside at intervals between basal cells. These cells produce melanin, a complex biopolymer derived from tyrosine which strongly absorbs visible light and UV radiation. Dendritic processes of the melanocytes interdigitate between keratinocytes and facilitate the transfer of melanin-containing granules, called melanosomes, into the keratinocytes. These melanosomes are carried outward within the keratinocytes, and ultimately, in more pigmented individuals, some melanin may be deposited in the stratum corneum. Racial differences in skin color are mostly due to variations in the productivity of melanocytes and not in the number or size of melanocytes. Absorption of UV radiation by melanin in the stratum corneum provides some protection against actinic damage to the skin. In general, the tendency to sunburn or to develop the most common forms of skin cancer is inversely related to how much melanin is present. Increased production of melanin (tanning or melanogenesis) is induced following sufficient exposure to UV radiation.

Langerhans cells are another specialized, dendritic cell found in the epidermis, long considered to be derived from, or even precursors of, the melanocyte. It is now known that these cells are of mesenchymal origin and form part of the macrophage–monocyte component of the immune system. The Langerhans cells form a network in the upper layers of the epidermis to screen antigens entering through the skin, process the antigen, and then probably transport and present it to immunologically competent cells in the dermis.

The dermis is much thicker than the epidermis (up to 4 mm), has fewer cells, and is mostly connective tissue or fibers. Blood vessels, lymphatics, and nerves course through the dermis. The dermis provides much of the substance of skin. The dermis is mostly a semisolid mixture of fibers, water, and a viscous gel containing mucopolysaccharides. There are three types of fibers present in the dermis: collagen, reticulum, and elastin. Collagen constitutes about 70% of the dry weight of dermis. Scattered fibroblasts produce the fibers, proteins, and viscous materials of the dermis. The complex gel and fibers of the dermis create a tissue with very high tensile strength and impressive resistance to compressive force. At the same time, the tissue remains pliable and movable. Leather is animal dermis which has been modified by dehydration and certain processes (tanning) that render it stable and resistant to decomposition or bacterial decay. Besides fibroblasts, other important cellular components of the dermis include lymphocytes and mast cells that are important in immediate and delayed immune responses. The deepest layer of the skin, the subcutaneous tissue, is mainly fatty tissue and acts as an insulator and a shock absorber.

From the point of view of metabolic need, the skin is vastly overperfused with blood. The mean blood flow is many times greater than the minimum flow necessary for skin cell nutrition because cutaneous blood flow serves as a heat regulator of the entire organism and is not governed solely by metabolic requirements of the organ. Depending on body and ambient temperature, as much as 10% of the total blood volume is in the skin and thus available for exposure to UV radiation. Prolonged exposure of the skin may make it possible to irradiate a larger portion of blood and blood cells as they course through superficial skin vessels. Effects of in vivo UV radiation on blood cells and blood-borne metabolites have been demonstrated in animals and humans.

ULTRAVIOLET RADIATION

The radiation region of the spectrum has been subdivided into several bands in terms of phenomenologic effects. The subdivisions are arbitrary and differ somewhat, depending on the scientific discipline involved. Dermatologic photobiologists generally divide the ultraviolet spectrum into three portions, called UVA, UVB, and UVC, in order of decreasing wavelength (Fig. 1-3). In this text, the wavelength range from 200 to 290 nm is called UVC. Radiation of wavelengths shorter than 200 nm is mostly absorbed by air, and solar radiation of wavelengths below 290 nm does not reach the earth's surface, because of absorption by ozone formed in the stratosphere. The band from 290 to 320 nm is called UVB, and the band from 320 to 400 nm is called UVA. The division between UVC and UVB is sometimes chosen as 280 nm, and 315 nm is sometimes chosen as the division between UVB and UVA.

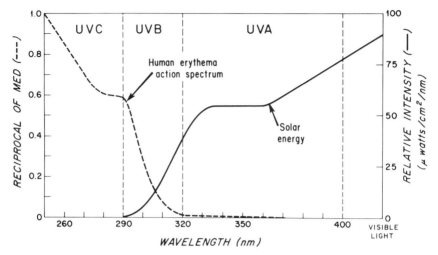

Fig. 1-3. Diagrammatic representation of human erythema action spectrum and terrestrial solar spectrum. These curves can roughly define the UV wavebands described in the text.

Because the divisions between UVC, UVB, and UVA are neither phenomenologically exact nor agreed upon, for critical work one should always define UV radiation in more rigorous spectroradiometric terms.

Radiation in the UVC band causes erythema of normal skin very efficiently and can cause photokeratitis. UVC is also called germicidal radiation because of its effectiveness in killing one-celled organisms. UVC is often called short-wave UV because the wavelengths in this region are the shortest UV radiation transmitted through air. This ultraviolet region is the furthest from the visible spectrum and is also called far-UV.

Solar UV radiation of wavelengths between 290 and 320 nm reaches the earth in relatively small quantities but is very efficient in causing sunburning of human skin. For this reason, it is often referred to as the sunburn spectrum or the erythema band. Radiation of wavelengths longer than 320 nm is relatively inefficient at causing redness of human skin. Because of its relative spectral position, UVB is also called middle-UV, mid-UV, or middle-wave-UV. The UVB portion of the spectrum has been shown to induce skin cancer in laboratory animals and mutations in bacteria. Epidemiologic evidence strongly suggests that solar UVB causes skin cancer in humans. Long-term UVB exposure is also thought to be at least partly responsible for producing the changes of exposed human skin that are commonly termed "premature" aging, or actinic degeneration.

Historically, much less attention has been paid to UV radiation of wavelengths longer than 320 nm (UVA, 320–400 nm). UVA is both melanogenic and erythemogenic, but the amount of energy required to produce an effect is orders of magnitude higher than for the UVB region. UVA is sometimes referred to as long-wave UV and is also called near-UV because of its proximity to the visible spectrum. This spectral region has also been called the blacklight region, because its principal use for many years was to excite fluorescent and phosphorescent substances that reradiate the absorbed energy as light in the visible spectrum. UVA has recently received more attention because high-intensity sources of UVA, including lasers, are now available and UVA has been shown to affect cells and microorganisms. UVA may potentiate or add to the biologic effects of UVB. Photosensitivity reactions in the skin are often mediated by UVA. There is experimental and epidemiologic evidence to suggest that solar UVA is one of the possible etiologic agents for certain kinds of cataracts in humans. UVA-induced photopolymerization and photochemical reactions are being used in industry to alter rubber, plastic, glass, metal, paper, and photographs. Photopolymerization of certain chemicals provides a convenient way to apply dental and orthopedic appliances and "photocure" them in place. The use of UVA in conjunction with photosensitizing drugs has opened up new therapeutic possibilities in chronic skin disorders.

PHOTOTOXICITY

Phototoxicity is a term sometimes used in a general way to describe cell injury or tissue alterations induced by nonionizing electromagnetic radiation, especially in the UV and visible ranges. The term has also been used with more specific meaning, but unfortunately the specific meaning varies with different texts or scientific disciplines. Some authors use the term only when chemical photosensitizers are involved, others only when no photosensitizer is present. In the context of describing in vivo use of chemical photosensitizers in complex organisms, the term is also used to separate nonimmunologic photobiologic (phototoxic) responses from those effects involving immune mechanisms (photoallergic). Phototoxicity is also used in medicine to describe acute and chronic alterations of skin by UV or visible radiation with or without the addition of chemical photosensitizers. The term is used by clinicians to describe gross morphologic changes and by pathologists to describe a complex of histologic changes induced by ultraviolet photosensitizers. Further confusion is caused by the use of the term "phototoxicity" when considering beneficial aspects of electromagnetic radiation. It is most likely, however, that phototherapy does work by injuring certain cells. Because of the confusion created by a wide variety of specific meanings for the term phototoxicity, we suggest clearly defining it when using it, avoiding using the term, or using it only in a general way to mean injury or toxicity by photons.

RESPONSE OF THE SKIN TO ULTRAVIOLET RADIATION

Multiple photochemical events occur upon absorption of ultraviolet photons within the skin. Alterations of bases in DNA have received much attention because of the importance of DNA in cell regulation and replication, the presence of nonredundant genetic sequences, and the relative stability of some of the DNA photoproducts, which makes them available for study. But many other photochemical changes occur in cells, affecting RNA, structural and enzymatic proteins, and membranes. Some of these alterations may have little effect on cells, while others may change cellular metabolism or survival or lead to the release of chemicals that later affect adjacent cells or tissues. In the first hours after radiation of skin cells, synthesis of DNA, RNA, and proteins is decreased, metabolism is altered, and histochemical evidence of cell injury is present. It is early in this period of decreased macromolecular synthesis that DNA repair is initiated. Subsequently, the cell either recovers, mutates, or dies. Expression of mutation or death may be immediate or delayed for several cell cycles.

The effects of killing individual, partially differentiated keratinocytes within the epidermis must be considered in the context of the normal structure and function of these skin cells. The most superficial living epidermal cells, which receive the highest exposure dose, are the cells that are already programmed to die as a final stage of their differentiation in becoming stratum corneum. Early death, abnormal differentiation, or malfunction of a portion of these cells may not create significant problems to the host. Presumably, mutation of the stem cells (basal layer) that supply the epidermal cell population is of greater concern because skin cancer may occur.

The response of the skin to UV exposure is, in general, a reparative and protective reaction. Over hours to days, changes in blood flow, cell kinetics, and pigment production cause grossly observable changes in the whole organ. Many of the immediate and most of the subsequent intracellular events remain unknown. Sunburn is an example of inflammation, a generalized, primitive, protective, pathophysiologic response designed to remove injurious agents. Many features of the response are similar to those caused by other irritating or toxic agents. However, UV exposure is one cause of inflammation in which no matter actually enters the tissue, often producing little heating and no physical trauma. The injurious agents of UV exposure must be certain photoproducts formed within the tissue.

Melanin pigmentation is a major defense of the skin against the acute and chronic effects of sun exposure. Constitutive pigmentation describes the individual's baseline color, and facultative pigmentation is the ability to tan in response to UV exposure. These characteristics are both genetically determined. Thickening of the epidermis is a generalized protective response often associated with inflammation. Increased proliferation of keratinocytes following UV exposure of skin leads to thickening of the epidermis and subsequently may be associated with a noticeable increase in desquamation or "peeling."

Repeated episodes of UV-induced skin injury over many years eventually cause skin cancer and the appearance of prematurely aged skin. Skin cancer is the most common malignant tumor affecting humans and comprises more than one-third of all cancers occurring in the United States—over 300,000 new cases are diagnosed and treated yearly. If properly diagnosed, most skin cancer can be removed or cured by a variety of techniques; however, these tumors still result in substantial discomfort, permanent disfigurement, and 1500 deaths annually. They also are responsible for millions of dollars in direct and indirect treatment costs. The evidence that UV radiation causes skin cancer is very convincing. Repeated experiments with animals and epidemiologic studies of humans have documented the causal relationship. Human skin cancer occurs mostly on sites of the body that are habitually exposed to sun and is more common in outdoor than indoor workers. Skin cancer in white persons is greatest in tropical climates and least in northern latitudes with little sunlight.

Repeated sun exposure over many years gradually alters the cells and fibers in the skin and leads to changes in the appearance of the skin: wrinkling and furrowing, irregular pigmentation, dilated tortuous blood vessels, and irregularly thin outer layer. It has not been shown that the microscopic, chemical, and molecular alterations of chronic sun exposure are the same as those occurring in the normal aging process. But because the cumulative sun-induced changes have come to be associated with aged appearance, the sun has been said to cause "premature aging" of skin. Any UV exposure sufficient to injure cells adds a small but finite contribution of this process. These changes occur most rapidly in persons with maximum sun exposure and little protective pigmentation. In our society, these changes may have marked impact because of our attitude toward youth and prejudice about the aged.

In contrast with all the protective, reparative, and deleterious responses of the skin to UV radiation, there is only one carefully documented, widely accepted beneficial response. Absorption of UV radiation is essential for the conversion of 7-dehydrocholesterol to previtamin D_3; the active metabolites of vitamin D are necessary for normal calcium metabolism.

Abnormal responses of the skin to the UV and visible radiation are many and include a special challenge to the photobiologist. Exaggerated or qualitatively abnormal responses occur if persons have too little protective pigment, have abnormal DNA repair, or produce or retain excess or abnormal endogenous photosensitizing chemicals such as porphyrins. Some persons also exhibit abnormal inflammation or immunologic reactions to UV or visible radiation.

Chemical photosensitivity is a term that embraces all forms of photo-sensitivity resulting from excitation of an identified chemical by electro-magnetic radiation. A wide variety of photosensitizing chemicals of thera-peutic, industrial, agricultural, or other origin may reach the skin directly or via the bloodstream, each having its own pattern of absorption, metabolism, and binding to skin components. A variety of photochemical and molecular mechanisms is involved. In general, the compounds possess highly resonant structures with a molecular weight of less than 500, and absorb radiation in the UV and visible range. Many are planar molecules.

SUNLIGHT VS. ARTIFICIAL ULTRAVIOLET SOURCES

"Artificial" or man-made sources are used more than sunlight for all forms of phototherapy and photochemotherapy of skin diseases. Booths, chambers, bed units, or cabinets are often designed to permit total-body radiation. There is a trend toward using home phototherapy units. These sources of UV radiation differ from sun in several aspects. All of these differences offer potential advantages as far as convenience and safety are concerned. Artificial sources are usually of higher intensity and the intensity is relatively constant. For example, the UVB irradiation from "sunlamps" is typically 10–20 times that of sun. This gives the advantage of inducing a given photobiologic response in relatively short exposure times. A 1-sec exposure to a UV laser or a 1-min exposure to fluorescent sunlamps may cause the same response as a 20-min sun exposure. The fact that the output is constant gives artificial sources a greater potential for accurate dosimetry. In sunlight, the intensity and spectral power distribution change with time of day, cloud cover, season, and degree of air pollution. Artificial UV sources usually emit a narrower waveband than does the sun. Omission of certain portions of UV radiation is used for selective effects such as "tan without burn" and omission of the large amounts of visible and infrared radiation normally present in sunlight reduces the heat load on the skin. The geometry of artificial radiators varies considerably and is usually quite different from sun. Booths used for phototherapy or photochemotherapy provide multidirectional radiation which allows exposure of front and back and sides at the same time. These features plus privacy and the convenience of location, and the fact that the sources are available day and night, through all weather and all seasons, offer an ease of access preferable to sun.

However, these same properties also create the potential for more harmful effects from artificial sources than from sunlight. The chief risk is overexposure. Because the UV radiation intensity is so much greater than that of sunlight, inexperienced persons are likely to overestimate the exposure time their skin can tolerate. The higher intensity also makes the regulation of exposure time more critical.

The narrow spectrum may eliminate hazardous or uncomfortable radiation normally present in sunlight, but in doing so it also eliminates some of the learned and physiologic mechanisms that protect us from solar UV radiation. Visible light can be seen, making us aware of the sun. The high intensity of visible light present in sun also protects our eyes by stimulating constriction of the pupils and by initiating an automatic response that makes us look away from extreme brightness. We can feel the heat caused by absorption of radiation from the sun. The total heat load caused by exposure to sunlight may cause us to seek the shade.

In the past it has been assumed that action spectra for sunburn, suntan, photocarcinogenesis, and premature aging were identical, but recent studies show this not to be the case. Because the action spectra for UV radiation-induced phenomena differ, the relative threshold or risk of these effects varies with wavelength. The threshold dose for acute inflammation (sunburn) is often used as a limit of exposure to UV radiation sources. Avoiding this response does not assure absence of cell injury. Also, with any change in spectral power distribution, a "sunburn" dose would carry a different likelihood of pigmentation and a different risk of cancer or other effects. For example, the threshold dose of 254-nm radiation required to induce a fixed degree of redness in skin may cause much more DNA damage than a dose of 297-nm or 313-nm radiation that induces the same redness.

The lower UV intensity of the sun relative to certain artificial sources limits UV radiation exposure in two additional ways. The total available UV dose is limited; only so much UV is present each day. Also, the effects of sunburn, although delayed in onset, may begin while sun exposure continues, signaling the victim to cease exposure.

An obvious but often overlooked danger of artificial ultraviolet sources is the fact that they are electrical equipment containing fragile and sometimes very hot glass. High voltages are necessary for the operation of the fluorescent bulbs used in most units. Fainting after standing for a long time in hot booths is another risk to be considered. Patients should be protected from the possibility of electrical shock and cuts from broken glass or metal edges.

There may be other biologic benefits or hazards related to the properties of artificial sources, but inadequate information exists. UV-induced delayed erythema is related to total exposure dose and not to intensity. That is, within wide limits, exposure to a high-intensity source for a short time or a low-intensity source for a long time results in the same degree of sunburn if the total UV dose is the same. Therefore, the high intensity itself has no effect on sunburn. This same dose–response relationship does not hold true for all cutaneous effects of UV radiation. In fact, there is evidence in animals that very low-intensity UV radiation causes more skin cancer than high-intensity radiation when the total dose is the same. It is not known how this relates to human skin cancer or how other long-term UV radiation effects relate to intensity or to elimination of other wavebands. Finally, artificial sources of

UVB generally emit some radiation of the shorter UVC wavelengths, which have not been present at the earth's surface during mammalian evolution.

THE FUTURE

Phototherapy

A variety of skin diseases will be alleviated with phototherapy as we learn more about the optical properties of human skin and how to alter these properties to selectively and spectrally increase and decrease radiation into normal and abnormal skin. Definition of precise action spectra for beneficial or harmful effects of radiation and advances in electronics and optics will permit the design of safer and more effective phototherapy. The study of waveband interactions may suggest ways to improve phototherapy of all kinds. It is unwise to assume that radiation effects caused by various wavebands making up action spectra of human cells are always additive. In complex human organs action spectra may be made up of many competing, augmentative, synergistic, and additive processes. Repair phenomena can be increased or decreased by previous, simultaneous, or subsequent electromagnetic radiation within or outside of the primary action spectrum for a given photobiologic response. Infrared radiation may modify several aspects of the sequence of events following in situ photochemistry. It is likely that photobiologic responses can be modified and risk/benefit ratios improved by increased knowledge of waveband interactions.

Photochemotherapy

Photochemotherapy is the combined use of drugs plus nonionizing electromagnetic radiation to treat disease; the site and nature of the in vitro photochemistry and subsequent photobiology are altered by supplying an exogenous chromophore. In the doses usually used, the drug alone or the electromagnetic radiation alone have no effect. Hematoporphyrin derivative is one example of a photosensitizer that selectively remains in higher concentration in malignant tissue, and has therefore been used to treat metastatic cancer. The hematoporphyrin derivative is also fluorescent, and can be used to detect tumor masses. Recently the known potent photosensitizing properties of psoralens have been better quantified and utilized to treat a variety of diseases, including psoriasis, mycosis fungoides, vitiligo and some forms of eczema.

The concept of photochemotherapy will probably prove to be more important than any specific example presently in use. Systemic delivery of photoactive chemicals is convenient and often achieves a more uniform, predictable distribution than usually permitted by percutaneous administration. In addition, the site of action of the systemically administered chemicals can be controlled at the time of subsequent photoactivation by nonionizing optical radiation, so that areas of the body not affected by disease can be shielded and spared. The depth of therapeutic action is influenced by the properties of the activating photons. Careful selection of the chemical, wavelength, timing, and intensity of exposure can produce specific effects on the viability and function of target cells, organelles, or molecules in selected body sites, including skin, blood, and organs of the body that are accessible to optical radiation using optical fibers. Photochemotherapy is a treatment modality in which specific chemical reactions can be produced in a controlled manner at specific tissue depths, in selected body sites, using photons as the activation energy.

Drug Delivery

Photochemical interactions may have considerable potential for refining the delivery of drugs, enzymes, and substrates to specific cells, tissues, and organs. For example, drugs or enzymes can be chemically bound in vitro to side chains that render them inactive. If the linking chemical bond is designed to be subsequently broken by photons absorbed in vivo after the drug has been given to the host, the drug can be subsequently released at designated tissue sites and depths by selecting appropriate wavebands of radiation.

There exists a large portion (roughly 320–800 nm) of the optical spectrum which has sufficient photon energy for activation or deactivation of chromophore-containing molecules, but may produce little effect when no chromophore is supplied. This region is therefore ideally suited for the rational design of new forms of photochemotherapy and other modalities employing photon–drug interactions. Fortunately, this same spectral region corresponds to a very broad range of penetration into the layers of skin, blood, and even internal organs. Because absorption and action spectra associated with many chromophores are broad, one can in principle set the tissue depth treated by a judicious choice of wavelength. These considerations argue strongly for use of this spectral region in designing such treatments.

Liposomes (microscopic vesicles made up of lipid bilayer membranes) can be synthesized in a way that they trap chemicals within them. Subsequent heating of these particles to the specific liquid–crystalline transition temperature induces molecular rearrangements in the membrane that allow the trapped drug to leak out. The transition temperature region varies with the lipid constitution of the liposome and can be a sharp transition within the physiologically tolerable temperature range. Liposomes filled with drug could be administered to the host and subsequent in vivo exposure to conducted heat, infrared, or high-irradiance visible or long-wave UV radiation could cause local release of drug. The timing, site, and tissue depth of the drug release is influenced by the source of the local heating and distribution of liposomes. Such therapy could be termed *thermochemotherapy*. Liposomes could be made with altered lipids that absorb in the UV spectrum that reaches blood vessels of the skin, or specific chromophores could be incorporated into the wall of the liposome. The in vitro incorporation of drug plus subsequent in vivo exposure to appropriate wavebands of nonionizing electromagnetic radiation could rupture the liposome and lead to local drug release (photochemochemotherapy). If heat-sensitive or photosensitive liposomes contained a photoactive drug, one waveband could cause release and a second waveband activate the drug at specific sites. Therefore, *thermophotochemotherapy* and *photochemophotochemotherapy* become possible selective forms of therapy. The use of heat, UVA or visible radiation, pharmacologic agents, and suction or pressure to modify local blood flow and vessel permeability add additional means of control for this type of drug delivery and activation.

Photoimmunology

This study of interactions of nonionizing radiation and the immune system is a new and comparatively unexplored area of research which promises to increase our understanding of certain diseases and certain forms of phototherapy. Exposure to UV radiation can suppress allergic contact dermatitis and classic delayed hypersensitivity, alter the immunologic response to UV-induced neoplasms, and delay skin allograft rejection. It may be possible in the future to selectively inhibit allergic reactions to antigens in the environment and alter components of the immune system so as to favorably influence diseases that have an immunologic basis.

Lasers

Diagnostic and surgical uses of lasers will expand as a function of growth in technology and increased knowledge of the optical properties of skin and blood. In addition, lasers may be used to induce nonlethal cellular changes, reversible tissue alterations, and selective destruction of specific structures or cells in skin and blood. Certain lasers may become more appropriate exposure sources for certain forms of phototherapy and photochemotherapy. The major present disadvantage of lasers for this use is their cost and limitations in treating the whole surface area of human skin. Most forms of phototherapy involve exposure of large areas of skin. If the laser beam is spread or swept over large areas, the average power is often decreased well below that available with less expensive sources. Coherence and impressive mono-chromaticity are not essential to most forms of phototherapy and photo-chemotherapy at present. However, our need for these characteristics may increase substantially as we learn more about the mechanisms and side effects of phototherapy. By careful use of the various photon densities and pulse widths made available with lasers, it may be possible to induce responses which deviate from the usual laws of reciprocity but which do not kill cells or destroy tissue. If therapeutic responses and undesirable side effects differ in their dependence on intensity, manipulation of exposure dose parameters makes it possible to make treatments more acceptable. As our understanding of both the optical and thermal properties of tissue improves, pulsed lasers may be designed specifically for microthermal destruction of blood vessels, pigmented cells, and unwanted cells or structures.

SUMMARY

The potentials of photomedicine are greatly enhanced by growth in several disciplines. Advances in electronics, physics, and optics have expanded the capabilities of optical diagnostics, photon dose delivery, and quantitative measurements of photobiologic endpoints. Many photobiologic principles, with particular emphasis on reciprocity and wavelength interactions, have been explored at the cellular and molecular levels by scientists working with plants, bacteria, and simple organisms and in the fields of photosynthesis and photochemistry. Understanding these principles makes the tasks in human photobiology less overwhelming. The effect of nonionizing optical electromagnetic radiation on mammalian cells in vitro is being defined. This information may make it possible for the creative photobiologist to improve our understanding of disease, refine our diagnostic skills, and aid in the development of new forms of treatment.

Photomedicine is photobiology applied to medicine. Human nonvisual photobiology is concerned predominantly with radiation of wavelengths 200–800 nm and with photochemical alterations in biomolecules that eventually affect the viability or function of cells. Electromagnetic radiation in the range of 200–800 nm passes into the skin and peripheral circulation. The general scope of modern photomedicine is broad and includes the manipulation of exposure dose parameters and the alteration of the host with exogenous agents to maximize the beneficial and/or minimize the adverse effects of nonionizing electromagnetic radiation. One specific aspect of photomedicine is the therapeutic use of in vivo photochemistry to change the properties of metabolites and to alter the viability and function of abnormal cells. Advances in chemistry, electrooptics, and photobiology make it possible to explore new forms of therapy that include light-sensitive drug-delivery systems.

ACKNOWLEDGMENTS. This work was supported by NIH Grant AM 25395-02 and by funds from the Arthur O. and Gullan M. Wellman Foundation.

II

Photophysics, Luminescence,
and Photochemistry

2

On Light, Colors, and the Origins of Spectroscopy

J. W. Longworth

PROLOGUE

The progress of science can be regarded as layers interconnected into an elaborate network:

1. Paradigms which summarize and predict data: the laws of science.
2. Experimental data: scientific research.
3. Technical devices and procedures: scientific instruments, methods, and materials.

A fourth layer could be included, a goal or inspiration.

My goal in this introductory article is to present a succession of histories which are connected into a network drawing from these three layers and which illustrate the present research practice of photobiology. The work of the pioneers often provides the crucial concepts in a clear way and one that is close to everyday experience. I hope the reader will capture, as I have, the inspiration in the spectacle of the rainbow, the iridescent glint of cobwebs, the brief brilliance of lightning. There is beauty in the spectrum created with a wedge of glass, the blue glow from a gin-and-tonic at a summer picnic, or the

J. W. Longworth • Biology Division, Oak Ridge National Laboratory, Oak Ridge, Tennessee 37830.

warmth of the sun on a spring day. These lead to the discovery of the dispersion of refraction defined in Snel's law, Stokes' law of fluorescence, and the existence of infrared radiation. Our tools are an apparent bending of a fishing line in a pond, a photographic plate, or an electric light. Inevitable with the development of a new tool, there is collection of data, which instigates a systematizing paradigm that may then account for the inspiration that led to the development of the tool or at least provides a fabric of understanding.

Photobiology has at its heart the exchange of energy between electromagnetic radiation and organic molecules. Photobiology applies the laws and methods of photophysics and utilizes spectroscopic instruments and photoelectric detectors. These then are the three layers. The fourth is the response of living organisms to light: vision, sunburn, photosynthesis, etc.

DISCOVERY OF THE SOLAR SPECTRUM

The rainbow must always have attracted interest and aroused curiosity as to its cause, but it remained mysterious until the studies of Issac Newton at his home of Woolsthorpe Manor in Colsterworth during January 1666 and later that summer in his rooms at Trinity College, Cambridge (1).

A crucial early step leading to the analysis of Newton was the rediscovery of the concept of one-point perspective in the Renaissance, lost since the Romans. This was first used by the Florentine architect Filippo Brunelleschi between 1410 and 1415 in a lost fresco and then in his drawings, but was applied to the full in a painting by Masaccio in his trinity fresco in the church of Sta. Maria Novella, Florence, painted in 1427. These principles of perspective were codified and written about in a widely read text from Leon Alberti (1a). In the mid-16th century a Sicilian optical physicist, Francesco Maurolico (2), used these same principles with a heliocentric perspective to account for the rainbow having a constant arc and being subject to rising and falling with the sun. Light travels in a straight line centered on the sun and describes a circular arc before the viewer, upon rain drops. There is in some manner a special angle for the "reflection" and this creates the rainbow with the sun behind and high in the sky. Maurolico had departed from the classical tradition which placed the observer at the center of the meteorological sphere and the sun on the periphery, which failed to give a constant arc. Maurolico also defined seven colors he could observe in the rainbow (Appendix A). Johannes Kepler (3), then working in Prague, in 1611 suggested that there were refractions and an internal reflection within the drops of rains, and that these would in some manner cause the appearance of a rainbow. Kepler was clearly seeking the basis for the special angle of Maurolico, but Kepler never was able to develop any law for refraction and unlike Maurolico he stayed with the mediaeval perspective. In the same year a Croatian, Marko Antonije

Dominis, then Archbishop of Split, suggested that a varying refraction angle and an internal reflection was responsible in some unspecified fashion for the appearance of colors; Dominis used the perspective of Maurolico. These then are the ingredients for a correct explanation (4).

An exact law for the refraction of light was determined by Willebrord Snel of Leiden in 1621. The results of Snel were published by Rene Descartes (5). Descartes applied Snel's law to two refractions and a reflection within a drop of rain. He carried out extensive calculations for many angles and Descartes discovered there was a maximum angle, and so convincingly demonstrated there was a special range of angles that will cause the appearance of a bright arc of reflection of the sun. But Descartes had no explanation for the color of the rainbow (5). All these works were known to Newton, who graduated from Cambridge at the age of 22 in the spring of 1665. Since the University closed for two years following Newton's graduation because of the plague, he began two years of studies in his home in the Lincolnshire countryside. These are the *anni mirabili* for the calculus, celestial mechanics, optics, and the science of human color vision. Newton purchased glass prisms at a countryside fair, since he knew that a glass wedge broke up light into colors and he wished to investigate this phenomenon. He first viewed a red and a blue strip of paper placed side-by-side through a prism and noticed there was an apparent displacement. Light of different colors is refracted to different extents; there is a dispersion in the value of the refractive index (Fig. 2-1).

Newton then let sunlight into a darkened room through a pinhole in a window shade and used a lens to form an image on a screen, passing the light through a prism. The earliest experiments did not use a lens. A continuous stripe of colored images was formed, with violet at the top and red at the bottom of the screen, creating "vivid and intense colors which was at first a very pleasing divertissement." Newton termed this a spectrum (Fig. 2-1). He concluded that solar radiation was a heterogeneous mixture which could be

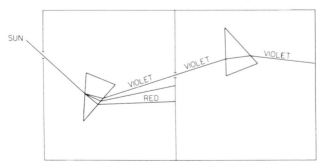

Fig. 2-1. Formation of the spectrum and demonstration of the heterogeneity of white light by Newton.

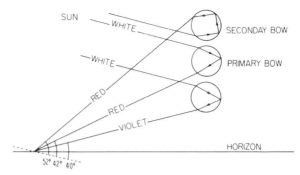

Fig. 2-2. Formation of a rainbow by reflection from raindrops, according to Descartes and Newton.

dispersed by the varying refraction. Further passage of a single color, isolated by another pinhole in the view screen, through a crossed prism only refracted the colored light further, without producing any new color (Fig. 2-1). This light was homogeneous, which he termed monochromatic. In describing has spectrum Newton said, "Strictly speaking light is not colored, rather it elicits the sensation of color in the human mind." By using a parallel prism he reconstituted white light, and this began his studies upon human color vision.

Newton could explain the colors of the rainbow and then used his newly developed method of calculus to determine the special angle or extremum. He could also now calculate the angle for the second bow and show why there is dark between the two bows (Fig. 2-2). A simple mathematical model fully describes a natural phenomenon, the origins of mathematical physics.

We now know that Newton failed to observe any dark regions within the solar emission spectrum. He realized that a pinhole would create a mixture of colors at a given location, and this could be minimized by using an oblong or slit as the source of sun radiation. With a slit source Newton still did not notice any dark lines; this must have been because of the poor optical quality of the surfaces and the glass, of which he made many complaints in his writings, though England in that period produced the best available quality of optical components. These studies were described in Newton's first scientific paper in 1672 (6). The spectroscope with a collimating lens and a pinhole source continued to be used by other workers for more than a hundred years.

Measurement of Radiation with Instruments

In 1800 William Herschel extended the range of radiation known for the solar spectrum by using an instrument, rather than the human eye, to detect the radiation. Knowing that a lens will focus the sun and burn paper, he placed a thermometer in the various colors in the solar spectrum. He found that the thermometer was heated the most by a region of the spectrum beyond the red light. This showed there is infrared radiation in solar emission (7). The next year (1801) a Jena physician, Johann Ritter (8), using the prior observations of Carl Scheele (9) of the blackening of silver chloride crystals by white light (8), investigated the effectiveness of different colors. He showed that radiation beyond the violet was most effective, and thus there is ultraviolet radiation emitted by the sun.

By the beginning of the 19th century, through the use of instruments, scientists were able to divide the solar emission spectrum into three regions: Ritter, Newton, and Herschel (ultraviolet, visible, and infrared). This was later extended to include gamma, x, and vacuum-ultraviolet radiation (Villard, 1900; Röntgen, 1895; Schumann 1893) in the high-energy region and millimeter and micrometer and radio radiation (Rubens and Nichols, 1897; Nichols and Tear, 1923; Hertz, 1887) in the low-energy range, comprising the electromagnetic radiation spectrum.

The studies of Herschel and Ritter set the stage for the development of photography. In 1802 Thomas Wedgewood worked with Humphry Davy to produce silhouettes on paper soaked in silver nitrate, but they were not permanent. Joseph Niépce (1826) produced a permanent image of a farmyard formed on the surface of an asphalt block. The black material absorbed the heat, and the evaporation hardened the illuminated areas, which were not dissolved by oil, while the unevaporated regions were. Thus a photoresist was produced which could be used to print an image, a photogravure print. In 1835 William Fox Talbot soaked paper in silver chloride, and the light darkening formed an image which he fixed by extracting unreacted silver chloride. Louis Daguerre, in 1837, coated a copper surface with silver, which was then exposed to iodine vapor. Using a method developed by John Herschel (1839) to fix the negative image, Daguerre extracted the unexposed silver iodine with sodium thiosulfate, and fixed the silver image with mercury to produce the dramatically detailed images which still impress today.

Instruments extend the range of the solar spectrum and allow permanent and quantitative measurement of radiation.

Measurement of Wavelength

It is obviously important to quantitatively define the colors that can be seen in the solar emission spectrum. Our story begins with the observations of a Bolognian physicist, Francesco Grimaldi. In 1660 Grimaldi (10) studied the shadow cast by an edge illuminated from a pinhole source of sunlight, a sunbeam. There was light within the shadow, which was tinted with the hues of the rainbow, forming a gradation of colored light or fringes. Light was not propagated strictly rectilinearly, but rather was diffracted by the edge. Grimaldi continued these observations by scratching a series of closely spaced lines upon a mirror; in viewing large angular reflections he noticed the formation of the colors seen in the rainbow. In 1664 Robert Boyle (11) described the color seen in reflections from thin films of mica or oil layers formed on the surface of water. These are the colors familiar in our childhood from bubbles of soap, or the weak supernumerary colored rings that occur inside the bright blue primary arc of the rainbow, or the atmospheric corona rings surrounding the sun viewed through rain. Boyle's assistant at the Royal Society, Robert Hooke, produced thin films of air by contacting two lenses of long focus. When viewed in reflection, an image with a complex sequence of colored rings is seen (black, blue, white, orange, red, violet, blue, green, yellow, orange, red, etc.) (12). Newton, learning of this work when he gave an account of his studies in London to the Royal Society in 1672, improved upon the observation of Boyle and Hooke. The thin film of air was produced by contacting a lens of large focus with a flat plate. With this precise geometry, Newton could calculate directly the thickness of the film or air associated with a particular colored ring (13). Newton noticed a central dark spot and a progression of colored rings with varying width. This procedure is still widely used to test the quality of optical surfaces.

The English physician Thomas Young explained the production of these colored effects in 1801 (14). He extended the work of Grimaldi by illuminating two adjacent slits with a light beam isolated by a narrow slit. A pattern of light and dark images was formed on a screen, which Young could account for by an interference between two waves. Light was described as a wave. In 1802 Young, (15) recognized that the colors of Boyle, Hooke, and Newton were the consequence of an interference of light reflected from the upper and lower surfaces of the air films or thin materials. Young calculated the wavelength of light for the seven colors recognized by Newton (violet, indigo, blue, green, yellow, orange, and red) (Appendix A). Young used the measurements of Newton (16), and the values he calculated are remarkably close to modern values.

A prism disperses radiation into a spectrum, but does not allow a direct measure of wavelength nor a measure that can be readily reproduced by other workers. Interference of light by thin films would provide a means to accurately measure wavelength when the thickness of the film is known. The magnitude and the need for flat surfaces was beyond the resources of the age. Today this is the method used to define a unit for length.

Another device was needed, and the germ for the idea lies in the observations of Grimaldi. David Rittenhouse, a Philadelphia astronomer, following Huygens, used spider cobwebs to create graticules for precision astronomical measurements. Perhaps he had noticed the iridescent glint of light reflected at large angles from a web. In 1788 he determined the angular diffraction of the spectral colors from an array of silk threads (4 threads/mm) (17). Joseph Fraunhofer, a Munich optical instrument designer, needed to quantitatively define the wavelength of light to better measure the index of refraction of optical glasses to be used in instruments. In 1821, he suspended thin silver wires between fine screws around their threads to form a framework of parallel wires or a grating (19 wires/mm) (18). With this device he measured the angular diffraction of his transmission grating and, using the procedure of Young, could directly calculate the wavelength. Applying a procedure originated with Grimaldi, Fraunhofer cut grooves onto a plate of glass with a diamond tool controlled by a precision screw, and by 1823 he could rule a diffraction grating with 300 lines/mm (19). He greatly praised the engine used to rule the diffraction gratings, though he never provided details of its design. With the diffraction gratings he fabricated, Fraunhofer was able to measure wavelengths extremely close to modern values in the solar spectrum or sodium light.

The diffraction grating provided the means to quantitatively measure the wavelength of radiation, though the prism spectroscope or photographic spectrograph provides an inexpensive survey tool which is still widely used.

Discovery of Absorption Spectrum

William Wollaston, working in his private laboratory in London in 1802, viewed the solar emission spectrum of a slit image rather than a pinhole (20). There was not a continuous gradation from one hue to the next; rather, there were dark regions of the spectrum, dark lines across the bright spectrum. He called these absorption lines "regions of the spectrum lacking light." Fraunhofer studied these lines extensively in 1817 and reported there were at least 754 lines (21). To achieve these results he greatly improved upon the Newton spectroscope by viewing the spectrum with a small telescope. He was able to measure the angles accurately, and the basic design of the prism spectroscope (collimator lens, prism, and telescope), has remained largely unaltered since then.

Discovery of Emission Spectrum

Another source of radiation besides the sun is flames, and the different colors of flames are exploited for entertainment with fireworks; a textbook on the art of using high temperatures and the color of flames to identify metals was published in the Renaissance (22). This ancient fact was not appreciated by early spectroscopists. Thomas Melvill, using a pinhole spectroscope, associated the bright yellow color of sodium flames with the presence of salt (23); this is the familiar yellow color of a candle. With his slit spectroscope, Wollaston (20) noted that there were various intensities and colors of emission from flames of different materials. The capability of the grating spectroscope was such that in 1823 Fraunhofer resolved the yellow sodium light into two closely similar wavelengths. There are characteristic emission lines emitted by elements in a flame. Moreover, Fraunhofer commented upon the identity of these two wavelengths and two absorption lines of the solar emission spectrum. This led him to suggest that in some way there must be sodium present in the sun—the beginnings of both astrochemistry and flame spectrophotometry. This suggestion removed an opinion of the pioneer sociologist Auguste Comte (1810) that we could never know the composition of stars because of their distance from earth.

DEVELOPMENT OF ARTIFICIAL LIGHT SOURCES

Introduction of modern artificial sources of light awaited the development of a convenient source of electricity. At first only electrodeless electrostatic discharges were used to create light. In 1791 Luigi Galvani, a Bolognian physician, pressed a copper hook into the spinal column of a frog and hung this hook from an iron rail; he noticed that muscle twitching occurred (24). The Pavian physicist Alessandro Volta realized in 1792 that the frog muscular contraction was acting only as an electroscope. He placed a copper coin and a zinc coin on opposite sides of his tongue and on connecting them with a copper wire sensed a salty taste (1797). Electricity was being produced by the dissimilar metals. Instead of his tongue, Volta then used a disk of paper soaked in salt solution, and he constructed a pile of coins (silver and zinc) separated with soaked disks. This pile was a source of high-current, low-voltage electricity—the voltaic pile (1800). Humphrey Davy demonstrated in 1808, at a Friday evening discourse in the Royal Institution, an electric discharge in air between two horizontal electrodes made from carbon. When he struck the arc with a third carbon rod to briefly reduce the electrode separation, a bow of light, or an arc discharge, occurred. This was an intense white source of radiation—artificial sun radiation. Such arc lights were introduced (1878) in use as street lighting and remained in the City of London until 1890 because of their resemblance to sunlight.

ORIGINS OF CHEMICAL SPECTROSCOPY

At the beginning of the 19th century, then, there were the essentials for spectroscopy: artificial sources of radiation (carbon arcs and gas flames), precision slits used as the source of radiation in spectrographs, ruled gratings to diffract light, and thermal and photochemical devices to detect radiation quantitatively. During this century the spectrographs were applied to chemical and biologic studies.

Newton had noticed that flames were mostly of similar color, and he concluded that all materials would produce the same color. He ignored fireworks and turned his back upon associating characteristic flame colors with specific chemicals. No doubt this was not helped by his inability to discern absorption lines in the solar emission spectrum. The prevalence of sodium as a contaminant in inorganic samples perpetuated this view. With improved purity and resolution, the abundance of calcium, carbon, and nitrogen provided additional complications.

Viewing the solar emission spectrum after it had passed through a sodium flame, Leon Foucault in 1848 noticed that the Fraunhofer D absorption line became darker. He suggested that sodium in the flame had absorbed that light. When the flame alone was viewed, there were two bright D emission lines. Gustav Kirchhoff in 1859 described the relationship between absorption and emission (25, 26) from thermodynamic considerations. Two bodies radiating the absorbing radiation will remain at the same temperature, so there must be an equivalent absorption associated with emission for the two sources. Realizing this relationship between the extents of absorption and emission, Kirchhoff joined his research with that of a chemist, Robert Bunsen, and together they began a study of the absorption and emission of the now available pure elements in gas flames (27, 28). The familiar tubular burner with a throttled base air inlet was designed by Michael Faraday. Bunsen and Kirchhoff described how specific elements had individual and characteristic emission and absorption spectra and that flame emission could be used to qualitatively and quantitatively determine the composition. Kirchhoff could now explain the origin of Fraunhofer's absorption lines. The absorption was a result of the elements in the cooler, outer regions of the sun absorbing emission from the hot, central region. He found sodium light of a bright flame was dimmed by passage through another flame (27, 28).

David Brewster used a slit-prism spectroscope to study the absorption properties of organic materials. He investigated several complex natural products that could be obtained with good purity, particularly chlorophyll, which was extracted by hot alcohol from nettle leaves (29). These studies in 1833 disclosed that light was absorbed in a characteristic way by natural products and the absorption occurred over a wide spectral interval, which he termed absorption bands. In 1862 William Miller (30) made quantitative measurements of absorption bands by using the newly developed (1851) wet photographic plate of Frederick Scott Archer and was able to extend the studies into the ultraviolet region. George Stokes used a fluorescent screen to visualize ultraviolet radiation (31) and in 1864 reported on the absorption bands of simple organic compounds in the ultraviolet region (32). In 1872 Walter Hartley in Dublin acquired the quartz prism spectrograph from Miller and also had the sensitive silver bromide gelatin dry plates just devised (1871) by R. L. Maddox and produced commercially by Joseph Swan (1877). A systematic photometric spectroscopy of simple organic materials was possible, and this took place during the rise of organic chemistry (33). Hartley associated a characteristc absorption spectrum with moieties that constituted a part of the organic compounds, with he called chromophoric groups (34).

Discovery of Phosphorescence

Vincenzo Cascariolo (1603), a Bolognian cobbler and alchemist, found that heavy spar, a barium sulfate mineral found near Bologna on Monte

Paterno, after being calcined (reduced with charcoal) to BaS, glowed yellow in the dark following a brief exposure to sunlight. The rock was known as lapis solaris and became an object for collection during the Grand Tour of Europe by the aristocracy. The existence of the stone achieved widespread knowledge after it was described by the Jesuit scientific reporter Athanasius Kircher of Fulda (35). He also described the fluorescence of Eysenhardtia wood extracts, which brought attention to fluorescence.

Phosphorescence from other substances, both organic and inorganic, was found as a result of a visit to a patient by the Bolognian physician Jacopo Beccari. The patient was resting in a shaded room during her lying-in and drew Beccari's attention to her diamond ring, which she said would glow brightly when moved into the shade. This observation had actually been made much earlier by Benvenuto Cellini (36). Returning home, Beccari discovered that one of his own diamonds had this property of glowing in the dark. Becarri had built a light-tight box into which he could enter and become dark-adapted. An entrance into the box made of a rotating turret allowed materials to be exposed to light, rapidly rotated into this dark room, and then observed by the dark-adapted human eye; this device was the Beccari box or phosphoroscope. Beccari quickly discovered that the exposure to sunlight need not be long to create phosphorescence, that sunlight was more effective than sky light, and that least effective was sunlight which had passed through a glass window. The phosphorescence of many materials was of short duration (37). The next year Beccari found that his freshly washed hands shone brightly when they were chilled by the frost that January (38). He had discovered the ultraviolet-excited phosphorescence of protein, which required cold material to reduce oxygen quenching. To achieve appreciable excitation, the urocanic acid which accumulates in human skin must be extracted with water (39). Our hindsight makes us realize the significance of direct January sun radiation, cold hands, and the fresh washing of the hands, together with the use of an extremely sensitive light detector.

Beccari relied upon the relatively long duration of phosphorescence to devise a mechanical means to move a sample from exposure to exciting radiation to observation of phosphorescence emisson. This principle is still used to isolate phosphorescence. Edmond Becquerel greatly improved upon the Beccari phosphoroscope by revolving two slotted disks on the same shaft with the sample between such that the sample is alternately excited and viewed (40). In an alternative design, a slotted can surrounds the sample and is rotated. With machines of this type, phosphorescence that exists from 100 μ sec to many seconds could be investigated. Becquerel was never able to detect phosphorescence from fluids. By varying the rotation and slotting of the disks he demonstrated that phosphorescence decays exponentially with time after cessation of excitation (41). Eilhard Wiedemann found that dyestuff solutions made extremely viscous by addition of gelatin or by forming a sucrose glass, a candy, emit both fluorescence and phosphorescence (42). James Dewar created rigid solutions by cooling fluids to liquid air temperature and discovered the presence of a strong phosphorescence (43). Wiedemann and Gerhart Schmidt emphasized that phosphorescence originated from metastable chemical species and that this species was associated with a new absorption. (44–47).

The association of fluorescence with a nanosecond exponentially decaying event and phosphorescence with a millisecond or longer exponential decay from organic dyestuffs is found in the studies of Sergei Vavilov and Vadim Levshin (48, 49). Fluorescence is a higher energy emission and of short duration; an energy level diagram summarizing these observations was first provided by Alexander Jablonski (50).

Phosphorescence from simple aromatic organic materials was observed by Eugen Goldstein (51, 52) and both fluorescence and phosphorescence were observed by Kowalski (53–55). Though both reported luminescence spectra in detail and both used liquid air to form alcohol glass solution, some of the emission spectra they described are now known to be from radicals created by the intense and long-duration exposures used to collect the emission spectra.

Gilbert Lewis and his co-workers suggested several possibilities concerning the nature of the metastable species that emits phosphorescence, among which they included a triplet state (56). Aleksandr Terenin made similar suggestions (57). Neither report, however, strongly favored the triplet state. Lewis pursued the possibility of phosphorescence coming from a triplet state, and in 1945 with Melvin Calvin he measured a photoparamagnetism (58). Doubts were cast upon the measurements (59), but the photoparamagnetic measurements were later shown to be substantially correct when Evans (60) reported that phosphorescence intensity and photoparamagnetism decayed with identical time durations. Phosphorescence was emission from the triplet state and fluorescence was emission from the singlet state of an organic molecule. Wiedemann and Schmidt, and later Lewis and co-workers, had noted the transient absorption accompanying the presence of the triplet state. Oxygen interacts strongly with triplet states and quenches or reduces their lifetime. In fluid media there is abundant oxygen, and effort has to be made to eliminate oxygen so that a phosphorescence can be observed but the intensity is still weak from triplet excimer quenching.

Pieter Musschenbroek, a Leiden physicist, and George Kleist, the Dean of Kamień Cathedral in Pomerania, independently discovered the air capacitor in 1745, and this provided a source of high-voltage electricity. Giovanni Beccaria, a priest at Turin, excited phosphors with radiation from a spark discharge from a Leiden jar, including some phosphors he obtained from Beccari (61). A more extensive study was performed by the mayor of Warsaw, Karl Körtum, in 1794; he excited many phosphors, following the work of Beccari, with radiation produced by capacitative spark discharge (62). The ultraviolet radiation is the predominant cause for these excitations of Beccaria and Kortum. In 1810 Jean Dessaignes (63) excited phosphors by a spark in an evacuated chamber, though he attributed the excitation to electricity and not ultraviolet radiation. Joseph Heinrich (64) realized in 1812 that it was radiation, and noted that phosphors that were excited by the ultraviolet radiation of the sun were also readily excited by spark discharges. Charles Wheatstone in 1835 produced intense pulses of radiation by discharging a bank of capacitors (65). In 1839 Becquerel (66) demonstrated that the ultraviolet radiation produced by spark discharges could be readily transmitted by quartz, but not by glass Joseph Henry (1845) found the aurora borealis would excite quinine fluorescence from its UV components. In 1852 Stokes found that lightning readily excited fluorescence and realized that a spark discharge was a brief and intense pulsed source of ultraviolet radiation. George Porter and Maurice Windsor (67) combined these concepts and produced short-duration and intense ultraviolet radiation pulses which rapidly form large concentrations of triplet states. The transient absorption of the triplet states was detected with an apparatus little altered in principle from those of Newton and Stokes, or the radiation sources of Kortum and Wheatstone.

Discovery of Fluorescence

A blue fluorescence from water contained in cups of fresh wood of the medicinally important Northern Mexican shrub *Eysenhardtia polystacha* (kidney wood) was first noticed by the early Spanish botanical explorer Nicholas Monardes in 1577 (68).* Cups of the wood were much sought after, and news of the blue fluorescence became well known through the reports of Kircher (35). Boyle (11) carefully studied the fluorescence and discovered that the blue color would disappear or quench in concentrated solutions or in solutions to which acid or alkali had been added. Brewster in 1833

(29) reported on the bright red fluorescence of alcohol solutions of chlorophyll, a more accessible natural product. He observed that the green solutions gave off a red color when a beam of sunlight passed through the solution and was viewed from the side. He found that this red emission was not polarized. John Herschel (69, 70) discovered in 1845 that concentrated solutions of

*Monardes comments briefly upon his observation of a blue fluorescence in a chapter entitled, "Of the Woode for the Evilles of the Raines and of the Urine." He wrote of a "white woode which gives a blue color" when placed in water that was good "for them that doeth not pisse liberally and for the paines of the Raines of the stone." The fluorophore is a complex isoflavanoid, agustlegorretosin, related to pterocarpin of red sandlewood (*Pterocarpus santalinus*) of the Philippines with similar fluorescent and medicinal properties (174). Similar compounds are found in cloves and pea and are fungicides; there is a similarity to rotenoid insecticides.

quinine sulfate gave off a blue fluorescence only from the irradiated surface of the liquid. The Irish physicist Stokes reinvestigated these studies of Boyle, Brewster, and Herschel and, in a 100-page paper, described all the principal characteristic features of fluorescence (71). Anders Angström unknowingly performed studies similar to Stokes (1855). He coined the word fluorescence*, which he then adopted throughout a short follow-up paper (72). Stokes identified fluorescence as an emission band, using the crossed prism spectroscope of Newton. The fluorescence emission band was always lower in energy than the absorption bands of the compounds, a feature now known as Stokes' law of fluorescence. Because of this property, fluorescene could be excited and viewed through complementary glass color filters, which is still the basis for simple fluorimeters. Stokes had placed a quinine sulfate solution by an open window and noticed that this colorless solution fluoresced stongly when irradiated by a lightning flash. Heinrich (64) and Becquerel (66) had found that there was an intense ultraviolet component in an electric spark discharge, so Stokes realized that ultraviolet radiation can be visualized by the brilliant blue emission of a quinine sulfate solution—a phenomenon, like the spectrum, which is always attractive. He also concluded from this observation that the existence time for the state that emits fluorescence must be brief. Becquerel (1843) visualized ultraviolet radiation with a powdered phosphor attached to paper with gum arabic, and in 1862 Stokes (31) used filter paper soaked in quinine sulfate or uranyl salt glasses to visualize ultraviolet radiation. In 1839 Becquerel had found that quartz transmitted radiation which excited phosphorus from electric discharges whereas glass did not (66). Stokes, using a fluorescent screen, showed that quartz was transparent to a large interval of ultraviolet radiation, and hence dispersing prisms and containers could be fabricated from quartz. He used Wheatstone's capacitor electric spark discharge to detect strong ultraviolet emission lines from many metal elements.

Development of Quantum Spectroscopy

A rigorous interpretation of the nature of fluorescence and phosphorescence required the development of quantum spectroscopy. Its origins stem from further exploration of the metal spark discharge emission (Schuster, 1877) and spectra from low-pressure gases (Plucker, 1859). A regular distribution of emission lines was noted in sodium and magnesium by Eluthère Mascart in 1869 (73). A similar regularity was noticed in H_2 by Stoney in 1870 (74), and in 1871 Louis Soret reported a mathematical relationship for the spectral emission lines of magnesium (75). The crucial

*Abbe Rene-Just Hauy, professor of minerology at the Museum National d'Histoire Naturelle in Paris, commented upon the blue coloration of crystals of fluorspar in light in 1801 (175). Stokes showed that fluorspar emitted a blue light and said, "I am inclined to coin a term and call it fluorescence, from fluorspar, as the analogous term opalescence is derived from the name of a mineral."

report was an ansatz which fitted the visible emission lines of H_2 that had been discovered by David Alter in 1854 (76, 77). This relationship was provided in 1885 by a Swiss mathematics teacher, Johann Balmer (78), and the ansatz accurately predicted the observed progression of lines from the red to a limit in the ultraviolet. The significance of the regularities became apparent with the Bohr (79) model for the atom.

Development of Artificial Light Sources for Spectroscopy

To further laboratory spectroscopic studies, an artificial source of radiation was essential, especially if the ultraviolet region was to be explored, and this is the spectral interval occupied by simple materials. Davy in 1822 noticed the intense greenish emission from an electric spark in mercury vapor (80). In 1836 Wheatstone (65) produced spark discharges between electrodes connected across air capacitors (Leiden jars) charged to a high voltage with an electrostatic generator engine similar to the Wimshurst machines of 1875— which charge up your hair in science museums. Wheatstone introduced mercury into the spark discharge and then into a carbon arc discharge and, like Davy, noted the brilliant light emitted. A sequence of steps followed, leading to the contemporary mercury arc radiation source. First the mercury was contained in a pool at one electrode of a carbon arc (Jackson, 1852); the electrodes were enclosed in a glass case (Binks, 1853); and a discharge in mercury vapor was reached by a partial vacuum (Dowsing and Keating, 1896). A major difficulty existed for mercury, as the heating that accompanied the operation increased the pressure and shut off the discharge. Peter Cooper-Hewitt (1900) devised envelopes that contained a condensing region which returned by gravity the cooled mercury to the cathode pool; the arc lamp did not quench. Techniques for the manufacture of fused silica by distillation of sand were devised, and now enclosures could be manufactured that would withstand the high pressures. Quartz–molybdenum seals were discovered, and so enclosures which contained tungsten electrodes with a short separation could be fabricated. In 1930 high-pressure mercury arcs were constructed that operated at high current.

The fused silica envelopes made it possible to explore other materials, and a source comparable to the sun spectrum was found to be emitted by xenon at high pressure (Paul Schulz, 1947).

An alternative artificial light source is an incandescent source. Thomas Drummond (1817) devised an intense point source of light by burning hydrogen and oxygen and applying the flame to a block of limestone—this was called lime light. This light source was used with a focus mirror in the geodetic survey of Ireland (1820). It was immediately used as a source of light in lighthouses, though electrolytic production of hydrogen from voltaic piles proved inconvenient in the remote places where lighthouses must be placed. In 1835 Drummond's lime light was first used in the theatre in Dublin. It gave an intense beam of light, a spot light, drawing attention to actors and allowing the creation of effects—lightning, moonlight, etc. The emission is a black body (yellow–white) and calcium lines (violet and red), a combination which favors the human complexion.

To eliminate the inconvenience of lime light, Joseph Swan (1860) passed electric current through a thin carbon fiber made by carbonizing a fiber of wood (paper). He enclosed the carbon fiber in an evacuated envelope, but the vacuum was insufficient to prevent oxidation; a water jet ejector pump was used. This proved to be an intense source of light. By 1878 the automated Sprengel mercury ejector pump became available, and both Swan and Thomas Edison attained adequate vacuums to sustain the light emission for many hundred of hours. Edison developed the technology of electric power distribution and the sale of the electric light by devising high-resistance filaments and supplying current with parallel distribution (September, 1882). Swan continued to develop the manufacture of the carbon fiber. Following a much earlier suggestion of Hooke on imitating the silkworm to produce a fiber, Swan, in 1883, extruded nitrocellulose and produced fine fiber. Then the chemically converted the nitrocellulose to cellulose and pyrolyzed it to produce carbon fiber filaments. Count Louis de Chardonnet took up Swan's principle in 1889 to manufacture in Bescancon artificial textile fibers—rayon. In 1905 William Coolidge devised a procedure to extrude tungsten by crystal drawing, and now a high-resistance coiled metal filament could be fabricated to replace carbon fibers. In 1918 Irving Langmuir developed the methods to operate at higher temperature by filling the envelopes with an inert gas, initially nitrogen and later argon. In 1958 Elmer Fridrich and Emmett Wiley included iodine within the envelope, which cyclically redeposited evaporated tungsten upon the filament. Ribbon filaments could now be contained within a fused quartz envelope and lamps operated at high current to provide an intense source of radiation. Quartz-tungsten lamps with radiation ranging from the ultraviolet are presently manufactured and used in car headlights, etc.

INTERACTION OF ELECTROMAGNETIC RADIATION WITH MATTER

The interaction of radiation with matter involves an exchange of energy. Our knowledge of the process consists of detailed theories which account for observed events. These theories constitute one of the major achievements of science. Theoretical models precisely predict the value, or the range of values, for the exchanged energy by atoms and molecules.

To be strict in usage, light is that part of the spectrum of electromagnetic radiation which is sensed by the normal human eye. Many use the word "light" to mean electromagnetic radiation which has sufficient energy to alter energies of electrons within atoms or molecules. This was once called actinic rays, and this would serve our purpose well if actinic did not also convey an antique sense.

Electromagnetic radiation is a field which propagates energy at a fixed velocity. It is describable as a transverse wave. When there is an exchange of energy between the radiation field and matter, it is necessary to treat the field as a particle with momentum rather than as a wave. Such a particle is termed a photon.

The energy of a photon can be defined through the wavelength of the radiation field it represents, or else by the corresponding frequency. Both wavelength and frequency are measurable quantities. The range of wavelength values can effect a change in the electronic energy of matter is 150–1200 nm [nano, n = 10^{-9}], corresponding to a frequency range 2.2 PHz–300 THz [Peta, P = 10^{15}; Tera, T = 10^{12}] and an energy range 700–100 kJ mol^{-1}.

The value for the energy is expressed for an amount of photons of a mole, which is the chemical unit of measure for energy. A mole of photons is the number of photons equal in value to Avogadro's constant.

Exposing molecules to radiation with the energy or wavelength equal in value to the difference in energy between two electron levels for that molecule will alter the energy of the electron within the molecule, and a photon will be annihilated. This event is termed the absorption of radiation. The molecule now has an electron in a more energetic level—this condition or state of the molecule is termed an excited state. Absorption of radiation creates an excited state and annihilates a photon.

The excited state is a distinct chemical species. It is different from the parent or ground unexcited state that absorbed the radiation.

The excited state has excess energy derived from the absorbed photon. This energy ultimately will be dissipated by the excited state. This conforms to the second law of thermodynamics that there is a unique Gibbs energy that is least in value for a system, matter and radiation. The pathways or channels for the dissipation of this excess energy from an excited state fall into three categories: (1) creation of molecular motion—vibrationless relaxation; (2) emission of radiation—luminescence; (3) reorganization of the molecule— photochemistry. Thus an excited state can dissipate electronic energy as heat, luminescence, or undergo chemical reaction. Photophysicists declare that there are radiationless, radiative, or photochemical decay channels. Each of these three categories of decay events proceeds at a given rate. Hence the excited state exists for a period of time governed by the three processes. The excited state is therefore only a transient chemical species produced after an absorption event.

The excited state is a chemical which can be characterized by the radiation it emits—its luminescence; the heat it liberates—photocalorimetry, especially photoacoustic effect; or analysis of the chemicals it becomes— photochemistry. Moreover, as a distinct chemical species it, too, will have a characteristic absorption, albeit different from that of the parental ground state, so the excited state can be studied by the transient absorption created after absorption by the parental ground state.

Molecules, like atoms, have many vibrations available to them. Motion of the nuclei of a molecule alters the precise value for a given electronic level. So, rather than a unique value for an electronic level, there is a range of values determined by the variation created by the molecular vibrations. In the study of the exchange of energy between a radiation field and a molecule— absorption of radiation—it is necessary to vary the energy of the exciting radiation. The distribution of photon energies comprises the absorption band first seen by Brewster in 1833 (29).

Phenomenologic Treatment of Absorption of Radiation

The absorption of radiation by a homogeneous sample of material placed in a (parallel) beam of radiation was first developed in 1729 by a priest at Le Havre, Pierre Bouguer (81, 82), and later elaborated by Johann Lambert in 1760 (83). They demonstrated that the proportion of radiation absorbed by a material is independent of the intensity of the radiation. Absorption depends only on the number of incident photons. The number of exchanges of energy is proportional to the number of photons: more photons, more exchanges of energy.

The decrease in light intensity dI on passage of a plane wave through a homogeneous layer of material after travel of a distance db is proportional to the incident intensity I (Fig. 2-3). This is expressed by

$$dI/I = -\alpha\, db$$

where α is the constant of proportionality. The negative sign reflects the decrease or absorption of radiation. This constant is characteristic for the material at a specific wavelength of radiation.

Upon integration we obtain

$$\int_{I_0}^{I} dI/I = -\alpha \int_0^b db$$

$$\ln I/I_0 = -\alpha b$$

$$I = I_0 e^{-\alpha b}$$

The Bouguer–Lambert law states that there is an exponential decrease in

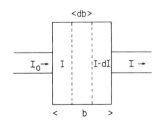

Fig. 2-3. Bouguer–Lambert absorption of radiation.

radiation intensity with the length of passage of radiation through a homogeneous material.

In 1852 August Beer (84) found that the transmission of radiation by a homogeneous material depends only upon the number of molecules through which the radiation travels. He showed that the number of exchanges of energy is directly proportional to the number of absorbing molecules n. The number of molecules in a volume V is given by the concentration, that is, the amount of substance per volume, c:

$$n = N_A c V$$

where N_A is Avogadro's constant of proportionality to mass and the number of interactions (dI) is proportional to $-In$.

Beer's law is

$$dI/I = -\beta \, dc$$

The Bouguer–Lambert law may be combined with Beer's law to provide the law of absorption for radiation absorbed in a cross section or area (Fig. 2-3) of homogeneous concentration

$$dI/I = -\kappa c \, db$$

and κ is the molar constant of proportionality for absorption; cross-sectional area $(n = \kappa c \, db)$. It follows that upon integrating over an entire path length (b) or concentration (c)

$$\int_{I_0}^{I} (dI/I) = -\kappa c \int_0^b db = -\kappa b \int_0^c dc$$

$$ln(I/I_0) = -\kappa c b$$

or

$$\ln(I_0/I) = \kappa c b$$

Thus

$$I = I_0 e^{-\kappa c b}$$

It is a curious footnote, but Beer never stated that radiation absorption is proportional to concentration when the length of passage for the radiation is a fixed, defined pathlength. This is a corollary to his observations and is the one

Table 2-1. Unit of Measure for ϵ

Traditional	International recommendation
$dm^3 mol^{-1} cm^{-1}$	$m^2 mol^{-1}$
$10^3 cm^2 mol^{-1}$	
$10 m^2 mol^{-1}$	
ϵ (traditional) $= 10\epsilon$ (recommended)	

we use today to estimate concentration from absorption photometry and invariably call Beer's law.

Bunsen and Henry Roscoe began the tradition in 1857 of using decadic logarithms (85):

$$\log_{10}(I_0 / I) = \kappa cb / \ln 10 = \epsilon cb$$

The molar constant of proportionality ϵ is the molar (decadic) absorptivity. It is characteristic of the absorbing chemical aspects at a specified wavelength, under declared conditions for the material, e.g., solution, solid, etc. In tabulations of molecular properties, the molar absorptivity has the virtue of being independent of both concentration and pathlength used. This proportionality constant was once widely called the "extinction" coefficient. Because this term implied that there was loss of radiation by diffusive scattering and not absorption, it is no longer in use.

The question of units of measure for molar absorptivity is awkward. International recommendations specify that the concentration, the amount of substance per volume, be expressed in mol m^{-3}, and the length in m. Biochemists and chemists measure concentration in mol l^{-1} (mol dm^{-3}) and the pathlength in cm for purposes of tabulation. Thus, rather obviously, the magnitude of ϵ depends upon the convention adopted for its unit of measure (Table 2-1 and Appendices B and C).

Measurement of the absorption of a material is often made upon solute dissolved in a transparent solvent and placed into containers fabricated from a material that is completely transparent to the radiation in the spectral interval of interest. The containers are also precisely fabricated to be equal in dimension and shape to allow interchange without change in the window transmission and reflections and light passage length.

It is the internal transmittance that is of concern, that is, the transmittance that disregards any influence of the container (transmission and reflections). To measure this quantity the transmittance T_0 of only the solvent is determined by

$$T_0 = I / I_0$$

The solvent is replaced by the solution of interest, and its corresponding transmittance is T_s. Hence the internal transmittance T of the material is

$$T = T_s / T_0$$

By two successive measurements, the influence of the container is removed, since it makes an equal contribution to T_s and T_0.

In chemical and biochemical studies a more useful quantity than transmittance is the transmission density A. This is defined as

$$A = \log_{10}(T_0 / T_s) = \log_{10} 1 / T$$

Transmission density was first proposed by Hurter and Driffield in 1890 (86) and became widely known as optical density. The term optical density is passing from usage and being replaced by the phrase transmission density. The convenience of transmission density is clear from the following relations:

$$A = -\log_{10} T = \epsilon c b$$

The linear additive property with concentration is the basis for its use in chemical analysis. When mixtures exist, measurements are made at a series of wavelengths where the molar absorption coefficients differ. The number of components can then readily be determined from the matrix as equal to the number of nonzero eigenvalues, and the amount of each component can be estimated by use of factor analysis for which least-squares solutions are known.

For application of the combined laws of Bouguer–Lambert and Beer, the absorption law, several critical assumptions enter, and their applicability must exist:

1. The radiation is monochromatic.
2. Absorption takes place in a volume of uniform cross section, i.e., the irradiating beam is parallel across the sample.
3. The absorption of radiation by a given species is independent of that of other species.

Diffuse Reflection

The treatment just given for light absorption applies only to the simplest of materials—homogeneous. Many biologic materials, e.g., skin or leaves, are far from homogeneous. There is no satisfactory treatment for the interaction of light with a heterogeneous material, but the broad outlines of procedures and interpretation can be given.

Lambert remarked in his treatise in 1760 (83) that a white wall appears equally bright at all angles of observation. Here radiation is scattered diffusively in all directions. This isotropic scattering, diffuse scattering, is known as Lambert's cosine law. Perhaps a more familiar illustration is the ability to see the place where a beam of light strikes a mirror. The beam is predominantly reflected, yet its spot on the mirror can be seen from the side as light is diffusively scattered from mirror material. The cosine law can be obtained by treating the material as composed of small platelets of the material that have all possible orientations. Light incident upon an individual platelet is reflected and transmitted according to Fresnel's equations. Part of the transmitted light can be absorbed, and this was analyzed by Joseph Fourier in 1817.

Light emitted by a black body also meets the cosine law. The appearance of the sun as a flat disk or the coil of an electric lamp as a strip is the direct consequence. The Lambert cosine law for blackbody emission, isotropic distribution of emission, is directly related to the second law of thermodynamics.

Diffuse reflection can be measured by enclosing the material with a sphere coated with a "white" diffusive reflector—no absorption, only scattering of all energies. Sumpner realized in 1892 that light emitted from a small hole in a sphere that had its interior coated with freshly deposited magnesium oxide would be equal for any direction after the interior was illuminated with a central source of radiation (87). Ulbricht (88) applied this principle to studies of reflectance by irradiating a sample of diffusively reflecting material surrounded by the sphere and measuring the radiation emitted from a small hole after diffusive scattering from the sample and throughout the sphere. Taylor (89, 90) developed a complete theoretical treatment to obtain the reflectance of the sample.

No rigorous theory of multiple scattering exists, but a phenomenologic treatment which includes absorption and scattering provides an ansatz with two parameters. One treats the radiation within the sample as to opposing beams. For a thick layer of material, Paul Kubelka and Peter Munk (91, 92) relate the reflectance R_∞ to absorption K and backward scattering S:

$$F(R_\infty) = (1 - R_\infty)^2 / 2R = K/S$$

The reflectance is measured with an Ulbricht sphere, and rather than an absolute measure, a reference standard is compared—typically a block of magnesium carbonate or a paint. Again, familiar experience suggests what is incorporated in the Kubelka–Munk relation—that a perfect white scatter, $K = 0$, is unattainable because a small absorption makes an appreciable reduction in reflectance.

The applicability of the Kubelka—Munk relation rests upon diffuse illumination. In facile procedures of measurement a directed irradiation beam is used to pass radiation into the sphere. For densely scattering samples multiple scattering will take place, and after a small penetration depth diffuse irradiation will prevail.

A more relevant assumption concerns the size of the scattering particle. It is assumed that the particle is large with respect to the wavelength of light. For particles that are small, scattering follows the treatment of John Strutt, Lord Rayleigh (1871); here scattering increases with decreasing size and with decreasing wavelength (the reason the sky is blue). The theory predicts partially polarized scattered radiation with equal forward and backward scattering. A result is that there is less penetration depth and thus less absorption. Colored crystals become paler as they are ground to smaller sizes.

Scattering of radiation by particles commensurate in size with the wavelength of light depends upon the size, shape, and refraction and is described by a sum of a series of Legendre polynomials in a theory developed by Gustar Mie (93). It predicts a greater forward scattering, and Mie was able to explain the various colors of solutions of gold particles of different size.

For dilute scattering solutions, the absorption can be determined by placing the material within an integrating sphere which determines the total scattering and transmission. By further measuring the transmission by selecting only a narrow beam at large distance from the material, Latimer and co-workers showed how it is possible to account completely for the scattering (94, 95), using either Mie scattering or anomalous diffraction described by van de Hulst.

Multiple scattering alters the forward-scattering Mie distribution, and though there is no exact solution reached, the scattering approaches an isotropic distribution—the familiar white color of clouds and fog (96). An effect of multiple scattering is to increase the apparent pathlength for absorption—the "detour" effect (97). The consequence of the scattering is to greatly intensify the absorption, up to several hundredfold.

Two alternative procedures to using an integrating sphere have been devised. The first illuminates the sample with diffusively scattered irradiation by transmitting the radiation beam through an opal quartz plate placed before the sample (98). All the transmitted radiation is detected by an end-window photomultiplier which responds with a large angular collection. A second alternative is to surround the sample with a fluorescence quantum counting screen (99, 100) and again use an end-window photomultiplier to detect the entire fluorescence emission.

An entirely distinct approach which applies to samples with large aggregations of chromophore in organelles (chloroplasts) is to neglect scattering. Here one is concerned only with the heterogeneous distribution of the chromophore. An individual beam of radiation passing through the sample may intersect less absorption than an adjacent parallel beam—the sieve effect. The result is an apparent flattening of the absorption, which is dependent upon particle size (101, 102). No satisfactory treatment with a small number of parameters has been devised to apply to densely scattering material such as skin.

LAWS OF PHOTOPHYSICS AND PHOTOCHEMISTRY

Six statements define basic properties in photophysics and photo-chemistry of organic molecules. They have at their heart the quantal basis for electromagnetic radiation. The laws are phenomenologic and strictly pertain only to interactions of matter and electromagnetic radiation that involve a single photon. Thus, these are restricted to moderate radiation intensities and not to intensities that can be reached with pulsed lasers.

1. Absorption law of Theodor Grotthus (1815) (103) and John Draper (1841) (104): Only radiation that is absorbed by a molecule can be effective in producing luminescence or a photochemical change in that molecule.

This law is considered the first law of photophysics. It is regrettable that it is not unheard of to listen to or even to read reports on luminescence or photochemical products in which this essential paradigm is not met.

2. Quantum law of Johannes Stark (1908) (105) and Albert Einstein (1912) (106): Each molecule that emits luminescence or is chemically altered by radiation absorbs one quantum of radiation.

This law applies to the primary absorbing event. A further development of this law is the principle of photophysical equivalence, stated by Einstein: The sum of quantum yields for each individual photophysical and photo-chemical process identified must be unity.

3. Reciprocity law of Robert Bunsen and Henry Roscoe (1859) (107): The total number of absorbed photons and not their energy content nor the rate at which they are absorbed determines the extent of a photophysical or photochemical process.

This is the extension of the Proust–Dalton law of definite combining proportions to include radiation photons. It emphasizes that the amount of photons is the quantity of importance. It implies the following three laws.

4. Emission energy shift law of Zanotti and Francesco Algarotti (1713) (108) [and later of Ritter (1803) (109) and Stokes (1852) (71)]: The peak energy of the emission spectrum for luminescence is less in energy than the exciting radiation energy.

This is a consequence of emission from the lowest vibronic level of the first excited state and results from vibrational relaxation in the ground state. It is further increased by alteration of molecular geometry in the excited state of solvent dipolar relaxation.

5. Invariance of luminescence emission spectrum law of Nicolai Zucchi (1652) (110)* [and later of Dessaignes (1810) (63), Stokes (1852) (71), and Nichols and Merritt (1904) (111)]: The luminescence spectrum is invariant with changes in the excitation radiation energy.

This law is a consequence of vibrational relaxation among higher excited levels and demonstrates sole emission from the lowest vibronic level of the first excited state.

6. Constancy of quantum yield of fluorescence law of Sergei Vavilov (1922) (112): The quantum yield of fluorescence is invariant with changes in the exciting radiation energy.

The law demonstrates that there is vibrational relaxation among the excited electronic levels.

These principles are combined in a useful quantity, the quantum yield Φ:

Φ_L = number of luminescent photons emitted/number of photons absorbed

Φ_P = number of molecules chemically altered/number of photons absorbed

It is often convenient to measure a rate rather than the amount of events, so a more frequent definition is

Φ = rate of luminescence or photochemical reaction/rate of absorption

Quantum Efficiency

Another useful quantity is the quantum efficiency q:

q = extent of effect/number of incident photons

= response/dose

= response rate/fluence (dose rate)

This quantity, quantum efficiency, is a product of two phenomena (absorption and the photoeffect) and a proportionality constant (the response coefficient R):

*Nicolai Zucchi (1586–1670), a teacher of mathematics at Collegio Romano in Rome, wrote *Optica Philosophia* in 1652. He found that barium sulfide phosphorescence was the same color whether exposed to white light or to light that had passed through glass of red, yellow, or green color. Francesco Maria Zanotti (1692–1777), President of the University of Bologna, worked with Count Francesco Algarotti, writer and connosseur, in 1713, and they confirmed the studies of Zucchi by using a prism to disperse sunlight. Zanotti and Algarotti showed that barium sulfide phosphor "shines by its own natural light, which is only kindled by foreign light" (108). Trace component luminescence complicated many studies which followed using the pioneering technique of Beccari. Jean Dessaignes, working with many new phosphors, was able to confirm the initial studies of Zucchi, and so emphasized the wide validity of this phenomenon (63).

q = fractional absorption · effect quantum yield · response coefficient

Action Spectrum of Quantum Response Spectrum

This is the spectrum for the wavelength dependence of the quantum efficiency. Its importance was first emphasized by Emil Warburg in 1920 (113). Because absorption spectra can characterize the chemical nature of the absorbing molecule, the action spectrum plays the crucial role in photobiologic studies of relating a photoevent to a molecular species:

$$q(\lambda) = f(\lambda)\Phi(\lambda)R$$

The quantum yield is most frequently independent of the exciting wavelength, and the action spectrum then is the fractional absorption spectrum of the photoreactive molecule.

Excitation Spectrum

Philipp Lenard (114) emphasized the importance of varying the energy of excitation to define the chemical nature of the absorbing species. When the fractional absorption of radiation is small, the action spectrum will resemble the absorption spectrum:

$$f \quad = 1 - e^{-(\ln 10)\epsilon cb}$$

$$f\big|_{f\to 0} = [(\ln 10)\epsilon cb]1/1! - [(\ln 10)\epsilon cb]2/2! + \dots$$

$$= (\ln 10)\epsilon cb$$

Thus for $f \to 0$, $q(\lambda) = A(\lambda)\Phi R$

The wavelength dependence of a photoeffect for small fractional absorption for a fixed quantal fluence will equal the variation in absorbance. It is thus necessary to measure only the incident quantal flux or fluence.

Excitation spectra are widely determined in photophysical studies where there can be direct experimental control of absorbance.

Response Spectrum or Effectiveness Spectrum

In practical situations, it is an effectiveness that is measured:

response = radiant exposure · quantum efficiency

where the radiant exposure is the incident amount of photons or dose or, if response rate is determined, the fluence. When the wavelength of excitation is altered, both the radiant exposure and quantum efficiency change. The variation of response with wavelength comprises the response spectrum. To obtain an excitation or action spectrum, it is necessary to determine in a separate experiment the variation of the radiant exposure, typically by using a quantum counting screen.

The variation in radiant exposure depends on the emittance spectrum of the radiation spectrum and the transmittance of the photon isolator, monochromator, or color filter. Thus the most effective wavelength need not be the wavelength with greatest quantum efficiency; appreciable differences frequently exist.

The devices used to isolate photons of differing energy do not separate radiation into monochromatic photons—photons with a single value of energy. Rather, they transmit a spectral interval. If in this interval there is a significant change in radiant exposure spectrum—the source intensity spectrum—then the response is a convolution or folding integral over that spectral interval

$$R(\lambda) = I(\lambda) * q(\lambda)$$

The effect of a convolution is difficult to realize, and is summarized in Appendix D. Convolution effects become dominant when color filters are used to isolate a spectral interval; with monochromators or interference filters, only small variation in source spectrum exists for a selected energy of excitation.

MEASUREMENT OF RADIATION INTENSITY

The measurement of the intensity of radiation is crucial for many biologic studies. The amount of incident and concomitant absorbed photons determines the number of events—amount of luminescence emitted or amount of altered chemicals produced.

Measurement of radiant intensity can be separated into two topics: the measurement of absolute radiant energy (radiation thermometry) and the measurement of photon flux at more than one photon energy (heterochromatic photometry).

Thermal Detection of Optical Radiation

William Herschel initiated the procedures for quantitative measurement of radiant intensity through thermal detection using a liquid expansion thermometer (7). Macedonio Melloni devised a sensitive thermometer from a thermocouple, based on a phenomenon studied by Thomas Seebeck in 1821 and discovered by Ritter in 1803. Seebeck noticed the movement of a magnet when a junction of dissimilar metal was heated. Melloni increased the sensitivity of the thermocouple by fabricating a series of bimetal junctions, which he termed a thermopile (115). He coated the thermopile with a metal black, either micrometer metal droplets condensed from a vapor, or microcrystallites electrolytically deposited. Such a metal black is a diffusive, matte surfaces which absorbs all incident photons at all wavelengths. The metal black permits heterochromatic photometric response, and a measurement of the temperature increase of the metal black provides the absolute measure of the radiant intensity.

Today, microcircuitry techniques are used to create an array of metal junctions, and these are embedded within a gold–black layer. This device can be calibrated through a resistive heating of the conductive metal black, most simply by applying current pulses derived from a precision generator, the number being determined with a scaler. Thermal detection, though moderately sensitive, has the drawback of responding slowly to changes and then needing careful attention for constant thermal surroundings to be created. The array is of necessity small in area. A typical thermopile is fabricated with an 8×8 array of bismuth–antimony junctions behind a 10 mm^2 metal black surface. Such a device can detect 100 nJ at 1-Hz detection bandpass.

Dutch merchants returned from Sri Lanka with toumaline. When toumaline is placed in hot ashes and then removed, ash sticks to it, but is repelled after it cools. Toumaline crystals were known as Ceylon magnets— electric equivalents to magnets. The Estonian physicist Franz Hoch (Aepinus) found in 1756 that opposite faces of toumaline have different polarities. David Brewster termed the phenomenon the pyroelectric effect and found synthetic salts which exhibit it (1823).

A comparable sensitivity is available, though with a smaller effective detection area, from pyroelectric crystals coated with a metal black point. Pyroelectric crystals have a spontaneous electric polarization created by oriented electric dipoles grouped into a ferroelectric domain. The domain structure is altered when the crystal dimensions changes through a change in temperature, modifying the spontaneous polarization creating an electric charge from stray sources which is measured with an electrometer. This phenomenon became known in Europe in 1703, but it has become exploited only in the last decade, in part because of the ready availability of suitable electrometer integrated circuit devices. The pyroelectric effect has the potential of rapid response, at the expense of sensitivity.

Fluorescence Screen Detection

A photon converter can improve upon the sensitivity of detection for radiation. It is a luminescent material which absorbs radiation of one energy and then reemits radiation of lesser energy but now in a spectral interval which can be detected through sensitive devices. Ultraviolet radiation can be detected by the luminescence of a crystalline phosphor material, which emits light readily sensed by the human eye. Ultraviolet radiation was first observed by using this technique by Johann Goethe working with Thomas Seebeck in 1792, after Goethe had visited Monte Paterno (1786) to collect a sample of heavy spar. Goethe published his observations many years later (116). Ritter reported similar observation in 1803 (109). These investigations mark the beginning of the development of the familiar domestic artificial light source, the fluorescent lamp. Edmund Becquerel powdered a phosphor and stuck it to paper with gum and was able to visualize the solar spectrum, including UV radiation, in 1843.

John Herschel (69, 70) found that concentrated solutions of quinine sulfate emit light only from a layer at the surface of the solution exposed to the radiation—epipolic fluorescence was his term. Stokes noticed the brilliant blue fluorescence from quinine sulfate solutions irradiated by a lightning flash and realized that fluorescence could be used to visualize ultraviolet radiation (71). He soaked paper in quinine sulfate solutions and made fluorescent screens to view ultraviolet radiation. He explored the emission of ultraviolet radiation from electric spark discharges of metals and gases and found that quartz was transparent to a large interval of ultraviolet radiation and so could be used to fabricate dispersing prisms, envelopes, and containers (31, 66).

Victor Henri replaced the human eye as the radiation detector with a photographic plate in 1921 (117). The photon converter extended the spectral range of the plate into the ultraviolet interval. Stokes had noted that the fluorescence spectrum did not alter when the exciting radiation was changed (71). This was investigated quantitatively by Edward Nichols and Ernest Merritt in 1910 (111); later they measured the fluorescence energy yield with a thermopile and found that it increased linearly with the energy of the exciting radiation (118). In 1922 Sergei Vavilov (112, 119) extended the spectral range and discovered that the proportionality constant was equal in value to Planck's constant. Vavilov had demonstrated that the quantum yield of fluorescence was independent of the exciting radiation energy. The intensity of fluorescence depends only upon the number of exciting photons. Fluorescence screens respond to the incident photon flux and can be used for heterochromatic photometry with photographic plates (120).

Bowen (121) realized the importance of detecting the surface fluorescence by viewing the fluorescence through the concentrated fluorophore solution. This had been implicit in the work of Henri and later of Anderson and Bird. In the concentrated solutions, the high-energy region of the fluorescence emission spectrum is reabsorbed, and to achieve a constant extent of re-absorption it is essential to allow the fluorescence radiation to pass through the solution. There will be variation in the depth of penetration of the exciting radiation at varying exciting energies, but this variation will be negligible compared with the length of travel through the solution, μm compared with cm ($1 : 10^{-4}$). Bowen described the fluorescence screen viewed from the rear as a quantum counting screen: the intensity of the output depends upon the quantal fluence and not the quantal energy. He used photocells, but we now

use a photomultiplier because of its greater sensitivity, attaining the ultimate—detection of individual photons. The dye solutions can be of several
materials (122) dissolved in transparent solvents which prevent dimerization,
or in solid polymer solutions (123). To create a detector that is insensitive to
radiant energy, polarization, and source position or change in radiation
direction, it is only necessary to surround the quantum counting screen with
an integrating sphere (124).

A monochromator can be used to isolate specific radiation energy, and
the emergent monochromatic radiation can be detected with a previously
calibrated photomultiplier or with a quantum counting screen. These
combinations permit spectroradiometry, absolute radiant intensity at specified wavelengths. Monochromators have a varying transmission depending
upon radiation energy. To determine this, recourse is taken to a substitution
method which originated with Gauss. A second monochromator is used to
isolate monochromatic radiation from the radiation source or a source which
emits over the spectral interval of interest. The monochromatic radiant
intensity is measured with a thermopile to provide an absolute value, and at
other wavelengths with a quantum counting screen. The monochromator to
be calibrated is now introduced and the radiation intensity remeasured. Thus
the transmission of the monochromator under calibration is determined by
ration (125). The spectral response of a photomultiplier can be determined as
readily. These calibration coefficients can be included on a PROM (pro-
grammable read-only memory module) available to a microcomputer which
controls the spectroradiometer so that a simple operation procedure is
inexpensively provided.

The heterochromatic photometric response of a thermopile that is crucial
in its use for absolute radiant intensity measurements can be determined by
use of a radiation source whose spectral distribution is calculable from theory,
a blackbody radiator (126, 127).

Though the devices and procedure to calibrate instruments and components for absolute spectroradiometry are simple, they are tedious and
require attention to details. An alternative is to use fluorescence spectra of
compounds that have previously reported calibrated fluorescence spectra
(128).

Polarization of Radiation

Newton did not provide a detailed interpretation of light but did state
that shining bodies emit energy which travels largely rectilinearly (he knew of
the work of Grimaldi) and that light was sensed by the human eye. He offered
as suggestions only that light was corpuscular or had a wavelike interaction
with bodies and materials. It was later workers who considered only the
corpuscular suggestion and attributed the concept to Newton. Boyle considered light a wave, and in 1657 Hooke tentatively suggested that the wave was

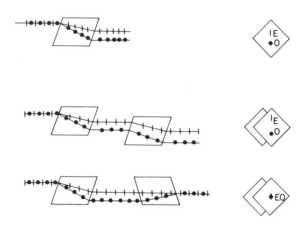

Fig. 2-4. Experiments on double refraction by Iceland spar by Huygens.

transverse to the propagation direction and was not like the longitudinal waves on water or in materials—the familiar ripples on the surface of a pond.

In 1670 Erasmus Bartholin reported on the double refraction of calcium carbonate crystals (calcite or Iceland spar): light passing through calcite produces two images (129). Christiaan Huygens gave a detailed description of how a wave nature for light could fully account for rectilinear propagation. He took up the discovery of Bartholin and working with two calcite crystals demonstrated that two beams produced by calcite were different in behavior by showing a difference in their response on passage through the second crystal (130); he demonstrated this by rotating the second rhomb with respect to the first (Fig. 2-4). Newton, in describing the double refraction, considered there was a polar interaction between light and the material of the crystals which depended upon two directions of vibration, essentially a transverse wave vibration for light (131), north–south vs. east–west.

Étienne-Louis Malus, seeking a prize on double refraction, viewed light reflected from the windows of the Luxembourg Palace in Paris in 1809 (132)

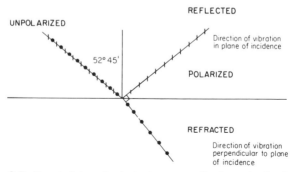

Fig. 2-5. Brewster's law of polarization upon reflection and refraction.

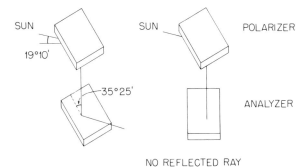

NO REFLECTED RAY

Fig. 2-6. Experiment by Malus on the transmission of polarized radiation by a polarizer.

through a calcite crystal rhomb, and he noticed the successive extinction for particular orientations of first one and then the other image which the crystal was rotated. There are orientations at right angles where only one image is produced. In detailed studies of light reflecting off a water surface, Malus found that at a specific angle (52° 45′) the reflected light behaved identically to one of the beams produced by a calcite rhomb (133) (Fig. 2-5). Light reflected at this specific angle was polarized. Malus analyzed the reflected light off a piece of glass at this angle (polarizer) by another reflection on a glass surface at the same angle (an analyzer) and studied the dependence on the orientation of the analyzer with respect to the polarizer ($\cos^2 \theta$), Malus law (134) (Fig. 2-6). He next noted that the light transmitted by the reflecting glass plate polarizer was partially polarized at right angles to the reflected light. Adding more reflection plates increased the extent of the polarization of the transmitted light—a pile-of-plates polarizer (135, 136). In 1812 Brewster investigated the dependence of polarizing angle on the nature of the material and discovered the dependence upon the refractive index, Brewster's law (137): there is a refraction angle when the reflected and refracted components are at right angles, and this is the angle for maximum polarization (Fig. 2-5).

Grimaldi had realized that light does not propagate rectilinearly but is diffracted by the edge of precision objects. In 1801 Young (14) convincingly demonstrated the wave nature of light, but initially interpreted the interference effects with longitudinal waves (ripples on connecting canals). In 1816 Augustin Fresnel repeated the two-slit experiments of Young using polarized light created with a pile-of-plates polarizer (138, 139). Francois Arago and Fresnel found there was no interference pattern produced between the polarized components. In 1817 Young interpreted Fresnel's experiments with a transverse wave for electromagnetic radiation (140). The existence of a transverse wave was fully explained by Fresnel in 1821. He gave the complete theory of reflection and refraction by transparent material in 1823 (141). This experimental journey from Newton to Fresnel and Young gives the principal properties of optical radiation.

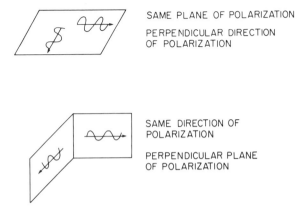

SAME PLANE OF POLARIZATION

PERPENDICULAR DIRECTION
OF POLARIZATION

SAME DIRECTION OF
POLARIZATION

PERPENDICULAR PLANE
OF POLARIZATION

Fig. 2-7. The inappropriateness of using the phrase "plane of polarization."

William Nicol (142) devised a procedure to cut calcite rhombs to fashion a prism that transmits only one polarized component, and other prisms were devised by Alexis Rochon (143) and Wollaston (144) that transmit two widely divergent, perpendicularly polarized beams. These prisms permit the design of optical instruments which can measure the extent of polarization or radiation.

William Thomson, Lord Kelvin, in 1884 (145) regarded polarization as an inept description since it leads to the phrase "plane of vibration of the electric vector of radiation" and the direction of propagation. This is entirely inadequate, as one can see by inspecting Fig. 2-7. Whenever one thinks about polarization of radiation, one should follow Thomson and use the phrase "direction of vibration" and refer to radiation as linearly, circularly, or elliptically polarized. One should never use the phrase "plane polarized" radiation. Few texts or reports maintain this needed clarity; Newton still is a powerful influence.

In 1833 Brewster found that the red fluorescence from alcohol solutions of chlorophyll was unpolarized, and Stokes confirmed this observation in his 1852 studies. Subsequently, unpolarized radiation was regarded as a property of fluorescence. Fritz Weigert and Gerhard Kappler (146–148) discovered that viscous glycerol solutions of fluorophoric dyes emit polarized fluorescence radiation. The degree of polarization of glycerol solutions varied with temperature (149, 150).

Vadim Levshin (151, 152) interpreted this variation as a dependence on viscosity and temperature created by Brownian rotatory motion. He used a plausible value for the molar volume and obtained a value for the lifetime of fluroescence that agreed with experimental values then being measured in the Warsaw laboratories by Ernesto Gaviola (153). Francis Perrin developed a detailed theory for Brownian rotation and directly determined the molar volumes by diffusion. He demonstrated the strict dependence of the rate of rotation on the ratio of viscosity to temperature, with the extent of depolarization being set by the ratio of the rates of fluorescence emission and disorientation (154, 155). There is now much interest in investigating the diffusionally controlled chemical rate dependence upon the temperature-viscosity ratio. In 1934 Mitra (156) increased the extent of polarization by quenching fluorescence, and this procedure is used today to measure the viscosity of membranes by including a quenching agent to increase the polarization of a membrane fluorophore. If the initial fluorescence decay rate and biomolecular quenching constants are known, the increase in polarization provides the viscosity.

Fluorescence Lifetimes

John Kerr applied a large electric field to certain materials, and this caused them to become birefringent (gain the property of double refraction) (157). This is an electrooptical effect. When cells containing materials with this property were placed between two polarizing prisms oriented to extinguish any light passage, application of an electric field permitted light to then pass. Light gates that respond to electric fields were possible. Heinrich Hertz in his studies (1885-1889) on radio radiation developed the pulsed light source, the electric spark gap. He generated radio radiation with a capacitor-spark discharge at the center of a metal mirror and detected radio radiation with a spark gap across an antenna receiver also at the focus of a metal mirror (a G structure). The received radiation created a spark discharge. The sparks were emitting nanosecond optical radiation as well as gigahertz radio radiation. In 1899 Abraham and Lemoine combined a Kerr light gate with a spark discharge, where the Kerr cell was also the storage capacitor and reflected the light with increasing light pathlength, to measure the velocity of light (158). The light gate now allowed a quantitative measure of the lifetime of fluorescence (159, 160), drawing on the realization of Stokes with regard to lightning and electric flash excitation. These devices are now used to measure picosecond times.

Photoelectric Effect

In 1887 Hertz (161) noticed that when he had placed one spark gap discharge immediately adjacent to another spark gap whose electrode separation was just sufficient to prevent breakdown, this gap began sparking. He realized that the ultraviolet radiation from the first spark had lowered the needed potential for breakdown of the second gap—this was the photoelectric effect, a liberation of electrons by metal exposed to radiation. Independently in 1899 both Joseph Thomson (162) and Lenard (163) directly detected the liberation of electrons from materials exposed to radiation. In 1902 Lenard found the maximum energy of the ejected electrons was independent of the

intensity of the radiation but did depend on the irradiation energy (164).*
Einstein (165, 166) proposed that by assuming the existence of quanta of
radiation one could completely explain the photoelectric effect. In 1908
Erich Ladenberg (167) showed that there was a linear dependence between
the energy of radiation and the maximum energy of the ejected electrons. Owen
Richardson and Karl Compton in 1912 measured the proportionality
constant, and they found that it equalled in value Planck's constant, amply
confirming Einstein's propositions (168). This development is paralleled by
the later studies on the quantal nature of fluorescence radiation.

The photoelectric effect provides the basis for an electronic device to
detect radiation. An electron beam impinging upon materials causes the
release of many electrons, secondary electron emissions, which can be used for
amplification (Joseph Slepian, 1919). By assembling a pile of secondary
emission electrodes, one can create a succession of these processes, which will
amplify an original photoelectron into a swarm of many that can readily be
detected by electronic devices (169). This device when combined with a
photoemission surface is the photoelectron multiplication tube or photomultiplier (170).

A photoelectric material composed of group III and group IV elements
(GaP, BaAs, InGaAs) strongly absorbs optical radiation and emits photo-
electrons with an incident quantum efficiency that is independent of the
exciting radiation energy. These materials provide a quantum counting
photomultiplier tube. Unfortunately, the devices can only be constructed with
a small area, but they are capable of detecting individual photons with
excellent heterochromatic photometric response.

APPENDIX A. SPECTRAL COLOR NAMES

Maurolico reported four primary colors in the rainbow (purple, blue,
green, and yellow) and three more transition colors. Newton likewise reported
seven colors (violet, indigo, blue, green, yellow, orange, and red). Most
observers today use six color names to describe the hues discernible in the
visible spectrum. Indigo is now considered as a mixture of blue and black. The
need to describe seven colors perhaps stemmed from alchemical beliefs;
Newton is known to have held Hermetic beliefs, among which are the concepts
of opposed forces, which may have led him to doubt the strict mechanical
models for natural phenomena adopted by his immediate predecessors.

Color names recognized by observers apply to hues over a spectral

*Lenard is also known for his xenophobic interpretation of natural science (176) and the
remarkable comment in 1933 that "The most important example of the dangerous influence of
Jewish circles in the study of nature has been provided by Einstein with his mathematically
botched up theories." On the contrary, any consideration of the development of science is a
document in praise of the breadth and diversity in the origin and experience of the contributors.

Table 2-2. Perception of Spectral Colors

Color name	Range, nm	Majority, nm	Width, nm^{-1}
Violet	400–440	439	230
Blue	440–500	472	270
Green	500–570	512	240
Yellow	570–590	577	80
Orange	590–610	598	40
Red	610–700	630	210

interval; the range, majority wavelength, and width are tabulated in Table 2-2. The relatively constant energy width except for yellow and orange is apparent. Obviously for violet and red there is a constant recognition after the majority wavelength to the limit of perception.

APPENDIX B. PHYSICAL QUANTITIES, UNITS, NUMERICAL VALUES, AND SYMBOLS FOR PHYSICAL QUANTITIES

Physical Quantities

A physical quantity is the product of a numerical value (a pure number, which is typically obtained by experiment) and a unit of measure.

Base Physical Quantity

Physical quantites are organized into a system in which each base quantity has a dimension, and a symbol is used to represent that base quantity which does not imply the unit of measure for that quantity (Table 2-3).

Derived Physical Quantity

All other physical quantities are regarded as derived from the base quantities by definitions involving multiplication, division, differentiation, and / or integration.

Table 2-3. Symbols for Base Physical Quantities

Base physical quantity	Symbol for quantity
Length	l
Mass	m
Time	t
Temperature	T
Amount of substance	n

Table 2-4. Units and Symbols

Physical quantity	Name of unit	Symbol for unit
Length	meter	m
Mass	kilogram	kg
Time	second	s
Temperature	Kelvin	K
Amount of substance	mole	mol

Recommended Names and Symbols

There has been considerable effort made to compile and suggest recommended names and symbols for quantities used in physical chemistry.

Units and Symbols for Units

An international system of base units of measure exists: meter, kilogram, second, Kelvin, and mole (Table 2-4).

There are appropriate derived units formed by multiplication and/or division of these base units.

There are decimal prefixes to construct multiples or submultiples (Table 2-5). Wherever possible, the use of multiples involving 10^3 is urged.

Printing of Numbers

The radix is accepted as a point of the line (.)

$$273.14$$

and a comma is used to group numbers in blocks of three for readability,

$$2,574,187.242,100$$

Table 2-5. Unit Prefixes

Multiple	Prefix	Symbol	Fraction	Prefix	Symbol
10	deca	da	10^{-1}	deci	d
10^2	hecto	h	10^{-2}	centi	c
10^3	kilo	k	10^{-3}	milli	m
10^6	mega	M	10^{-6}	micro	μ
10^9	giga	G	10^{-9}	nano	n
10^{12}	tera	T	10^{-12}	pico	p
10^{15}	peta	P	10^{-15}	femto	f
10^{18}	exa	E	10^{-18}	atto	a

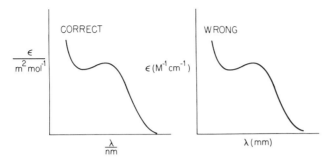

Fig. 2-8. Labels for graphs (Guggenheim's grammar).

Grammar of Scientific Notation

Operations involving physical quantities, units, and numerical values follow ordinary laws of algebra:

physical quantity = numerical value $\times$ unit of measure

The numerical value is a pure number. The symbol used to denote a physical quantity must never imply a particular choice of unit.

Text. One writes in a text: "The temperature T was 298 K (Kelvin)."

Table headings. Following the rules of ordinary algebra, the expression

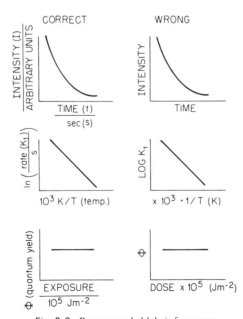

Fig. 2-9. Recommended labels for graphs.

Table 2-6. Temperature Analysis

	Physical quantity	Unit of measure
$\ln(F/a)$ vs. 10^3 K$/T$	F, fluorescence intensity	a, arbitrary
	T, temperature	K, Kelvin

placed at the head of a column of numerical values for a physical quantity presented in a table must be a pure number. This is the quotient for the symbol representing a physical quantity and the symbol for the unit of measure used. Thus typical table headings are:

K, nm for wavelength, nanometer
ϵ, m^2 mol^{-1} for molar absorption coefficient

Graph labels. It follows that expressions used to define physical quantities plotted upon a graph must also be pure numbers (Fig. 2-8).

The advantage of taking the care to use this grammar is found when numerical multiples of the reciprocal of base units are plotted. A frequently encountered example is an Arrhenius temperature analysis, in which relative fluorescence intensity is graphed against the reciprocal of temperature (Fig. 2-9; Table 2-6).

APPENDIX C. AMOUNT OF SUBSTANCE

The amount of substance n is proportional to the number of specified elementary particles of that substance. The elementary unit may be a molecule, ion, radical, electron, photon, or even organelle. The proportionality constant to mass is the same for all substances and is called Avogadro's constant (N_A for solids and liquids, after Avogadro, 1811; N_L for gases, after Loschmidt, 1865).

The unit measure in the international sysem is the mole. The mole is the amount of substance that contains as many elementary units as there are atoms in 0.012 kg of carbon-12. Avogadro's constant is 6.0220978 ± 1.05 ppm × 10^{23} mol^{-1}. It is now known to 1 ppm, and with a potential improvement to 0.01 ppm it may provide a more objective standard for mass than the current international artifact and perhaps even define the ampere.

Chemists have never developed a term for the phrase "amount of substance," though dose is used by radiobiologists for the amount of photons and by physicians for the amount of pharmaceutical.

Molar, an adjective used before an extensive physical quantity, which means "divided by amount of substance," is a poor choice because of ready association with the particular unit called the mole.

A frequently used quantity is the molar mass, mass per amount of substance $M = m/n$ kg mol^{-1}. Biochemists sometimes use an alternative physical quantity, which they call dalton, for an elementary unit mass. Dalton is defined as N_A^{-1} g mol^{-1}, where the physical quantity is the reciprocal of Avogadro's constant and the unit is g mol^{-1}. The dalton is *not a unit*, but is a physical quantity like concentration and is measured in the unit g mol^{-1}.

Molecular weight is a dimensionless number which means the relative molecular mass of a substance, M_r.

The physical quantity concentration c_B or [B] is the amount-of-substance density, where the international unit of measure is mol m^{-3}. This unit has no name, nor is it one widely used today. Chemists have always used mol dm^{-3} as the unit for concentration, which they term molar, M. There are considerable grounds for confusion with other uses for the term "divided by amount of substance" and for the accepted symbols. Unless the context is clear, specification of the unit of measure will be needed for clarity.

APPENDIX D. CONVOLUTION

The convolution or integral folding of two functions is a concept that describes many important physical effects. The most familiar example is the

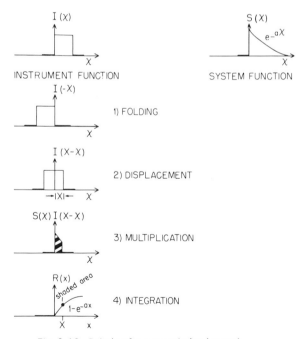

Fig. 2-10. Solution for a convolution integral.

response spectrum of photobiologic process, the folding of a source spectrum with an action spectrum.

The convolution integral is a mathematical relationship which is difficult to realize. A mathematical statement for it is

$$R(X) = \int_{-\infty}^{+\infty} S(x) \, I(X - x) \, dx$$

This is often described in a compact notation

$$R(X) = S(X) * I(X)$$

where the symbol * is the convolution process. $R(X)$ is the response function, the measured effect; $S(X)$ is the system response, the process desired; and $I(X)$ is the instrument response, which must be measured in a separate experiment.

For evaluation of this integral two X functions $S(x)$ and $I(X - x)$ are required. $S(x)$ and $I(x)$ are simply $S(X)$ and $I(X)$, where X is replaced by x. The function $I(-x)$ is the image of $I(x)$ created by folding about the ordinate axis, and $I(X - x)$ is simply the function $I(-x)$ shifted by the quantity X. To compute the integral it is necessary to multiply the shifted function by $S(x)$ and integrate: the area under the product $I(X - x)$ and $S(x)$ is the value of the convolution at x. To summarize:

1. *Folding.* Take mirror image of $I(x)$ about the ordinate axis.
2. *Displacement.* Shift $I(-x)$ by the amount X.
3. *Multiplication.* Multiply the shifted function $I(X - x)$ by $S(x)$.
4. *Integration.* Area under the product of $I(X - x)$ and $S(x)$ is the value of the convolution at x.

The details of a solution to a convolution are tedious (Fig. 2-10).

REFERENCES

1. Westfall, R. S. (1980): *Never at Rest: A biography of Isaac Newton.* Cambridge Univ. Press, Cambridge.
1a. Alberti, L. B. (1435): *Della pittora.* Firenze. [Translated by J. R. Spenser (1967); *On Painting,* Yale University Press, New Haven.]
2. Maurolico, F. (1553): *Photismi de Lumine et Umbrae ad Perspectivam et Radiorum Incidentiam Facientes.* Venice. [Translated by H. Crew. (1940): *Photismi de Lumine of Maurolico. A Chapter in Late Mediaeval Optics.* American Book Company, New York.]
3. Kepler, J. (1611): *Dioptrice.* Prague. (Reprinted 1962, Cambridge University Press, Cambridge.)
4. Dominis, M. A. (1611): *De Radiis Visus et Lucis in Vitris Perspectivis et Iride Tractatus.* Venice. [Summary in C. B. Boyer. (1959): *The Rainbow, from Myth to Mathematics.* Yoseloff Press. New York.]

5. Descartes, R. (1637): *Discours de la methode pour bien conduire sa raison et chercher la verite dans les sciences.* Appendix I: *La Dioptrique.* Appendix III: *Les Meteores.* Paris. [Translated by P. J. Olscamp. (1965): *Discourse on Method, Optics, Geometry and Meteorology.* Indiana Univer. Press. Indianapolis.]

6. Newton, I. (1672): A new theory about light and colours. *Phil. Trans. R. Soc. Lond.* **6:**3075–3087.

7. Herschel, W. (1800): Experiments on the refrangibility of invisible rays of the sun. *Phil. Trans. R. Soc. Lond.* **90:**255–283, 284–292, 293–326.

8. Ritter, J. W. (1801): *Physisch-chemische Abhandlungen,* Vol. 2. Leipzig.

9. Scheele, C. W. (1779): Untersuchung des Flusspathes und dessen Saure. *Crell's Chem. J.* **2:**192–203.

10. Grimaldi, F. M. (1664): *Physico-Methesis de Lumine, Coloribus et iride* Bologna. [The Physics of Light, Colours and the Rainbow. Dawson Publications. Hamden CT.]

11. Boyle, R. (1664): *Experiments and Considerations Touching Colours.* London. (Reprinted 1964, Johnson Reproductions, New York.)

12. Hooke, R. (1665): *Micrographia, or Some Physiological Descriptions of Minute Bodies Made in Magnifying Glasses.* London. (Reprinted 1961, Dover Press, New York.)

13. Newton, I. (1675): *An examination of colour phenomena in thin films and an Hypothesesis Explaining the Properties of Light. Phil. Trans. R. Soc. Lond.* **9:**515–533. [Refs. 6 & 13 reproduced in I. B. Cohen: (1978). *Isaac Newton's Papers and Letters on Natural Philosophy.* 2nd ed. Harvard University Press. Cambridge.]

14. Young, T. (1802): On the theory of light and colours. *Phil. Trans. R. Soc. Lond.* **92:**12–48.

15. Young, T. (1802): An account of some cases of the production of colours not hitherto described. *Phil. Trans. R. Soc. Lond.* **92:**387–397.

16. Newton, I. (1730): *Opticks: A Treatise on the Reflections, Refractions, Inflections and Colours of Light.* 4th ed. London. (1st ed., 1704.) (Reprinted 1952. Dover Press. New York.)

17. Rittenhouse, D. (1786): *An Optical Problem. Trans. Am. Phil. Soc.* Philadelphia. **2:**202–206. [Reproduced in T. D. Cope. (1932): Rittenhouse diffraction grating. J. Franklin Inst. **214:**99–104.]

18. Fraunhofer, J. (1821): Formation of spectrum upon diffraction from a framework of wire. *Denkschr. Konig Akad. Wiss., Munchen* **8:**1–76. [Refs. 18, 19, & 21 Reproduced in J. S. Ames (1898): *Prismatic and Diffraction Spectra.* Harper, New York.]

19. Fraunhofer, J. (1823): Kurzer Bericht von den Resultaten neuerer Versuche über die Gesetze des Lichtes und die Theorie derselben. *Ann. Physik* **74:**337–378.

20. Wollaston, W. H. (1802): A Method of examining refractive and dispersive powers by prismatic reflection. *Phil. Trans. R. Soc. Lond.* **92:**365–380.

21. Fraunhofer, J. (1817): Bestimmung des Brechungs- und Forbenzerstreuungs-Vermögens Verschiedener Glasarten, in Bezug auf die Vervollkommnung achromakscher Fernröhre. *Ann. Physik* **56:**264–313.

22. Biringuccio, V. (1540): De la pirotechnia. Venice. Trans. 1966. MIT Press. Cambridge.

23. Melvill, T. (1752): *Physical and Literary Essays.* Edinburgh. [Reprinted in *J. R. Astron. Soc. Canada* **8:**231 (1914).]

24. Galvani, L. (1791): *De viribus electricitatis in motu musculori commentarius.* Bologna. [Translated by R. M. Green. (1980): *Commentary on the Effect of Electricity on Muscular Motion.* Williams and Wilkins. Baltimore.]; A. Volta (1793): Account of some discoveries made by Galvani. *Phil. Trans. R. Soc., Lond.* **90:**403–431.

25. Kirchhoff, G. R. (1860): Ueber die Franunhofer'schen Linien. *Ann. Physik* **109:**148–150.

26. Kirchhoff, G. R. (1860): Ueber das Verhältniss zwischen dem Emissionsvermögen und dem Absorptionsvermögen der Körper für Wärme und Licht. *Ann. Physik* **109:**275–301.

27. Kirchhoff, G. R., and Bunsen, R. W. (1860): Chemische Analyse durch Spectral Beobachtung, I. *Ann. Physik* **110:**161–189.

28. Kirchhoff, G. R., and Bunsen, R. W. (1861): Chemische Analyse durch Spectral Beobachtung, II. *Ann. Physik* **113**:338–381.

29. Brewster, D. (1833): On colours of natural bodies. *Trans. R. Soc. Edinburgh* **12**:538–545.

30. Miller, W. A. (1862): Photographic detection of the ultraviolet emission of characteristic spectra from metal sparks. *Phil. Trans. R. Soc. Lond.* **152**:861–887.

31. Stokes, G. G. (1862): On the long spectrum of the electric light. *Phil. Trans. R. Soc. Lond.* **152**:599–619.

32. Stokes, G. G. (1864): On the application of the optical properties to detection and discrimination of organic substances. *J. Chem. Soc.* **22**:303–318.

33. Hartley, W. N. (1882): Note on certain photographs of the ultra-violet spectra of elementary bodies. *J. Chem. Soc.* **41**:84–90.

34. Hartley, W. N. (1884): Researches on spectrum photography in relation to new methods of quantitative chemical analysis. *Phil. Trans. R. Soc. Lond.* **175**:49–62.

35. Kircher, A. (1646): *Ars Magna Lucis et Umbrae.* in mundo-Rome.

36. Cellini, B. (1568): *Due trattati dell'Orificera.* Firenze. [Translated by C. R. Ashbee. (1966): Dover Press. New York.]

37. Beccari, J. B. (1745): De adamante aliisque rebus in phosphorium numerum referendis. *Comm. Accad. Bonon.* **2**(1):274–303.

38. Beccari, J. B. (1746): De quam plurinis phosphoris nunc primum detectis. *Comm. Accad. Bonon.* **2**(2):136–179.

39. Anderson, R. R., Levine, M. J., and Parrish, J. A. (1980): Selective modification of the optical properties of psoriatic vs. normal skin. In: *8th International Congress on Photobiology, Strasbourg.* Book of Abstracts, p. 152.

40. Becquerel, E. (1858): Recherches sur divers effects lumineux. Mémoires I, II and III. Action de la lumiere sur les corps. *C. R. Acad. Sci. (Paris)* **45**:815–819; **46**:969–975.

41. Becquerel, E. (1861): Recherches sur divers effets lumineux. IV Mémoire. Intensité de la lumiere emise. *Ann. Chim. Phys.* **62**:5–100.

42. Wiedemann, E. (1888): Über Fluorescenz und Phosphorescenz. *Ann. Physik* **34**:446–449.

43. Dewar, J. (1894): Phosphorescence and photographic action at the temperature of boiling liquid air. *Chem. News* **70**:252–253.

44. Wiedemann, E. (1889): Zur Mechanik der Leuchtens. *Ann. Physik* **37**:177–248.

45. Wiedemann, E., and Schmidt, G. C. (1895): Über Liminescenz. *Ann. Physik* **54**:604–625.

46. Wiedemann, E., and Schmidt, G. C. (1895): Über Luminescenz von festen Korpern und festen Losungen. *Ann. Physik* **56**:18–26.

47. Wiedemann, E., and Schmidt, G. C. (1895): Uber Lichtemission organischer Substanzen im gasformingen, flussigen und festen Zusrand. *Ann. Physik* **56**:201–254.

48. Vavilov, S. I., and Levshin, V. L. (1926): Die Beziehung zwischen Fluoreszenz und Phosphoreszenz fester und flüssiger Medien. *Z. Physik* **35**:920–936.

49. Vavilov, S. I., and Levshin, V. L. (1927): Die Beziehung zwischen Fluoreszenz und Phosphoreszenz fester und flüssiger Medien. *Z. Physik* **44**:539.

50. Jablonski, A. (1935): Über der Mechanismus der Photolumineszenz von Farbstoffphosphoren. *Z. Physik* **94**:38–46.

51. Goldstein, E. (1904): *Uber die Emissionspektren Aromatischer Verbinduggen. Ver. Dtsch. Phys. Ges.* **6**:156–170; Discontinuous luminous spectra from solid organic bodies. *Ver. Dtsch. Phys. Ges.* **6**:185–190.

52. Goldstein, E. (1911): Uber die Untersuchung der Emissionsspektren fester aromatischer Substanzen mit den ultraviolet Filter. *Phys. Z.* **12**:614–620.

53. Kowalski, J. (1910): La phosphorescence progressive a basse température. *C. R. Acad. Sci. (Paris)* **151**:810–812.

54. Kowalski, J., and Dzierzbicki, J. (1910): Le spectre de phosphorescence progressive des composés organique à basse température. *C. R. Acad. Sci. (Paris)* **151**:943–945.

55. Kowalski, J., and Dzierzbicki, J. (1911): Influence des groupements fontionels sur le spectre de phosphorescence progressive. *C. R. Acad. Sci.* (*Paris*) **152**:83–85.

56. Lewis, G. N., Lipkin, D., and Magle, T. T. (1941): Reversible photochemical processes in rigid media. A study of the phosphorescent state. *J. Am. Chem. Soc.* **63**:3005–3018.

57. Terenin, A. (1943): Photochemical processes in aromatic compounds. *Acta Physicochem.* (*USSR*) **18**:210–241.

58. Lewis, G. N., and Calvin, M. (1945): Paramagnetism of the phosphorescent state. *J. Am. Chem.Soc.* **67**:1232–1233.

59. Lewis, G. N., Calvin, M., and Kasha, M. (1949): Photomagnetism. Determination of the paramagnetic susceptibility of a dye in its phosphorescent state. *J. Chem. Phys.* **17**:804–812.

60. Evans, D. F. (1955): Photomagnetism of triplet states of organic molecules. *Nature* **176**:777–778.

61. Beccari, G. B. (1753): *Dell 'Electricismo Artificale e Naturale.* Turin. [*A Treatise upon Electricity.* London (1776).]

62. Körtum, K. (1794): Resultate einer Reihe electrische phosphorische Eigenschaft verscheidner Körper zu beobachten. *Voigt's Mag. Neueste an Physik Natur* **9**:1–44.

63. Dessaignes, J. P. (1810): Mémoire sur les phosphorescence. *J. Physique* **70**:109–128.

64. Heinrich, J. (1812): Traité de la phosphorescence des corps. *J. Physique* **74**:307–315.

65. Wheatstone, C. (1836): On the prismatic decomposition of the electric light. *Phil. Mag.* **7**:299–300.

66. Becquerel, E. (1839): Recherches sur le rayonnement calorifique de l'étincelle électrique. *C. R. Acad. Sci.* (*Paris*) **8**:334–337, 493–497; (1843): Des effects produits sur les corps par les rayons solarires. *Ann. Chem. Phys.* **9**:257–322.

67. Porter, G., and Windsor, M. W. (1954): Triplet states in solution. *J. Chem. Phys.* **21**:2088.

68. Monardes, N. (1574): *La Historia Medicinal de las Cosas que se Traen de Nuestras Indians Occidentales que Sirvem al Usos de Medicina.* [Translated by J. Frampton, *Joyful Newes out of the Newe Founde Worlde.* London (1577). Reprinted 1925, Knopf, New York.]

69. Herschel, J. F. W. (1845): On a case of superficial colour presented by a homogeneous liquid, internally colourless. *Phil. Trans. R. Soc. Lond.* **135**:143–145.

70. Herschel, J. F. W. (1845): On the epipolic dispersion of light. *Phil. Trans. R. Soc. Lond.* **135**:147–153.

71. Stokes, G. G. (1852): On the change of refrangibility of light, I. *Phil. Trans. R. Soc. Lond.* **142**:463–562; A. J. Angstrom (1855) Optische Untersuchungen. *Ann. Physik.* **94**:141–164.

72. Stokes, G. G. (1853): On the change of refrangibility of light, II. *Phil. Trans. R. Soc. Lond.* **143**:385–396.

73. Mascart, E. (1869): Sur les spectres ultra-violet. *C. R. Acad. Sci.* (*Paris*) **69**:337–338.

74. Stoney, G. J. (1870): On the cause of the interrupted spectra of gases. *Phil. Mag.* **41**:291–296.

75. Soret, J. L. (1871): On harmonic ratios in spectra. *Phil. Mag.* **42**:464–465.

76. Alter, D. (1854): On certain physical properties of light of the electric spark within certain gases, as seen by a prism. *Am. J. Sci.* **18**:55–57.

77. Alter, D. (1855): On certain physical properties of light of the electric spark within certain gases, as seen by a prism. *Am. J. Sci.* **19**:213–214.

78. Balmer, J. J. (1885): Notiz über die Spectrallinien des Wasserstoff. *Ann. Physik* **25**:80–87.

79. Bohr, N. (1913): Constitution of atoms and molecules, I and II. *Phil. Mag.* **26**:1–25, 476–502.

80. Davy, H. (1822): On the electrical phenomena exhibited in vacuo. *Phil. Trans. R. Soc. Lond.* **112**:64–75.

81. Bouguer, P. (1729): *Éssai d'Optique sur la Graduation de la Lumière.* Le Havre.

82. Bouguer, P. (1760): *Traité D'Optique sur la Graduation de la Lumière*. Paris. (Opus posthum.) [Translated by W. E. K. Middleton. (1961): University of Toronto Press. Toronto.]

83. Lambert, J. H. (1760): *Photometria Siva de Mensura et Gradibus Luminis, Colorum et Umbrae*. Augsberg.

84. Beer, A. (1852): Bestimmung der Absorption des rothen Lichts in farbigen Flüssigkeiten. *Ann. Physik* **86**:78–88.

85. Bunsen, R. W., and Roscoe, H. E. (1857): Photo-chemical researchers. Part 3, Optical and chemical extinction of the chemical rays. *Ann. Physik* **102**:235–263.

86. Hurter, F., and Driffield, V. C. (1890): Photo-chemical investigations and a new method of determinations of the sensitiveness of photographic plates. *J. Soc. Chem. Ind. (Lond.)* **9**:455–469.

87. Sumpner, W. E. (1892): *Proc. R. Soc.* **12**:10.

88. Ulbricht, R. (1900): Photometer for mean spherical candle-power. *Elektrotech. Z.* **21**:595–597.

89. Taylor, A. H. (1920): Measurement of absolute reflecting powers. *J. Opt. Soc. Am.* **4**:9–23.

90. Taylor, A. H. (1931): Measurement of reflection factors in the ultraviolet. *J. Opt. Soc. Am.* **21**:776–784.

91. Kubelka, P., and Munk, F. (1931): Reflection characteristics of paints. *Z. Tech. Physik* **12**:593–601.

92. Kubelka, P. (1948): New contributions to the optics of intensely light scattering materials. *J. Opt. Soc. Am.* **38**:448–457.

93. Mie, G. (1908): Contributions to the optics of turbid media, especially colloidal metal solutions. *Ann. Physik* **25**:377–445.

94. Latimer, P. (1959): Influence of selective light scattering on measurements of absorption spectra of chlorella. *Plant Physiol.* **34**:193–199.

95. Bryant, F. D., Secher, B. A., and Latimer, P. (1969): Absolute optical cross sections of cells and chloroplasts: Total scattering and absorption. *Arch. Biochem. Biophys.* **135**:97–108.

96. Theissing, H. H. (1950): Macrocontribution of light scattered by dispersions of spherical dielectric particles. *J. Opt. Soc. Am.* **40**:232–243.

97. Butler, W. L. (1962): Absorption of light by turbid materials. *J. Opt. Soc. Am.* **52**:292–299.

98. Shibata, K. (1957): Simple absolute method for measuring diffuse reflectance spectra. *J. Opt. Soc. Am.* **47**:172–175.

99. Amesz, J., Duysens, L. N. M., and Brandt, D. C. (1961): Methods for measuring and correcting absorption spectrum of scattering suspensions. *J. Theor. Biol.* **1**:59–74.

100. Dorman, B. P., Hearst, J. E., and Maestre, M. F. (1973): UV absorption and circular dichroism measurements on light scattering biological specimens; fluorescent cell and related large-angle light detection techniques. *Methods Enzymol.* **27**:767–796.

101. Duysens, L. N. M. (1956): The flattening of absorption spectrum of suspensions, as compared to that of solutions. *Biochem. Biophys. Acta* **19**:1–12.

102. Felder, B. (1964): The dependence of light absorption on particle size in heterogeneous systems. I. Theoretical considerations. *Helv. Chim. Acta* **47**:488–497.

103. Grotthus, (1815): Über einen neuen Lightsauger nebst einigen allegemeinen Betrachtungen über die Phosphoreszenz und die Farben. *J. Chem. Physik* **14**:133–192.

104. Draper, J. W. (1841): On some analogies between phenomena of chemical rays and those of radiant heat. *Phil. Mag.* **19**:195–210.

105. Stark, J. (1908): Further remarks upon thermal and chemical absorption in the band spectrum. *Z. Physik* **9**:889–894. See also Ann. Phys. 38:407–430 (1912).

106. Einstein, A. (1912): Thermodynamic foundation of the law of photochemical equivalents. *Ann. Physik* **37**:832–838.

107. Bunsen, R., and Roscoe, H. E. (1859): The laws of photochemical action. *Phil. Trans. R. Soc. Lond.* **149**:876–926.

108. Zanotti, F. M. (1748): De lapide bononiensi. *Comm. Accad. Bonon.* **1**:181–205.

109. Ritter, J. W. (1803): Bemerkungen zu vorstehender Abhandlung der Herrn Carl Wunch. *J. Chem. Physik* **6**:633–719.

110. Zucchi, N. (1652): *Optica Philosophica Experimentis et Ratione a Fundamentis Constituta.* Lugduni.

111. Nichols, E. L., and Merritt, E. (1910): Distribution of energy in fluorescence spectra. *Phys Rev.* **30**:328–346.

112. Vavilov, S. I. (1922): The dependence of the intensity of fluorescence of dyes on the wavelength of exciting light. *Phil. Mag.* **43**:307–320.

113. Warburg, E. (1920): Quanten theoretische Grundlagen der Photochemie. *Z. Elektrochem.* **26**:54–59.

114. Lenard, P. (1910): Über Lichtemission und deren Erregung. *Ann. Physik* **31**:641–685.

115. Melloni, M. (1833): Memoire sur la transmission libre de la chaleur rayonnante par differents corps solides et liquides. *Ann. Chim. Phys.* **55**:5–73. [See also E. S. Barr (1962): Infra Red Pioneers. II. Melloni. *Infrared Physics* **2**:67–73.

116. Goethe, J. W. (1810): *Zur Farbenlehre.* Weimar. [Translation MIT Press (1970).]

117. Henri, V. (1922): Étude des spectres d'absorption et de fluorescence du benzène. *J. Physique* **3**:181–214.

118. Nichols, E. L., and Merritt, E. (1910): The specific exciting power of different wavelengths of the visible spectrum in the case of eosin and resorufin. *Phys. Rev.* **32**:381–387.

119. Vavilov, S. I. (1922): Die Fluoreszenz ausbeute von Farbstofflösungen. *Z. Physik* **22**:266–272.

120. Anderson, W. L., and Bird, L. F. (1928): The measurement of ultraviolet quanta by fluorescent photometry. *Phys. Rev.* **32**:293–297.

121. Bowen, E. J. (1936): Heterochromatic photometry of the ultraviolet region. *Proc. R. Soc.* **154**:349–353.

122. Taylor, D. G., and Demas, J. N. (1979): Light intensity measurements. 1. Large area bolometers with microwatt sensitivities and absolute calibration of rhodamine B counter. *Anal. Chem.* **51**:712–717; 2. Luminescent quantum counter comparator and evaluation of some luminescent quantum counters. *Anal. Chem.* **51**:717–722.

123. Mandel, K., Pearson, T. D. L., and Demas, J. N. (1980): Luminescent quantum counters based on organic dyes in polymer matrices. *Anal. Chem.* **52**:2184–2189.

124. Mielenz, K. D., Mavrodineanu, R., and Cehelnik, E. D. (1975): Efficient averaging spheres for visible and ultraviolet wavelengths. *Applied Optics* **14**:1940–1947.

125. Teale, F. W. J., and Weber, G. (1957): Ultraviolet fluorescence of the aromatic amino acids. *Biochem. J.* **65**:476–482.

126. Christensen, R. L., and Ames, I. (1961): Absolute calibration of a light detector. *J. Opt. Soc. Am.* **51**:224–236.

127. Perkampus, H. H., Körtum, K., and Bruns, H. (1969): Calibration of fluorescence apparatus. *Appl. Spectrosc.* **23**:105–110.

128. Lippert, E., Nagele, W., Seibold-Blankenstein, I., et al. (1959): Measurement of fluorescence spectra with spectrophotometers and comparison standards. *Z. Anal. Chem.* **170**:1–18.

129. Bartholin, E. (1670): *Experimenta Crystalli Islandici Disdiaclastici Quibus Mira et Insolita Refractio Detegetur.* Copenhagen.

130. Huygens, C. (1690): *Traité de la lumiere, avec un discours de la cause de la pesanteur.* Paris. (Translated 1966. Dawson Press. Hamden, CT.)

131. Newton, I. (1704): *Opticks* (Question 29, Book III). London.

132. Malus, É.-L. (1809): Sur une propriété de la lumière réfléchie. *M. Soc. Arceuil* **2**:143–158.

133. Malus, É.-L. (1809): Sur une propriété des forces repulsives qui agissent sur la lumière. *Mem. Soc. Arceuil* **2**:254–267.

134. Malus, É.-L. (1810): Mémoire sur nouveaux phénomènes d'optique. *Mem. Inst. France* **11**:105–111.

135. Malus, E.-L. (1810): Mémoire sur les phénomenès qui accompagnent la reflection et la réfraction de la lumière. *Mem. Inst. France* **11**:112–120.

136. Arago, D. F. J. (1811): Sur une modification remarquable qu'éprouvent les rayons lumineaux dans leur passage a travers certain corps diaphanes, et sur quelques autres nouveaux phénomènes d'optique. *Mem. Inst. France* **12**:93–134.

137. Brewster, D. (1815): On the laws which regulate the polarization of light by reflection from transparent bodies. *Phil. Trans. R. Soc. Lond.* **105**:125–159.

138. Fresnel, A. J. (1816): Sur la diffraction de la lumière, ou l'on examine particulaièrement le phénomène des franges colorées que présentent les ombres dans corps éclairés par un point lumineux. *Ann. Chim. Phys.* **1**:239–281.

139. Arago, D. F. J., and Fresnel, A. J. (1819): Memoire sur l'action que les rayons polarises exercent les uns sur les autres. *Ann. Chim. Phys.* **10**:288–305.

140. Young, T. (1817): Chromatics, In: *Supplement to Encyclopaedia Britannica*, 6th ed. (1824). London.

141. Fresnel, A. J. (1825): Mémoire sur la double réfraction que les rayons lumineux éprouvement en traversant les aiguilles de cristal de roche suivant des directions paralleles a l'axe. *Ann. Chim. Phys.* **28**:263–279.

142. Nicol, W. (1828): On a method of so far increasing the divergence of two rays of calcareous-spar that only one image may be seen at a time. *Edinb. N. Phil. J.* **6**:83–84.

143. Rochon, A. M. (1811): Expériences sur la formation de la double image, et sur sa disparition dans le spath d'Islande et dans le cristal de roche, appliquées au perfection-nement de tous les micromètres composés de ces deux substances. *J. Physique* **72**:319–332.

144. Wallaston, W. H. (1820): On the methods of cutting rock crystals for micrometers. *Phil. Trans. R. Soc. Lond.* **110**:126–131.

145. Thomson, W. (Lord Kelvin) (1904): *Baltimore Lectures on Physics (1884)*. Cambridge University Press, Cambridge.

146. Weigert, F. (1922): Über polarisierte Fluoreszenz. *Phys. Z.* **23**:232–233.

147. Weigert, F., and Kappler, G. (1924): Polarisierte Fluoreszenz im Farbstofflösungen, I. *Z. Physik* **25**:99–117.

148. Weigert, F., and Käppler, G. (1925): Polarisierte Fluoreszenz im Farbstofflösungen, II. *Z. Physik* **33**:801–802.

149. Vavilov, S. I., and Levshin, V. L. (1922): Zur Frage uber polarisierte Fluoreszenz von Farbstofflosüngen, I. *Phys. Z.* **23**:173–176.

150. Vavilov, S. I., and Levshin, V. L. (1923): Zur Frage über polarisierte Fluoreszenz von Farbstofflösungen, II, *Z. Physik* **16**:135–154.

151. Levshin, V. L. (1924): Über polarisiertes Fluoreszenzlicht von Farbstofflösungen. *Z. Physik* **26**:274–284.

152. Levshin, V. L. (1925): Polarisierte Fluoreszenz und phosphoreszenz dur Farbstofflösungen. *Z. Physik* **32**:307–326.

153. Gaviola, E. (1926): Die Abklingungszeiten der Fluoreszenz von Farbstofflösungen. *Z. Physik* **35**:748–756.

154. Perrin, F. (1926): Polarisation de la lumière de fluorescence. Vie moyenne des molécules dans l'état excite. *J. Physique* **7**:390–401.

155. Perrin, F. (1929): Fluorescence des solutions. Induction moléculaire, polarisation et durée d'emission, et photochemie. *Ann. Physique* **12**:169–275.

156. Mitra, S. M. (1934): Über den Einfluss des K I auf die Polarization der Fluoreszenz von im Lösung befindlichen Farbstoffen. *Z. Physik* **92**:61–63.

157. Kerr, J. (1875): A new relation between electricity and light; dielectrified media birefringence. *Phil. Mag.* **50**:337–348.

158. Abraham, H., and Lemoine, J. (1899): Kerr phenomena. *C. R. Acad. Sci. (Paris)* **129**:206–208.

159. Wood, R. W. (1921): The time interval between absorption and emission of light in fluorescence. *Proc. R. Soc.* **A99**:362–371.

160. Gottling, P. F. (1923): Determination of the time between excitation and emission for certain fluorescent solids. Barium cyanoplatinate and rhodamine. *Phys. Rev.* **22**:566–573.

161. Hertz, H. R. (1887): Über einen Einfluss des ultravioletten Lichtes auf die electrische Entladung. *Ann. Physik* **31**:983–1000.

162. Thomson, J. J. (1899): On the masses of ions in gases at low pressures. *Phil. Mag.* **48**:547–567.

163. Lenard, P. (1900): The production of cathode rays by ultraviolet light. *Ann. Physik* **2**:359–375.

164. Lenard, P. (1902): Light electric effect. *Ann. Physik* **8**:149–198.

165. Einstein, A. (1905): Über einen die Erzeugung und Verwandlung des Lichtes betreffenden heuristisches Gesichtspunkt. *Ann. Physik* **17**:132–148.

166. Einstein, A. (1906): Zur Theorie die Lichterzeugung und Lichtabsorption. *Ann. Physik* **20**:199–206.

167. Ladenberg, E. (1908): On the initial velocity and number of photoelectric electrons produced by light of different wavelengths. *Phys. Z.* **8**:590–594.

168. Richardson, O. W., and Compton, K. T. (1912): The photoelectric effect. *Phys. Rev.* **34**:393–396.

169. Farnsworth, P. T. (1934): An electron multiplier. (A new type of cold-cathode tube of high current amplifying ability marks another step toward the solution of television problems.) *Electronics* **7**:242–243.

170. Rajchman, J. A., and Snyder, R. L. (1940): An electrically-focused multiplier phototube. *Electronics* **13**:20–23.

171. Newton, E. Harvey (1957): *A History of Luminescence*. The American Philosophical Society, Philadelphia.

172. Pringsheim, Peter (1949): *Fluorescence and Phosphorescence*. Interscience, John Wiley, New York.

173. Wood, Robert (1934): *Physical Optics*. Macmillan, New York.

174. Deminguez, X. A., Franco, F., and Diaz Viveros, Y. (1978): *Rev. Latinam. Quim.* **9**:209.

175. Haüy, René-Just (1801): Traité de Minerologie. Paris.

176. Lennard, P. (1935): *German Physics*. Berlin.

3

Introduction to Fluorescence Diagnosis

S. S. West

The fluorescence phenomenon offers many possibilities for visual and instrumental aid to diagnosis at the solution and cellular levels. This chapter will focus on some aspects of the fluorescence phenomenon exhibited by the fluorescent dye acridine orange (AO), which already gives strong promise of clinical usefulness and can serve as the basis for many additional applications. Though AO is dealt with specifically, the methodology utilized for determining some basic properties of the complexes it forms with various biopolymers is applicable to other fluorescent dyes chosen for use as biologic stains.

Acridine orange is a vital dye which can also serve as a molecular probe. Fluorescent molecular probes complex with a limited number of intracellular biopolymers. Such dyes display alterations in their optical and other properties as a function of environmental factors, including the nature of the complexing substrate molecule. Given the appropriate phenomenologic approach, it is possible to identify and localize particular biopolymers in an intact unfixed cell. This also holds true for fixed material, provided the effects of the fixation process are duly taken into account. Generally, instrumental methods are required. Although these are usually manual to begin with, the data obtained may lead to strategies for automation. Instrumental analysis is required because visual observation cannot provide either spectroscopic analysis or reproducible quantitation of fluorescence intensity, both of which are generally necessary. Similarly, fading of fluorescence cannot be visually

S. S. West • Division of Engineering Biophysics, School of Public Health, University of Alabama in Birmingham, Birmingham, Alabama 35294.

quantitated and induced optical activity (1, 2) cannot even be visually detected. (The latter is not treated in this chapter.) However, these can be additional means for characterizing or identifying particular cellular biopolymers or particular clinical entities. Despite the need for instrumental analysis, visual examination of cytologic material is of fundamental importance. Until such time as a sufficiently unique set of criteria has been established which is judged characteristic of the clinical entity under consideration, visual identification of the material which is the source of the data is essential.

Emphasis has been placed on the cell because of the present and growing importance of cytopathology. Also, the intact cell presents a much more difficult problem than a solution containing a purified cellular extract. Nevertheless, such solutions play an important fundamental role in developing knowledge of cellular biochemistry. The quantities of material present in a single cell are too small to be analyzed by any known biochemical techniques. Biochemical analysis of large numbers of cells provides qualitative and quantitative analysis which is only true for each cell present when the population of cells is perfectly homogeneous. This is rarely the case. Further, if the cell type of interest is a distinct minority in the cell population, its contribution to the biochemical analysis may not be detected. Conversely, when it is detected its contribution is assigned to all the cells present.

Fluorescent molecular probes provide a means for qualitative and quantitative comparison and correlation between data obtained from solutions and data obtained from cells. Fluorescence is a very sensitive phenomenon which makes possible detection and characterization of the extremely small quantities of biopolymer present in a single cell. Fluorescent molecular probes such as AO also form complexes with biochemically characterized biopolymers in solution. Given appropriate standards of measurement for the analytical techniques employed, data obtained from cells can be qualitatively and quantitatively compared with data obtained from solutions subjected to the same analytical techniques. This enables the identification of intracellular biopolymers in situ in the cell with particular macromolecules the biochemist has isolated, named, and studied in solution. Thus fluorescent molecular probes can serve to link biochemistry to cytochemistry. In addition, where a biochemical characterization of a given clinical entity exists, it may be detected in individual cells provided a probe that complexes with the telltale biopolymer is available and the distinguishing characteristics of the probe–biopolymer complex have been established.

The above briefly presents some of the attributes of fluorescence analyses of fluorochrome–cell and biopolymer complexes. However, from the standpoint of aid to diagnosis it is worthwhile to list a set of conditions which are required by an ideal diagnostic system, particularly one that is to be automated. Suggested systems can then be compared with this set of criteria.

IDEAL CRITERIA FOR AUTOMATED CYTOPATHOLOGY

1. Have knowledge of a biochemical marker(s) which is uniquely characteristic of the clinical entity of interest. This includes both qualitative and quantitative aspects.

2. Localization within the cell of the marker biopolymer(s) is specified.

3. Absolute physical optical and physical chemical characteristics of the fluorochrome marker–biopolymer complex which distinguishes it from other dye–biopolymer complexes are known.

4. Means are provided for absolute quantitation of the amount of marker biopolymer present whenever such quantitation is of importance.

5. Means must be provided for producing absolute data of sufficient accuracy to enable intra- and interlaboratory comparison of results. Absolute data, independent of instrumental characteristics, also greatly facilitate the design of automated instrumentation. The need for absolute data simply points to a need for absolute standards which can be stored for reference and can also be readily disseminated to all users.

6. The validity and accuracy of the methodology is in keeping with the epidemiologic characteristics of the disease in question. This is especially important for automated systems.

7. The cell or cells which produced an instrumental indication of the possible presence of the disease in question should be available for visual examination by the cytotechnologist and the cytopathologist. (In the case of flow systems, not treated here, this is ordinarily not possible. The entire diagnostic burden rests upon the instrumentation.)

8. The instrumental strategy for automated cytology depends upon prior explicit, detailed qualitative and quantitative information couched in instrument-compatible form.

The above criteria are entirely general and can, conceivably, be satisfied by various phenomenologic approaches in addition to fluorescence. However, fluorescence has already been employed in this manner and can provide a specific example which also serves to illustrate application of the principles involved. It is worth emphasizing that the principles are quite general, can be applied to any fluorochrome and its complexes, and in some instances are not limited to fluorescence. The discussion is carried forward with automated cytology as a goal, as this presents the severest problem. But the biophysical aspects apply equally to measurements taken with manual instrumentation under visual control as well as to solutions.

ACRIDINE ORANGE—A VITAL FLUOROCHROME AND MOLECULAR PROBE

Acridine orange is a vital fluorescent dye which exhibits marked metachromasy whenever conditions are such that dye molecules can interact with each other. This occurs in aqueous solution when concentrations of the dye in excess of approximately 2×10^{-6} M exist. It is observed by fluorescence spectroscopy or by the departure from linearity of the change in fluorescence intensity of the dye monomer as a function of dye concentration. The monomer of the dye emits green fluorescence with a peak at approximately 540 nm. The dimer and higher polymers of the dye emit red fluorescence with a peak of approximately 660 nm. When AO complexes with biopolymers it may be constrained to emit only green fluorescence, only red fluorescence, or some combination of both, depending upon the nature of the biopolymer and the dye-to-polymer ratio. Salt concentration, and pH also play a role. The green fluorescence emission band can be identified with a long-wavelength absorption band having a peak at approximately 490 nm. The red fluorescence emission band can be identified with a short-wavelength absorption band having a peak at approximately 455 nm. The peaks of both the fluorescence bands and the absorption bands may shift slightly when the dye complexes with biopolymers. In the presence of a biopolymer that binds the dye, the organization of the dye molecules with respect to each other is mediated by the nature of the biopolymer. The properties of each such complex are dependent upon the nature of the complexing biopolymer and consequently may enable the identification of that particular biopolymer even when it is present in a mixture. Thus, though AO stains a number of biopolymers within the cell, it is possible to distinguish each polymer from all the others provided the appropriate background information is available. One source of such data is provided by the studies of dye–polymer complexes in solutions of the purified substance. Another very useful source is cells that store large quantities of a particular macromolecule, e.g., as in mucopolysaccharidoses and other storage diseases. In the case of the storage diseases, extracts from cells must be analyzed to identify the cellular biopolymer. Analysis of tissue samples leaves indeterminate whether the biopolymers found are intracellular or extracellular.

Among the properties of the dye–macromolecular complex that can be determined are equilibrium thermodynamic binding constants (3–6), absorption and fluorescence spectra, induced optical activity usually observed as circular dichroism (CD) or optical rotatory dispersion (ORD) [ORD spectra (2, 7) have been obtained from individual AO-stained cells], and the kinetics of fluorescence fading (8–11). All of these properties must be explored as a function of either dye-to-polymer ratio in solution or as a dye-to-cell (12, 13) ratio when dealing with suspensions of cells. (For quantitative investigations, staining of cells is ordinarily carried out with cell suspensions.) Dye-to-cell ratio is employed because, ordinarily, there is no a priori knowledge of the amount of a particular biopolymer present in each cell in a suspension. The dye-to-cell ratio, expressed in moles of dye per cell, is an approximation that has proved useful. It has provided excellent agreement with results obtained from solution studies when the cell population is fairly homogeneous with respect to the biopolymers that complex with the dye. This has been demonstrated for DNA in AO-stained unfixed mouse leukocytes, and heparin in AO-stained neoplastic mast cells (5, 11). Note that concentration of dye with respect to the solvent is of secondary importance.

METHODOLOGY

Solution studies may require severe restriction of the salt concentration to obtain results that match those obtained from cells. Formation of the red-fluorescing molecular species on the substrate biopolymer is inhibited as a function of salt concentration. Consequently, in most of our solution experiments, the concentration of buffer has been limited to 0.003 M and sodium chloride has been omitted. When staining unfixed cells, physiologic saline is employed and the buffer concentration kept to a minimum so that the ionic strength of the solution remains within physiologic limits. The behavior of the dye within the cell does not appear to be affected by the external salt concentration. The staining reaction must be allowed to continue until equilibrium is reached, i.e., until no further dye is lost to the cells from the staining solution. This is generally a matter of approximately 20 min. After equilibration, no further changes in the staining reaction will occur as long as the cells retain their integrity and temperature is held constant.

For quantitative studies, adsorption of AO on the glassware must be prevented by using Teflon or fused quartz that is scrupulously clean. The plastic tips for automatic pipeters also show no appreciable adsorption of AO. Standard glassware may also be treated with "Desicote," "Siliclad," or similar agents, but this does not always prevent adsorption. The amount of dye adsorbed on glassware is a function of AO concentration, length of time the surface is in contact with dye solution, and probably other factors. Adsorption is a reversible phenomenon, so that the amount of AO adsorbed on the surface of a particular piece of glassware will change if the AO concentration in the solution changes. Thus it is no simple matter to compensate for adsorption. The much preferred procedure is to prevent its occurrence.

It is very important to check everything for adsorption of dye, even fused quartz and Teflon. Adsorption will occur on the latter two surfaces if they are not perfectly clean. The check consists in exposing the surface to a solution of AO in distilled water (we use deionized distilled water) for at least the length of time solutions will be stored in the course of an experiment. Containers that will be used for long-term storage can be assayed after 24 hr. After the surface has been exposed to the solution for the required length of time the containers are emptied and rinsed four or five times with deionized or distilled fluorescence-free water. The container is then rinsed with spectral-grade fluorescence-free acetone, which is then assayed in a fused quartz fluorescence cuvette for fluorescence. The acetone will show no fluorescence when adsorption is absent.

Purified AO should always be used.* Purified dye is essential for scientific investigations that seek to develop detailed understanding of the underlying chemical mechanisms. Purified dye is also necessary for reproducible results in other applications. Purity of AO can be ascertained by absorption spectroscopy (ϵ_{492} = 74,000 in ethanol) and by thin-layer chromatography on cellulose using the ethanol/water/acetic acid (56:43:1) system of Appel and Zanker (14).

FLUORESCENCE EMISSION SPECTROSCOPY (12, 13, 15)

The fluorescence emission spectra of the dye and its complexes are necessary for maximizing sensitivity by the use of appropriate optical parameters in instrumentation, to display all the spectroscopic species present and their respective behaviors, to display differences among the various complexes formed with the dye, and to serve the analytical requirements of the physical chemist as he seeks to provide a mechanistic explanation, referred to the molecular level, for experimental observations. For a given substance all wavelengths shorter than some long-wavelength limit will excite fluorescence. The intensity of the resulting fluorescence will depend upon the spectral composition of the radiation produced by the light source, by the transmittance, bandwidth, and spectral position of the fluorescence-exciting filter, and on the absorption spectrum of the fluorescing species. Thus, when using a high-pressure mercury lamp, isolating the 436-nm line and neighboring spectral components in the radiation from the lamp will usually produce the brightest fluorescence of AO and its complexes despite the fact that one of its absorption bands has a maximum at approximately 490 nm. This is due to the fact that the 436-nm Hg line is relatively very intense and AO has sufficient absorbance in this spectral region to make this exciting wavelength very effective. Changing the exciting wavelength does not change the fluorescence emission spectrum. However, if two fluorescing species are present, one may have a longer wavelength cutoff for fluorescence excitation than the other. Such is the case for red-fluorescing and green-fluorescing species of AO. In this instance, excitation by the 546-nm (green) Hg line will only excite red fluorescence. Conversely, 436-nm Hg line excitation will excite both the green-and the red-fluorescing species. Thus, since the fluorescence emission spectrum has constant shape over broad ranges of excitation spectra, there is usually no particular need to vary the exciting wavelength in studying the

*Purified AO is available from Polysciences, Inc., Warrington, PA 18976.

fluorescence behavior of a particular dye. But the nature of the exciting radiation should always be reported. There are, of course, instances where the exciting wavelength is changed. A continuous variation is used to obtain an excitation spectrum. A change to a longer wavelength may be made to isolate one of the fluorescing species. Fading of the red fluorescence of AO–mucopolysaccharide complexes is frequently carried out with 546-nm excitation. Aside from eliminating green fluorescence, the much smaller extinction coefficient is very advantageous for fluorescence fading kinetics, where the assumption is made that the absorbance is negligible. Excitation at 546 nm provides an excellent approximation.

In order to be meaningful, fluorescence emission spectra must be corrected for all spectroscopic distortions introduced by the instrumentation. Such spectra are termed "corrected spectra." Uncorrected spectra generally vary considerably among laboratories and even within the same laboratory. Uncorrected spectra in the literature can be misleading, particularly at the red end of the spectrum, or when ratios of the amplitudes at two wavelengths are given. Additionally, fluorescence emission spectra should be recorded rapidly enough that fading has no appreciable effect on the shape or on the amplitude. The fading rates of the spectroscopic species present in a given fluorescence emission spectrum generally differ from each other. Consequently, a slow spectroscopic scan will distort the spectrum to some extent. A rate of approximately 1 sec for a scan ranging from 400 to 700 nm is usually sufficiently rapid. But there do exist molecular species with faster fading rates, necessitating a more rapid scan.

In the case of fluorochrome-stained cells, identifying the biopolymers that have complexed with the dye may be facilitated by the metachromasy exhibited by the dye. AO is very strongly metachromatic. The green- and red-fluorescing spectroscopic species are widely separated, vary independently in their behavior, and can be detected individually even with simple optical filters. Also, both the green and the red fluorescence emission bands may shift their positions in the spectrum as a function of the substrate biopolymer. Spectroscopy with the microscope ordinarily employs relatively low resolution spectroscopic systems, particularly for fluorescence. As a consequence, when shifts in the position of a fluorescence emission band are small, additional properties of the dye–polymer complexes must be employed, such as the thermodynamic binding constants, the behavior of the complexes formed as a function of dye-to-cell ratio, and the fluorescence fading behavior, where this is applicable. Also, an important aid to identifying a dye–biopolymer complex is visual localization of the source of spectroscopic information. A variable diaphragm in an image plane that can be superimposed over the image of the cell can be used to permit radiation only from a selected area within the cell to contribute to the recorded fluorescence emission spectrum (e.g., Leitz MPV systems). When the nucleus is so selected, the spectra recorded are due to the complex of AO with the intranuclear nucleic acids (NA). Fluorescing cytoplasmic inclusions, vesicles, or organelles can be optically isolated in the same fashion. This serves to greatly reduce the number of molecular species responsible for the spectrum and greatly simplifies the analysis.

During the manipulations that are entailed in optically isolating a cell or a portion thereof, fading of fluorescence will occur. Such fading would invalidate the subsequent measurements. It can be entirely prevented by illuminating the specimen with yellow light. Any sharp cutoff yellow filter that prevents fluorescence-exciting wavelengths from striking the sample will do. Microscopes that have provision for two light sources can employ a high-pressure Hg lamp (100 W) dedicated to fluorescence excitation, and a tungsten or halogen light source for viewing the specimen while arranging for the optical isolation of the area from which measurements are to be taken. Epi-illumination cannot be used with yellow light, as a very poor image of the specimen results. Transillumination must be used along with such aids to visualization as interference contrast or phase microscopy. We have found the former to be preferable. Data are taken immediately upon switching to fluorescence-excitation.

Cells stained with the low concentrations (10^{-7}–10^{-5} M approximately) of AO that should be used exhibit very little absorbance, particularly in yellow light. This makes it difficult at first to identify cytoplasmic organelles or vesicles that contain the AO complexes of interest. Thus, there will be occasions when the optically isolated structure does not display the presence of the dye complexes of interest. However, experience with a given cell type in time provides some clues for the observer that greatly reduce the frequency of such occurrences. The nucleus, of course, is usually recognized quite easily. There are occasions, though, when storage granules appear to have merged, when discerning the nucleus with yellow light may be difficult. Here again experience can be a great help.

SOME INDICATIVE RESULTS

A few examples of results emphasize the importance of the principles given above.

1. The red fluorescence frequently observed in cytoplasmic granules is probably due to AO complexes with glycosaminoglycans (mucopolysacchardies) (GAG). The GAG can be distinguished from each other by the kinetics of their fading behavior both in the cell and in solution. Interestingly, all GAG except hyaluronic acid produce only a red fluorescence emission band. In contrast, hyaluronic acid, when complexed with AO, exhibits only green fluorescence even at large dye-to-cell or -polymer ratios.

2. The nucleic acids exhibit still different behavior (13, 15, 16). At low dye-to-polymer ratios only a green-fluorescing molecular species is present. As the dye-to-cell ratio is increased, the green-fluorescing molecular species saturates when approximately 20% of the available sites (phosphates) are occupied. As the green-fluorescing species approaches saturation a red-fluorescing spectroscopic species begins to make its appearance. With further increases in the dye-to-cell ratio the green species, as just stated, will saturate and the red species will continue to increase in intensity without further effect upon the green-fluorescing species. This behavior is observed in cells. In solution, the formation of the red-fluorescing species may occur at the expense of the green-fluorescing species. Also, in the cell, the dye does not distinguish between DNA and RNA. As a consequence, nucleoli are not distinguishable in AO-stained nuclei except in instances where the dye-to-cell ratio is very large. Under the latter conditions the nucleoli appear as reddish bodies in the nucleus, while the rest of the chromatin is yellow-orange. Other than this extreme, which frequently represents a dye-to-cell ratio toxic to the cell, AO does not distinguish between RNA and DNA. The properties of the red-fluorescing species that forms on complexing AO with nucleic acids (NA) are markedly different from those evidenced by the red-fluorescing AO–GAG complexes. The latter generally fade more slowly and have appreciably larger thermodynamic binding constants (11, 17). In the cell these values are found to be quite similar to those in solution. Heparin in rat mast cells, however, fades more slowly in cells than in solution; but biochemical analysis confirms that it is heparin in the mast cell granules. It is these characteristics that are the basis for judging that most red-fluorescing cytoplasmic granules probably contain AO–GAG complexes.

3. Fading of fluorescence shows several promising potentials. Fading of the red-fluorescing AO–GAG complex follows second-order kinetics both in cells and in solution. Second-order kinetics is evidenced when a plot of the inverse of fluorescence intensity vs. time yields a straight line. If the intensity of fluorescence-exciting radiation is measured in absolute units (e.g. w/m^2), an absolute number, the fading constant r'' (k'' in our earlier papers) can be derived which is characteristic of the substrate biopolymer (8). In our experience there is a different r'' for each of the GAGs. Since, with the exception of heparin, r'' obtained for an intracellular complex agrees with the r'' of the purified GAG in solution, this represents a method for identifying intracellular GAGs so that the identity is consonant with the biochemical identification.

Fluorescence fading can also serve as a means for measuring the intensity of fluorescence-exciting radiation in absolute units of measurement, if it is so calibrated. It is the only known example of a natural actinometer. This is accomplished by finding the slope r' of the replotted experimental data after taking account of initial fluorescence intensity. The value of r' varies linearly with intensity of fluorescence-exciting radiation. The wavelength and bandwidth and the emission spectrum of the light source must be specified. For specified conditions, a graph of r' vs. absolute values of fluorescence-excitation intensity provides a means for determining the irradiance produced by an unknown light source.

There is also preliminary evidence that r'' may be related to the activity of heparin. While additional work is required to firmly establish this relationship and seek understanding of the underlying chemistry, the initial results appear very promising indeed (9, 18).

QUANTITATION

Quantitation can be of fundamental importance for diagnostic applications and for increasing knowledge of the biochemistry underlying a particular clinical abnormality. It is useful to treat quantitation in two separate domains. These two domains are: (a) the instrumentation, and (b) the fluorescence properties of material that is to be evaluated. These two domains are interrelated since the nature of the instrumentation depends upon the particular property of the material that is to be detected and measured. Conversely, since biologic and biochemical preparations are frequently sensitive to environmental influences, the effect the instrumentation can have on the material must be accounted for. This clearly implies adequate knowledge of, in this instance, the fluorescence properties of the material to be examined coupled with qualitative identification. For cells, the latter condition requires identification as to type, while for solutions purification to some agreed upon level is necessary. Similarly, instrumentation artifacts must be taken into account and eliminated or corrected. In short, what must be sought is meaningful measurements truly related to the material under consideration.

The measurements one chooses to make must be intelligible to others as well as accurate and reproducible. This requires the use of standards. In the case of fluorescence, though it is possible to make absolute measurements by methods already described in the literature (19, 20), they are cumbersome and have not been generally employed. Hence, the state of affairs is described by one investigator as "fluorescence measurements are all over the lot." The use of the fading of AO–GAG complexes as a natural actinometer, described above, offers the possibility of a simpler means for absolute measurement of the intensity of fluorescence-exciting radiation. Also, since fading of fluorescence is irreversible, the measurements can be made more convenient by using a phosphor screen or a phosphor particle as a transfer standard (15).

Calibration and maintainence of the quantitative accuracy of any fluorometer requires two independent standards. This is due to the fact that the instrument light source and the photoelectric detector are independent of each other. Reference fluorescent materials cannot be used for calibration except when the same substance is to be assayed or only relative measurements are desired. Not only does the fluorescence emission spectrum vary from substance to substance, but the intensity of fluorescence it produces depends upon the spectral composition and the intensity of the fluorescence-exciting radiation. The readings produced by a fluorometer are entirely arbitrary unless suitable calibration of both the fluorescence-exciting radiation and the photoelectric detector is carried out.

Calibration of the fluorescence-exciting radiation has been discussed above. A phosphor screen (for solution instruments) and a phosphor particle (for microscope fluorometers) are convenient means for checking and maintaining calibration of the fluorescence-exciting radiation. The fluorescence of the phosphors is detected and measured by the instrument photoelectric detector. Thus, for the phosphors to be useful in maintaining calibration of the instrument, the calibration of the photoelectric detector must be assured. Another function the phosphors can perform is to enable measurement of the stability and noise content of the fluorescence-exciting radiation, since the phosphors, when dry, are nonfading fluorescent sources. In our experience the 100-W, high-pressure Hg concentrated arc lamp operated from the power supply described by West (13) is a very stable light source with regard to arc position as well as intensity. A stable light source is important for fluorescence. The small amount of light frequently available from fluorescent samples makes double-beam systems undesirable. Other methods of compensating for lamp instability add complexity and may not be entirely satisfactory. Also, lamp life is extended considerably with the West power supply, which could be an important consideration given the present price of lamps.

The photoelectric detector, generally a photomultiplier (PMT), must be characterized with respect to its spectral response and with respect to its sensitivity. The spectral response can be obtained by using a calibrated thermopile, a monochromator, and a suitable set of calibrated neutral density filters. A PMT has much greater sensitivity than a thermopile and should not be exposed to high light intensities. The PMT response will probably be nonlinear and the photocathode may be damaged. Exposure of a photo-cathode to too much light, even for a short interval, may produce permanent damage. A photocathode damaged by exposure to too much light is evidenced by nonlinear behavior of the PMT at any light level. The response of the PMT may also become sluggish. The spectral response of the PMT is obtained by substitution. A correction curve or a set of correction factors can be calculated which is utilized for producing corrected spectra. The PMT is calibrated in absolute units by comparison with the calibrated thermopile and the attenuation of the neutral density filters. The sensitivity of the PMT is maintained by using a radioactively stimulated light source. This consists of an inorganic phosphor mixed with tritium, the radioactive decay of which causes fluorescence of the phosphor. This is a constant light source over which we have no control. However, it decreases in intensity at a rate given by the half-life of the radioactive substance utilized to stimulate the emission from the phosphor. Since this occurs at a fixed rate, a calibration curve for this light source can be drawn as a function of time. Tritium has a half-life of 12.45 yr.

Sensitivity of the PMT may vary with time and consequently should be checked continuously during its use. Good practice is to check it at the beginning and end of an experimental run. Such practice also will detect a photocathode impaired by exposure to too much light. A check for PMT linearity should also be performed regularly. This consists of interposing a 0.3 or other known value neutral density filter somewhere in the optical train to see whether the response of the PMT is decreased by a factor equivalent to the attenuation of the neutral density filter. In general, because of reflection losses, the reduction of the PMT response will be somewhat greater than the attenuation factor of the neutral density filter. Appreciable departures, either more or less, from the attenuation introduced by the neutral density filter indicate a nonlinear PMT. Replacement of the PMT is the proper corrective measure.

The spectral characteristic is ordinarily quite stable and does not have to be obtained directly again. Once the spectral response of a given PMT has been obtained and a set of correction factors stored in a computer or in the curve-follower (15), additional PMTs can be calibrated by substituting them for the calibrated PMT in a scanning instrument. The differences between the two results that are obtained can be utilized to provide a new set of correction factors for the new PMT. It is also possible to obtain a spectral response curve by requesting it from the manufacturer.

The radioactively stimulated light source is calibrated when a calibrated PMT is exposed to its emission. A narrowband filter should be interposed. Once so calibrated, the radioactively stimulated light source can be used to provide absolute calibration for other PMTs provided the spectral response curves are known. When these calibrations are carried out for the fluorescence excitation and the detection portions of the fluorometer the instrument can be used as an absolute fluorometer, and quantum yield of fluorescence can be obtained. This procedure has been described in detail for a microspectro-fluorophotometer (21). In applications such as the measurement of fluorescence fading, absolute calibration of the PMT is not required, but constant sensitivity is. This can be checked by using the radioactively stimulated light source.

Data taken by a fluorometer calibrated in absolute units of measurement can be compared qualitatively and quantitatively with data taken with any other fluorometer that is so calibrated. It is by this means that the data obtained from solution studies can be compared directly with data taken from individual cells with the microscope.

FLUORESCENCE AS AN AID TO DIAGNOSIS

The first consideration in deciding to pursue an automated or semi-automated system as an aid to diagnosis is to examine the epidemiology of the disease under consideration. If the incidence is high, then the methodology employed can afford some number of false positives and false negatives without unduly overloading or interfering with the health-care delivery system. (Obviously, the number of patients subjected to false-positive or false-negative diagnoses should always be kept as small as possible for reasons of compassion.) The population as a whole should be considered, as automation is usually directed at screening large numbers of individuals; otherwise the cost effectiveness may be very poor except in instances where automation provides new, necessary information that will benefit the patient. Therefore, one must examine the incidence of a given disease in the general population or, in selected instances of industrial exposure, in populations at risk. The epidemiologic aspects of a given disease determine the validity and accuracy that instrumentation, automated or manual, must have in order to be cost effective and avoid overloading the health-care delivery system. Validity refers to how well the detection criteria upon which the instrumentation operates serve to separate individuals with the disease of interest from all other individuals. Accuracy refers to the performance of the instrumentation, given an adequate sample. Thus, it is possible to have perfect instrument performance with regard to detection of the chosen marker characteristics of samples supplied to it. Yet the validity may be poor if the marker(s) chosen are common to other clinical entities in addition to the disease of interest. This is most serious when normal individuals are identified as being afflicted with the disease for which the instrumentation is supposedly screening. Potential accuracy can be determined theoretically and confirmed in the laboratory. Determination of validity requires a clinical trial.

Cancer of the cervix and bladder cancer can serve as examples. The incidence of cancer of the female reproductive system was 141 per 100,000 or 0.14% of the total U.S. female population in 1975. Carcinoma in situ and nonmalignant tumors are excluded. Incidence of cancer of the urinary system in males was 29 per 100,000 or 0.03% of the total U.S. male population. For females the incidence of cancer of the urinary system was 12 per 100,000 or 0.01% of the total U.S. female population. These data are also for 1975 (22). Cancer of the female cervix and bladder cancer are subsets of these populations, so that the values for incidence would be even smaller. However, for the purposes of analyzing the effectiveness of an automated system, such differences are of no consequences since the values for incidence given above are already so small.

The incidence of cervical cancer is so small that any instrumentation used for screening must have perfect accuracy and the results must be perfectly valid. In the case of an industrial population at risk for bladder cancer because of exposure to a carcinogen in the work place, the expectation might be that approximately 10% of these individuals will develop bladder cancer. However, the latency period may be as long as 30 yr, so that the incidence per year can still be quite small. Thus even here, essentially perfect performance of the instrumentation is required.

Whether such performance of instrumentation can be obtained by statistically treating arbitrary measurements taken on the patient samples remains problematic. There is, however, a more certain approach to achieve the results that epidemiology dictates are required. This entails having a marker or markers that are considered definitive and which can be described in instrument-compatible terms. However, not to be lost sight of is the fact that authoritative identification of cell types and their reference to cancer are based upon visual examination by appropriately trained observers.

Image analysis has not yet succeeded in replacing the human observer to the extent that is can be applied to routine clinical use. This is not surprising when one considers the number of years required for the training of a competent cytopathologist or cytotechnologist. In the case of cancer, and cervical cancer in particular, the lists of characteristics that have been developed are still not sufficient by themselves to train a cytologist. Time spent at the microscope with a sufficient amount of material is the only known route for developing competence in the human observer. Hence, since the human observer is more intelligent and more versatile than any machine, it is unreasonable to expect that a set of morphologic criteria can be listed which will without fail and in every instance identify a malignant or premalignant cell. By the same token, classifying cells by machine into the various groupings used by pathologists presents even greater problems when depending on morphologic criteria alone.

In contrast, aneuploidy of chromosome number or of DNA content is considered an excellent correlate of malignancy (23). Karyotyping is a complex, time-consuming process which is also frequently plagued by a scarcity of material. Microspectrophotometric measurement of the DNA content of a nucleus is much more attractive. Measurements can be made on every cell in the preparation. Also, microphotometry lends itself much more readily to instrumental analyses with automated systems (16,24). Classically these measurements have been made after staining by means of the Feulgen reaction using manual microspectrophotometers. Scanning microscopes for quantitating the amount of DNA per nucleus, after treatment with the Feulgen reaction, have also been built, but have not found clinical application. The careful, meticulous manual absorption measurements of nuclei subjected to the Feulgen reaction have helped to establish the concept of the constancy of DNA content in normal nuclei. Such measurements have also demonstrated DNA aneuploidy and provide the basis for the strong correlation between DNA aneuploidy and malignancy (23). It has been suggested that the pathologist should resort to the Feulgen reaction in those instances where the diagnosis of the sample is indeterminate. In general, this suggestion has not been acted upon; few laboratories are equipped with absorption microspectrophotometers and the expertise to make the measurement.

The Feulgen reaction, whether measured by absorbance or fluorescence, yields self-consistent results in any single staining run, but the absolute values of absorbance or fluorescence vary from staining run to staining run. Such variability is difficult for automated instruments to cope with.

The fluorescence of AO-stained nuclei presents attractive possibilities in the solution of this problem. As mentioned earlier in this chapter, AO complexes with NA in the green-fluorescing form to the point where approximately 20% of the available sites are bound. Further addition of dye results in the appearance of a red-fluorescing species with no further alterations in the fluorescence of the green-fluorescing species (16). Thus, when red fluorescence is present in the nucleus (yellowish appearance to the eye) a stoichiometric amount of dye has complexed with the NA of the nucleus and the intensity of its fluorescence is a measure of the amount of NA present. Compared with DNA, RNA is a minor component of the nucleus. Also, the interest here is in detecting cells that are suspected of being malignant or cancer-related, not in absolute quantitation of the DNA per se. Note that fluorescence will always be observed when a fluorochrome is complexed with a macromolecule to which it can bind. However, the amount of fluorescence that is produced is not representative of the amount of substrate macromolecule present unless some end point is reached which indicates binding of the stoichiometric amount of dye. The AO–NA system displays this very nicely by the appearance of a new, red-fluorescing spectroscopic species. (Parenthetically, it can be pointed out that in the complexing of AO with GAG a green-fluorescing species does not appear, but a red-fluorescing species occurs immediately upon binding of the dye. It is not yet clear as to what indicator can be used to show that a stoichiometric amount of dye has bound to the substrate GAG. In the present state of knowledge, it is not possible to quantitate the amount of GAG present in a cell by the intensity of the fluorescence that is observed. Relative differences of course can be seen, or measured, but absolute quantitation is not yet possible.) The green fluorescence is separated by considerable distance, spectroscopically, from the red fluorescence band. It is easily isolated with a monochromator or a simple optical filter.

Using the AO methodology, a simple microspectrophotometer employing a green-transmitting filter of sufficiently narrow bandwidth to eliminate the red fluorescence band, means for optically isolating the nucleus, and a PMT tube are all that is necessary. Of course, the necessary associated electronics must be provided. A phosphor particle is employed as an arbitrary absolute unit of measurement. The intensity of fluorescence produced by any nucleus is expressed in phosphor particle units (ppu).

Measurements taken from normal and abnormal cells in this manner demonstrate that normal cells never produce nuclear fluorescence intensity beyond some maximum value. In terms of the ppu we employ as a standard, this is approximately 0.6 ppu. In contrast, in every population of cells taken from patients with a malignancy or an atypia a continuous distribution of fluorescence intensity (NA content) per nucleus has been found, which extends to considerably larger values than have ever been observed for normal nuclei. These results immediately suggest a strategy for an automated instrument (25). It is only necessary to recognize the nucleus, measure the total green fluorescence it produces, and decide whether the value obtained is greater than or less than the highest intensity ever produced by the fluorescence of a normal nucleus. Calibration of the instrument can be accomplished with the phosphor particle standard. The image analysis problem of finding and identifying each nucleus in the field of the microscope is not a difficult one and is aided by the appreciably greater brightness of nuclear fluorescence compared to cytoplasmic fluorescence. The instrument should be an automated scanning microscope. As such, any green-fluorescing object it detects should be brought to the attention to the cytotechnologist/ cytopathologist either by sounding an alarm and halting the scan, or by recording the coordinates of each alarm to permit recall and visual examination after the scanning pattern is completed. Thus, in all instances the instrument brings only *suspicious* objects to the attention of the attending personnel. The instrument need make no further attempt at diagnosis. The cytotechnologist and/or cytopathologist can examine the object that caused the alarm either directly through the microscope or by means of a color photograph of the suspicious object. The color photograph can also serve as a permanent record of suspicious cells. The term "object" is used because extraneous material, clumps of leukocytes or bacteria, as well as cancer-related cells can cause an alarm to be sounded. Scanning instrumentation contains a television-type display monitor. The cytotechnologist can recognize many of the false alarms as such from the monitor display. In the case of a truly suspicious cell, the cytotechnologist, with confirmation by the cytopathologist, makes the identification by direct microscopic examination. Such a strategy for automated instrumentation relieves the cytotechnologist and the cytopathologist of the burden of examining normal samples, which constitute an overwhelming majority of the slides. Instead, they, and the cytotechnologist in particular, need only be concerned with abnormal cells selected by the instrument. This strategy guards against artifacts and false positives. The false-positive rate depends upon the competance of the cytotechnologist and the cytopathologist, just as it does for the examination of PAP-stained material. The false-negative rate depends upon the performance of the instrumentation and the validity of the marker—DNA aneuploidy in this instance.

This approach offers distinct promise of performance which is in keeping with the constraint imposed by the epidemiology of the disease. The accuracy of the instrumentation can be assessed prior to its construction and can be tested in the laboratory. This was indeed done with an early model of the Leitz Texture Analyzing System (TAS). This model had no provision for quantitating the integrated fluorescence from each nucleus. But the essentially constant morphology of normal cervical epithelial cells permitted an approximation which depended upon size criteria as well as upon the intensity of the signal exceeding the threshold set by normal cells as the nucleus was scanned. This approximation will not do for bladder cells, because of the morphologic variability characteristic of normal cells.

Results reported for this system using the TAS were based upon samples from 65 patients (25). Of these patients 29 were normal and 36 were abnormal. The results obtained with the TAS showed zero false negatives and zero false positives. However, some cells called suspicious by the instrument showed inflammatory changes on visual examination. Although these are considered negative with regard to cancer, they are not considered false positives from the standpoint of the patient. The inflammatory cells do indicate that further medical attention is required. Additional patient samples have been assayed since the above referenced publication, which brings the total number of patients to 150, of which 72 were positive, 14 showed inflammatory changes, and 65 were normal. The results are comparable to those given in the published report, i.e., zero false positives (inflammatory cells are considered true positives) and one false negative. The false negative was an atypia with small nuclei that fell outside the size criterion. However, manual measurements of such cells have demonstrated integrated nuclear fluorescence in the abnormal range. Therefore, this false negative can be attributed to the inability of the particular instrument to perform a true integration of the fluorescence produced by each nucleus. This instrumental deficiency is eliminated in the current model of the TAS. All positives for cancer were confirmed by the normal practices of the pathology laboratories.

These results clearly demonstrate that the accuracy which this strategy predicts can be achieved in practice and is in keeping with the epidemiologic requirement. The detection of inflammation is considered a desirable attribute. The results also indicate that this strategy may be valid. However, a clinical trial is required to properly establish validity.

The increased nuclear fluorescence exhibited by inflammatory cells is interesting. Is it due to increased intranuclear content of DNA, RNA, or some other biopolymer that complexes with AO? It could also be some combination of these possibilities. If due to an increase in DNA content, is this cancer-related (26)? Future investigations, which will include longitudinal studies, will explore these possibilities.

Thus far studies on bladder cancer have been limited to manual microspectrofluorophotometer (MSF) measurements, as a scanning instrument capable of quantitating integrated nuclear fluorescence has not been available to us. However, the results obtained are essentially the same as those that have been obtained for cervical samples. Intensity of fluorescence from normal cell nuclei does not exceed 0.6 ppu and the abnormal cell nuclei show a continuous range of intensities which extends considerably beyond 0.6 ppu. Since the measurements are instrumental, whether taken manually with the MSF or on the automated TAS, they can be judged for accuracy. At the same time, indications of validity become clearly evident. Validity remains in some doubt because the limited number of patients who participate in preliminary trials may not provide adequate assurance that all possible interferences that may exist in the population at large have been encountered. A clinical trial, properly planned with regard to biostatistical and epidemiologic considerations, can provide the best test for the validity of a given approach as an aid in diagnosis or screening.

Another important consideration in evaluating a system is whether the new methodology is an aid to diagnosis because it provides additional important information. Here the fluorescence metholodogy that has been outlined appears to offer some advantages.

1. With respect to cancer, fluorescence can quickly and easily give evidence of the presence or absence of DNA aneuploidy. This information is not available from PAP-stained material.

2. Cytologic samples are dispersed and stained in solution. This effects a randomization of the sample components which is generally not the case in smear preparations. This randomization, coupled with the quantitative examination of every cell in the optical fields presented to the microscope in the automated system, may reduce errors due to the inhomogeneous distribution of cells in a smear preparation.

3. The clear delineation of morphology, the high-contrast image, and the randomization of the cell population on a slide may prove to be effective aids to visual examination. Indeed, this has been the experience in our laboratory.

4. This quantitative fluorescence methodology may provide early detection of malignant or premalignant cells. Koss et al. (26, 27) have shown that abnormal cytology suggestive or diagnostic of cancer may precede by months or years the appearance of a clinical lesion. Cancer of the cervix also shows a long latency period during which cytologic abnormalities can be observed. Koss et al. also point out that carcinoma in situ may mimic inflammatory changes. Thus, based on morphology alone, cytology can provide early indication of the occurrence of a cancerous or precancerous lesion. The fluorescence approach may provide even earlier detection of abnormal cells suggestive of cancer. In our studies of bladder cancer four cells from three patients were found which exhibited abnormally high nuclear fluorescence intensity, but which were normal morphologically. Of these three patients, two had undergone operations for bladder cancer four months and eight months, respectively, prior to our cytologic examination of their urine sediments. The third is suspected of having a ureteral tumor, but will permit

no surgery. In our experience cells with abnormal nuclear fluorescence intensity and normal morphology have never been found in patients with no history of cancer. The significance of this finding will be pursued in longitudinal studies. It may be, and this is not unreasonable, that DNA aneuploidy occurs prior to the appearance of abnormal cell morphology and that the fluorescence methodology can make this evident. Should this prove to be the case, opportunity for therapeutic intervention could occur even earlier in the pathogenesis of the disease than detection based on morphologic cytology.

5. Usefulness for screening a population at large or a population at risk cannot be adequately judged until a proper clinical trial has been carried out and evaluated. The primary concern must be with whether the number of false positives is small enough to preclude both overloading the health-delivery system and driving up the cost. False negatives do not have the same deleterious effects on screening, despite the undesirable consequences for the patient. Given an adequately small number or percentage of false positives, other considerations which must underlie a decision to screen or not to screen can be given attention. Only costs are mentioned here, as cost/benefit ratios and the criteria on which they may be based are properly left to the epidemiologists, biostatisticians, and health economists. Cost of automated equipment, rate of sample processing, and consequent cost per sample can, of course, easily be calculated from estimates provided by manufacturers of equipment. It shoud be strongly cautioned, however, that such initial estimates may be far higher than will later be the case when specialized, dedicated equipment becomes available. For good commercial reasons the equipment initially is designed to have great versatility and to perform many functions. Quite frequently, it is such equipment that is used initially to automate cytopathology. Naturally, such equipment is expensive, yet it is much less so than comparable equipment designed and built in the research laboratory. But, as manufacturers perceive a potential market, simpler, specialized, dedicated equipment will appear that is more suitable for the clinical laboratory and will also be less expensive. Such future costs are very difficult to judge. It is therefore suggested that the health benefits that can result from screening be given primary emphasis in reaching decisions with regard to screening programs.

SUMMARY

The principles underlying absolute qualitative and quantitative data from fluorochrome-stained cells have been presented. Such investigations can yield fundamental scientific information. The scientific findings can be applied to clinical cytologic samples to yield a strategy and a means for aiding in diagnosis or screening for particular clinical entities. A set of criteria has been given for an ideal system for automated cytopathology. Application of the absolute quantitative fluorescence methodology to cervical and bladder cancer has been given. Comparison of the automated system for detection of cervical cancer with the criteria for an ideal system shows that all the criteria are satisfied, with the exception that validity of the analysis, while strongly indicated, still requires a clinical trial to be fully established. It thus appears that fluorescence, using dyes such as AO to stain cells, and taking data from cells and solutions in such fashion that AO becomes a molecular probe, holds a great deal of promise for many fundamental investigations and clinical applications. Such methodology not only enables correlation of solution studies with cytochemical investigations, but also bridges the gap between basic scientific investigations and clinical applications.

It must also be emphasized that there are additional phenomena associated with AO–biopolymer and AO–cell complexes, such as fluorescence fading and induced optical activity. These may prove useful in analyzing the biochemical content of a cell, which may help in understanding the metabolic role of particular cellular macromolecules, and which may also serve as aids to diagnosis and means for following the course of therapy. A given problem may benefit from more than one phenomenologic approach. Finally, since identification of cytologic material depends upon visual examination, the capability of fluorescent dyes such as AO to yield biochemical, biophysical, and physical chemical data from cells without destroying the morphology must be considered among its most important attributes. This system should conceivably prove useful in screening for any tumor that displays DNA aneuploidy.

ACKNOWLEDGMENTS. This work was supported in part by U.S. Public Health Service Research Grant HL22402, Heart, Lung, and Blood Institute, National Institutes of Health. The author also thanks Ms. B. Perkins for her careful typing of the manuscript.

REFERENCES

1. West, S. S. (1969): Quantitative microscopy in bacteriology. *Ann. N.Y. Acad. Sci.* **157**:111–122.

2. West, S. S. (1970): Optical rotatory dispersion and the microscope. In: *Introduction to Quantitative Cytochemistry—II*, edited by G. L. Wied and G. F. Bahr, pp. 451–475. Academic Press, New York.

3. Menter, J. M., Hurst, R. E., and West, S. S. (1977): Thermodynamics of mucopolysaccharide-dye binding. II. Binding constant and cooperativity parameters of acridine orange–dermatan sulfate system. *Biopolymers* **16**:695–702.

4. Menter, J. M., Hurst, R. E., Nakamura, N., et al. (1979): Thermodynamics of mucopolysaccharide-dye binding. III. Thermodynamic and cooperativity parameters of acridine orange–heparin system. *Biopolymers* **18**:493–505.

5. West, S. S. (1970): The microscope, spectra, and automated analysis. *Clin. Chem.* **16**:643–650.

6. West, S. S., Hurst, R. E., and Menter, J. M. (1977): Thermodynamics of mucopoly-

saccharide-dye binding. I. Identification of free and bound dye via membrane filtration; acridine orange–dermatan sulfate system. *Biopolymers* **16**:685–693.

7. West, S. S., and Lorincz, A. E. (1973): In: *Fluorescence Techniques in Cell Biology*, edited by A. A. Thaer and M. Sernetz, pp. 395–407. Springer-Verlag, Berlin/New York.

8. Menter, J. M. Golden, J. F., and West, S. S. (1978): Kinetics of fluorescence fading of acridine orange–heparin complexes in solution. *Photochem. Photobiol.* **27**:629–633.

9. Menter, J. M. Hurst, R. E. Corliss, D. A., et al. (1979): Structural basis for the anticoagulant activity of heparin. 2. Relationship of anticoagulant activity to the thermodynamics and fluorescence fading kinetics of arcidine orange–heparin complexes. *Biochemistry* **18**:4288–4292.

10. Menter, J. M., Hurst, R. E., and West, S. S. (1979): Photochemistry of heparin–acridine orange complexes in solution: photochemical changes occurring in the dye and polymer on fluorescence fading. *Photochem. Photobiol.* **29**:473–478.

11. Nakamura, N., Hurst, R. E., West, S. S., et al. (1980): Biophysical cytochemical investigations of intracellular heparin in neoplastic mast cells. *J. Histochem. Cytochem.* **28**:223–230.

12. West, S. S. (1965): Fluorescence microspectroscopy of mouse leukocytes supravitally stained with acridine orange. *Acta Histochem.* (Jena) **1965 (Suppl. 6)**, 135.

13. West, S. S. (1969): In: *Physical Techniques in Biological Research*, Vol. 3C, edited by A. W. Pollister, pp. 253–321. Academic Press, New York.

14. Appel, W., and Zanker, V. (1958): Über die Bildung reversibler Assoziate des Acridinorange Metachromasie durch Heparin. *Z. Naturforsch.* **B13**:126–134.

15. Golden, J. F., and West, S. S. (1974): Fluorescence spectroscopic and fading behavior of Ehrlich's hyperdiploid mouse ascites tumor cells supravitally stained with acridine orange. *J. Histochem. Cytochem.* **22**:495–505.

16. Golden, J. F., West, S. S., Echols, C. K., et al. (1976): Quantitative fluorescence spectrophotometry of acridine orange-stained unfixed cells. Potential for automated detection of human uterine cancer. *J. Histochem. Cytochem.* **24**:315–321.

17. West, S. S., Golden, J. F., Menter, J. M., et al. (1976): Quantitation of fluorescence fading phenomena for identifying intracellular biopolymers. *J. Histochem. Cytochem.* **24**:59–63.

18. Hurst, R. E., Menter, J. M., West, S. S., et al. (1979): Structural basis for the anticoagulant activity of heparin. 1. Relationship to the number of charged groups. *Biochemistry* **18**:4283–4287.

19. Melhuish, W. H. (1973): *Absolute Spectrofluorometry*. National Bureau of Standards (U.S.) Special Publication #378, pp. 137–150.

20. Parker, C. A. (1968): *Photoluminescence of Solutions*. Elsevier, New York.

21. Corliss, D. A., West, S. S., and Golden, J. F. (1980): Calibration of a microspectrofluorophotometer in absolute units of radiation. *Applied Optics* **19**:3290–3294.

22. Hartunian, N. S., Smart, C. N., and Thompson, M. S. (1980): The incidence and economic costs of cancer, motor vehicle injuries, coronary heart disease, and stroke: a comparative analysis. *Am. J. Public Health* **70**:1249–1260.

23. Bohm, N., and Sandritter, W. (1975): DNA in human tumors: a cytophotometric study. *Curr. Top. Pathol.* **60**:151–219.

24. Al, I., and Ploem, J. S. (1979): Detection of suspicious cells and rejection of artefacts in cervical cytology using the Leyden Television Analysis System. *J. Histochem. Cytochem.* **27**:629–634.

25. Golden, J. F., West, S. S., Shingleton, H. M., et al. (1979): A screening system for cervical cancer cytology, *J. Histochem. Cytochem.* **27**:522–528.

26. Koss, L. G., Melamed, M. R., Ricci, A., et al. (1965): Carcinogenesis in the human urinary bladder. Observations after exposure to para-aminodiphenyl. *N. Engl. J. Med.* **272**:767–770.

27. Koss, L. G., Melamed, M. R., and Kelly, R. E. (1969): Further cytological and histological studies of bladder lesions in workers exposed to para-aminodiphenyl: progress report. *J. Natl. Cancer Inst.* **47**:233–243.

4

Ultraviolet-Induced Damage and Its Repair in Human DNA

W. L. Carrier, R. D. Snyder, and J. D. Regan

Electromagnetic radiation of appropriate wavelength and intensity can induce damage in cellular macromolecular structures. Ultraviolet (UV) radiation can, for example, damage many cellular structures, including membranes, protein, RNA, and, of course, DNA. Almost all cells, including human cells growing in tissue culture, show a striking lowering of viability after moderate doses of UV irradiation. There is evidence suggesting that damage to DNA is the primary event responsible for UV-induced cell degeneration and death (1–3). Although cause and effect has not been definitely established, a number of experimental correlations support the theory that UV-induced DNA pyrimidine dimers represent one of the principal causative agents in the death and mutation of mammalian cells. Certainly, the identification of dimers as inactivating agents in human cells has provided us with the best insight available into an understanding of the role of cellular DNA repair processes in environmental carcinogenesis.

Dimers may produce their effects by altering a variety of cellular processes. Good evidence now exists that UV radiation blocks both transcription and translation and that above certain critical doses this block is irreversible and must therefore lead to cell death (4, 5). Thus, while it is true that organisms or cell strains showing decreased ability to remove UV radiation photoproducts from their DNA often show an associated altered

W. L. Carrier, R. D. Snyder, and J. D. Regan • Biology Division, Oak Ridge National Laboratory, Oak Ridge, Tennessee 37830.

By acceptance of this article, the publisher or recipient acknowledges the U. S. Government's right to retain a nonexclusive, royalty-free license in and to any copyright covering the article.

survival curve for UV radiation, one must be careful in interpreting this phenomenon.

In addition to the study of effects of chemical carcinogens on DNA, there has been for many years a concentrated effort to study the effects of nonionizing and ionizing radiation on DNA. The basis of this intense interest in DNA damage lies in the following points: Physical and chemical carcinogens induce DNA damage, and practically all procaryotic and eucaryotic organisms have evolved mechanisms to remove or neutralize these damages. Maintenance of these repair systems thus implies that the damages in the DNA must have some biologic significance. Moreover, the vast majority of carcinogens tested have proved to be mutagens, suggesting that the interaction of the substances with DNA might be the primary event in the sequence leading to carcinogenesis. Finally, individuals with genetically defective repair systems have a greatly increased risk of cancer, as evidenced by studies of the disease xeroderma pigmentosum among others. Taken together, these observations suggest that in photocarcinogenesis the primary event leading to the development of the cancerous state is a sunlight-induced lesion in the DNA of skin cells. Much work has been carried out in the elucidation of the types of lesions induced in cellular DNA by UV radiation.

The pyrimidine dimer has received far more attention in terms of research effort than all of the other UV-induced lesions for two reasons, the first of which relates to the biologic significance of the pyrimidine dimer. In systems where it can be adequately examined, reversal of pyrimidine dimers by a photoreactivating enzyme system at least partially restores such biologic parameters as colony-forming ability, transcriptional capacity, semiconservative DNA synthesis, and normal low mutagenesis rates. The second reason is a technical one relating to the relatively large numbers of these lesions induced in DNA by a given dose of UV radiation (as compared to some of the other lesions) and to the availability of assays that allow quite accurate quantitation of the dimers. Therefore, the many experiments published on pyrimidine dimers not only reflect the biologic significance of the dimer, but also the ease with which these lesions may be analyzed.

In general, most organisms have evolved three mechanisms for dealing with DNA damage (Fig. 4-1). The first of these, photoreactivation, is a light-dependent process requiring a single enzyme that is capable of reconstituting thymine in situ without DNA strand breakage or resynthesis. Photoreactivation has been observed to occur in practically every phylum of plants and animals, but although several accounts of this phenomenon in human cells have been published (6), other reports indicate only low and inconsistent photoreactivation in human cells (7). Dimers pose an immediate threat to the cell's DNA synthetic process in that a dimer is a block to chain growth. The cell must either remove the dimer or, failing in that effort, somehow bypass the impeding structure. The second process, that of

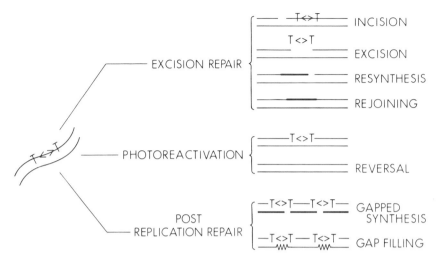

Fig. 4-1. Mechanisms for repair of DNA containing UV-induced pyrimidine dimers in human cells.

postreplication repair in human cells, is poorly understood but evidently allows restoration of DNA synthesis without dimer removal. It seems clear that postreplication repair occurs when gaps left in the daughter strand are slowly filled in by de novo synthesis (8, 9). Evidence exists for other modes of repair, such as a recombinational mechanism (10–12) or a simple read-through of the dimer. The most thoroughly studied of the three modes of repair is the excision repair process, in which a battery of enzymes act in a sequential fashion (see Fig. 4-1), resulting in the removal of the lesion and subsequent resynthesis of the DNA (13–16).

The first part of this chapter will be devoted to the induction and fate of pyrimidine dimers: specifically, those aspects relating to the wavelength dependence of induction, dose–response relationships, and the analyses of various methodologies aimed at understanding the mechanisms and kinetics of the excision repair process in human cells. For further information on the processes of photoreactivation and postreplication repair, the interested reader is referred to the review by Cleaver (15). In the second part of the chapter, we will deal with other UV photoproducts and their repair.

INDUCTION OF DIMERS IN CELLULAR DNA

UV radiation causes a linkage of adjacent pyrimidines in DNA, giving rise to thymine–thymine, thymine–cytosine, and cytosine–cytosine (T$<>$T, T$<>$C, C$<>$C) dimers. It is estimated that about 90% of the damage induced in DNA by UV radiation occurs with the formation of these types of dimers.

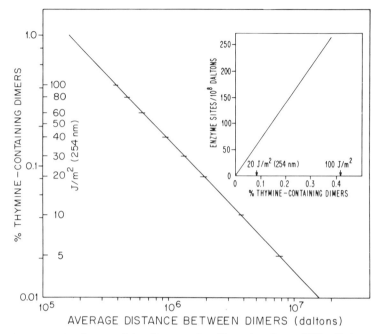

Fig. 4-2. Percent thymine-containing dimers produced by various doses of UV radiation and the average distance in daltons between dimers. Inset shows the relationship between percent dimers and the number of UV-endonuclease-sensitive sites.

Using the procedures of two-dimensional paper chromatography (17) and an assay of UV-endonuclease-sensitive sites (ESS) (18), one may quantitate dimers following various doses, each representing a different wavelength of UV radiation. The ordinate axis of Fig. 4-2 shows that the percent thymine in dimers increases with increase in dose of 254-nm radiation. The linearity of this relationship at low doses is seen clearly in the inset, where a determination of ESS is plotted against the dose of 254-nm radiation. Assuming a random distribution of dimers in the DNA, one can then estimate the average distance between dimers. As seen in Fig. 4-2, this estimate of the distance between dimers based on chromatographic data is substantiated by the ESS analysis.

If one exposes cells to longer UV wavelengths, much higher doses are needed to create the same number of dimers in the DNA. Figure 4-3 demonstrates that increasing the wavelength from 254 to 313 nm requires a 2000-fold increase in dose to produce one million dimers per cell. In experiments reported by Trosko et al. (19), human cells in culture exposed to 100 min of July sunlight in East Lansing, Michigan, produced about the same

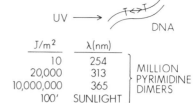

UV ⟶ DNA

J/m²	λ(nm)	
10	254	
20,000	313	MILLION PYRIMIDINE DIMERS
10,000,000	365	
100'	SUNLIGHT	

Fig. 4-3. Numbers of pyrimidine dimers represented by T<>T in tissue culture cells following irradiation at various wavelengths of light.

number of dimers as 10 J m^{-2} of 254-nm radiation. However, it is estimated that only about 10% of the wavelengths around 300 nm would penetrate the skin to the sensitive basal layers (20), so that one could conclude that a biologically significant dose of 254-nm radiation might be in the neighborhood of 1–5 J m^{-2}.

However, since essentially no 254-nm radiation reaches the earth's surface, it is desirable to extend our observations to include studies with a source more closely approximating the wavelengths of natural solar light. We have conducted studies using a Westinghouse FS40 sunlamp that produces mostly near-UV but some wavelengths in the far-UV as well. The spectral irradiance of the cellulose acetate (Kodacel)-filtered lamps closely simulates sunlight (21, 22). Figure 4-4 shows that, as in the case of 254-nm radiation, there is a linear increase in dimers with increase in exposure time. Filtering out lower wavelengths with various filters reduces the dimerization drastically. A

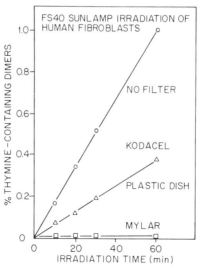

Fig. 4-4. The percentage of thymine-containing dimers induced in human fibroblast DNA after irradiations with an FS40 Westinghouse sunlamp filtered with either two layers of Kodacel TA-401 (5 ml; 0.13 mm) plastic film, a plastic culture dish top, or one layer of Mylar type A (10 ml; 0.25 mm) plastic film. The dose rate for Kodacel-filtered light samples was 1.6 J m^{-2} sec^{-1}.

thin film of Mylar effectively masks all wavelengths below about 315 nm, with the result that essentially no dimers are induced at these doses.

A more detailed study of wavelength dependence on dimer formation has recently been conducted by Rothman and Setlow (23). Their results with the Chinese hamster V-79 cell system are consistent with our results in human cells.

In addition to ascertaining the total number of dimers induced in DNA by various wavelengths of UV radiation, we determined the relative proportions of the three pyrimidine dimer types. Labeling of both thymidine and cytosine in human cells using $[^{14}C]$uridine as a precursor allows one to quantitate all three dimers by using two-dimensional paper chromatography (24). After 50 J m^{-2} of 254-nm radiation, the ratio of C<>C, C<>T, T<>T in human cellular DNA is 16:24:60. In contrast, this ratio is 24:38:38 in *Escharichia coli*. Due to the absorption characteristics of cytosine, not only are fewer C<>C dimers produced, but, in addition, their incidence levels off more at lower doses thar. does that of the other forms. For example, while thymine-containing dimers may be induced to a level of about 10% of the total pyrimidines, the C<>C dimer will make up only 0.05% of that total. Cytosine-containing dimers, however, make up a large proportion of the total dimers when cells are irradiated with low biologically relevant doses of the wavelengths contained in sunlight. A low dose of filtered FS40 radiation produces dimers at a ratio of 20:40:40 (C<>C, C<>T, T<>T) in human cells. The number and kinds of pyrimidine dimers induced in DNA by UV radiation are related to the DNA base ratio, the wavelength of UV radiation, and the total dose. In human cells after low biologic doses of 254-nm radiation, the thymine-containing dimers comprise about 75% of the total dimers; after "sunlight" the number is reduced to 60%. Whether or not this difference in the kinds of dimers seen at different wavelengths is biologically significant is at present unclear.

METHODS FOR STUDYING DNA EXCISION REPAIR

Table 4-1 lists a number of different methods for the study of excision repair. The majority of the information on human dimer excision presented in this chapter has been derived in our laboratory utilizing three of these methods: (1) two-dimensional paper chromatography of pyrimidine dimers; (2) enzymatic assay on UV–ESS; and (3) bromodeoxyuridine photolysis. These methods are briefly described this section.

Chromatographic Analysis of Thymine-Containing Dimers

Pyrimidine dimers removed from the DNA of UV-irradiated cells during excision repair may be observed directly by paper chromatographic analysis

Table 4-1. Methods of Studying Excision Repair

I. Loss of dimers from DNA
    A. Dimer chromatography (17, 25)
    B. Dimer-specific enzyme-sensitive sites (18)
II. Repair replication
    A. Unscheduled DNA synthesis (26)
    B. Bromodeoxyuridine photolysis (27)
    C. Bromodeoxyuridine incorporation plus
        isopycnic gradient analysis (28–30)
    D. BND–cellulose chromatography (31)
III. Strand Breakage
    A. Alkaline sucrose sedimentation (32)
    B. Alkaline elution (33)
    C. Alkaline strand separation plus
        hydroxylapatite chromatography (34)
    D. Nucleoid sedimentation (35)
IV. Immunologic analysis (36)
V. Inhibition of repair (37–39)

---

of radioactive thymine in DNA hydrolysates. The number of dimers remaining after a postirradiation incubation period under visible light or in the dark is an indication of the cell's capacity to perform either photoreactivation repair or excision repair. The procedure for the measurement of the repair of thymine-containing dimers involves these steps: (1) growth and labeling of the DNA of cells with radioactive thymine; (2) UV-irradiation and postirradiation incubation; (3) cell lysis, DNA isolation, and fractionation on the basis of insolubility in 5% trichloracetic acid; (4) DNA hydrolysis in 98% formic acid to free bases and photoproducts; (5) separation of the labeled thymine and thymine–thymine and thymine–cytosine dimers; and (6) calculation of the percentage radioactivity contained in thymine-containing dimers. The resolution of the radiochromatographic technique is difficult at UV doses below 5 J m^{-2}. In contrast to other ways of studying DNA repair, such as bromodeoxyuridine photolysis and techniques measuring repair replication, this method as well as the ESS methods described below allow determination of the fate of a specific biologically relevant lesion in cells, i.e., the pyrimidine dimer. Other methods measure every DNA lesion that elicits repair replication.

Enzymatic Assay of UV-Irradiated DNA

The first evidence for the presence of specific enzymes capable of producing incisions in UV—damaged DNA was obtained by Strauss (40). He discovered that extracts of *Micrococcus luteus* could degrade UV-irradiated transforming DNA, but not untreated DNA. Carrier and Setlow (41) showed that this same extract from *M. luteus* was able to excise thymine-containing dimers from irradiated DNA. While dimer-specific enzymes have been isolated from bacterial sources, attempts to purify them from human cells have been unsuccessful. [For a review of the use of enzymes capable of producing single-strand nicks into UV-irradiated DNA see Paterson (18)].

This in vitro method measures the number of enzyme-sensitive sites (pyrimidine dimers) contained in UV-irradiated DNA. This assay is performed as follows: Separate cultures of diploid fibroblasts having the DNA labeled with $[^3H]$- or $[^{14}C]$thymidine are exposed to UV irradiation. The ^3H-labeled cells are incubated in medium, allowing cellular processes to remove dimers from the DNA. Since the enzyme produces less than 0.1 nonspecific break per 10^8 daltons of DNA in unirradiated cells, these cells are not required for the assay. After the cells have been allowed to repair, they are mixed with unincubated but irradiated ^{14}C-labeled cells. The combined DNAs are then coextracted by a modification of the chloroform–isoamyl alcohol procedure of Marmur (42). The cells are lysed, treated with pronase and RNase, shaken with chloroform–isoamyl alcohol, centrifuged, and a small aliquot of the collected DNA is precipitated with 95% ethanol. The samples are dissolved in the enzyme assay buffer and analyzed immediately or frozen for assay at a more convenient time. This isolated enzyme-untreated DNA has a molecular weight of $\sim 20 \times 10^6$ daltons and is easily discernible on sucrose gradients from the enzyme-treated 2×10^6 daltons DNA resulting from cells given 20 J m^{-2} of 254-nm radiation. After treatment of the two DNA samples with enzyme they are co-sedimented in a 5–20% alkaline sucrose gradient. Fractions are collected on paper strips and the acid-soluble radioactivity is determined in a scintillation counter (43). Then the distribution of counts is converted to average molecular weights by a computer program. If one assumes that the breaks are distributed randomly, then $M_n = M_w/2$. The number of breaks per unit molecular weight is $1/M_n$, and the change in $1/M_n$ is a result of degradation by the treatment and represents the number of enzyme-sensitive sites (pyrimidine dimers) per dalton.

Until recently it was thought that nicks produced in UV-irradiated DNA at dimer sites were performed by a single enzyme, i.e., UV-endonuclease. It has now been shown (44, 45) that the action of the *M. luteus* and T4 enzymes are the result of one enzyme that ruptures the glycosylic bond of the 5′-pyrimidine of the dimer and another enzyme that cleaves the phosphodiester backbone between the resulting apyrimidinic site and the 3′-pyrimidine of the dimer. This finding, however, in no way alters the validity or sensitivity of the above assay.

Bromodeoxyuridine (BrdU) Photolysis

The bromouracil photolysis assay (27) is based on the incorporation of BrdU into areas of DNA undergoing repair synthesis and the subsequent scission of these areas when cells are irradiated with 313-nm radiation. From the kinetics of appearance of strand breaks with increasing fluence of radiation, one can calculate the number of repaired areas per unit length of DNA and, more importantly, the average number of residues inserted per repaired area. From an analysis of these patch sizes, much information can be obtained relating to molecular mechanisms of repair and to comparisons between UV radiation and various carcinogenic chemical agents with respect to lesion recognition.

To perform the assay, human cells growing in vitro are labeled overnight with $[^3H]$- or $[^{14}C]$thymidine. The cells are then irradiated with UV and placed in medium containing the thymidine analog BrdU. During the repair period, the UV-induced pyrimidine dimers are removed along with long patches of undamaged nucleotides. These long (60–100 nucleotides) open gaps are then filled in with nucleotides by the repair polymerase. When large amounts $(10^{-4} M)$ of BrdU are present in the medium, this thymidine analog is incorporated into the DNA at each site in the repaired region ordinarily occupied by thymidine. Absorption of 313-nm radiation by bromouracil-substituted DNA results in the production of alkaline-labile regions that are detectable as DNA single-strand breaks in alkaline sucrose gradients. The number of strand breaks observed in the DNA is a measure of the number of regions repaired during the incubation period. By delivering increasing doses of 313-nm radiation, one can estimate the size of the average repaired region, since long patches of BrdU-containing DNA will be photolysed by lower doses of 313-nm radiation, while the shorter patches offer a smaller target for the 313-nm radiation and thus will require higher doses.

EXCISION REPAIR

It is not the intention of this chapter to provide an exhaustive review of the literature concerning excision repair of UV-induced pyrimidine dimers, since many excellent reviews are already in print. Instead we wish to focus attention on certain aspects of UV damage repair that seem important in terms of their biologic implications and possible medical significance.

In 1968, we first described the excision of dimers from the DNA of human cells (46). In these experiments, we monitored the loss of pyrimidine dimers from TCA-insoluble cell fractions as a function of time following UV irradiation of various cell lines. Within the error of determination, there was no difference in the repair of dimers in human amnion cells, HeLa cells, or a human diploid fibroblast cell strain (WI-38). It was concluded at that time that even though dimer loss could be clearly seen in all of the cell lines, thus suggesting an excision process, complete loss of those dimers did not occur. Instead it appeared that the higher the dose of UV radiation administered, the lower the percent of dimers removed. Modifications of two-dimensional paper chromatography techniques have allowed more accurate determination of dimer amounts following low doses of UV radiation and have led to the demonstration, as detailed below, that most dimers are, in fact, excised at low doses. However, a saturation of the excision system seems to occur at higher doses and, even at times of up to 72 hr after irradiation, not all dimers are removed from cellular DNA. Improvements in the sensitivity of the chromatographic assay allowed us to show that rodent cells, previously thought to lack any excision repair of dimers, did, in fact, possess a repair system capable of removing dimers to about 10–15% of normal human levels.

The important observation made by Cleaver (30) that cells from patients with xeroderma pigmentosum (XP) showed very low levels of repair replication and unscheduled DNA synthesis following UV irradiation led us to a study of the dimer removal in these XP lines. In collaboration with Setlow and German (47), we showed that cells of classical XP patients exhibited essentially no loss of dimers from their DNA, possibly due to a defect in the incision process.

The so-called chromosome-breakage syndromes have also been of particular interest to workers in the area of DNA repair because of the many spontaneous chromosome aberrations seen in these cell lines. Abnormal cytogenetics in Bloom syndrome, Fanconi anemia, and Louis–Barr syndrome (ataxia-telangiectasia) suggest that a defect exists in DNA replication and/or DNA repair processes in these cells (48). Although our studies demonstrate no deficiency in dimer removal in these cell strains as far as the excision of dimers from cellular DNA is concerned, recent evidence suggests that repair of other lesions may be deficient. Paterson et al. (49), for example, have shown that ataxia-telangiectasia cells may be defective in their ability to remove gamma-ray-induced lesions from their DNA. Recent reports, using a more sensitive technique, found no deficiency in the rate of DNA-strand rejoining of these cells (50). Remsen and Cerutti (51) have demonstrated an altered capacity of fibroblasts from both ataxia-telangiectasia and some Fanconi anemia patients to remove gamma-ray products of the dihydroxydihydrothymine type.

The details of the time course and extent of excision repair of pyrimidine dimers in human tissue culture cells continue to be controversial. The reason for the observed discrepancies may be due to the use of different cell types and/or different methods of determining repair. It is also true that the reliability of different methods may depend upon the extent of damage and, indeed, measure different steps of the process. The direct measurement of pyrimidine dimers by paper chromatography is most reliable at doses above 10 J m^{-2} of 254-nm irradiation. At the biologically relevant doses of 254 nm $(10–100 \text{ J m}^{-2})$ discrepancies in results have been reported among studies using a variety of human cell types. Some investigators have reported little or no excision during the first few hours after irradiation, while others have found excision restricted to the first few hours (52, 53). Most agree that only about half of the dimers produced by $10–30 \text{ J m}^{-2}$ of 254-nm irradiation are excised within 24 hr (46, 54–60). Results from several assay methods show that during the first 3 hr following irradiation, repair replication occurs at the maximum rate (61). Other investigators, using other assay methods, find little or no excision repair occurring within this time. Satisfactory interpretation of these different results on a molecular basis has not yet been achieved. However, the method of determining excision repair may be involved. Chromatographic methods allow determination of the release of small acid-soluble oligonucleotides from the DNA. Enzymatic methods determine the number of dimers remaining in DNA of the size of 10^7 daltons. Some of the other methods used involve the uptake of isotopic label or halogenated analogs into any DNA lesion that elicits repair synthesis. The contribution of lesions other than dimers to the level of repair synthesis immediately following irradiation has not been ascertained.

Many experiments involving the repair of UV-radiation damage are performed on tissue culture cells using 20 J m^{-2} of 254 nm. This dose approaches saturation and allows adequate characterization of the extent of repair by a number of assay methods. DNA excision repair is thought to result from the action of several enzymes acting in a coordinated fashion. One line of evidence for this is that very few incision breaks are observed at any one time in mammalian cells undergoing repair. It has been postulated that complexes of repair enzymes systematically scan the DNA strand, repairing each lesion before moving further along the strand to the next lesion. The release of dimers from DNA in vitro occurs more efficiently under conditions allowing repair replication (62, 63). In mammalian cells, the evidence suggests that excision and resynthesis may be coupled processes (64).

We have carried out various experiments (55, 65, 66) aimed at determining the relationship between the rate and extent of dimer removal and the frequency of UV-induced pyrimidine dimers in human skin fibroblasts. It will become apparent in the following sections that the kinetics of repair is complex, varying both with respect to the time at which cells are examined after irradiation and with the particular radiation dose.

In order to study the sensitivity and reliability of different assay methods we irradiated human cells with UV and followed excision repair by two different assay methods. As evidenced by data in Fig. 4-5, kinetics of dimer loss as measured by chromatography and kinetics of loss of endonuclease-sensitive sites are similar at times of up to at least 48 hr. It is seen, however, that endonuclease-sensitive sites do begin to decrease relative to dimer content at times beyond 24 hr. This difference, which becomes more marked at higher doses and at later times postirradiation, manifests itself as DNA strand breaks. The protracted dimer removal process is shown better in Fig. 4-6, where dimers are plotted against dose delivered to the cells as a function of time after irradiation. At low doses (2.5 J m^{-2}), dimer removal goes almost to completion at relatively short times after irradiation (24–48 hr), while at

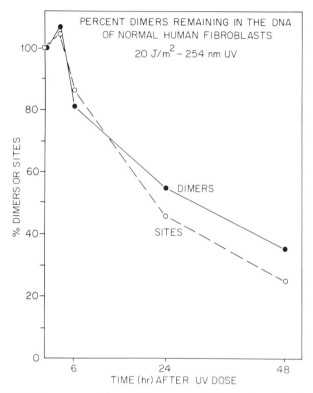

Fig. 4-5. Rate of dimer removal from cells as measured by two-dimensional paper chromatography or UV-endonuclease-sensitive sites.

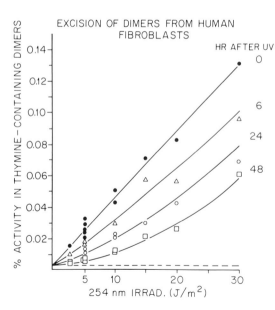

Fig. 4-6. The amount of dimers remaining in the DNA of cultured human fibroblasts as a function of time after irradiation and UV dose [From Regan et al. (55).]

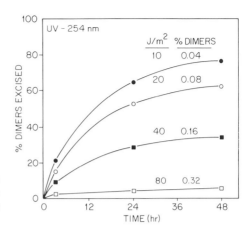

Fig. 4-7. The relationship between the number of pyrimidine dimers induced by various doses of 254-nm radiation and the percent excised with time.

higher doses, excision is not complete by 48 hr. In fact, about 72 hr is needed to remove most of the dimers following the insult of 5–10 J m^{-2} of UV radiation. At 30 J m^{-2}, the highest dose shown in these experiments, only about one-half of the total dimers are removed by 48 hr. An extension of these studies is shown in Fig. 4-7, where removal of dimers, expressed as percent dimers excised, is plotted as a function of time following doses of up to 80 J m^{-2}. At the highest dose employed, there is very little dimer excision by 48 hr and, as the dose decreases, a greater percentage of dimers induced are excised in a given amount of time. That these results are interpretable as an inhibition of repair at higher doses is more clearly shown in Fig. 4-8, where both the percentage of dimers excised and absolute numbers of dimers excised are plotted as functions of time and dose. The results show that at doses of up to about 40 J m^{-2} the percentage of dimers excised increases with time and with dose. At doses above this, however, the absolute number of dimers removed in a given period of time is either the same (as in the case of 60 J m^{-2}) or is actually less (as in the case of 80 J m^{-2}). The maximum number of dimers that can be excised in normal cells over a 24-hr period after irradiation does not exceed 0.05% (counts in dimers/counts in thymine times 100) or about one million dimers per cell. Since the absolute number of dimers excised decreases at 80 J m^{-2} as compared to 40 J m^{-2}, one must hypothesize that an actual inhibition of excision repair is occurring. The basis of this inhibition is not clear, but two explanations seem possible. The first of these is presented graphically in Fig. 4-2, which shows that the number of endonuclease-sensitive sites does not saturate even at doses as high as 100 J m^{-2}. Since it has already been shown that removal of dimers reaches saturation at much lower doses, it seems possible that the observed inhibition at high doses of UV radiation results from an uncoupling of the incision step from the rest of the repair sequence. This, in turn, may be due to the limited number of repair enzymes or to the inadequacy of some regulatory function. Since it has also been established

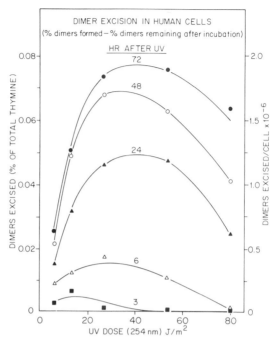

Fig. 4-8. Removal of pyrimidine dimers from human cells as a function of time and UV-radiation dose. Percent dimers removed is actually percent dimers formed minus percent dimers remaining after incubation. Dimers excised/cell was calculated according to the method of Williams and Cleaver (56) with the assumption of 2.4×10^{12} daltons DNA/cell. The points are the averages of 8–20 experiments.

that high doses of UV radiation cause substantial cross-linking of DNA to chromosomal protein (67), one can envision this uncoupling resulting from a tying up of repair components by binding to the DNA. Although it has been demonstrated that this cross-linking is repairable with time and thus should be reversible, our data show no such reversal of inhibition. A second explanation is suggested by the finding of Kantor and Hull (4), who showed that blocks to transcription or translation occur at high UV-radiation doses. These blocks could inhibit the synthesis of short-lived repair enzymes, leading to an abnormal saturation of repair. Studies by Gautschi et al. (68), however, suggest that maintenance of steady levels of repair synthesis following UV irradiation requires no de novo protein synthesis for at least 8 hr after insult and is reduced by only 35% even after 20 hr.

As we have discussed earlier in the section on induction of dimers, 254-nm radiation does not entirely simulate a biologic system with respect to the effective wavelengths of UV radiation encountered in sunlight. Therefore, it is of some interest to evaluate dimer removal following irradiation simulating a "natural" source. If one uses an FS40 sunlamp filtered with cellulose acetate to screen out wavelengths below 290 nm and the appropriate dose is given to human cells, dimers may be easily quantitated and the kinetics of their removal determined. Fig. 4-9 shows that the relationship between dose (as represented by percentage of thymine-containing dimers) and the amount of dimers removed in 24 hr is the same for both 254-nm irradiation and FS40 irradiation. Our results using "sunlight" wavelengths suggest that there is no excision repair sensitivity relative to 254 nm. One may conclude from this that the source of the insult to the cells is not an important factor in determining the rate of dimer removal. Moreover, if and when other photoproducts are formed by wavelengths between 290 and 400 nm (e.g., thymine glycols), the possible repair of these photoproducts does not inhibit the excision of pyrimidine dimers.

We have also examined pyrimidine dimer excision from a more mechanistic standpoint. Using the technique of BrdU photolysis developed in collaboration with R. B. Setlow, we have demonstrated two distinctly different modes of repair in human cells (69). A "short-patch" type repair is characterized by the insertion of fewer than 10 nucleotides into a repaired region and is exemplified by gamma-irradiation repair and, to a certain extent, by repair following alkylation damage. "Long-patch" repair involves insertion of 60–100 nucleotides into the repaired areas and is very easily demonstrated following insult of the cells with UV radiation or UV-mimetic carcinogenic chemicals. A typical experiment is shown in Fig. 4-10, which shows that with increasing exposure of the cells to the bromouracil-

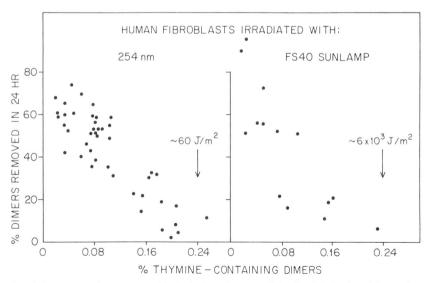

Fig. 4-9. Percent dimers removed in 24 hr from human cellular DNA following either various doses of 254-nm or sunlight-simulating Kodacel-filtered Westinghouse FS40 sunlamp irradiation.

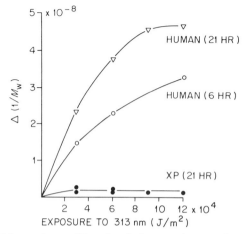

Fig. 4-10. Typical bromodeoxyuridine photolysis curves (see text for description of experimental procedures) for normal human or xeroderma pigmentosum fibroblasts that had been exposed to 20 J m^{-2} of 254-nm irradiation and then incubated in the presence of bromodeoxyuridine for 6 or 21 hr prior to 313-nm irradiation. Some of the data shown are from Regan and Setlow (70).

photosensitizing 313-nm radiation, the DNA becomes smaller until it reaches an apparent saturation. At this point increasing the fluence of radiation produces no additional breaks in the DNA. From kinetic analyses of this type one can calculate directly the average patch size per repaired region. It is also important to note from this figure that XP cells fail to show this characteristic response to 313-nm radiation—a fact consistent with the theory that they are deficient in one or more steps of excision repair of UV-induced dimers. That XP cells also respond in this fashion to a variety of known UV-mimetic agents as compared to normal human cells has become a useful criterion in the screening of carcinogens, thus serving as a double check on the mode of repair induced by these agents. While the factors that determine "long-" vs. "short-patch" repair are at present not known, we are pursuing several approaches toward an investigation of these questions.

NONDIMER PHOTOPRODUCTS

Nondimer damage in DNA caused by UV irradiation is the subject of a recent and extensive review by Rahn (71). Previous reviews have also covered the chemical properties and possible biologic consequences of many nondimer photoproducts in some detail (72, 73). We will deal only with those types of photoproducts that have been studied in human or other mammalian cells and that may conceivably be of some medical significance. Although cytosine hydrate and thymine glycol are the most prevalent lesions, they are induced at a level of only 10–20% of pyrimidine dimers. DNA–protein cross-linking is difficult to quantitate. Estimates have ranged from between 30 per cell to 60,000 per cell per 5 J m^{-2} UV-radiation treatment (67).

Thymine Glycol

Hariharan and Cerutti (74) studied the formation of thymine lesions of the 5,6-dihydroxydihydrothymine type in UV-irradiated HeLa cells. Upon irradiation of the cells with monochromatic radiation of 240, 265, 280, and 313 nm, the yield of these lesions (thymine glycols) increased appreciably relative to pyrimidine dimers at the higher wavelengths. It was proposed that these glycols represent minor DNA lesions at the lower far-UV wavelengths but major ones in the near-UV wavelengths, particularly at 300–305 nm. Setlow (2) has suggested that this latter wavelength is in the region that possesses maximum effectiveness for induction of actinic carcinoma.

Remsen and Cerutti (75) found that the capacity of whole-cell homogenates or nuclear preparations from two of four patients with Fanconi anemia was significantly below normal in ability to remove photoproducts of the thymine glycol type following gamma irradiation.

Cytosine Hydrate

The formation of cytosine hydrate (6-OH-5,6-dihydrocytosine) in irradiated solutions of cytosine or in DNA has been assayed by several methods. The most specific of these assays has been that of borohydride reduction. At a fluence of 5.8×10^3 J m^{-2}, Cerutti and Vanderhoek (76) found a 6:1 ratio of thymine dimers to cytosine hydrates. In another study, Setlow and Carrier (77) found a tenfold higher yield of cytosine hydrates when single-stranded DNA was irradiated rather than native DNA. This higher formation of cytosine hydrates in single-standard DNA could be significant in light of the recent findings of Bjursell et al. (78) demonstrating long regions of single-stranded DNA in human cells.

Apurinic Sites

Apurinic (or apyrimidinic) sites are found in irradiated cells in relatively low numbers as compared to some of the other photoproducts. Nevertheless, human cells contain apurinic endonucleases that nick the DNA at these sites (79). The possible significance of these depurinated DNA sites in light-induced disease is unknown, but it may be more than coincidence that certain XP complementation groups with a predisposition toward light-induced skin cancer lack an apurinic endonucleolytic activity (80).

DNA–DNA Cross-Links

These cross-links can be induced by UV radiation, although relatively high doses are required to produce substantial numbers. Cells from patients with Fanconi anemia are sensitive to cross-linking agents such as psoralen plus radiation and mitomycin-C (81). Thus a deficiency in ability to repair UV-induced DNA cross-links may play a role in producing the complex symptomatology of Fanconi anemia.

DNA–Protein Cross-Links

While we know of no direct experiments testing the medical significance of these lesions, it is to be expected that failure to remove proteins bound to the DNA would lead to inhibition of DNA replication and transcription and other DNA metabolic processes and would therefore contribute directly to UV-induced cell death. Several investigators have examined the question of cellular repair of these lesions, however, and have found no strong evidence for the existence of such repair (67).

SUMMARY

Clearly, cells from normal individuals possess the ability to repair damage to DNA. Numerous studies indicate that individuals deficient in DNA repair are prone to cancer. Although not all cancers arise from defects in DNA repair, evidence is abundant that events leading to malfunctions in DNA replication and repair create a high potential for malignant transformation.

The biologic relevance of induction and repair of DNA damage should properly emerge from a correlation of such damage and repair with (a) mutation, (b) cell killing, and (c) environmental carcinogenesis. It is encouraging that some correlations have been made and are consistent with the idea that more DNA damage and/or less repair lead to more mutation and cell killing (82). With regard to correlation of DNA damage and repair and environmental carcinogenesis, the problem is more complex, in that experimental carcinogenesis is properly studied in the whole animal while DNA damage and cellular response are most conveniently done in cell culture.

Invaluable tools which would contribute to the understanding of the repair process in human cells would be either the development of specific mutant cell lines defective in the different steps of repair, or a clear characterization of the biochemical significance of the seven complementation groups found in XP (48, 83). The meaning of the multiple complementation groups of XP is unclear. Do seven genes control incision, the first step of excision repair? Or do these groups represent mutations in genes controlling different enzymatic steps in the repair pathway?

It is hoped that continued studies on the control of cellular processes, detailed kinetic analyses of the mechanisms involved in DNA damage and its repair, and further clarification of the correlations between biochemical events and changes in cell behavior will lead to the understanding and subsequent control of carcinogenesis.

ACKNOWLEDGMENTS. Postdoctoral Investigator supported by Training Grant T32-CA09336 from the National Cancer Institute. Research sponsored jointly by the Office of Health and Environmental Research, U.S. Department of Energy, under contract W-7405-eng-26 with the Union Carbide Corporation, NASA Agreement #40-565-76; and NCI Agreement #40-5-63.

REFERENCES

1. Setlow, R. B., and Setlow, J. K. (1972): Effects of radiation on polynucleotides. *Rev. Biophys. Bioeng.* 1:293–346.
2. Setlow, R. B. (1974): The wavelengths in sunlight effective in producing skin cancer: a theoretical analysis. *Proc. Natl. Acad. Sci. U.S.A.*, 71:3363–3366.
3. Elkind, M. M., Han, A., and Chang-Liu, C. (1978): Sunlight induced mammalian cell killing: A comparative study of ultraviolet and near-ultraviolet inactivation. *Photochem. Photobiol.* 27:709–715.
4. Kantor, G. J., and Hull, D. R. (1979): Effects of ultraviolet light on RNA and protein synthesis in non-dividing human diploid fibroblasts *Biophys. J.* 27:359–370.
5. Sauerbier, W. (1976): Ultraviolet light damage at the transcriptional level. *Adv. Radiat. Biol.* 6:49–106.
6. Sutherland, B. M. (1978): Photoreactivation in mammalian cells. In: Aspects of Genetic Action and Evolution, edited by G. H. Bowine and Danielli, *Int. Rev. Cytol.* 1978 (Supplt 8):301–333.
7. Mortelmans, K., Cleaver, J. E., Friedberg, E. C., et al. (1977): Photoreactivation of thymine dimers in UV-irradiated human cells: Unique dependence on culture conditions. *Mutat. Res.* 44:433–446.
8. Lehmann, A. R. (1975): Postreplication repair of DNA in mammalian cells. *Life Sci.* 15:2005–2016.
9. Buhl, S. N., Setlow, R. B., and Regan, J. D. (1972): Steps in DNA chain elongation and joining after ultraviolet irradiation of human cells. *Int. J. Radiat. Biol.* 22:417–425.
10. Waters, R., and Regan, J. D. (1976): Recombination of UV-induced pyrimidine dimers in human fibroblasts. *Biochem. Biophys. Res. Commun.* 72:803–807.
11. Meneghini, R., and Hanawalt, P. (1976): T4-endonuclease V-sensitive sites in DNA from ultraviolet-irradiate human cells. *Biochim. Biophys. Acta* 425:428–437.
12. Lehmann, A. R., and Krik-Bell, S. (1978): Pyrimidine dimer sites associated with the daughter DNA strands in UV-irradiated human fibroblasts. *Photochem. Photobiol.* 27:297–307.
13. Setlow, R. B., and Carrier, W. L. (1964): The disappearance of thymine dimers from DNA: An error-correcting mechanism. *Proc. Natl. Acad. Sci. U.S.A.* 51:226–231.
14. Boyce, R. P., and Howard-Flanders, P. (1964): Release of ultraviolet light-induced thymine dimers from DNA of *E. coli. Proc. Natl. Acad. Sci. U.S.A.* 51:293–300.
15. Cleaver, J. E. (1974): Repair processes for photochemical damage in mammalian cells. *Adv. Radiat. Biol.* 4:74.

16. Hanawalt, P. C., Cooper, P. K., Ganesan, A. K., et al (1979): DNA repair in bacteria and mammalian cells. *Ann. Rev. Biochem.* **48**:783–836.

17. Carrier, W. L., and Setlow, R. B. (1971): The excision of pyrimidine dimers (The detection of dimers in small amounts). In: *Methods in of Enzymology*, edited by L. Grossman and K. Moldave, Vol. XX, Part D. Academic Press, New York.

18. Paterson, M. C. (1978): Use of purified lesion-recognizing enzymes to monitor DNA repair *in vivo*. *Adv. Radiat. Biol.* **7**:1–53.

19. Trosko, J. E., Krause, D., and Isoun, M. (1970): Sunlight-induced pyrimidine dimers in human cells *in vitro*. *Nature* **228**:358–359.

20. Strickland, P. T., Burns, F. J., and Albert, R. D. (1979): Induction of skin tumors in rats by single exposure to ultraviolet radiation. *Photochem. Photobiol.* **30**:683–688.

21. Sisson, W. B., and Caldwell, M. M. (1975): Lamp/filter systems for simulation of solar UV irradiance under reduced atmospheric ozone. *Photochem. Photobiol.* **21**:453–456.

22. Krizek, D. T., and Koch, J. E. (1979): Use of regression analysis to estimate UV-spectral irradiance from broad band radiometer readings under FS40 fluorescent sunlamps filtered with cellulose acetate. *Photochem. Photobiol.* **30**:483–489.

23. Rothman, R. H., and Setlow, R. B. (1979): An action spectrum for cell killing and pyrimidine dimer formation in Chinese hamster V-79 cells. *Photochem. Photobiol.* **29**:57–61.

24. Unrau, P., Wheatcroft, R., and Cox, B. S. (1972): Methods for the assay of ultraviolet light-induced pyrimidine dimers in *Saccharomyces cerevisia*. *Biochim. Biophys. Acta* **269**:311–321.

25. Goldmann, K., and Friedberg, E. C. (1973): Measurement of thymine dimers in DNA by thin-layer chromatography. *Anal. Biochem.* **53**:124.

26. Rasmussen, R. E., and Painter, R. B. (1964): Evidence for repair of ultraviolet damaged deoxyribonuclease acid cultured mammalian cells. *Nature* **203**:1360–1362.

27. Regan, J. D., Setlow, R. B., and Ley, R. D. (1971): Normal and defective repair of damaged DNA in human cells: A sensitive assay utilizing the photolysis of bromodeoxyuridine. *Proc. Natl. Acad. Sci. U.S.A.* **68**:708–712.

28. Pettijohn, D., and Hanawalt, P. (1964): Evidence for repair replication of ultraviolet damaged in bacteria. *J. Mol. Biol.* **9**:395–410.

29. Rasmussen, R. E., and Painter, R. B. (1966): Radiation-stimulated DNA synthesis in cultured mammalian cells. *J. Cell Biol.* **29**:11–19,

30. Cleaver, J. E. (1968): Defective repair replication of DNA in xeroderma pigmentosum. *Nature* **218**:652–656.

31. Scudiero, D., and Strauss, B. (1974): Accumulation of single–stranded region in DNA and the block to replication in a human cell line alkylated with methyl methanesulfonate. *J. Mol. Biol.* **83**:17–34.

32. McGrath, R. A., and Williams, R. W. (1966): Reconstruction *in vivo* of irradiated *Escherichia coli* deoxyribonucleic acid: The rejoining of broken pieces. *Nature* **212**:534–535.

33. Kohn, K. W., Erickson, L. C., Weig, R. A. G., et al. (1976): Fractionation of DNA from mammalian cells by alkaline elution. *Biochemistry* **15**:4629–4637.

34. Ahnstrom, G., and Edwardsson, K. A. (1974): Radiation-induced single-strand breaks in DNA determined by rate of alkaline strand separation and hydroxylopatite deromatography: An alternative to velocity sedimentation. *Int. J. Radiat. Biol.* **26**:279–292.

35. Cook, P. R., and Brazell, I. A. (1976): Conformational constraints in nuclear DNA. *J. Cell. Sci.* **22**:287–302.

36. Vunakis, H. V. (1980): Immunological detection of radiation damage in DNA. *Photochem. Photobiol. Rev.* **5**:293–311.

37. Dunn, W. C., and Regan, J. D. (1979): Inhibition of DNA excision repair in human cells by arabinofuranosyl cytosine: Effect on normal and xeroderma pigmentosum cells. *Mol. Pharmacol.* **15**:367–374.

38. Collins, A. R. S., Schor, S. L., and Johnson, R. T. (1977): The inhibition of repair in UV irradiated human cells. *Mutat. Res.* **42**:413–432.

38. Synder, R. D., Carrier, W. L., and Regan, J. D. (1981): Application of Arabinofuranosyl cytopine in the kinetic analysis and quantitation of DNA repair in human cells after ultraviolet irradiation. *Biophys. J.* **35**:339–350.

40. Strauss, B. S. (1962): Differential destruction of the transforming activity of damaged deoxyribonucleic acid by a bacterial enzyme. *Proc. Natl. Acad. Sci. U.S.A.* **48**:1670–1675.

41. Carrier, W. L., and Setlow, R. B. (1966): Excision of pyrimidine dimers from irradiated deoxyribonucleic acid *in vivo. Biochim. Biophys. Acta* **129**:318–325.

42. Marmur, J. (1961): A procedure for the isolation of deoxyribonucleic acid from micro-organisms. *J. Mol. Biol.* **3**:208–218.

43. Carrier, W. L., and Setlow, R. B. (1971): Paper strip method for assaying gradient fractions containing radioactive macromolecules. *Anal. Biochem.* **43**:427–431.

44. Haseltine, W. A., Gordon, L. K., Lindan, C. P., et al (1980): Cleavage of pyrimidine dimers in specific DNA sequences by a pyrimidine dimer DNA-glycosylase of *M. luteus. Nature* **285**:634–460.

45. Radany, E. H., and Friedberg, E. C. (1980): A pyrimidine dimer-DNA glycosylase activity associated with the *v* gene product of bacteriophage T4. *Nature* **286**:182–185.

46. Regan, J. D., Trosko, J. E., and Carrier, W. L. (1968): Evidence for excision of ultraviolet-induced pyrimidine dimers from the DNA of human cells *in vitro. Biophys. J.* **8**:319–325.

47. Setlow, R. B., Regan, J. R., German, J., et al. (1969): Evidence that xeroderma pigmentosum cells do not perform the first step in the repair of ultraviolet damage to their DNA. *Proc. Natl. Acad. Sci. U.S.A.* **64**:1035–1041.

48. Friedberg, E. C., Ehmann, U. K., and Williams, J. I. (1979): Human diseases associated with defective DNA repair. *Adv. Radiat. Biol.* **8**:85–160.

49. Paterson, M. C., Smith, B. P., Lohman, P. H. M., et al. (1976): Defective excision repair of gamma-ray damaged DNA in human (Ataxia telangiectasia) fibroblasts. *Nature* **260**:444–447.

50. Fornace, A. J., Jr., and Little, J. B. (1980): Normal repair of DNA single-strand breaks in patients with Ataxia telangiectasia. *Biochim. Biophys. Acta* **607**:432–437.

51. Remsen, J. F., and Cerutti, P. A. (1976): Deficiency of gamma-ray excision repair in skin fibroblasts from patients with Fanconi's anemia. *Proc. Natl. Acad. Sci. U.S.A.* **73**:2419–2423.

52. Isomura, K., Nikaido, O., Horikawa, M., et al. (1973): Repair of DNA damage in ultraviolet-sensitive cells isolated from HeLa S3 cells. *Radiat. Res.* **53**:143–152.

53. Amacher, D. E., Elliott, J. A., and Lieberman, M. W. (1977): Differences in the removal of acetylaminofluorine and pyrimidine dimers from the DNA of cultured mammalian cells. *Proc. Natl. Acad. Sci. U.S.A.* **774**:1553–1557.

54. Ehmann, U. K., Cook, K. H., and Friedberg, E. C. (1978): The kinetics of thymine dimer excision in ultraviolet-irradiated human cells. *Biophys. J.* **22**:249–264.

55. Regan, J. D., Carrier, W. L., Smith, D. P., et al. (1979): Pyrimidine dimer excision in human cells and skin cancer. *Natl. Cancer Inst. Monogr.* **50**:141–143.

56. Williams, J. I., and Cleaver, J. E. (1978): Excision repair of ultraviolet damage in mammalian cells. Evidence for two steps in the excision of pyrimidine dimers. *Biophys. J.* **22**:265–279.

57. Ahmed, F. E., and Setlow, R. B. (1978): Kinetics of DNA repair in ultraviolet-irradiated and *N*-acetoxy-2-acetylaminofluorene-treated mammalian cells. *Biophys. J.* **24**:665–674.

58. Ahmed, F. E., and Setlow, R. B. (1979): Saturation of DNA repair in mammalian cells. *Photochem. Photobiol.* **29**:983–989.

59. Inoue, M., and Takebe, H. (1978): DNA repair capacity and rate of excision repair in UV-irradiated mammalian cells. *Jpn. J. Hum. Genet.* **58**:285–295.

60. Konze-Thomas, B., Levinson, J. W., Maher, V. M., et al (1979): Correlation among the rates of dimer excision, DNA repair replication and recovery of human cells from potentially lethal damage induced by ultraviolet radiation. *Biophys. J.* **28**:315–326.

61. Edenberg, H. J., and Hanawalt, P. C. (1973): The time course of DNA repair replication in ultraviolet irradiated HeLa cells. *Biochim. Biophys. Acta* **324**:206–217.

62. Friedberg, E. C., and Lehman, I. R. (1974): Excision of thymine dimers by proteolytic and

amber fragments of *E. coli* DNA polymerase I. *Biochem. Biophys. Res. Commun.* **58**:132–139.

63. Masker, W. E. (1977): Deoxyribonucleic acid repair *in vitro* by extracts of *Escherichia coli. J. Baceriol.* **129**:1415–1423.

64. Cleaver, J. E. (1978): DNA repair and its coupling to DNA replication in eukaryotic cells. *Biochim. Biophys. Acta* **516**:489–516.

65. Regan, J. D., Smith, D. P., and Carrier, W. L. (1979): Excision of pyrimidine dimers from the DNA of human cells exposed to 254 nm radiation or to simulated sunlight from an FS40 lamp. Abstract, 7th Annual Meeting of the American Society for Photobiology, Asilimar.

66. Carrier, W. L., and Regan, J. D. (1980): The number and fate of near-UV (FS40 sunlamp) and far-UV (254 nm) induced pyrimidine dimers in the DNA of human fibroblasts. *Radiat. Res.* **83**:424.

67. Todd, P., and Han, A. (1976): Ultraviolet-induced DNA to protein cross-linking in mammalina cells. In: *Aging, Carcinogenesis and Radiation Biology. The Role of Nucleic Acid Addition Reactions,* edited by K. C. Smith, pp. 83–104. Plenum Press, New York.

68. Gautschi, J. R., Young, B. R., and Cleaver, J. E. (1973): Repair of damaged DNA in the absence of protein synthesis in mammalian cells. *Exp. Cell Res.* **75**:87–94.

69. Regan, J. D., and Setlow, R. B. (1974): Two forms of repair in the DNA of human cells damaged by chemical carcinogens and mutagens. *Cancer Res.* **34**:3318–3325.

70. Regan, J. D., and Setlow, R. B. (1973): Repair of chemical damage to human DNA. In: *Chemical Mutagens: Principles and Methods for Their Detection,* edited by A. Hollaender, pp. 151–170. Plenum Press, New York.

71. Rahn, R. O. (1979): Non-dimer damage in deoxyribonucleic acid caused by ultraviolet radiation. In: *Photochemical and Photobiological Reviews,* Vol. 4, edited by K. C. Smith, pp. 267–330. Plenum Press, New York.

72. Varghese, A. J. (1972): Photochemistry of nucleic acids and their constituents. In: *Photophysiology,* Vol. VII, edited by A. C. Giese, pp. 207–274. Academic Press, New York.

73. Patrick, N. H., and Rahn, R. (1976): Photochemistry of DNA and polynucleotides: *Photoproducts.* In: *Photochemistry and Photobiology of Nucleic Acids,* Vol. II, edited by S. Y. Wang, pp. 35–95. Academic Press, New York.

74. Hariharan, P. V., and Cerutti, P. A. (1977): Formation of products of the 5,6-dihydro-xythymine type by ultraviolet light in HeLa cells. *Biochemistry* **16**:2791–2795.

75. Remsen, J. F., and Cerutti, P. A. (1977): Excision of gamma-ray induced thymine lesions by preparations from Ataxia telangiectasia fibroblasts. *Mutat. Res.* **43**:139–146.

76. Cerutti, P. A., and Vanderhoek, C. (1976): Photochemistry of DNA and polynucleotides: Photoproducts. In: *Photochemistry and Photobiology of Nucleic Acids,* Vol. II, edited by S. Y. Wang, pp. 83–87. Academic Press, New York.

77. Setlow, R. B., and Carrier, W. L. (1970): Cytidine photoproducts in DNA. *Biophys. Soc. Abtracts* **10**:255a.

78. Bjursell, G. E., Gussander, E., and Lindahl, T. (1979): Long regions of single-stranded DNA in human cells. *Nature* **280**:420–423.

79. Brent, T. P. (1972): Repair enzyme suggested by mammalian endonuclease activity specific for ultraviolet-irradiated DNA. *Nature [New Biol.]* **239**:172–173.

80. Kuhnlein, V., Penhoet, E., and Linn, S. (1976): An altered apurinic endonuclease activity in xeroderma pigmentosum fibroblasts. *Proc. Natl. Acad. Sci. U.S.A.* **73**:1169–1173.

81. Sasaki, M. S., and Tonomura, A. (1973): A high susceptibility of Fanconi's anemia to chromosome breakage by DNA cross-linking agents. *Cancer Res.* **33**:1829–1836.

82. Maher, V. M., and McCormick, J. J. (1976): Effect of DNA repair on the cytotoxicity and mutagenicity of UV irradiation and of chemical carcinogens in normal and xeroderma pigmentosum cells. In: *Biology of Radiation Carcinogenesisy,* edited by J. M. Yuhas, R. W. Tennant, and J. D. Regan, pp. 129–145. Raven Press, New York.

83. Keijzer, W., Jaspers, N. G. J., Abrahama, P. J., et al. (1979): A seventh complementation group in excision-deficient xeroderma pigmentosum. *Mutat. Res.* **62**:183–190.

5

Photodynamic Reactions in Photomedicine

J. D. Spikes

According to standard evolutionary theory, the early atmosphere of the earth was reducing and the first living organisms thus evolved in the absence of free molecular oxygen (1). With the appearance of plants capable of using water as a hydrogen source in photosynthesis, molecular oxygen began to accumulate in the atmosphere, finally reaching its present concentration of approximately 20%. Although this event made possible the highly efficient aerobic respiration reactions and provided a substantial shield against short-wave solar ultra-violet (UV) radiation via ozone formation, it also posed a severe problem to the existing organisms, since oxygen and certain of its derivatives are highly toxic. Some of these derivatives are produced by metabolic reactions, and, of special pertinence to this chapter, several are produced in good yield by sensitized photobiologic processes involving visible and near-UV radiation.

Although the phenomenon was clearly observed earlier, we usually regard experimental studies on photosensitization in biologic systems as starting with the work of Oscar Raab published in 1900 (2). Raab, a medical student working in the laboratory of von Tappeiner in Munich, found that low concentrations of certain acridines and of eosin, which had no effect in the dark, led to the rapid killing of the protozoan paramecium on illumination. This observation came at a time when there was a great deal of interest in the effects of light on living systems and it stimulated a very large amount of research. During the next few years it was shown that enzymes could be inactivated, and that many kinds of cells and small animals could be killed on

---

J. D. Spikes • Department of Biology, University of Utah, Salt Lake City, Utah 84112.

illumination in the presence of a variety of photosensitizers; in general, molecular oxygen was required for these reactions. It was suggested at the time that these reactions were simply sensitized photooxidation processes. This interpretation did not appeal to biomedical scientists, and in 1904 von Tappeiner and Jodlbauer (3) coined the term "photodynamic action" to distinguish these photobiologic phenomena from physical chemical phenomena such as the photosensitization of photographic plates by dyes. This term is now implanted in biologic thought and literature so firmly that there is little possibility of changing it. Blum (4) suggested that the term photodynamic action be applied only to those photosensitized reactions in biologic systems in which molecular oxygen is consumed; the term will be used in that sense in this chapter. Most of the known photosensitized reactions in biology and medicine appear to be of this type. There are several notable exceptions, however. For example, psoralens (furocoumarins), which are used in the photochemotherapy of certain skin diseases (see Chapter 22), can photosensitize some kinds of reactions (such as photobinding to DNA) in the absence of oxygen (5, 6). They can also sensitize the photoinactivation of some enzymes by reactions that involve oxygen (7, 8). Chlorpromazine, a phototoxic phenothiazine drug used in psychotherapy, photosensitizes in some systems by reactions requiring oxygen. However, it can also sensitize the photokilling of bacteria under anaerobic conditions; in the process the drug photobinds to cellular protein, and to a lesser extent, to DNA (9). Chlorpromazine and the phototoxic antidepressant protriptyline sensitize the anaerobic photohemolysis of red blood cells (10).

There is a rather large literature on photosensitization phenomena in biology and medicine. My purpose in this chapter is to review photodynamic reactions in an extensive rather than intensive manner in order to illustrate the scope of the field. In most cases I will use recent papers to illustrate the points I wish to make; these can be consulted for entries into the literature. Fortunately, many reviews on various aspects of photosensitized reactions in biology and medicine have been published. The literature prior to 1940 has been nicely reviewed in Blum's monograph (4); subsequent reviews are listed in the reference section of this chapter in chronologic order (11–78). In addition, considerable information pertinent to photodynamic reactions may be found in several recent books and proceedings of conferences (79–81).

MECHANISMS OF PHOTODYNAMIC REACTIONS

The basic photochemical aspects of photosensitized reactions are considered in Chapter 1 of this book. In brief, molecules that act as photosensitizers have two types of electronically excited states. On illumination, the ground state sensitizer S is converted to a singlet excited state ^1S, which typically has a very short lifetime. In most efficient photodynamic sensitizers, the excited singlet state undergoes conversion to another energy-rich form, the triplet state ^3S. This state has a much longer lifetime and therefore has a much greater probability of undergoing chemical reaction. Almost all photodynamic reactions are mediated by the triplet state. Thus,

$$S \xrightarrow{\text{light}} {}^1S \longrightarrow {}^3S \longrightarrow \text{photodynamic reactions} \qquad (1)$$

In typical photodynamic systems the excited sensitizer is not consumed in the reaction and is restored to the ground state, where it can function again; under certain conditions, some sensitizers are slowly destroyed by side reactions on illumination. In simple photodynamic systems (in nonreactive solvents), the triplet sensitizer can react in two major ways, i.e., by electron or hydrogen transfer processes (Type I or free radical reactions) or by energy transfer processes (Type II reactions) (28, 57, 64). The relative participation of the two types of processes depends on the chemical nature of the sensitizer and substrate as well as on the reaction conditions (pH, solvent, concentrations of components).

Type I (Electron Transfer) Photodynamic Processes

Several alternative pathways are possible in Type I processes, depending on the sensitizer, etc. For example, the triplet sensitizer can abstract an electron or a hydrogen atom from a reducing substrate RH (most common in biologic systems), giving a semireduced form of the sensitizer $SH\cdot$ and a semioxidized form of the substrate $R\cdot$ as follows:

$$^3S + RH \longrightarrow SH\cdot + R\cdot \qquad (2)$$

The free radicals thus formed can react further in a variety of ways in the presence of oxygen, typically giving an oxidized form of the substrate and ground state sensitizer as the final products. For example, some semireduced sensitizers such as flavins can dismutate, giving ground state and fully reduced sensitizer; the latter can react with oxygen to give hydrogen peroxide and ground state sensitizer:

$$SH\cdot + SH\cdot \longrightarrow S + SH_2 \qquad (3)$$

$$SH_2 + O_2 \longrightarrow S + H_2O_2 \qquad (4)$$

Some semireduced sensitizers can also react with oxygen, giving ground state sensitizer and the oxygen superoxide radical $O_2^-\cdot$ (or its conjugate acid, $HO_2\cdot$):

$$SH\cdot + O_2 \longrightarrow S + HO_2\cdot \qquad (5)$$

Triplet sensitizers in some cases can react with oxidants to give a semioxidized form of the sensitizer and a reduced oxidant. Finally, triplet sensitizers can also react by transferring an electron to ground state oxygen, giving semioxidized sensitizer and oxygen superoxide; this process is very inefficient, however. In summary, then, Type I processes can, depending on the reactants and the reaction conditions, produce semioxidized biologic substrates (which can then react further to give fully oxidized species) and significant amounts of semireduced and semioxidized sensitizer, hydrogen peroxide, and oxygen superoxide. Not much is known about the interactions of the free radical forms of sensitizers with biologic substrates, although there is some evidence that semioxidized eosin can oxidize tyrosine, tryptophan, and related compounds [see (82) for references]. Hydrogen peroxide oxidizes a wide variety of biologically important compounds, and superoxide oxidizes dihydroxyphenylalanine, epinephrine, and related compounds (82, 83).

Type II (Energy Transfer) Photodynamic Processes

In this type of reaction, triplet sensitizer most commonly reacts with ground state oxygen (which, unlike most molecules, is in the triplet state) by an energy transfer process to give an electronically excited singlet state of oxygen $^1O_2$ and ground state sensitizer:

$$^3S + {}^3O_2 \longrightarrow S + {}^1O_2 \tag{6}$$

Ground state oxygen $^3O_2$ does not directly oxidize most biomolecules at appreciable rates under ordinary conditions, because they are typically in the singlet state; however, singlet excited oxygen reacts rapidly with a wide variety of simple organic compounds and compounds of biologic importance. Typical reactions include: (a) "ene"-type processes in which singlet oxygen reacts with substituted olefins giving hydroperoxides (for example singlet oxygen reacts with unsaturated fatty acids to give lipid peroxides); (b) reactions of singlet oxygen with compounds containing heteroatoms (for example, methionine is oxidized to the sulfoxide); and (c) 1,4-addition reactions of singlet oxygen with dienes and heterocyclic compounds with the formation of endoperoxides (57, 64, 72).

In summary, the illumination of a photodynamic system induces a large variety of possible reactions; the relative participation of the different reaction pathways and reactive intermediates depends on the sensitizer, the substrate, and the reaction conditions. Actually, by changing the reaction conditions, the major pathway in some sensitized photooxidations can be shifted from Type I to Type II, or vice versa. For example, with flavin sensitizers, methionine in water is photooxidized largely by a Type I process, giving an aldehyde (methional) as the main organic photooxidation product. In contrast, with alcohols as solvent, the reaction is mainly Type II, giving methionine sulfoxide as the only final product (31).

Diagnostic Methods for Photodynamic Reactions

In studying the mechanisms of photodynamic processes, it is important to be able to determine the relative participation of the different reaction pathways. There are several ways to access the probable participation of singlet oxygen (64, 68, 72); unfortunately, none of them is completely unambiguous [see comments by Foote (84)]. One promising technique is to determine the structural pattern of the photooxidation products. For example, the oxidation of cholesterol with singlet oxygen gives a characteristically different product from that observed in a radical-type oxidation [see references in (85)]. Another way is to compare photooxidation rates in water and in deuterium oxide (D_2O). The lifetime of the Δ_g singlet state of oxygen (the most important form in photodynamic reactions) is at least 10 times longer in D_2O than in H_2O (86). Thus, if the rate of a photodynamic reaction is increased significantly in D_2O, this indicates the involvement of singlet oxygen (87); this approach is valid only under certain conditions, depending on substrate concentration and the rate constants for the reaction of substrate with singlet oxygen and for the decay of singlet oxygen in the solvent employed [see (64) and comments by Foote (84)]. Another technique is to examine the effect of compounds, such as sodium azide (88), which quench singlet oxygen with very high efficiency and which are not themselves good substrates for free radical Type I reactions; unfortunately, there are no water-soluble quenchers that are completely specific for singlet oxygen. However, reasonably reliable data can be obtained with azide if reaction conditions are used that give simple competition between azide and substrate for the singlet oxygen being produced (89). Finally, the flash photolysis technique has been used in attempts to determine the relative participation of Type I and Type II processes [see (82) for references]. In summary, then, it is not an easy matter to establish the detailed mechanism of the primary processes in a photodynamic reaction even in rather simple systems; it is usually necessary to do detailed kinetic and biochemical studies using multiple approaches.

The Chemistry of Photodynamic Sensitizers

Many compounds absorbing in the visible and near-UV regions act as photodynamic sensitizers. The most recent compilation (46) includes over 400 compounds which have been shown to sensitize, but there must be many more. Thus it is important that compounds that are proposed to be used in foods (90), medicines (41, 91, 92), cosmetics (93), etc., be carefully tested to establish that they are not effective sensitizers. Many naturally occurring pigments, including chlorophyll and related compounds, other noniron porphyrins such as protoporphyrin IX, flavins (lumiflavin, 3-methyl lumiflavin, riboflavin, FMN; but not FAD), and polycyclic plant pigments such as hypericin are efficient photodynamic sensitizers. Thus photodynamic sensitizers must be listed among the types of potentially toxic agents that occur naturally in foods (53). Many kinds of synthetic organic compounds act as photosensitizers, including acridines (proflavin, acridine orange, etc.), anthraquinones, azine dyes (safranines), many ketones, thiazine dyes (methylene blue, thionine, toluidine blue), thiopyronine, and xanthene dyes (eosin Y, rose bengal, etc.). In contrast, azo dyes, indophenols, nitro dyes, nitroso dyes, oxazine dyes, and triarylmethane dyes are usually not effective sensitizers. The structures of several representative photosensitizers are shown in Fig. 5-1; consult (94) for the structures of synthetic dyes.

The rates of many photodynamic reactions can be decreased, often significantly, by compounds which interact physically or chemically (quenchers) with the excited or reactive intermediates described above. For example, carotenoids such as beta-carotene (one of the best-studied quenchers) quench singlet oxygen with very high efficiency and triplet-state photosensitizers with reasonably high efficiency [(26, 55, 64, 66); also see Chapters 13 and 14]. Depending on the photosensitizer and substrate, some photodynamic reactions are inhibited by paramagnetic metal ions, iodide ion, various antioxidant compounds (including such naturally occurring compounds as ascorbic acid and alpha-tocopherol), etc. [see references in (95)].

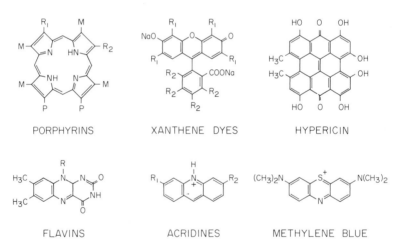

Fig. 5-1. Structural formulas of typical photodynamic sensitizers. In the porphyrin formula, M and P represent methyl and propionic acid groups, respectively; for hematoporphyrin, R_1 and R_2 are hydroxyethyl groups, while in protoporphyrin they are vinyl groups. The xanthene dye nucleus is shown as the disodium salt. Several xanthene dyes are potent photodynamic sensitizers, including eosin Y, where R_1 is bromine and R_2 is hydrogen, and rose bengal, where R_1 is iodine and R_2 is chlorine. Hypericin is a polycyclic hydrocarbon found in the leaves of some kinds of plants. The flavin nucleus is shown; in lumiflavin, R is a methyl group; in riboflavin it is a ribityl group, and in FMN it is a ribityl-5'-phosphate group. The acridine nucleus is also shown; in proflavine R_1 and R_2 are amino groups, while in acridine orange they are dimethylamino groups. Methylene blue is shown as the cation; thiopyronine has a very similar structure, with a carbon atom replacing the nitrogen atom in the middle ring.

Although some organisms show natural photodynamic sensitivity [see references in (27, 34, 35)], living material is, in general, well designed to minimize the occurrence of photodynamic processes involving endogenous sensitizers. Chlorophyll (a porphyrin containing the nonparamagnetic metal zinc) is an excellent photodynamic sensitizer, yet photosynthetic organisms that contain large amounts of chlorophyll are ordinarily highly resistant to photodynamic damage. This is due in part to the highly organized structure of the photosynthetic organelles, which results in the very fast transfer of chlorophyll singlet excitation to a "trap" where the electron transfer reactions of photosynthesis start; as a result, only a very small fraction of the photoexcitations of the chlorophyll lead to triplet production which could drive photodynamic reactions. Photosynthetic organelles contain very high concentrations of carotenoids, which efficiently quench chlorophyll triplets and any singlet oxygen that may be produced; as a result (unless deprived of carbon dioxide), very little photodamage occurs in photosynthetic organisms even though they contain high concentrations of a potent sensitizer [see (26, 64, 66) and Chapter 13]. Essentially all other porphyrins in living organisms, such as the heme (ferric protoporphyrin IX) of hemoglobin and most other hemoproteins, contain a paramagnetic iron atom. This effectively renders the porphyrin inactive as a photodynamic sensitizer, apparently by decreasing the triplet lifetime to such an extent that little if any singlet oxygen can be formed (61, 96). However, if hemin, for example, is converted to a low-spin derivative by ligation with cyanide ions, it becomes a photodynamic sensitizer (97). Porphyrins are usually regarded as singlet oxygen sensitizers (96, 98); however, it has been shown recently that the illumination of protoporphyrin produces at least some superoxide (99).

In summary, then, a number of factors are involved in the efficiencies of photodynamic reactions. A good photodynamic sensitizer must do more than merely absorb light with high efficiency; the quantum yield of triplet formation must be high, and the triplet must be long-lived. The physical state of the sensitizer can also be of importance. Many sensitizers are highly efficient free in solution. However, in cells and tissues, most dyes would tend to be bound to or associated with macromolecular structures rather than existing as free molecules. Bound sensitizers often show altered photochemical properties (23). For example, bilirubin is a very poor photodynamic sensitizer in solution. However, it sensitizes the photoinactivation of several membrane enzymes when incorporated into isolated human red cell membranes (100). Illumination of 1:1 complexes of bilirubin with human and bovine serum albumin results in the destruction of histidyl, tryptophyl, and tyrosyl residues (101). In contrast, some sensitizers lose activity on binding, while others show little change (102, 103). In attempts to better approximate cell level systems, considerable work has been done recently in model systems with sensitizers incorporated into surfactant micelles (104, 105), films and monolayer assemblies (106), and liposomes [see (85, 107, 108) for references].

PHOTODYNAMIC STUDIES WITH MULTICELLULAR ORGANISMS

It was shown by Hausmann in 1908 that mice injected with the photosensitizer hematoporphyrin were killed on exposure to light. In 1913 the German physician Myer-Betz injected himself intravenously with 200 mg of hematoporphyrin; on limited exposure to light he suffered a marked erythema and edema and remained light-sensitive for several months. Large mammals such as sheep and cattle can be rendered highly light-sensitive by the ingestion of certain sensitizers which occur in plants. Isolated organs and tissues from animals can also be photosensitized, as can all parts of multicellular plants. It would appear, then, that any multicellular animal or plant (or parts thereof) can be sensitized to photodynamic injury and killing (4, 11).

Photodynamic Studies with Mammals Other than Humans

Photosensitization in humans will not be considered, here since this topic is covered in Chapters 11 and 12 [also see (41, 44)]; actually, nonhuman mammals probably show most of the same kinds of photosensitized light responses described in those chapters. Small mammals injected with a photosensitizer exhibit a characteristic pattern of responses on exposure to light, including apparent skin itching, hyperactivity, and skin damage (edema, erythema, cell death, and necrosis). The immediate reaction appears to be of the histamine-release type. With more sensitizer and/or light, generalized responses occur, including decreased blood pressure, intestinal hemorrhage, circulatory collapse, and death. These responses probably result from the photodynamic formation of toxic materials in the skin, which are then transported to all parts of the body in the blood stream (4). There is a considerable literature on photosensitization using photodynamic sensitizers such as porphyrins in the usual small laboratory mammals, including mice, rats, guinea pigs, and rabbits; in those cases that have been examined, oxygen is necessary for the reaction [see (61) for references]. In addition to the usual phototoxic responses, guinea pigs, like humans, show a photoimmunologic type of response with some photosensitizing drugs [see (109) and Chapter 11].

Grazing animals often become photosensitive as a result of eating plants containing photodynamic sensitizers. In particular, many species of plants of the genera *Hypericum* (which contain a group of potent photosensitizers, the hypericins; see Fig. 5-1) and *Fagopyrum* (the buckwheats, which contain similar sensitizers, the fagopyrins, fortunately not in the seeds) have posed a serious problem in many parts of the world (4, 11, 35). Under some conditions, sheep and goats show serious light sensitivity due to the accumulation of phylloerythrin. This is a porporphyrin produced from chlorophyll by bacterial action in the gut of the animal. Normally it is excreted in the bile; if bile discharge is interfered with, however, the sensitizer accumulates in the blood, leading to serious photodynamic injury (4, 35). Other chlorophyll derivatives can also sensitize; for example, chlorophyllide *a* and pheophorbide *a* are potent photosensitizers in the rat (110). If the bile duct in sheep is ligated, photosensitivity develops when the animal is on a diet of green plants; when fed grain or when protected from light, no symptoms develop (4, 11, 35). Experimentally, guinea pigs on a green-plant diet show light sensitivity as a result of carbon tetrachloride-induced liver damage, or if the common bile duct is ligated (111). Strains of cattle have been found which show hereditary porphyrias; animals with this disease ("pink tooth") have red-colored teeth, bones, and urine and often become highly photosensitive in unpigmented areas of the skin (4, 11, 35, 112).

Small mammals can be protected to some extent against photodynamic injury by various chemicals. For example, thiols protect photosensitized mice (113). Mathews (114) showed that beta-carotene protects mice against hematoporphyrin-sensitized photoinjury [also see (115) and Chapter 13], an observation that led to the use of carotene as a photoprotective agent for patients with erythropoietic protoporphyria (see Chapter 14).

Photodynamic Studies with Other Multicellular Animals

The lower vertebrates have not been used to any great extent for photodynamic investigations. Some work was carried out earlier with fish and amphibians, as reviewed by Blum (4). Tadpoles (116) and newts (117) can be killed by photodynamic treatment, and frog muscle has been used in studies on the photodynamic stimulation of contraction (118). Further, very little has been done with the more primitive invertebrates, although Blum (4) does mention some early work with hydra and rotifers. The photodynamic stimulation of the adductor muscle of larval mussels has been examined; contraction appears to be stimulated in a process that does not involve nervous tissue (119). The miracidia and cercaria (larval stages) of the blood fluke *Schistosoma mansoni* are killed on illumination in the presence of acridine orange or methylene blue; miracidia lose the ability to infest mice after a very brief photodynamic treatment (120). A number of polycyclic aromatic hydrocarbon carcinogens sensitize the photodynamic immobilization of brine shrimp nauplii (121).

The insects have received somewhat more attention from photodynamic investigators. Graham (39) reviewed the earlier work in this area and made some interesting speculations on the possible role of photodynamically active pigments in natural foods on the evolution of insects as well as on the possible role of such pigments in the resistance of plants to insects. Some of the earlier work on photosensitization of mosquito larvae suggested the use of photodynamic reactions in mosquito control. Polycyclic hydrocarbons sensitize the photodynamic killing of mosquito larvae roughly in proportion to their effectiveness as chemical carcinogens (122). More recently several insects (including the housefly, the imported fire ant, and the boll weevil) have been shown to be highly sensitive to photodynamic treatment [see (123) for references], suggesting the use of photodynamic dyes incorporated into appropriate foods as insecticides for destroying positively phototactic insects. The behavioral patterns of insects following photodynamic treatment indicate effects on the nervous system, perhaps mediated by the inactivation of acetylcholinesterase; this mechanism has not been established, however.

Photodynamic Studies with Multicellular Plants

Relatively few studies have been made with multicellular plants. However, any part of a plant can probably be injured or killed by photodynamic treatment since leaves, roots, and rootlets have been shown to be injured on illumination after permitting the organs to take up sensitizing dyes (4, 12). Sensitized roots show a positive phototropism on unilateral illumination (4) and the rate of the hormone-controlled growth of pea stem sections is decreased on illumination in the presence of riboflavin (124). Photodynamic treatment inhibits protoplasmic streaming in plant cells (125). Finally, if leaves are exposed to very high intensities of light in the absence of carbon dioxide, chlorophyll-sensitized photooxidations occur which bleach and kill them (126).

Photodynamic Carcinogenesis

It was demonstrated in 1937 (13, 45), using albino mice, that subcutaneous injections of photodynamic sensitizers such as hematoporphyrin promote skin-tumor formation when the animals are subsequently exposed to light. These sensitizers are not themselves chemical carcinogens. This phenomenon has not been demonstrated in humans, although it has been proposed that skin cancer in older humans might involve, in part, photosensitized reactions resulting from the gradual accumulation of porphyrin photosensitizers in the skin with age (13, 45). Under proper conditions, illumination with long-wavelength UV radiation accelerates the development of skin tumors in mice treated with the chemical carcinogen 3,4-benzpyrene (45, 127); this compound is a good photodynamic sensitizer. The mechanism of the phenomenon is not known, although it has been shown that photodynamic treatment with 3,4-benzpyrene increases the frequency of chromosome breaks in plant cells (45). A number of chemical carcinogens, including 3,4-benzpyrene, are degraded by photodynamic treatment (128); whether such reactions are significant in the conversion of precarcinogens in the environment into active forms is not known. There is a generally high correlation between the effectiveness of polycyclic hydrocarbons as chemical carcinogens and their ability to act as photodynamic sensitizers (13). The reason for this is not known, although theories suggesting the involvement of singlet oxygen in sensitized photocarcinogenesis have been advanced (64, 129). It should also be pointed out that tumors can be selectively destroyed by photodynamic treatment as described in Chapter 23.

PHOTODYNAMIC STUDIES WITH UNICELLULAR ORGANISMS AND CELLS

A large amount of the published work on photodynamic action has been carried out with unicellular organisms and cells from multicellular organisms. Mechanistic studies of photodynamic processes at this level are difficult because of the complexity of cells and the fact that most sensitizers tend to bind or localize (and thereby concentrate) in certain regions of cells (77); in most cases the precise location of these regions of high sensitizer concentration is not known. Further, as discussed above, binding can alter the photochemical properties of many sensitizers. Because of the characteristic differences in structure of procaryotic and eucaryotic microorganisms, photodynamic studies of the two groups will be considered separately; cells from multicellular organisms will be considered as a third category. Only a few references can be cited here. The earlier literature is covered in many of the reviews listed among the references, and an excellent analytical review of photodynamic mechanisms at the cellular level was published recently (77). The photodynamic degradation of biomembranes also has been reviewed (73).

Photodynamic Studies with Procaryotic Microorganisms

A number of types of photodynamic studies have been carried out with bacteria; the observed effects often depend on the species and strain of organism used as well as on the sensitizer, reaction conditions, and the physiologic state of the cells (20, 27, 77, 130). Effects can result from photodynamic damage to nucleic acids, to proteins, to membrane components (lipids, proteins), to ribosomes, etc. Many kinds of bacteria (20, 27) as well as some mycoplasmas (131) are killed (i.e., lose colony-forming ability) on illumination in the presence of photodynamic sensitizers. In many cases the sensitizer binds to or penetrates into the cell; however, *Escherichia coli* is also inactivated by externally generated singlet oxygen as produced by the illumination of rose bengal bound to polystyrene beads (132). Various metabolic activities in bacteria, including protein synthesis, respiration, glycolysis, etc., can be inhibited by photodynamic treatment; some cellular enzymes are destroyed (20, 27). The respiratory system in cell membranes isolated from *Sarcina lutea* is inactivated by photodynamic treatment with toluidine blue (133), while treatment of *Proteus mirabilis* increases the sensitivity of the cell envelope to lysis (134). Ribosomes isolated from *E. coli* are inactivated by photodynamic treatment (135); both protein and RNA are altered. *E. coli* ribosomal proteins are covalently cross-linked to ribosomal protein on photodynamic treatment with methylene blue (136). Some strains of bacteria show dark repair (77, 134). Photodynamic treatment of bacteria results in the efficient production of DNA–protein cross-links [see references in (137, 138)]. Mutations of different types are produced in several strains of *E. coli, Salmonella typhimurium*, etc., by photodynamic treatment with a number of sensitizers, including acridine orange, methylene blue, and phenothiazine tranquilizers (20, 27, 30, 49, 77, 139–141). It is well known that carotenoids protect bacteria against photodynamic damage involving both endogenous and exogenous sensitizers [see references in (66)]. The toluidine blue-sensitized photodynamic killing of a colorless mutant of *S. lutea* is enhanced in D_2O, while histidine and azide have a protective effect (142); these experiments suggest the involvement of singlet oxygen in the photodynamic killing of bacteria (77). Finally, it should be pointed out that many kinds of bacteria are "naturally" photosensitive due to the presence of endogenous sensitizing compounds (34, 143). It has been suggested that bacteria be used as experimental objects in the screening of compounds for phototoxic activity (144).

Photodynamic treatment has a characteristic pattern of effects on the swimming behavior of bacteria such as *S. typhimurium*. These bacteria normally swim in straight lines (smooth swimming) interrupted at intervals by brief periods of "tumbling" in which the direction of motion abruptly changes. In the presence of oxygen and a photodynamic sensitizer such as proflavine, short periods of low-intensity illumination cause smooth-swimming bacteria to tumble (145); longer periods of illumination lead to smooth swimming and finally to loss of motility.

Very little work has been done with procaryotic organisms other than bacteria; however, it was recently shown that acridine sensitizes the photodynamic inactivation and mutagenesis of the blue-green alga *Anacystis nidulans* (146).

Photodynamic Studies with Eucaryotic Microorganisms

A number of kinds of eucaryotic microorganisms have been used for photodynamic studies, in particular, yeast and paramecia. The work on yeast will be reviewed first, since this represents perhaps the most sophisticated area of photodynamic study at the cellular level. Ito (77) recently reviewed the mechanisms of photodynamic effects on yeast cells; this paper may be consulted for references. He concludes that sensitizers may act in three ways, depending on their physical chemical properties, as follows: (a) the dye remains outside the cell and illumination produces damage via singlet oxygen, primarily at the cell surface, (b) the dye penetrates the cell membrane, remains in the cytoplasm, and illumination produces mainly cytoplasmic damage (to enzymes, RNA, etc.), and (c) the dye binds to DNA in the nucleus, with DNA being the principal target of damage on illumination. Toluidine blue and other thiazine dyes operate mainly by the first mechanism and eosin Y and rose bengal primarily by the second mechanism; thiopyronine also appears to act primarily at the cytoplasmic level by inactivating respiration and fermentation (147). DNA-binding acridine dyes, such as acridine orange, act by the last mechanism; such dyes can produce genetic changes on illumination. In all three mechanisms, singlet oxygen appears to be the main mediator of photodynamic change (77, 148). Acridine orange binds to DNA in two different ways, by stacking on the outside of the molecule and by intercalation; the two kinds of complexes have different absorption peaks. Illumination at the peak of the intercalation complex induces mutations with greater efficiency than illumination at the stacking complex peak; however, illumination at the stacking complex peak produces singlet oxygen with higher efficiency (148).

RNA synthesis by a cell-free transcriptional system from yeast is inhibited by photodynamic treatment; this results from the photooxidation of both DNA and the RNA polymerase (149). Protein synthesis by a complete polyribosomal cell-free system from yeast is inhibited by photodynamic treatment with thiopyronine; the mechanism involves ribosomal damage and destruction of proteins such as aminoacyl-tRNA-synthetases rather than damage to tRNA (150). However, it should be pointed out that many other dyes do sensitize the photodynamic degradation of tRNA. Little work has been done on the genetic basis of photodynamic sensitivity in eucaryotic microorganisms; recently, however, mutants of yeast sensitive or resistant to photodynamic killing with thiopyronine have been isolated (151). The mechanism of resistance/sensitivity is not known. Both nuclear and cytoplasmic mutations have been produced photodynamically with thiopyronine in a haploid, photodynamically sensitive strain of yeast (152); no significant mutation occurred with a photodynamically resistant strain. Because of the simplicity of the measurements, it has been suggested that yeast be used as a screening organism to assess the probable phototoxicity to humans of drugs; however, there are discrepancies in the photodynamic killing response of yeast with some sensitizers as compared to the phototoxic response with albino mice (153).

A considerable amount of photodynamic research has been carried out with protozoa, starting with the pioneering studies of Raab (2). Paramecium has been the most generally used organism, although some work has been done with *Tetrahymena* and other protozoans. For example, paramecia have been used extensively in the photodynamic assay of polycyclic hydrocarbon air pollutants (154) and for detecting photosensitizing drugs (155). Paramecia sensitized with xanthene dyes can show photobehavioral responses, i.e., positive or negative phobophototaxic behavior, depending on dye concentration, light intensity, and oxygen concentration (156). Several dyes sensitize the photodynamic killing of dermatophyte fungi (157); under some conditions photodynamic treatment substantially reduces skin lesion formation in guinea pigs inoculated with such fungi (also see Chapter 20). Unicellular green plants (algae) can be killed by photodynamic treatment (27); however, they have not been used to any great extent in photodynamic studies.

Photodynamic Studies with Cells and Cell Organelles from Multicellular Animals

Many photodynamic studies have utilized "free" cells from multicellular animals, including sperm cells, egg cells, and various kinds of blood cells. Sperm cells typically show a sharp decrease in motility on treatment (158), while a variety of effects are noted with eggs from marine invertebrates, including the initiation of cell division and the suppression of fertilization membrane formation (27).

It was shown in 1908 that rabbit erythrocytes were hemolysed on illumination in the presence of porphyrin sensitizers (4). Since then, erythrocytes have been used extensively in photodynamic studies because of their relatively simple structure [photodynamic damage is expressed largely as membrane effects; see review by Lamola (73)] and because of the existence of certain kinds of porphyrias in humans in which photosensitizing porphyrins accumulate in the red blood cells (4, 61, 73). For example, a fraction of the erythrocytes in individuals with the rare hereditary condition erythropoietic protoporphyria contain high levels of protoporphyrin; on illumination, these cells rapidly hemolyse. Oxygen is required for this reaction, indicating that it is a typical photodynamic process [see references in (61, 73)]. Normal erythrocytes can be photohemolyzed following treatment with a wide variety of sensitizers. Photodynamic treatment of red blood cells with protoporphyrin markedly increases the passive cation permeability of the membrane, leading to an efflux of K^+ and an influx of Na^+. Unsaturated fatty acids, cholesterol, proteins, and enzymes in the membranes of erythrocytes and in isolated erythrocyte membranes (ghosts) are photooxidized on photodynamic treatment [see references in (73)]. There is also an extensive photo-cross-linking of membrane proteins (159, 160); it has been suggested that a secondary reaction between free amino groups and a photooxidation product of histidine, tryptophan, or tyrosine is involved in the photodynamic cross-linking (161). These results suggest that protein alteration may be involved in the lysis phenomenon. However, the photooxidation product of cholesterol in red cell membranes (3-β-hydroxycholest-6-ene 5α-hydroperoxide) has been demonstrated to lyse normal red blood cells (73). As would be expected for a singlet oxygen-mediated process, the antioxidant alpha-tocopherol, beta-carotene, etc., protect red blood cells from patients with erythropoietic protoporphyria against hemolysis on illumination; artificially sensitized red blood cells are also protected by beta-carotene [see references in (61, 73)].

Cells and tissues isolated from multicellular animals as well as cells in tissue culture have been used extensively for photodynamic studies. For example, the fibers in isolated rat diaphragm lose K^+ and gain Na^+ on illumination in the presence of rose bengal; the fibers twitch vigorously on illumination (162). Membrane-mediated effects are also observed in the photodynamic treatment of neurons [see references in (163)]. Many kinds of photodynamic responses have been studied using normal and neoplastic cells from humans and other mammals in tissue culture. These include killing, diminution of the ability to support virus growth, interference with protein synthesis and nucleic acid replication, interference with the normal pattern of cell division, etc. (27, 61, 164, 165); direct effects on DNA have been reported [(166–168); Chapter 4]. Light from ordinary fluorescent lamps is often injurious to mammalian cells growing in the usual tissue culture media. Effects include loss of cloning efficiency, production of chromosomal aberrations, production of mutations, decreased growth rate, etc. These effects are usually attributed to the riboflavin-sensitized formation of hydrogen peroxide and of toxic photoproducts from tryptophan and tyrosine in the culture medium [see references in (169)]. The tryptophan photo-oxidation product and metabolite N-formylkynurenine is a potent photosensitizer (170). In some strains of cells in culture, intracellular flavins and/or porphyrins apparently act as photodynamic sensitizers; damage to such cells on illumination is decreased by antioxidants such as alpha-tocopherol and ascorbic acid (171–173). The retina in many mammals is damaged by visible light; it has recently been suggested that retinal in the visual cells sensitizes such photodamage by a singlet oxygen mechanism (174). Very few measurements on the quantum requirements for photodynamic injury to animal cells have been reported. Blum (4) found that a photosensitized erythrocyte must absorb approximately 10^{10} photons for hemolysis to occur. More recently it was determined that 3.0×10^9 quanta of 620-nm light must be absorbed by TA-3 mouse mammary carcinoma cells containing 0.6 mM hematoporphyrin in order to obtain a 90% kill (175).

Many studies have been carried out in attempts to determine the site(s) of photodynamic damage in animal cells. Cells can be stained generally and then illuminated in a localized region with a microbeam of light. Cells can be treated with dyes that localize in a particular type of organelle and then the whole cell can be illuminated, and, finally, cell organelles can be isolated, purified, and studied outside the cell (176). The various techniques used for the microirradiation of cells have been discussed (37, 177). In some cases, fluorescence microscopy permits the observation of dye localization in living cells. Acridine orange, for example, localizes in the nuclei of many kinds of cells. The lysosomes of mammalian cells accumulate certain porphyrins; on illumination, lysosomal enzymes are released into the cytoplasm, causing cell injury and death (178). Isolated rat liver lysosomes release large quantities of enzymes on photodynamic treatment (179). Some dyes, such as rose bengal, accumulate in the external cell membrane of tissue culture cells; subsequent illumination leads to changes in membrane permeability and integrity. Illumination of isolated rat liver mitochondria in the presence of various sensitizers induces a rapid swelling of the mitochondria; in addition, various mitochondrial enzymes are inactivated (176, 180, 181). Fibroblasts in cell culture exhibit two patterns of photosensitization with hematoporphyrin; a brief exposure to the porphyrin sensitizes the cells to membrane damage, while prolonged exposure sensitizes them to cytoplasmic damage; preincubation with beta-carotene protects the cells against both types of damage (182). If sarcoplasm reticulum vesicle membranes prepared from rabbit skeletal muscle are illuminated in the presence of xanthene dyes, the rate of calcium ion uptake into the vesicles is decreased and the ATPase activity associated with the membranes is destroyed (183). Photodynamic treatment of isolated rat liver microsomes inactivates the mixed function oxidase system and peroxidizes membrane lipids, apparently by a singlet oxygen mechanism (184).

PHOTODYNAMIC STUDIES WITH VIRUSES

The photodynamic inactivation of viruses has been studied extensively. Some investigations have been concerned with the elucidation of fundamental photodynamic mechanisms, some with the use of the photodynamic technique as a probe of the molecular structure of viruses, some with the use of photodynamically inactivated viruses as antigens in the preparation of vaccines and antisera, and, especially in recent years, some in which photodynamic reactions are used in the treatment of superficial viral infections in humans. Work on animal viruses began with Herzberg's observation in 1931 that vaccinia virus eruptions on the skin of the rabbit could be suppressed by photodynamic treatment with methylene blue (4). Since that time, studies have been carried out with many different animal viruses, including rabies virus, adenoviruses, and influenza viruses. The earlier work has been extensively reviewed (17, 30, 42). Many animal viruses are quickly inactivated on illumination in the presence of sensitizers; others, such as polio virus, must be grown in the presence of certain kinds of dyes in order to become sensitized. Incubating many types of resistant viruses with the sensitizer at high pH renders them light-sensitive, apparently as a result of a pH-induced increase in the permeability of the protein coat of the virus (17). Although little direct evidence is available, it has been generally assumed that photodynamic effects on animal viruses involve the viral nucleic acid (42); for example, photodynamic treatment of polio virus RNA produces stable mutant varieties of the virus (17). However, in the case of the Moloney mouse leukemia virus, the RNA-dependent DNA polymerase component of the virus is the site of photodynamic damage (185).

A great deal of research has been done on the use of photosensitizing dyes plus light in the treatment of herpes simplex viral infections [(74, 186) and Chapter 19]. The risk/benefit relationships and the efficacy of this photo-chemotherapeutic approach to viral infections are somewhat controversial at present, especially in view of reports that photodynamically treated viruses can transform mammalian cells (187, 188). This topic is treated in detail in Chapters 19, 20, and 21. Very recently the hydrophobic dye acridine has been shown to be a very effective sensitizer for the photodynamic inactivation of herpes simplex and other lipid-containing viruses (189); the inactivating mechanism may not involve the viral nucleic acid. The proflavine-sensitized photodynamic induction of SV40 virus can take place within a virus–host system (190). The complexity of such interactions is indicated by the report that the transformation of thymidine kinase-deficient mouse cells is increased by the proflavine-sensitized photodynamic treatment of the cells (191).

Many studies have been made of photodynamic effects on bacteriophages (see 30, 192, 193). A number of compounds (in particular, the thiazine, acridine, and oxazine dyes) are effective photosensitizers; however, the mechanism of viral inactivation may be different with different sensitizers (194). The sensitivity of a given bacteriophage often depends on the permeability of the protein head membrane of the virus. A number of photodynamically inactive dyes (especially crystal violet and other triphenyl-methane dyes), which bind strongly at the bacteriophage nucleic acid, protect the virus against photodynamic inactivation, as do a variety of polyamines (192). Both proteins and nucleic acids can be destroyed in photodynamically treated bacteriophage. Nucleic acid is probably the major site of damage; polynucleotide strands are broken, and cross-linking between DNA and protein occurs (195). The N-formylkynurenine-photosensitized inactivation of bacteriophage is mediated in part by singlet oxygen and in part by direct interactions of the excited sensitizer with the bacteriophage; the singlet oxygen pathway apparently involves the protein tail and the purines in the head DNA (196). Mutations are readily produced in bacteriophage and in single-stranded DNA from bacteriophage by photodynamic treatment (49, 197). Photodynamically inactivated bacteriophage can be repaired in appro-priate host bacteria [see (197), for example].

Some photodynamic studies have been carried out with plant viruses (30); most of this work has been done with tobacco mosaic virus. The infectious RNA from tobacco mosaic virus is photoinactivated faster and more completely than the intact virus, suggesting that the protein coat can play a protective role as with many bacteriophages. With some sensitizers, the formation of a complex between the sensitizer and the viral RNA appears to be necessary for efficient photodynamic inactivation. Guanine appears to be the main site of damage in tobacco mosaic virus-RNA. Photodynamic mutations have been produced in tobacco mosaic virus-RNA (30, 49). As a final point it should be mentioned that photodynamic treatment with methylene blue has been suggested for the disinfection of tapwater, sea water, and treated sewage; preliminary laboratory studies involving polio virus appear promising (198).

PHOTODYNAMIC DEGRADATION OF BIOMOLECULES

Photodynamic damage to living material results from the photodynamic degradation of essential biomolecules. The molecules that make up protoplasm vary widely in their sensitivity to photodynamic treatment, depending on their chemical structure, the sensitizer, and the reaction conditions. Many categories of organic compounds found in or used in living material can be photooxidized, including acids, alcohols, aldehydes, amines, bilirubin, carbohydrates, drugs such as chlorpromazine and codeine, esters, growth factors and vitamins (such as ascorbic acid, alpha-lipoic acid, and alpha-tocopherol), ketones, nitrogen heterocyclics, nucleic acids (and certain of their component purines, pyrimidines, nucleosides, and nucleotides), olefins, phenols, proteins (and certain of their component amino acids), pyrroles, steroids, etc. (22, 30, 57, 64).

Carbohydrates and other alcohols are only moderately sensitive to photodynamic degradation [see references in (32, 64)]. Hexitols such as sorbitol are photooxidized first to the hexose and finally to the corresponding hexonic acid with quinone and ketonic sensitizers. Most of the research concerning photodynamic effects on carbohydrates has been carried out with cellulose, since many dyes sensitize the "phototendering" of cotton and other plant textile fibers; this is a photodegradative process which involves the consumption of oxygen and which decreases the mechanical strength of the dyed fibers. Cellulose appears to be photooxidized almost entirely by free radical mechanisms. The mucopolysaccharide hyaluronic acid (the major component of the jelly like vitreous humor of the eye as well as the ground substance of the animal tissue) is depolymerized on illumination in the presence of a number of photodynamic sensitizers; the rate is increased by the presence of ascorbic acid [see references in (32)]. Evidence from studies with hyaluronic acid as well as with the closely related polysaccharide sodium alginate indicates that free radicals are generated by photochemical reactions which in turn abstract hydrogen atoms from the polymers, leading to chain scission; singlet oxygen does not appear to be involved in the process (199). What role might be played by the photodepolymerization of hyaluronic acid by endogenous sensitizers in the mammalian eye in vivo is not known.

Unsaturated fatty acids and their esters (including triglycerides) can be photooxidized with a variety of sensitizers. The photooxidation of esters of unsaturated fatty acids by methylene blue and erythrosine proceeeds via singlet oxygen mechanisms to give hydroperoxide products (64, 200, 201). With riboflavin as sensitizer, the photooxidation proceeds largely by free radical mechanisms (200); both pathways appear to be involved with hematoporphyrin as the sensitizer (202). Unsaturated food oils such as olive oil and soybean oil are photooxidized in the presence of photosensitizers (203, 204). The flavor of potato chips, corn chips, and other snack foods marketed in transparent containers often deteriorates rapidly on exposure to the high light intensities found in the usual supermarkets. This probably results from the sensitized photooxidation of the cooking oils used (205); attempts are being made to extend the shelf life of these products by the incorporation of photodynamic quenchers such as carotenoids.

With very few exceptions, proteins are photooxidized rapidly on illumination in the presence of oxygen and photodynamic sensitizers. The sites of damage are cysteinyl, histidyl, methionyl, tryptophyl, and tyrosyl residues in the protein; in general, peptide and disulfide bonds are not broken and amino groups are not usually oxidized. These amino acids are also photooxidized in the free state, while the other amino acids typically found in proteins are resistant. The photooxidation of proteins, small peptides, and the sensitive amino acids has been the subject of a number of reviews (30–32, 40, 47, 58, 62, 64, 67, 70) which can be consulted for original references. The mechanism of the photooxidation of amino acids depends on the amino acid, the sensitizer, the solvent, the reactant concentrations, and, in particular, the pH. Cysteine can be photooxidized to cystine, while the imidazole ring of histidine is cleaved, yielding a large number of products, most of which have not been identified. The pH dependence of the photooxidation of histidine indicates that only the unprotonated molecule is sensitive. With singlet oxygen sensitizers, methionine is photooxidized to dehydromethionine, which in turn is converted into methionine sulfoxide; the mechanisms are complex and depend on the pH (206). In contrast, methionine is deaminated and decarboxylated on illumination in the presence of flavin sensitizers to yield the aldehyde methional (31). This latter reaction occurs in beer (31) and in milk (207) on illumination, resulting in the production of so-called sunlight flavor; for this reason beer is usually packaged in bottles of colored glass which do not transmit blue light. The photooxidation of tryptophan results in a mixture of products, one of which (*N*-formylkynurenine) is itself an efficient photodynamic sensitizer [(170); also see (208)]. Finally, the photooxidation of tyrosine involves the rupture of the phenol ring, giving products which have not been well characterized (82); the reaction is much faster at high pH, indicating that only the anionic form is photooxidized rapidly. The formation and disappearance of primary amine groups in amino acids during photooxidation have been followed using specific reagents such as fluorescamine (209).

In proteins, the rate of photooxidation of amino acid residues depends on their location; i.e., in general, a susceptible residue exposed at the surface will be photooxidized more rapidly than a residue buried in the interior of the protein molecule. By varying the reaction conditions and the dye, selective photooxidation of different residues in proteins can be obtained (31, 50). Photodynamic reactions can be used as probes of the three-dimensional structures of proteins in solution. In this approach, sensitizers are used that bind to specific and known sites in the protein molecules. On subsequent illumination only those sensitive amino acid residues located near the bound sensitizer will be altered (50). In a few cases, proteins contain natural photosensitizing moieties located at specific sites. For example, in many pyridoxal-dependent enzymes, such as 6-phosphogluconate dehydrogenase, the pyridoxal acts as a photosensitizer and illumination leads to the modification of amino acid residues located near the binding site for the cofactor (50). The heme group can be removed from some hemoproteins, such as horseradish peroxidase, apoleghemoglobin, etc., and replaced with a photosensitizing porphyrin (such as hematoporphyrin, protoporphyrin IX, etc.); illumination then leads to the destruction of residues in the heme-binding pocket (210, 211). Protective agents that bind at known sites can be used in conjunction with unbound sensitizers to probe protein structure; in this approach, specific limited regions of the protein will be protected from photodynamic damage (58).

Many types of physicochemical alteration occur in proteins as a result of photodynamic treatment, including changes in charge, conformation, digestibility by proteolytic enzymes, heat sensitivity, mechanical properties, molecular aggregation, optical rotation, solubility, viscosity, etc. [see (30, 31) for reference); some of these changes undoubtedly result from the photodynamic cross-linking of the protein (212). Changes in the biologic activity are also observed, including loss of activity of enzymes and of protein hormones such as insulin, loss of ability to bind cofactors, alteration of antibody activity and antigenic properties, and loss of toxicity of bacterial toxins and snake venoms [see (30, 31) for references].

In studies of the sensitized photooxidation of purines, pyrimidines, nucleosides, and nucleotides it is found that guanine and its derivatives are photooxidized most rapidly (at approximately neutrality). Thymine and its derivatives are oxidized more slowly, while the other bases and their derivatives are oxidized only very slowly with most sensitizers [see (30, 32, 43, 48, 51, 52, 64, 193, 213) for references]. In general, the rates of oxidation of the nucleic acid bases increase sharply with increasing pH, suggesting that the anions are much more sensitive than the neutral bases. The sensitized photooxidation of purines and pyrimidines typically leads to a complex mixture of reaction products; little is known of the primary products of photooxidation or of the subsequent transformations, although it has been suggested recently that epoxides may be the initial photooxidation products of pyrimidines (214). The array of reaction products produced during the methylene blue-sensitized photooxidation of guanosine is different, in part, from the products resulting from oxidation with singlet oxygen produced by a radiofrequency discharge; this suggests that both Type I and Type II processes are involved in the photodynamic reaction (215). Similar conclusions were reached in experiments using singlet oxygen quenchers and D_2O as mechanistic probes (216).

A large amount of work has been done on the sensitized photooxidation of nucleic acids in solution. With most sensitizers, guanine residues in DNA are preferentially destroyed; in many cases, binding of the sensitizers to nucleic acids increases the efficiency of photodynamic damage (52, 217). Free radicals are produced in the DNA moiety of DNA–sensitizer complexes on illumination (218). A variety of physical chemical changes is observed in photodynamically treated DNA molecules, including spectral shifts, increased sensitivity to enzymatic attack, conformational changes, changes in flexibility, chain cleavage, production of alkali-labile bonds, changes in sedimentation coefficients, etc. (30, 32, 219–221). Photodynamic treatment with ethidium bromide as sensitizer is used for the controlled production of "nicks" in DNA (222). Photodynamic treatment of DNA with methylene blue followed by treatment with piperidine specifically cleaves the chain at each guanine residue (223); this reaction can be used in nucleic acid sequencing strategies. Photodynamic treatment also alters the biologic properties of nucleic acids; for example, bacterial DNA-transforming principle is destroyed, template activity of both procaryotic and eucaryotic DNA is lost, as is the infectivity of RNA from tobacco mosaic virus (30, 32, 52, 224). In vivo studies indicate that guanine residues of cellular DNA are also selectively destroyed on photodynamic treatment. For example, fluorescent antibodies specific for unpaired cytosine residues in DNA have been used to demonstrate the selective photooxidation of guanine residues in the methylene blue-sensitized photodynamic treatment of human cells growing in culture (225). There is also some evidence that photodynamic treatment can produce chain breaks in DNA in vivo (226).

SUMMARY

We now have a fairly good understanding of the initial processes involved in photodynamic reactions, i.e., the production of light-excited states of sensitizer molecules and the interaction of excited sensitizers with substrate (hydrogen and / or electron transfer processes) and with molecular oxygen (by an energy transfer process to give singlet oxygen). In most cases our knowledge of the mechanistic organic chemistry of the sensitized photooxidation of substrate molecules (such as amino acids, proteins, nucleic acids and their bases, etc.) is poor. Finally, we have only hazy ideas as to the details of photodynamic reactions at the cellular and organismal levels.

Fundamental studies of photodynamic processes as described in this chapter are justifiable in their own right in terms of increasing our understanding of this important biologic phenomenon. A better understanding of the mechanisms of photodynamic reactions should also permit improvements in photochemotherapy techniques and in the treatment of phototoxic conditions in humans.

A better understanding should also permit the use of photodynamic reactions in more applied ways in the future. For example, such techniques have been suggested for use in destroying pollutants in industrial waste waters; preliminary studies have been made of the feasibility of using photodynamic sensitizers to photooxidize phenols, an important type of toxic water pollutant (103). It has also been suggested that biologic contaminants such as viruses and bacteria could be destroyed in the same way (198). Cellulose-containing wastes accumulate in large amounts from industrial and agricultural sources; photodynamic sensitizers have been shown to increase the rate of degradation of cellulose cattle feed lot wastes (227). Solar UV radiation degrades many pesticides and herbicides in the environment (228); it may become feasible to insert photosensitizing (or photoprotective) groupings into herbicide and pesticide molecules to control their persistence in the environment more precisely. Finally, it should be pointed out that photosensitized reactions can be used to generate chemical reagents rapidly and conveniently; such reactions are beginning to be used in analytical measurements. For example, photosensitized assays have been described for riboflavin (229), ascorbic acid, caffeine, epinephrine, and nicotine (230).

REFERENCES

1. Oparin, A. I. (1968): *Genesis and Evolutionary Development of Life.* Academic Press, New York.
2. Raab, O. (1900): Über die Wirkung fluorescirender Stoffe auf Infusorien. *Z. Biol.* **39**:524–546.
3. von Tappeiner, H., and Jodlbauer, A. (1904): Über die Wirkung der photodynamischen (fluorescierenden) Stoffe auf Protozoen und Enzyme. *Dtsch. Arch. Klin. Med.* **39**:427–487.
4. Blum, H. F. (1941): *Photodynamic Action and Diseases Caused by Light.* Reinhold, New York (Reprinted 1964, Hafner, New York).
5. Musajo, L., and Rodighiero, G. (1972): Mode of photosensitizing action of furocoumarins. *Photophysiology* **7**:115–147.
6. Rodighiero, G., and Dall'Acqua, F. (1976): Biochemical and medical aspects of psoralens. *Photochem. Photobiol.* **24**:647–653.
7. Poppe, W., and Grossweiner, L. I. (1975): Photodynamic sensitization via the singlet oxygen mechanism. *Photochem. Photobiol.* **22**:217–219.
8. Singh, H., and Vadasz, J. A. (1978): Singlet oxygen: A major reactive species in the furocoumarin photosensitized inactivation of *E. coli* ribosomes. *Photochem. Photobiol.* **28**:539–545.
9. Rosenthal, I., Ben-Hur, E., Prager, A., et al. (1978): Photochemical reactions of chlorpromazine; chemical and biochemical implications. *Photochem. Photobiol.* **28**:591–594.

10. Kochevar, I., and Lamola, A. A. (1979): Chlorpromazine and protriptyline phototoxicity: Photosensitized, oxygen independent red cell hemolysis. *Photochem. Photobiol.* **29**:791–796.

11. Clare, N. T. (1956): Photodynamic action and its pathological effects. In: *Radiation Biology*, Vol. III, edited by A. Hollaender, pp. 693–723. McGraw-Hill, New York.

12. Fowlks, W. L. (1959): The mechanism of the photodynamic effect. *J. Invest. Dermatol.* **32**:233–247.

13. Santamaria, L. (1960): Photodynamic action and carcinogenicity. In: *Recent Contributions to Cancer Research in Italy,* Vol. I, edited by P. Bucalossi and U. Veronesi, pp. 167–288. Casa Editrice Ambrosiana, Milan.

14. McLaren, A. D., and Shugar, D. (1964): *Photochemistry of Proteins and Nucleic Acids.* Macmillan, New York.

15. Santamaria, L., and Prino, G. (1964): The photodynamic substances and their mechanism of action. In: *Research Progress in Organic, Biological and Medicinal Chemistry,* Vol. I, edited by U. Gallo and L. Santamaria, pp. 260–336. Società Editoriale Farmaceutica, Milan.

16. Spikes, J. D., and Glad, B. W. (1964): Photodynamic action. *Photochem. Photobiol.* **3**:471–487.

17. Wallis, C., and Melnick, J. L. (1965): Photodynamic inactivation of animal viruses: A review. *Photochem. Photobiol.* **4**:159–170.

18. Berg, H. (Ed.), (1967): *Molecular Mechanismen photodynamischer Effekte.* Proceedings of the Fourth Jenaer Symposium. *Studia Biophys.* **3**:1–289.

19. Bourdon, J., and Schnuriger, B. (1967): Photosensitization of organic solids. In: *Physics and Chemistry of the Organic Solid State,* Vol. III, edited by D. Fox, M. M. Labes, and A. Weissberger, pp. 59–131. Interscience, New York.

20. Harrision, A. P. (1967): Survival of bacteria. Harmful effects of light, with some comparisons with other adverse physical agents. *Annu. Rev. Microbiol.* **21**:143–156.

21. Simon, M. I. (1967): Photosensitization. In: *Photobiology, Ionizing Radiation,* Vol. 27 in *Comprehensive Biochemistry,* edited by M. Florkin and E. H. Stotz, pp. 137–156. Elsevier, Amsterdam.

22. Spikes, J. D., and Straight, R. (1967): Sensitized photochemical processes in biological systems. *Annu. Rev. Phys. Chem.* **18**:409–436.

23. Bellin, J. S. (1968): Photophysical and photochemical effects of dye binding. *Photochem. Photobiol.* **8**:383–392.

24. Foote, C. S. (1968): Photosensitized oxygenations and the role of singlet oxygen. *Accts. Chem. Res.* **1**:104–110.

25. Foote, C. S. (1968): Mechansims of photosensitized oxidation. *Science* **162**:963–970.

26. Krinsky, N. I. (1968): The protective function of carotenoid pigments. *Photophysiology* **3**:123–195.

27. Spikes, J. D. (1968): Photodynamic action. *Photophysiology* **3**:33–64.

28. Grossweiner, L. I. (1969): Molecular mechanisms in photodynamic action. *Photochem. Photobiol.* **10**:183–191.

29. Smith, K. C., and Hanawalt, P. C. (1969): *Molecular Photobiology* (Inactivation and Recovery), Chapter 9, Photodynamic Action, pp. 179–191. Academic Press, New York.

30. Spikes, J. D., and Livingston, R. (1969): The molecular biology of photodynamic action: Sensitized photoautoxidations in biological systems. *Adv. Radiat. Biol.* **3**:29–121.

31. Spikes, J. D., and MacKnight, M. L. (1970): Dye-sensitized photooxidation of proteins. *Ann. N.Y. Acad. Sci.* **171**:149–161.

32. Spikes, J. D., and MacKnight, M. L. (1970): The dye-sensitized photooxidation of biological macromolecules. In: *Photochemistry of Macromolecules,* edited by R. F. Reinisch, pp. 67–83. Plenum, New York.

33. Wilson, T., and Hastings, J. W. (1970): Chemical and biological aspects of singlet excited molecular oxygen. *Photophysiology* **5**:50–95.

34. Eisenstark, A. (1971): Mutagenic and lethal effects of visible and near-ultraviolet light on bacterial cells. *Adv. Gen.* **16**:167–198.
35. Giese, A. C. (1971): Photosensitization by natural pigments. *Photophysiology* **6**:77–129.
36. Politzer, I. R., Griffin, G. W., and Laseter, J. L. (1971): Singlet oxygen and biological systems. *Chem. Biol. Interact.* **3**:73–93.
37. Cameron, I. L., Burton, A. L., and Hiatt, C. W. (1972): Photodynamic action of laser light on cells. In: *Concepts in Radiation Cell Biology,* edited by G. L. Whitson, pp. 245–258. Academic Press, New York.
38. Chandra, P. (1972): Photodynamic action: a valuable tool in molecular biology. In: *Research Progress in Organic, Biological and Medicinal Chemistry,* Vol. 3, edited by U. Gallo and L. Santamaria, pp. 232–258. North-Holland, Amsterdam.
39. Graham, K. (1972): Entomological, ecological, and evolutionary implications in photodynamic action. *Can. J. Zool.* **50**:1631–1636.
40. Grossweiner, L. I., and Kepka, A. G. (1972): Photosensitization in biopolymers. *Photochem. Photobiol.* **16**:305–314.
41. Harber, L. C., and Baer, R. L. (1972): Pathogenic mechanisms of drug-induced photosensitivity. *J. Invest. Dermatol.* **58**:327–342.
42. Hiatt, C. W. (1972): Methods for photoinactivation of viruses. In: *Concepts in Radiation Cell Biology,* edited by G. L. Whitson, pp. 57–89. Academic Press, New York.
43. Knowles, A. (1972): The dye-sensitized degradation of nucleotides. In: *Research Progress in Organic, Biological and Medicinal Chemistry,* Vol. 3, edited by U. Gallo and L. Santamaria, pp. 183–213. North-Holland, Amsterdam.
44. Magnus, I. A. (1972): Photodynamic action in the skin. In: *Research Progress in Organic, Biological and Medicinal Chemistry,* Vol. 3, edited by U. Gallo and L. Santamaria, pp. 561–600. North-Holland, Amsterdam.
45. Santamaria, L. (1972): Further considerations on photodynamic action and carcinogenicity. In: *Research Progress in Organic, Biological and Medicinal Chemistry,* Vol. 3, edited by U. Gallo and L. Santamaria, pp. 671–687. North-Holland, Amsterdam.
46. Santamaria, L., and Prino, G. (1972): List of the photodynamic substances. In: *Research Progress in Organic, Biological and Medicinal Chemistry,* Vol. 3, edited by U. Gallo and L. Santamaria, pp. XI–XXXV. North-Holland, Amsterdam.
47. Spikes, J. D., and MacKnight, M. L. (1972): Photodynamic effects on molecules of biological importance: amino acids, peptides and proteins. In: *Research Progress in Organic, Biological and Medicinal Chemistry,* Vol. 3, edited by U. Gallo and L. Santamaria, pp. 124–136. North-Holland, Amsterdam.
48. Wacker, A. (1972): Molecular mechanisms of photodynamic compounds. In: *Research Progress in Organic, Biological and Medicinal Chemistry,* Vol. 3, edited by U. Gallo and L. Santamaria, pp. 107–123. North-Holland, Amsterdam.
49. Zelle, M. (1972): Genetic effects of photodynamic action. In: *Research Progress in Organic, Biological and Medicinal Chemistry,* Vol. 3, edited by U. Gallo and L. Santamaria, pp. 280–296. North-Holland, Amsterdam.
50. Jori, G. (1973): Photosensitized oxidation of biomolecules as a tool for elucidating three-dimensional structure. *Anais Acad. Brasil. Cien.* **45**:33–44.
51. Löber, G., and Kittler, L. (1973): Photochemie und Photobiologie von Nukleinsäuren und Nukleinsäurebausteinen. *Studia Biophys.* **41**:91–153.
52. Lochmann, E.-R., and Micheler, A. (1973): Binding of organic dyes to nucleic acids and the photodynamic effect. In: *Physico-Chemical Properties of Nucleic Acids,* Vol. 1, edited by J. Duchesne, pp. 223–267. Academic Press, New York.
53. Scheel, L. D. (1973): Photosensitizing agents. In: *Toxicants Occurring Naturally in Foods,* 2nd ed., pp. 558–572. National Academy of Sciences, Washington, D.C.
54. Foote, C. S. (1974): Photooxidation: In: *Phototherapy in the Newborn: An Overview,* edited by G. B. Odell, R. Schaffer, and A. P. Simopoulos, pp. 21–33. National Academy of Sciences, Washington, D.C.

55. Krinsky, N. I. (1974): The protective functions of carotenoid pigments against aerobic sensitivity. In: *Progress in Photobiology,* edited by G. O. Schenck. Deutsche Gessellschaft für Lichtforschung, Frankfurt.

56. Berg, H. (1975): Photopolarographe und photodynamie. *Sitzunber. Akad. Wiss. Leipzig* 111:5–19.

57. Gollnick, K. (1975): Chemical aspects of photodynamic action in the presence of molecular oxygen. In: *International Congress of Radiation Research, 5th, Seattle, 1974,* edited by O. F. Nygaard, H. I. Adler, and W. K. Sinclair, pp. 590–611. Academic Press, New York.

58. Jori, G. (1975): Photosensitized reactions of amino acids and proteins. *Photochem. Photobiol.* 21:463–467.

59. Knowles, A. (1975): The effects of photodynamic action involving oxygen upon biological systems. In: *International Congress of Radiation Research, 5th, Seattle, 1974,* edited by O. F. Nygaard, H. I. Adler, and W. K. Sinclair, pp. 612–622. Academic Press, New York.

60. Laustriat, G., and Hasselman, C. (1975): Photochemistry of proteins. *Photochem. Photobiol.* 22:295–298.

61. Spikes, J. D. (1975): Porphyrins and related compounds as photodynamic sensitizers. *Ann. N. Y. Acad. Sci.* 244:496–508.

62. Choughuley, A. S. U., and Chadha, M. S. (1976): Reactions of singlet oxygen with amino acids, purines and pyrimidines. In: *Singlet Molecular Oxygen,* pp. 153–168. Bhabha Atomic Research Center, Bombay.

63. Elad, D. (1976): Photoproducts of purines. In: *Photochemistry and Photobiology of Nucleic Acids,* Vol. II, edited by S. Y. Wang, pp. 357–381. Academic Press, New York.

64. Foote, C. S. (1976): Photosensitized oxidation and singlet oxygen: consequences in biological systems. In: *Free Radicals in Biology,* Vol. II, edited by W. A. Pryor, pp. 85–133. Academic Press, New York.

65. Grossweiner, L. I. (1976): Photochemical inactivation of enzymes. In: *Current Topics in Radiation Research,* Vol. II, edited by M. Ebert and A. Howard, pp. 141–199. North-Holland, Amsterdam.

66. Krinsky, N. I. (1976): Cellular damage initiated by visible light. In: *The Survival of Vegetative Microorganisms* (Society for General Microbiology Symposium, Vol. 26), edited by T. R. G. Gray and J. R. Postgate pp. 209–239. Cambridge Univ. Press, Cambridge.

67. Matsuura, T., and Saito, I. (1976): Photooxidation of heterocyclic compounds. *Gen. Heterocycl. Chem. Ser.* 4:456–523.

68. Nilsson, R. (1976): The role of singlet state excited oxygen in photodynamic action. In: *Phototherapie* (Verhandlungsber. Dtsch.-Schwed. Symp. Photomedizin, 1975), edited by E. G. Jung, pp. 33–41. Schattauer, Stuttgart.

69. Rosenthal, I. (1976): Recent developments in singlet molecular oxygen chemistry (Yearly Review). *Photochem. Photobiol.* 24:641–645.

70. Singhal, G. S. (1976): Sensitized photooxidation of proteins. In: *Singlet Molecular Oxygen,* pp. 125–136. Bhabha Atomic Research Centre, Bombay.

71. Feitelson, J. (1977): The role of oxygen in photosensitized reactions of proteins and nucleic acids. In: *Research in Photobiology,* edited by A. Castellani, pp. 235–243. Plenum Press, New York.

72. Krinsky, N. I. (1977): Singlet oxygen in biological systems. *Trends Biochem. Sci.* **1977** (February).

73. Lamola, A. S. (1977): Photodegradation of biomembranes. In: *Research in Photobiology,* edited by A. Castellani, pp. 53–63. Plenum Press, New York.

74. Melnick, J. L., and Wallis, C. (1977): Photodynamic inactivation of herpes simplex virus: A status report. *Ann. N.Y. Acad. Sci.* 284:171–181.

75. Spikes, J. D. (1977): Photosensitization. In: *The Science of Photobiology,* edited by K. C. Smith, pp. 87–112. Plenum Press, New York.

76. Bartlett, P. D. (1978): Free radical aspects of photooxidation. *ACS Symp. Ser.* **69**(Org. Free Radicals):15–32.

77. Ito, T. (1978): Cellular and subcellular mechanisms of photodynamic action: The $^1O_2$ hypothesis as a driving force in recent research. *Photochem. Photobiol.* **28**:493–508.

78. Lochman, E. R., and Micheler, A. (1979): Molecular and biochemical aspects of photodynamic action (Yearly Review). *Photochem. Photobiol.* **29**:1199–1204.

79. Ranby, B., and Rabek, J. F. (1978): *Singlet Oxygen Reactivity with Organic Compounds and Polymers.* Wiley, Chichester.

80. Singh, A., and Petkau, A. (1978): International Conference on Singlet Oxygen and Related Species in Chemistry and Biology. *Photochem. Photobiol.* **28:(4/5)**:429–933.

81. Wasserman, H. H., and Murray, R. W. (eds) (1979): *Singlet Oxygen.* Academic Press, New York.

82. Rizzuto, F., and Spikes, J. D. (1977): The eosin-sensitized photooxidation of substituted phenylalanines and tyrosines. *Photochem. Photobiol.* **25**:465–476.

83. Jahnke, L. S., and Frenkel, A. W. (1978): Photooxidation of epinephrine sensitized by methylene blue—evidence for the involvement of singlet oxygen and superoxide. *Photochem. Photobiol.* **28**:517–523.

84. Spikes, J. D., and Swartz, H. M. (1978): International Conference on Singlet Oxygen and Related Species in Chemistry and Biology: Review and General Discussion. *Photochem. Photobiol.* **28(4/5)**:921–933.

85. Suwa, K., Kimura, T., and Schaap, A. P. (1978): Reaction of singlet oxygen with cholesterol in liposomal membranes. Effect of membrane fluidity on the photooxidation of cholesterol. *Photochem. Photobiol.* **28**:469–473.

86. Merkel, P. B., Nilsson, R., and Kearns, D. R. (1972): Deuterium effects on singlet oxygen lifetimes in solution. A new test of singlet oxygen reactions. *J. Am. Chem. Soc.* **94**:1030–1031.

87. Nilsson, R., and Kearns, D. R. (1973): A remarkable deuterium effect on the rate of photosensitized oxidation of alcohol dehydrogenase and trypsin. *Photochem. Photobiol.* **17**:65–68.

88. Nilsson, R., Merkel, P. B., and Kearns, D. R. (1972): Kinetic properties of the triplet states of methylene blue and other photosensitizing dyes. *Photochem. Photobiol.* **16**:109–116.

89. Kraljić, I., and Sharpatyi, V. A. (1978): Determination of singlet oxygen rate constants in aqueous solutions. *Photochem. Photobiol.* **28**:583–586.

90. Chan, H. W.-S. (1975): Artificial food colours and the photooxidation of unsaturated fatty acid methyl esters: The role of erythrosine. *Chem. Ind.* **1975**:612–614.

91. Ljunggren, B., and Moller, H. (1978): Drug phototoxicity in mice. *Acta Derm. Venereol. (Stockh.)* **58**:125–130.

92. Schothorst, A. A., Suurmond, D., and de Luster, A. (1979): A biochemical screening test for the photosensitizing potential of drugs and disinfectants. *Photochem. Photobiol.* **29**:531–537.

93. Vinson, L. J., Borselli, V. F., Oleniacz, W. S., et al. (1969): Laboratory and clinical procedures for assessing photosensitizing potential of topical agents. *Toxicol. Appl. Pharmacol., Suppl.* **3**:103–112.

94. Conn, H. J. (1961): *Biological Stains,* 7th ed. Williams & Wilkins, Baltimore.

95. Rizzuto, F., and Spikes, J. D. (1975): Mechanisms involved in the chemical inhibition of the eosin-sensitized photooxidation of trypsin. *Radiat. Environ. Biophys.* **12**:217–232.

96. Cauzzo, G., Gennari, G., Jori, G., et al. (1977): The effect of chemical structure on the photosensitizing efficiencies of porphyrins. *Photochem. Photobiol.* **25**:389–395.

97. Cannistraro, S., Jori, G., and Van de Vorst, A. (1978): Photosensitization of amino acids by di-cyan-hemin: kinetic and EPR studies. *Photochem. Photobiol.* **27**:517–521.

98. Cannistraro, S., and Van de Vorst, A., and Jori, G. (1978): EPR studies on singlet oxygen production of porphyrins. *Photochem. Photobiol.* **28**:257–259.

99. Buettner, G. R., and Oberley, L. W. (1979): Superoxide formation by protoporphyrin as seen by spin trapping. *FEBS Lett.* **98**:18–20.

100. Girotti, A. W. (1976): Bilirubin-sensitized photoinactivation of enzymes in the isolated membrane of the human erythrocyte. *Photochem. Photobiol.* **24**:525–532.

101. Rubaltelli, F. F., and Jori, G. (1979): Visible light irradiation of human and bovine serum albumin–bilirubin complex. *Photochem. Photobiol.* **29**:991–1000.

102. Schapp, A. P., Thayer, A. L., Blossey, E. C., et al. (1975): Polymer-based sensitizers for photooxidation. *J. Am. Chem. Soc.* **97**:3741–3745.

103. Seely, G. R., and Hart, R. L. (1977): Photosensitized oxidation by stained alginate beads. *Photochem. Photobiol.* **26**:655–659.

104. Miyoshi, N., and Tomita, G. (1979): Effects of indole and tryptophan on furan oxidation by singlet oxygen in micellar solutions. *Photochem. Photobiol.* **29**:527–530.

105. Bagno, O., Soulignac, J. C., and Joussot-Dubien, J. (1979): pH dependence of sensitized photooxidation in micellar anionic and cationic surfactants, using thiazine dyes. *Photochem. Photobiol.* **29**:1079–1081.

106. Horsey, B. E., and Whitten, D. G. (1978): Environmental effects on photochemical reactions: contrasts in the photooxidation behavior of protoporphyrin IX in solution, monolayer films, organized monolayer assemblies and micelles. *J. Am. Chem. Soc.* **100**:1293–1295.

107. Copland, E. S., Alving, C. R., and Grenan, M. M. (1976): Light-induced leakage of spin label marker from liposomes in the presence of phototoxic phenothiazines. *Photochem. Photobiol.* **24**:41–48.

108. Delmelle, M. (1978): Retinal sensitized photodynamic damage to liposomes. *Photochem. Photobiol.* **28**:357–360.

109. Harber, L. C., and Shalita, A. R. (1977): Immunologically mediated contact photosensitivity in guinea pigs. *Adv. Mod. Toxicol.* **4**:427–439.

110. Tapper, B. A., Lohrey, E., Hove, E. L., et al. (1975): Photosensitivity from chlorophyll-derived pigments. *J. Sci. Food Agric.* **26**:277–284.

111. Bremner, D. P. (1974): Hepatogenous photosensitization. Induction and study in guinea pigs. *J. Comp. Pathol.* **84**:555–568.

112. Burnham, B. F. (1969): Metabolism of porphyrins and corrinoids. In: *Metabolic Pathways,* 3rd ed., edited by D. M. Greenberg, Vol. 3, pp. 403–490. Academic Press, New York.

113. Harber, L. C., Hsu, J., Hsu, H., et al. (1972): Studies of photoprotection against porphyrin photosensitization using dithiothreitol and glycerol. *J. Invest. Dermatol.* **58**:373–380.

114. Mathews, M. M. (1964): Protective effect of β-carotene against lethal photosensitization by haematoporphyrin. *Nature* **203**:1092.

115. Mushell, A. N., and Bjornson, L. (1977): Protection in erythropoietic protoporphyria: Mechanism of protection by beta carotene. *J. Invest. Dermatol.* **68**:157–160.

116. Urbani, E. (1945): Photodynamic action in relation to oxidation on amphibian larvae. *Pontifica Acad. Sci. Acta* **8**:131–137 [*Chem. Abstr.* **45**:6760g (1951)].

117. Frankston, J. E. (1940): The photodynamic action of neutral red on *Triturus viridescens viridescens* (Rafinesque). *J. Exp. Zool.* **83**:161–190.

118. Sazonenko, M. K. (1963): On the photodynamic stimulation of frog skeletal muscle. *Biofizika* **8**:681–687.

119. Labos, E. (1966): Energetic aspects of the photosensitization of embryonic muscle by xanthene dyes. *Comp. Biochem. Physiol.* **17**:353–362.

120. Lacaz, P. S., and Holanda, E. J. C. (1974): Photodynamic effects on the miricidium and cercaria of *Schistosoma mansoni. Bol. Acad. Nac. Med. (Brazil)* **145**:43–58.

121. Morgan, D. D., and Warshawsky, D. (1977): The photodynamic immobilization of *Artemia salina* nauplii by polycyclic aromatic hydrocarbons and its relationship to carcinogenic activity. *Photochem. Photobiol.* **25**:39–46.

122. Matoltsy, G., and Fabian, Gy. (1946): Measurement of the photodynamic effect of cancerogenic substances with biological indicators. *Nature* **158**:877–878.

123. Fondren, J. E., Jr., Norment, B. R., and Heitz, J. R. (1978): Dye-sensitized photooxidation in the house fly, *Musca domestica*. *Environ. Entomol.* 7:205–208.

124. Galston, A. W. (1950): Riboflavin, light and the growth of plants. *Science* 111:619–624.

125. Keul, M., and Lazar-Keul, G. (1973): Photodynamic effect of erythrosin B and visible light on the rotation current in the root hairs of barley (*Hordeum vulgare*) and the protective effect of ATP on the photodynamic damage of cells. *Stud. Univ. Babes-Bolyai, Ser. Biol.* 18:55–61 [*Chem. Abstr.* 79:122244j (1973)].

126. Franck, J., and French, C. S. (1941): Photooxidation processes in plants. *J. Gen. Physiol.* 25:309–324.

127. Santamaria, L. (1974): Photodynamic action and skin cancer. In: *Progress in Photobiology,* edited by G. O. Schenck, paper no. 014. Deutsche Gesellschaft für Lichtforschung, Frankfurt.

128. Greenstock, C. L., and Wiebe, R. H. (1978): Photosensitized carcinogen degradation and the possible role of singlet oxygen in carcinogen activation. *Photochem. Photobiol.* 28:863–867.

129. Khan, A. U., and Kasha, M. (1970): An optical-residue singlet-oxygen theory of photocarcinogenicity. *Ann. N.Y. Acad. Sci.* 171:24–33.

130. Matsumoto, S. (1974): Photodynamic inactivation of *Escherichia coli* cells after starvation for required amino acid or chloramphenicol treatment. *Jpn. J. Genet.* 49:275–279.

131. Chaudhuri, U., Das, J., and Maniloff, J. (1978): Photodynamic inactivation and its repair in mycoplasmas. *Biochim. Biophys. Acta* 544:624–633.

132. Bezman, S. A., Burtis, P. A., Izod, T. P. J., et al. (1978): Photodynamic inactivation of *E. coli* by rose bengal immobilized on polystyrene beads. *Photochem. Photobiol.* 28:325–329.

133. Prebble, J., and Huda, A. S. (1973): Sensitivity of the electron transport chain of pigmented and non-pigmented *Sarcina* membranes to photodynamic action. *Photochem. Photobiol.* 17:255–264.

134. Jacob, H. -E. (1977): Photodynamically produced damages in *Proteus mirabilis* and their repair. *Studia Biophys.* 61:129–134.

135. Singh, H., and Ewing, D. D. (1978): Methylene blue sensitized photoinactivation of *E. coli* ribosomes: Effect on the RNA and protein components. *Photochem. Photobiol.* 28:547–552.

136. Zook, D. E., and Fahnestock, S. R. (1978): Covalent cross-linking of ribosomal RNA and proteins by methylene blue-sensitized photooxidation. *Biochim. Biophys. Acta* 517:400–406.

137. Smith, K. C. (1976): Radiation-induced cross-linking of DNA and protein in bacteria. In: *Aging, Carcinogenesis, and Radiation Biology,* edited by K. C. Smith, pp. 67–81. Plenum Press, New York.

138. Jori, G., and Spikes, J. D. (1978): Mapping the three-dimensional structure of proteins by photochemical techniques. *Photochem. Photobiol. Rev.* 3:193–275.

139. Basu, S., and Bagchi, B. (1978): Mutation in *Escherichia coli* during photodynamic inactivation and subsequent holding in buffer. *FEBS Lett.* 96:26–30.

140. Hass, B. S., and Webb, R. B. (1979): Photodynamic effects on bacteria. III. Mutagenesis by acridine orange and 500-nm monochromatic light in strains of *Escherichia coli* that differ in repair capability. *Mutat. Res.* 60:1–11.

141. Jose, J. G. (1979): Photomutagenisis by chlorinated phenothiazine tranquilizers. *Proc. Natl. Acad. Sci. U.S.A.* 76:469–472.

142. Mathews-Roth, M. M. (1977): Photosensitization in *Sarcina lutea*: Different mechanisms of exogenous and endogenous photosensitizers. *Photochem. Photobiol.* 25:599–600.

143. Webb, R. B. (1977): Lethal and mutagenic effects of near-ultraviolet radiation. *Photochem. Photobiol. Rev.* 2:169–261.

144. Kobayashi, F., Wada, Y., and Mizuno, N. (1974): Comparative studies on phototoxicity of chemicals. *J. Dermatol.* 1:93–98.

145. Taylor, B. L., and Koshland, D. E., Jr. (1976): Perturbation of the chemotactic tumbling of bacteria. *J. Supramol. Struct.* 4:343–353.

146. Sarma, T. A. (1978): Optimal conditions for photodynamic mutagenesis in *Anacystis nidulans*. *Indian J. Microbiol.* **18**:19–21.

147. Nishiyama-Watanabe, S. (1976): Photodynamic action of thiopyronine on the respiration and fermentation in yeast. *Int. J. Radiat. Biol.* **30**:501–509.

148. Kobayashi, K., and Ito, T. (1977): Wavelength dependence of singlet oxygen mechanism in acridine orange-sensitized photodynamic action in yeast cells: Experiments with 470 nm. *Photochem. Photobiol.* **25**:385–388.

149. Micheler, A., and Nishiyama-Watanabe, S. (1977): Thiopyronine-sensitized photodynamic inactivation of RNA synthesis *in vitro*. *Int. J. Radiat. Biol.* **31**:35–43.

150. Nishiyama-Watanabe, S., and Schultz-Harder, B. (1977): Photodynamic action of thio-pyronine on polyribosomes and cell-free protein synthesis in yeast. *Int. J. Radiat. Biol.* **31**:113–119.

151. Roth, R., Papierniak, K. J., and Anderson, J. M. (1978): Mutations in *Saccharomyces cerevisiae* affecting sensitivity to photodynamic action. *Photochem. Photobiol.* **27**:795–798.

152. Kenter, D., and Laskowski, W. (1978): Induction of mutations by photodyamic action of thiopyronine in *Saccharomyces cerevisiae*. *Radiat. Environ. Biophys.* **15**:379–385.

153. Ison, A. E., and Davis, C. M. (1969): Photoxicity of quinoline methanols and other drugs in mice and yeast. *J. Invest. Dermatol.* **52**:193–198.

154. Epstein, S. S., Mantel, N., and Stanley, T. W. (1968): Photodynamic assay of neutral subfractions of organic extracts of particulate atmospheric pollutants. *Environ. Sci. Tech.* **2**:132–138.

155. Barth, J., and Arnold, T. (1976): The paramecium test for the detection of photosensitizers. *Dermatol. Monatsschr.* **162**:900–904.

156. Metzner, P. (1921): Zur Kenntnis der photodynamischen Erscheinung: Die induzierte Phototaxis bei Paramaecium caudatum. *Biochem. Z.* **113**:145–175.

157. Propst, C., and Lubin, L. (1978): *In vitro* and *in vivo* photosensitized inactivation of dermatophyte fungi by heterotricyclic dyes. *Infect. Immun.* **20**:136–141.

158. Van Duijn, C., Jr. (1975): Toxic and photodynamic effects of vital staining with cresyl blue on bull spermatozoa. *Mikroskopie* **31**:14–22.

159. Girotti, A. W. (1976): Photodynamic action of protoporphyrin IX on human erythrocytes: Cross-linking of membrane proteins. *Biochem. Biophys. Res. Commun.* **72**:1367–1374.

160. Dubbelman, T. M. A. R., de Goeij, A. F. P. M., and van Steveninck, J. (1978): Protoporphyrin-sensitized photodynamic modification of proteins in isolated human red blood cell membranes. *Photochem. Photobiol.* **28**:197–204.

161. Dubbelman, T. M. A. R., de Goeij, A. F. P. M., and van Steveninck, J. (1978): Photodynamic effects of protoporphyrin on human erythrocytes. Nature of the cross-linking of membrane proteins. *Biochim. Biophys. Acta* **511**:141–151.

162. Parkin, A. C., Duncan, C. J., and Bowler, K. (1976): Studies of the effect of oubain, ethacrynic acid and photooxidation on cation and water balance of mammalian muscle. *Comp. Biochem. Physiol.* **55C**:11–16.

163. Pooler, J. F., and Valenzeno, D. P. (1978): Kinetic factors governing sensitized photo-oxidation of excitable cell membranes. *Photochem. Photobiol.* **28**:219–226.

164. Speck, W. T., Chen, C. C., and Rosenkranz, H. S. (1975): *In vitro* studies of effects of light and riboflavin on DNA and HeLa cells. *Pediatr. Res.* **9**:150–153.

165. Sery, T. W. (1979): Photodynamic killing of retinoblastoma cells with hematoporphyrin and light. *Cancer Res.* **39**:96–100.

166. Regan, J. D., and Setlow, R. B. (1977): The effect of proflavin plus visible light on the DNA of human cells. *Photochem. Photobiol.* **25**:345–346.

167. Speck, W. T., Santella, R. M., and Brem, S. (1979): Alteration of human cellular DNA by neutral red in the presence of visible light. *Mutat. Res.* **66**:95–98.

168. Hoffmann, M. E., and Meneghini, R. (1979): DNA strand breaks in mammalian cells exposed to light in the presence of riboflavin and tryptophan. *Photochem. Photobiol.* **29**:299–303.

169. Wang, R. J., and Nixon, B. T. (1978): Identification of hydrogen peroxide as a photoproduct toxic to human cells in tissue-culture medium irradiated with "daylight" fluorescent light. *In Vitro* **14**:715–722.

170. Pileni, M. -P., Santus, R., and Land, E. J. (1978): On the photosensitizing properties of *N*-formylkynurenine and related compounds. *Photochem. Photobiol.* **28**:525–529.

171. Jacobson, E. D., Krell, K., Dempsey, M. J., et al. (1978): Toxicity and mutagenicity of radiation from fluorescent lamps and a sunlamp in L5178Y mouse lymphoma cells. *Mutat. Res.* **51**:61–75.

172. Parshad, R. P., Sanford, K. K., Taylor, W. G., et al. (1979): Effect of intensity and wavelength of fluorescent light on chromosome damage in cultured mouse cells. *Photochem. Photobiol.* **29**:971–975.

173. Cheng, L. Y. L., and Packer, L. (1979): Photodamage to hepatocytes by visible light. *FEBS Lett.* **97**:124–128.

174. Delmelle, M. (1979): Possible implication of photooxidation reactions in retinal photo-damage. *Photochem. Photobiol.* **29**:713–716.

175. Dougherty, T. J., Gomer, C. J., and Weishaupt, K. R. (1976): Energetics and efficiency of photoinactivation of murine tumor cells containing hematoporphyrin. *Cancer Res.* **36**:2330–2333.

176. Haga, J. Y., and Spikes, J. D. (1972): Effects of photodynamic treatment on mitochondria. In: *Research Progress in Organic, Biological and Medicinal Chemistry,* Vol. 3, edited by U. Gallo and L. Santamaria, pp. 464–479, North-Holland, Amsterdam.

177. Berns, M. W. (1974): *Biological Microirradiation.* Prentice-Hall, Englewood Cliffs, N. J.

178. Allison, A. C., Magnus, I. A., and Young, M. R. (1966): Role of lysosomes and of cell membranes in photosensitization. *Nature* **209**:874–878.

179. Williams, D. S., and Slater, T. F. (1973): Photosensitization of isolated lysosomes. *Biochem. Soc. Trans.* **1**:200–202.

180. Obata, F. (1974): Photodynamic action of phloxine on mitochondrial respiration. *Chem. Pharm. Bull.* (Tokyo) **22**:1285–1290.

181. Aggarwal, B., Avi-Dor, Y., Tinberg, H. M., et al. (1976): Effect of visible light on the mitochondrial inner membrane. *Biochem. Biophys. Res. Commun.* **69**:362–368.

182. Fritsch, P., Gschnait, F., Honigsmann, H., et al. (1976): Protective action of beta-carotene against lethal photosensitization of fibroblasts *in vitro. Br. J. Dermatol.* **94**:263–271.

183. Kondo, M., and Kasai, M. (1974): Photodynamic inactivation of sarcoplasmic reticulum vesicle membranes by xanthene dyes. *Photochem. Photobiol.* **19**:35–41.

184. Rahimtula, A. D., Hawco, F. J., and O'Brien, P. J. (1978): The involvement of $^1O_2$ in the inactivation of mixed function oxidase and peroxidation of membrane lipids during the photosensitized oxidation of liver microsomes. *Photochem. Photobiol.* **28**:811–815.

185. Munson, B. R., and Fiel, R. J. (1977): Hematoporphyrin-sensitized photodynamic inactivation of viral RNA-dependent DNA polymerase. *Res. Commun. Chem. Pathol. Immunol.* **16**:175–178.

186. Melnick, J. L., Khan, N. C., and Biswal, N. (1977): Photodynamic inactivation of *Herpes simplex* virus and its DNA. *Photochem. Photobiol.* **25**:341–342.

187. Rapp, F., and Kemeny, B. A. (1977): Oncogenic potential of *Herpes simplex* virus in mammalian cells following photodynamic inactivation. *Photochem. Photobiol.* **25**:335–337.

188. Oxman, M. N. (1977): The clinical evaluation of photodynamic inactivation for the therapy of recurrent *Herpes simplex* virus infections. *Photochem. Photobiol.* **25**:343–344.

189. Snipes, W., Keller, G., Woog, J., et al. (1979): Inactivation of lipid-containing viruses by hydrophobic sensitizers and near-ultraviolet radiation. *Photochem. Photobiol.* **29**:785–790.

190. Bockstahler, L. E., and Cantwell, J. M. (1979): Photodynamic induction of an oncogenic virus *in vitro. Biophys. J.* **25**:209–213.

191. Verwoerd, D. W., and Rapp, F. (1978): Biochemical transformation of mouse cells by herpes simplex virus type 2: Enhancement by means of low-level photodynamic treatment. *J. Virol.* **26**:200–202.

192. Yamamoto, N. (1972): Genetic damage by photodynamic action and recombination of bacteriophage. In: *Research Progress in Organic, Biological and Medicinal Chemistry,* Vol. 3, edited by U. Gallo and L. Santamaria, pp. 297–319. North-Holland, Amsterdam.

193. Kittler, L., and Löber, G. (1977): Photochemistry of nucleic acids. *Photochem. Photobiol. Rev.* 2:39–131.

194. Piette, J., Calberg-Bacq, C. M., and Van de Vorst, A. (1978): Photodynamic activity of dyes with different DNA binding properties. II. T₄ phage inactivation. *Int. J. Radiat. Biol.* 34:223–232.

195. Jaffe-Brachet, A., Henry, N., and Errera, M. (1971): The photodynamic inactivation of λ bacteriophage particles in the presence of methylated proflavine. *Mutant. Res.* 12:9–14.

196. Walrant, P., Santus, R., Redpath, J. L., et al. (1977): *N'*-Formylkynurenine-photosensitized inactivation of bacteriophage. *Int. J. Radiat. Biol.* 30:189–192.

197. Piette, J., Calberg-Bacq, C. M., and Van de Vorst, A. (1978): Photodynamic effect of proflavine φX174 bacteriophage, its DNA replicative form and its isolated single-stranded DNA: Inactivation, mutagenesis and repair. *Molec. Gen. Genet.* 167:95–103.

198. Gerba, C. P., Wallis, C., and Mellnick, J. L. (1977): Application of photodynamic oxidation to the disinfection of tapwater, seawater and sewage contaminated with poliovirus. *Photochem. Photobiol.* 26:499–504.

199. Davies, A. K., Howard, K. R., McKellar, J. F., et al. (1976): Photochemical interaction between methylene blue and L-ascorbic acid in absence and presence of biological molecules. In: *Excited States of Biological Molecules,* edited by J. B. Birks, pp. 106–115. Wiley, London.

200. Chan, H. W. -S. (1977): Photo-sensitized oxidation of unsaturated fatty acid methyl esters. The identification of different pathways. *J. Am. Oil. Chem. Soc.* 54:100–104.

201. Terao, J., and Matsushita, S. (1977): Reactivities and products in photosensitized oxidation of unsaturated triglycerides. *Agric. Biol. Chem.* 42:667–668.

202. Cannistraro, S., and Van de Vorst, A. (1977): Photosensitization by hematoporphyrin: ESR evidence for free radical induction in unsaturated fatty acids and for singlet oxygen production. *Biochem. Biophys. Res. Commun.* 74:1177–1185.

203. Clements, A. H., Van Den Engh, R. H., Frost, D. J., et al. (1973): Participation of singlet oxygen in photosensitized oxidations of 1,4-dienoic systems and photooxidation of soybean oil. *J. Am. Oil Chem. Soc.* 50:325–330.

204. Carlsson, D. J., Suprunchuk, T., and Wiles, D. M. (1976): Photooxidation of unsaturated oils: effects of singlet oxygen quenchers. *J. Am. Oil Chem. Soc.* 53:656–660.

205. Radtke, R. (1974): Storage behavior of potato chips exposed to light and in dark. 1. Analysis of alterations of frying oils caused by light. *Fette Seifen Anstrichmittel* 76:540–546.

206. Sysak, P. K., Foote, C. S., and Ching, T. -Y. (1977): Chemistry of singlet oxygen—XXV. Photooxygenation of methionine. *Photochem. Photobiol.* 26:19–27.

207. Sattar, A., and deMan, J. M. (1975): Photooxidation of milk and milk products: A review. *Crit. Rev. Food Sci. Nutr.* 7:13–49.

208. Smith, G. J. (1978): Photooxidation of tryptophan sensitized by methylene blue. *J. Chem. Soc., Faraday Trans. 2* 74:1350–1354.

209. Straight, R., and Spikes, J. D. (1978): Sensitized photooxidation of amino acids: Effects on the reactivity of their primary amine groups with fluorescamine and *o*-phthalaldehyde. *Photochem. Photobiol.* 27:565–569

210. Kang, Y. -J., and Spikes, J. D. (1976): The porphyrin-sensitized photooxidation of horseradish apoperoxidase. *Arch. Biochem. Biophys.* 172:565–573.

211. Pertillä, U., and Ellfolk, N. (1978): Photooxidation of soybean apoleghemoglobin with protoporphyrin IX, heme and dye. *Eur. J. Biochem.* 91:335–338.

212. Girotti, A. W., Lyman, S., and Deziel, M. R. (1979): Methylene blue-sensitized photo-oxidation of hemoglobin: Evidence for cross-link formation. *Photochem. Photobiol.* 29:1119–1125.

213. Lober, G., and Kittler, L. (1977): Selected topics in photochemistry of nucleic acids: Recent results and perspectives. *Photochem. Photobiol.* **25**:215–233.

214. Ryang, H. -S., and Wang, S. Y. (1978): α-Diketone sensitized photooxidation of pyrimidines. *J. Am. Chem. Soc.* **100**:1302–1303.

215. Kornhauser, A., Krinsky, N. I., Huang, P. -K. C., et al. (1973): A comparative study of photodynamic oxidation and radiofrequency-discharge-generated $^1O_2$ oxidation of guanosine. *Photochem. Photobiol.* **18**:61–69.

216. Saito, I., Inoue, K., and Matsuura, T. (1975): Occurrence of the singlet-oxygen mechanism in photodynamic oxidations of guanosine. *Photochem. Photobiol.* **21**:27–30.

217. Walrant, P., Santus, R., and Charlier, M. (1976): Role of complex formation in the photosensitized degradation of DNA induced by N'-formylkynurenine. *Photochem. Photobiol.* **24**:13–19.

218. Piette, J., Calberg-Bacq, C. M., Cannistraro, S., et al. (1978): Photodynamic activity of dyes with different DNA binding properties. I. Free-radical induction in DNA. *Int. J. Radiat. Biol.* **34**:213–221.

219. Gutter, B., Speck, W. T., and Rosenkranz, H. S. (1977): The photodynamic modification of DNA by hematoporphyrin. *Biochim. Biophys. Acta* **475**:307–314.

220. Triebel, H., Bär, H., Jacob, H. -E., et al. (1978): Sedimentation analysis of DNA photooxidized in the presence of thiopyronine. *Photochem. Photobiol.* **28**:331–337.

221. Berg, H. (1978): Redox processes during photodynamic damage of DNA. II. A new model for electron exchange and strand breaking. *Bioelectrochem. Bioenerg.* **5**:347–356.

222. Martens, P. A., and Clayton, D. A. (1977): Strand breakage in solutions of DNA and ethidium bromide exposed to visible light. *Nucleic Acids Res.* **4**:1393–1407.

223. Friedmann, T., and Brown, D. M. (1978): Base-specific reactions useful for DNA-sequencing: Methylene blue-sensitized photooxidation and osmium tetraoxide modification of thymine. *Nucleic Acids Res.* **5**:615–622.

224. Kuratomi, K., and Kobayashi, Y. (1976): Photodynamic action of lumiflavin on the template DNA of RNA polymerase. *FEBS Lett.* **72**:295–298.

225. Gutter, B., Nishioka, Y., Speck, W. T., et al. (1976): Immunofluorescence for the detection of photochemical lesions in intracellular DNA. *Exp. Cell Res.* **102**:413–416.

226. Jacob, H. -E. (1971): *In vivo* production of DNA single-strand breaks by photodynamic action. *Photochem. Photobiol.* **14**:743–745.

227. Eskins, K., Bucher, B. L., and Sloneker, J. H. (1973): Sensitized photodegradation of cellulose and cellulosic wastes. *Photochem. Photobiol.* **18**:195–200.

228. Rabson, R., and Plimmer, J. R. (1973): Photoalteration of pesticides: Summary of workshop. *Science* **180**:1204–1205.

229. Clausen, E. (1975): Simple and fast assay method for riboflavine. *Lab. Pract.* **24**:161–162.

230. White, V. R., and Fitzgerald, J. M. (1975): Dye-sensitized continuous photochemical analysis: Identification and relative importance of key experimental parameters. *Anal. Chem.* **47**:903–908.

III

Photobiology of Normal Human Skin

6

Optical Properties of Human Skin

R. R. Anderson and J. A. Parrish

Despite the many years since optical spectra from human skin were first obtained, only recently have quantitative models of cutaneous optics been applied. This chapter aims to present the optics of human skin conceptually and quantitatively, to examine the structures and pigments that modify cutaneous optics, and to discuss current research in this area and its applications to photomedicine. Introductory sections on the structure of skin and on optical phenomena in turbid media are included in addition to the general introduction below. This chapter does not offer an exhaustive review of all studies related to the optics of human skin, but attempts to include those reliable studies pertinent to its goals. The interested reader can find thorough and more historical reviews in (1–3).

Unlike most other organs, the skin is accessible for visual inspection. Consequently, humans have learned to judge each other, in part, on the basis of pigmentation, texture, and cosmetic appearance of skin. The accessibility of skin often allows the dermatologist to diagnose and follow its condition simply by visual inspection. Specific local or generalized changes in skin color are most often due to abnormal structures or depositions of pigmented substances within the skin. As such, an understanding of the optical properties of the skin is helpful in explaining such changes and can be useful in diagnosis of skin or systemic disease. Quantitative optical measurements of skin in vivo can be used to quantify, monitor, and diagnose certain cutaneous and systemic conditions. For example, in phototherapy or photochemotherapy, in vivo spectral measurements of diffuse reflectance (remittance) can quantify

R. R. Anderson and J. A. Parrish • Department of Dermatology, Harvard Medical School, Massachusetts General Hospital, Boston, Massachusetts 02114

the vascular and pigmentary responses of skin, and might also be used as an aid in determining optical dosimetry. Neonatal serum bilirubin levels can be monitored noninvasively by a similar technique. Patterns of visible auto-fluorescence of pigmented skin can be used to deduce the locality of abnormal quantities of melanin pigmentation.

In addition to making such diagnostic techniques feasible, a quantitative understanding of the optics of skin yields knowledge of the optical radiation doses received by different cell layers within the skin, by cutaneous blood, and by internal organs, when humans are exposed to optical radiation. Different wavelengths across the optical spectrum, defined here as approximately 250 nm in the ultraviolet to approximately 3000 nm in the infrared, reach vastly different depths within tissue. Because most photobiologic effects are both wavelength- and dose-dependent, the rational design and explanation of the effects of various phototherapies require knowledge of *internal optical dosimetry*. Our rapidly increasing knowledge of cellular and molecular photobiology gained from in vitro bacterial and tissue culture studies can in theory be related to observed responses of cells in situ by comparing the dose-related effects of optical radiation in vitro to those in vivo. Conversely, on the basis of knowing the practical upper limits of spectral radiant exposure doses experienced by cell layers, blood, or other structures in vivo, one can then concentrate on basic studies of repair, mutation, and metabolic changes induced by equivalent doses in vitro. The use of laser irradiation for selective thermal destruction of optically absorbing structures in skin, and control of the tissue depth affected by various forms of photochemotherapy, are examples in which understanding cutaneous optics allows selectivity and control of the damage induced.

Describing "the" optics of human skin is somewhat like describing "the" weather; it can be measured and understood, but cannot be considered static. The skin is a highly dynamic organ capable of withstanding, and mounting protective responses to, a host of deleterious environmental treatments and agents. As such, the optical properties of skin are also dynamic. Many different physical structures and chromophores (optically absorbing molecular structures) within different layers of the skin influence its optical properties over different spectral regions. Changes in vasodilatation, vascular permeability, oxygenation of cutaneous blood, bile pigments, carotenoids, melanin pigmentation, and thickness of any of the various layers of skin affect cutaneous optics. The simple act of bathing alters the optics of the stratum corneum to make one more sensitive to certain ultraviolet wavelengths. A 10-min exposure on a sunny day is sufficient in many persons to cause immediate pigment darkening—a photochemical oxidation reaction of melanin—subsequent delayed hyperpigmentation (tanning), and epidermal hyperplasia. Systemic and cutaneous pathologic conditions can markedly alter cutaneous optics as well.

The microscopically complex structure of the skin makes an entirely rigorous analysis of its optics virtually impossible. The situation is not, however, too complicated to allow useful quantitative study of the optics of skin. On the macroscopic scale, phenomenologic theories of radiation transfer in turbid media can be applied to model the optics for each skin layer. Major optical variables within each layer in vitro have been studied, allowing one to conceptually consider the skin as a definable multilayered optical system. Optical interactions between each definable layer can then be considered, to produce a general and quantitative description of cutaneous optics. Fortunately, many of the major chromophores are normally confined to a single layer. Melanin, for example, is confined to the epidermis and stratum corneum, whereas the various forms of hemoglobins are confined to vessels of the dermis, and only indirectly exert any influence on optical radiation within the overlying epidermis. Considering the absorption spectra and localization of the major cutaneous pigments, and optical scattering for each layer, it is possible to arrive at mathematical descriptions of cutaneous optics which include most of the major variables in vivo. It must be emphasized, however, that a truly precise yet general quantitative model of cutaneous optics is lacking.

STRUCTURE OF THE SKIN

A thorough review of the anatomy of the skin and its structures is not within the scope of this chapter (4–7); however, an overview of skin as an optical medium is presented here. Figure 1-1 of Chapter 1 is a diagrammatic cross section of the skin showing three major tissue layers; the epidermis, the dermis, and the subcutaneous tissue. The thin outermost epidermis can be considered a sheet of epithelial cells called keratinocytes stacked 10–15 high. These cells continually migrate outward from a germinative layer toward the surface. In the process, they flatten, die, and cement together to form a proteinaceous, thin and tough outer layer called the stratum corneum. The stratum corneum attenuates ultraviolet (UV) radiation before it reaches living cells. The dermis is much thicker than the epidermis, has fewer cells, and is connective tissue. Blood vessels, lymphatics, and nerves course through the dermis. The deepest layer, the subcutaneous tissue, is mainly fatty tissue and acts as an insulator and a shock absorber.

Epidermis (Fig. 6-1)

The epidermal keratinocytes produce keratin, the fibrous protective lipoproteins of the skin. As keratinocytes differentiate and migrate outward, they flatten, and granules appear within the cytoplasm, forming the stratum

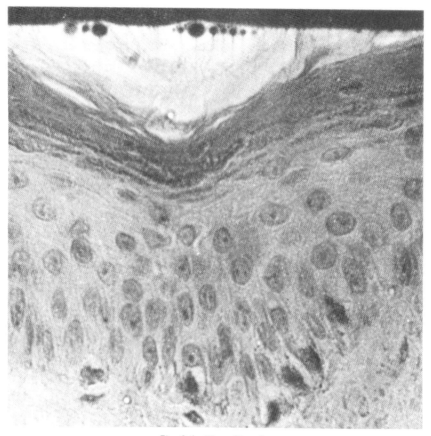

Fig. 6-1. The epidermis.

granulosum. Finally, these cells lose their nuclei, dehydrate, and flatten out into dead, polygonal cells with a surface area about 25 times that of the basal cells. The close packing and cementing of these flat, dead cells laden with keratin form the tough stratum corneum, and the cells are called corneocytes. In normal skin, it may take up to 14 days for a daughter cell of the basal layer to reach the stratum corneum and another 1–2 weeks before it is sloughed off from the skin surface.

Epidermal Melanin Pigmentation

The earliest scientific studies in pigmentation are attributed to Marcel Malpighi (8) and Johann Pechlin (9), who discovered in the 17th century that most of the blackness of Ethiopian cadaver skin was localized in a layer (the basal cell layer of the epidermis) between the white corium (dermis) and an outer "scarf" (the upper epidermis and stratum corneum). It is now known that this pigment is melanin, an amorphous complex polymer of tyrosine oxidation products and proteins. Specialized cells called melanocytes, derived from neural crest tissue, reside in the basal cell layer of the epidermis and produce melanin-containing granules called melanosomes, which are transferred through dendritic processes to the keratinocytes of the epidermis. As the keratinocytes migrate outward, some melanin is carried toward the surface of the skin, eventually appearing in the stratum corneum. Despite the continuous outward migration of melanin, its greatest concentration, as noted by Malpighi, is in the basal cell layer. This is primarily due to the presence of heavily pigmented melanocytes and resting basal cells in this germinative layer.

Melanin strongly absorbs shorter wavelength visible light and UV radiation because of extensively conjugated double bonds within the polymer. The protection against sunburn afforded by melanization of the skin has long been recognized and is experienced seasonally by most people. Thompson (10) and others (11–14) have shown, in excised human epidermis, that melanin pigmentation is a greater factor in determining the transmission of UV radiation through the epidermis than is variation in epidermal thickness. Protection by melanin and melanin's effects on skin color must be related not only to the quantity of melanin, but to where it is and how it is dispersed. In addition to inducing delayed melanogenesis, epidermal cell kinetics can be markedly altered by UV radiation (15, 16). Given that the quantity and distribution of melanin within the epidermis is dependent upon the dynamic equilibrium among its rate of production, its rate of transfer to keratinocytes, and its rate of loss as determined by keratinocyte and corneocyte cell kinetics, any perturbance of this dynamic equilibrium results in alteration of both the distribution and total amount of melanin. Hence, melanin's effects upon optics of the skin and sunburn protection are determined by a complex of factors, and vary over time.

Precise dose–response, action spectrum, or photoprotective-effect studies for single exposures or for multiple exposures leading to steady-state equilibria of this interesting photoinducible, photoprotective system are lacking. The action spectrum for induction of melanogenesis grossly resembles that for induction of delayed erythema, but at longer wavelengths in the near-UV or visible spectral regions, melanogenesis can be induced by suberythemogenic exposure doses (17, 18). Tanning induced by UVA (320–400 nm) radiation may be less protective against UVB (290–320 nm) radiation than UVB-induced tanning (19), but if true, the mechanism for this difference is unknown.

Dermis

The dermis is an optically turbid, semisolid mixture of fibers, cells, and vessels embedded in a viscous gel of water and mucopolysaccharides. There are three major types of fibers present: collagen, reticulum, and elastin. Collagen is a long protein molecule woven into fibrils that allow stretching and contraction while maintaining tensile strength. Collagen makes up about 70% of the dry weight of the dermis, and is optically birefringent. The scattering of light by collagen is an important feature of the optics of the dermis. The finely branched reticulum fibers serve to link bundles of collagen together, and the scattered elastin fibers presumably lend an elastic quality to the dermis as a whole. Scattered cells called fibroblasts produce the fibers, proteins, and viscous materials of the dermis.

The uppermost dermal layer, the papillary dermis, contains an extensive plexus of capillaries, lymphatics, and nerves. Scattered lymphocytes leave the blood vessels of this layer, giving it more cellular appearance than the underlying reticular dermis. The reticular dermis is more fibrous, contains larger vessels, and has fewer cells and less ground substance than the papillary dermis. The dermis normally contains no melanin. The structure of skin is summarized in Table 6-1.

AN OVERVIEW OF SKIN OPTICS

The *transmittance* of a planar sample is defined as that fraction of the radiation incident upon one side of the sample that passes through and

Table 6-1. Skin Layers

Layer	Typical thickness, μm	Basic structure
Stratum corneum	8–15	Ten to 20 single-cell layers of densely packed, flattened, dead keratinocytes, in remarkably regular arrangement; rich in the lipoprotein keratin; contains melanin granules, carotens
Stratum granulosum	3	Granular cells between viable epidermis and stratum corneum; two to four cell layers
Stratum malpighii	50–150	Ten to 20 cell layers of keratinocytes, which produce the materials of the stratum corneum as they differentiate and become flattened, moving outward
Germinative layer	5–10	Single-cell layer of columnar basal cells, which divide to produce a continuing supply of keratinocytes; melanocytes also present, which produce melanin pigment granules and transfer these melanosomes into keratinocytes
Dermis	1000–4000	Connective tissue composed of collagen, reticulum, and elastin fibers and ground substance (gel); few cells compared to epidermis; outermost dermis (papillary dermis) contains many capillaries, lymphatics, and nerves

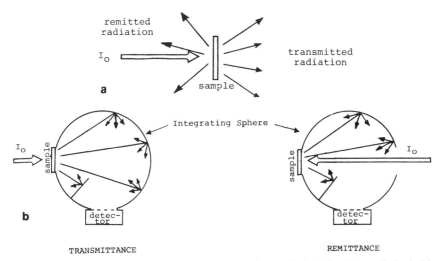

Fig. 6-2. (a) Transmittance is defined as (total transmitted radiation)/(incident radiation). (b) Measurement of transmittance (T) and remittance (R) of a sample, using an integrating sphere. The interior surface of the sphere is coated with BaSO₄ or MgO, which have nearly 100% diffuse remittance over the entire optical spectrum.

emerges from the other side of the sample. *Remittance* is defined as that fraction of the radiation incident upon one side of a sample that returns from or through the same side. The term "diffuse reflectance" is often used synonymously with remittance; however, the implication that the remitted radiation is truly diffuse (spatially isotropic) can sometimes be misleading. In order to measure the transmittance or remittance of skin layers, or of any turbid sample or sample with nonplanar surfaces, one must in general capture and measure all radiation entering each hemisphere on either side of the sample. This is most easily accomplished by using an integrating sphere, although other methods may also be used (1). These simple concepts and definitions are depicted in Fig. 6-2.

Initially, it is helpful to schematize the optics of normal skin as shown in Fig. 6-3. Upon encountering the skin at near-normal (nearly perpendicular) incidence, a small fraction of the incident radiation is reflected due to the step change in refractive index between air ($n_D = 1.00$) and stratum corneum ($n_D \approx 1.55$) (20). For normally incident radiation, this *regular reflectance* of an incident beam from normal skin is always between 4% and 7% over the entire spectrum from 250 to 3000 nm, for both Caucasoid and Negroid skin (1, 21). At larger angles of incidence, regular reflectance may reach higher values, as described by Fresnel's equations and shown graphically in Fig. 6-4 for a planar interface between air and a medium of refractive index 1.55. Although the skin surface is not strictly planar, the value of the regular reflectance from skin behaves similarly to that shown in Fig. 6-4 as the macroscopic angle of

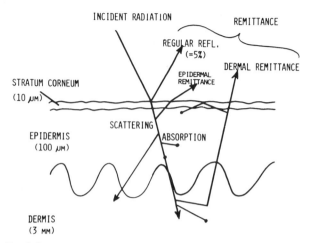

Fig. 6-3. Schematic representation of optical pathways in human skin.

incidence is varied. The main effects of the nonplanar surface topology of the stratum corneum are: (1) that the regular reflectance from skin is not specular, i.e., skin reflectance does not maintain an image, as does the reflectance of a mirror or a window; and (2) that collimated incident radiation, upon passing through this surface and into the skin, is refracted and therefore made somewhat more diffuse by this rough surface. These effects are conceptually similar to those that make a piece of ground glass translucent, compared with the transparency of polished glass.

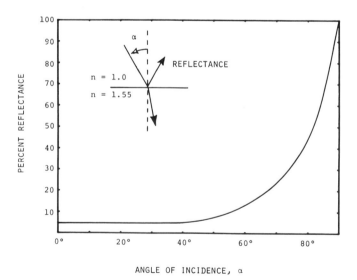

ANGLE OF INCIDENCE, α

Fig. 6-4. Regular reflectance at a planar interface of a material with refractive index 1.55.

Referring again to Fig. 6-3, and denoting the 4–7% regular reflectance as R_{reg}, we have that the fraction of normally incident radiation entering the skin is simply $1 - R_{reg}$, or 93–96%. Within any of the layers of skin, this radiation may be *absorbed* or *scattered*. These two processes taken together essentially determine the penetration of radiation into the skin. The remittance of the skin is also a function of both scattering and absorption within the various tissue layers to which the radiation penetrates.

Most of the absorbed radiation is rapidly converted by nonradiative deexcitation to heat, which is then dissipated. All biologic effects of optical radiation result directly or indirectly from either photochemical reactions or radiant heating, or both. Heating is initially localized near the pigments that absorb the radiation, but thermal diffusion rapidly spreads the heating over large volumes of tissue. A small fraction of the absorbed radiation, particularly in the UV region, leads to fluorescence, phosphorescence, and the photochemistry that initiates photobiologic responses. All of these three "nonthermal" means of dissipating the electronic excitation produced by photons are of interest in photobiology, but from a functional point of view, photochemistry is most important. The wavelengths producing photobiologic responses (i.e., the action spectrum) are theoretically those that are absorbed by specific molecules or chromophores that initiate the photochemical events leading to the observed biologic responses. An action spectrum may therefore correlate with the absorption spectra of chromophores involved (22), but account must be taken of the optical properties of the tissue itself. Knowing the quantitative transfer of incident radiation to a biologically significant layer or volume, one may correct the biologic action spectrum for tissue optics. Unfortunately, the location of chromophores initiating important responses is often a mystery.

Optics of Turbid Media

Photons (optical quanta) have a rest mass of zero. When a photon is absorbed, its energy is invested in the chromophore molecule, and the photon ceases to exist. Most scattering, on the other hand, is an elastic interaction between optical radiation and matter in which only the direction of photon propagation is altered. Some types of scattering are inelastic and result in a change of wavelength as well; these are of minor consequence in the present discussion. Scattering results from inhomogeneities in a medium's refractive index, corresponding to physical inhomogeneities. The spatial distribution and intensity of scattered light depend upon the size and shape of the inhomogeneities relative to the wavelength, and upon the difference in refractive index between the medium and the inhomogeneities. For molecules or small particles with dimensions less than roughly one-tenth of the wavelength, scattering is generally weak, nearly isotropic (equally distributed spatially), polarized, and varies inversely with the fourth power of wavelength. The molecular scattering of sunlight by the sky is the most common example of this kind of scattering, called *Rayleigh scattering*. For particles with dimensions on the same order as the wavelength, scattering is many orders of magnitude stronger than Rayleigh scattering, more forward-directed, and, while varying inversely with wavelength, is not such a strong inverse function. Scattering of a beam of light by cigarette smoke is a common example of this type of scattering. When the particle size greatly exceeds the wavelength, scattering is highly forward-directed and essentially independent of wavelength (so-called Mie scattering). Clouds are a common example of large-particle scattering. They are white or grey because of the lack of wavelength dependence of scattering by their condensed water droplets, which are very large compared with the wavelengths of light. Red or orange clouds appearing at sunset are colored not because of scattering in the clouds, but because Rayleigh scattering along an increased atmospheric path has removed much of the blue, shorter wavelength radiation from the sunlight. Figure 6-5 shows the intensity of scattering by spherical particles of a given size and refractive index for these various situations.

Within the skin all of these general types of scattering occur, but, quantitatively, scattering by structures with dimensions on the order of optical wavelengths or somewhat larger must dominate over Rayleigh scattering. In particular, scattering by collagen fibers largely determines the penetration of optical radiation within the dermis (21).

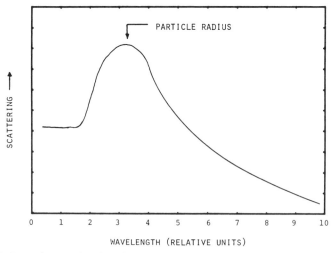

Fig. 6-5. Scattering as a function of wavelength for spherical particles with a refractive index relative to that of their surroundings of 1.3. Scattering is greatest when the wavelength and particle radius are approximately equal. The Rayleigh scattering region (wavelength much greater than particle size; scattering $\propto 1/\lambda^4$) extends infinitely beyond the right-hand side of the figure.

In a nonscattering medium, absorption of monochromatic, collimated, normally incident radiation follows the Lambert–Beer law, which states that the transmission of radiation varies inversely and exponentially with thickness of the medium and concentration of the absorber. The spectral transmittance of a thickness x of the medium is $T(\lambda) = 10^{-\epsilon(\lambda)cx}$, where $\epsilon(\lambda)$ is the molar extinction coefficient at wavelength λ, and c is the molar concentration of the absorbing chromophore. The absorbance of optical density (OD) of a sample is simply $-\log T(\lambda)$, or $OD = \epsilon(\lambda)cx$. When scattering is also present, however, the effective pathlength of radiation within the medium is increased, which generally increases the likelihood of absorption, and in addition some radiation may be backscattered such that remittance also occurs. Thus, the measured optical density of a scattering sample containing a given amount of absorbing chromophore is always greater than that of a nonscattering but otherwise equivalent sample. The effect of scattering upon radiation transfer within a sample is dependent upon both the degree of scattering and the spatial distribution of the scattered radiation, as described above. Analysis of this situation, especially when a variety of absorbers and types of scattering are present, is highly complex.

If scattering is marked (a highly turbid medium), most photons experience multiple scattering before being absorbed or backscattered from the sample. In this case, the spatial distribution of the radiation as it passes through the sample quickly becomes isotropic (i.e., perfectly diffuse), regardless of the spatial distribution obtained for a single scattering. Furthermore, isotropic radiation cannot be "reorganized" to become non-isotropic by scattering of any type. If the radiation is isotropic, one can show that the average pathlength of photons along an infinitesimal path dx in any one direction is simply $2\,dx$ (23). For perfectly diffuse (isotropic) radiation, the situation therefore becomes somewhat simplified, and one can derive absorption and scattering coefficients for diffuse radiation, equal to twice those for collimated radiation because of the pathlength argument given above, in terms of measurements of transmittance and remittance. The most popular model for this analysis is that derived by Kubelka and Munk (24–26), which is a special case of the general theory originally proposed by Schuster (27). An overview of this model, and its modification for application to skin, is presented below; the interested reader is referred to Kortüm (23), Wedlandt and Hecht (28), and Atkins (29) for exhaustive description of this and related radiation-transfer models. The differential (continuous) model proposed by Kubelka and Munk is certainly not the most elegant or thorough model of optical radiation transfer, but is simple and can be most readily applied to skin. In general, the more physically rigorous theories of radiation transfer require knowledge of structure and optical parameters which are difficult if not impossible to obtain for skin.

The Kubelka–Munk theory assumes that: (1) the sample has inhomogeneities causing scattering, which are small compared with the sample

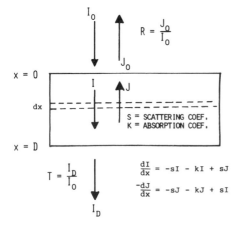

Fig. 6-6. The Kubelka–Munk model for radiation transfer in a scattering, absorbing medium. I and J are defined as diffuse fluxes, and S and K are backscattering and absorption coefficients for diffuse radiation, respectively.

$$T = \frac{I_D}{I_0}$$

$$\frac{dI}{dx} = -sI - kI + sJ$$

$$\frac{-dJ}{dx} = -sJ - kJ + sI$$

thickness; (2) the incident radiation is diffuse; and (3) differences in refractive index between the sample and external medium, causing regular reflectances, are neglected. Radiation within the sample is broken simply into two opposing diffuse fluxes, I and J in Fig. 6-6. The sample's backscattering (S) and absorption (K) coefficients for diffuse radiation are defined by two differential equations as the fraction of diffuse radiation either backscattered or absorbed per unit differential pathlength of the sample. These differential equations are

$$dI = (-KI - SI + SJ)\,dx \qquad (1)$$

$$-dJ = (-KJ - SJ + SI)\,dx \qquad (2)$$

which simply state that the change dI in flux I over some layer of thickness dx is equal to that fraction of I removed by absorption and backscattering plus some fraction contributed to I by backscattering from J. The second differential equation is an analogous statement for flux J. The minus sign in Eq. (2) is necessary because J is defined as positive in the minus x direction.

The differential equations (1) and (2) are solved to give a general solution of the form

$$I = A(1 - \beta)e^{\alpha x} + B(1 + \beta)e^{-\alpha x} \qquad (3)$$

$$J = A(1 + \beta)e^{\alpha x} + B(1 - \beta)e^{-\alpha x} \qquad (4)$$

where $\alpha = [K(K + 2S)]^{1/2}$ and $\beta = [K(K + 2S)]^{1/2}$.

The boundary conditions are that $T = I_d/I_0$, $R = J_0/I_0$, $I_0 = I_0$, and $J_d = 0$, where R and T are remittance and transmittance of the sample, respectively, and the subscripts represent values of x. Substitution of these boundary conditions gives a particular solution, which can then be rearranged to express S and K (our two unknowns) in terms of R and T (our measurable quantities). Written in the forms derived by Kubelka and Munk, these are

$$\frac{K}{S} = \frac{1 + R^2 - T^2}{2R} - 1 \tag{5}$$

$$S = \frac{1}{d} \left(\frac{K}{S(K/S + 2)} \right)^{-1/2} \coth^{-1} \frac{1 - R(K/S + 1)}{R[K/S(K/S + 2)]^{1/2}} \tag{6}$$

Because a minimum of two different measurements is always necessary to determine two unknowns, measurement of both remittance and transmittance (or, alternatively, remittance with two different reflective "backgrounds" of different reflectance behind the sample) is required. In order to use this model practically, one must also account for regular reflection occurring at both sample boundaries and adhere to the use of diffuse incident radiation. This has been accomplished for dermal samples in vitro (21), and S and K for human dermis devoid of blood have been calculated. In vivo, blood exerts major influence upon K, which thus far has been only crudely estimated from in vivo remittance spectra of depigmented skin. Once S and K are known, the two fluxes I and J can be reconstructed via Eq. (3) and (4). The total density of optical radiation at a given depth is the algebraic sum of I and J at that depth; it is this sum that determines optical dosimetry within the layer. For an infinitely thick sample (in practice, a sample for which T approaches zero), $A = 0$ and $B = 1/(1 + \beta)$ in Eq. (3) and (4). The sum of I and J is therefore

$$I + J = \frac{2e^{-\alpha x}}{1 + \beta} \tag{7}$$

and the depth at which the radiation density is attenuated to $1/e$, or 37%, of its incident value is

$$d(37\%) = \frac{1}{\alpha} \left(1 + \ln \frac{2}{1 + \beta} \right) \tag{8}$$

Near the front surface of a scattering sample, the sum of I and J can easily exceed I_0, the incident density of optical radiation. In the extreme case, I plus J just inside the surface of a sample with 100% remittance is twice I_0, since $I_0 = I_0$ at the surface. Thus the density of optical radiation in the superficial layers of a scattering sample can easily exceed that of the incident beam. As shall be seen, this is often the case for fair Caucasian skin, especially over the visible and near-infrared regions.

In the Kubelka-Munk model, variations in the coefficients S and K are essentially independent of one another if the absorbing chromophores scatter weakly compared with surrounding nonabsorbing but strongly scattering structures. Fortunately, the structures of skin that lead to strong scattering, and hence determine S, are in general different than those chromophores present that determine K. For any given layer of skin, K is compositely determined by the concentration and distribution of those chromophores present. This is convenient because in normal skin certain chromophores, such as hemoglobins, bilirubin, and melanin, change rapidly, causing changes in absorption coefficients, whereas scattering coefficients should not change significantly until some gross alteration of structure occurs. As such, scattering coefficients are relatively constant compared with absorption coefficients, even between individuals. In particular, we shall use this basic model to describe radiation transfer within the dermis.

The Kubelka–Munk model also illustrates important concepts concerning the remittance and transmittance of samples with different relative degrees of absorption and scattering and of different thicknesses. In the case of a nonscattering sample, $S = 0$ and Eq. (3) reduces to give the Lambert-Beer law, stating that radiation traveling through a purely absorbing sample is attenuated as a simple exponential function of an absorption coefficient times the pathlength. When $K = 0$, there is no absorption and Eq. (5) reduces to $R + T = 1$, indicating that no radiation is lost. If a sample is infinitely thick, or simply thick enough that T approaches zero, one can rewrite Eq. (5) as

$$\frac{K}{S} = (R - 1)^2 / 2R \qquad (9)$$

That is, the remittance of a thick sample depends solely upon the ratio of its absorption and scattering coeffients. This dependence is shown graphically in Fig. 6-7. Fortunately, the dermis is sufficiently thick that, for all optical wavelengths less than 600 nm, its transmittance is essentially zero. Therefore, for wavelengths less than 600 nm, the dermis can be thought of as a semi-infinite optical medium, greatly simplifying the analysis of skin remittance spectra as related to changes in dermal pigments. Finally, it is apparent that as the thickness of any particular sample decreases, R always decreases and T always increases. Indeed, it makes intuitive sense that, for a given turbid medium, very thin samples would transmit more and remit less radiation than thick samples. It shall be seen in the case of the stratum corneum, and to a large extent the entire normal human epidermis, that the layer is thin enough and has a high enough value of K/S that its direct contribution to remittance (other than the regular reflectance discussed above) can be essentially neglected over the entire visible and near-infrared spectral regions (21).

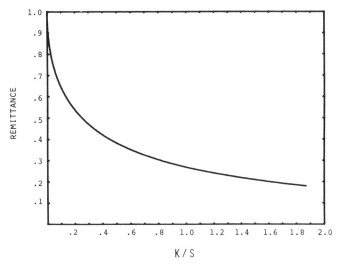

K / S

Fig. 6-7. Remittance of an infinitely thick sample as a function of K/S, according to the Kubelka–Munk theory. In practice, a sample may be considered infinitely thick whenever its transmittance is close to zero.

Optics of the Stratum Corneum and Epidermis

Many studies of the transmission of UV radiation through excised human epidermis and stratum corneum have been reported since the original work of Hasselbalch (30). Much of the early work, however, failed to account accurately for the diffuse nature of transmission through skin samples, largely because of inadequate instrumentation (30–36). Since the advent of commercially available spectrophotometers with integrating spheres, however, several groups have measured and published total transmission spectra of human epidermis (11, 37). Everett et al. (11) compared epidermal samples obtained by cantharadin blisters in vivo, by heat-and-stretch separation in vitro, and by suction in vivo. They also compared stratum corneum samples obtained from sunburn-induced vesicles (parakeratotic stratum corneum plus stratum granulosum) and by mild trypsinization of previously separated epidermis. As had been seen in previous studies, the UV-visible transmission of Caucasian stratum corneum or epidermis qualitatively resembles that of a solution of protein containing the aromatic amino acids tryptophan and tyrosine, with a minimum in transmittance near 275 nm due to absorption by these and other aromatic chromophores. Nucleic acids, with an absorption maximum near 260 nm, and numerous small aromatic molecules, especially urocanic acid, with an absorption maximum at 277 nm at pH 7.4, also contribute to the broad 275-nm absorption band seen in epidermis and stratum corneum. Finally, melanin content and distribution play a major role in determining the transmission of optical radiation through the stratum corneum and epidermis. The high absorbance of epidermis and stratum corneum for wavelengths less than 240 nm is largely due to peptide bonds.

Two technical problems have plagued all previously reported epidermal or corneal transmission spectra, however. First, the tissue is autofluorescent, primarily because of aromatic amino acids (38) and perhaps melanin as well (39). A broad excitation band centered near 280 nm is associated with an emission band between 330 and 360 nm, consistent with tryptophan or tyrosine fluorescence (R. R. Anderson, unpublished observations). This emission band is of sufficient intensity to cause suspicion of epidermal transmission spectra taken with integrating spheres equipped with broadband (UV–visible-sensitive) photomultiplier detectors, as in essentially all standard commercially available systems. The portion of absorbed 260–290-nm radiation which is emitted as fluorescence at 330–360 nm is falsely recorded by the broadband detector as transmittance at 260–290 nm. The comparatively high epidermal transmittance at the 330–360-nm fluorescence emission band can cause order-of-magnitude errors in the measurement of 260–290-nm epidermal transmittance, especially if the samples are heavily pigmented. Second, if the epidermal sheet is simply suspended in air or placed against a quartz slide at the entrance port of an integrating sphere, as has been the case in previous studies of epidermal transmittance, some total internal reflection of forward-scattered off-axis rays can occur, which are then lost for measurement purposes.

The autofluorescence error has been overcome by using a "solar-blind" detector, which is insensitive to wavelengths longer than 320 nm. The problem of total internal reflection has been overcome by building a chamber in which epidermal samples are floated over a hemispherical-shaped quartz chamber containing normal saline. This apparatus is shown diagrammatically in Fig. 6-8. Representative fair-skinned Caucasian epidermal and stratum corneum transmission spectra taken with this system, and expressed in absorbance or optical density (OD $= -\log T$) units, are presented in Fig. 6-9 and compared with conventional spectra not corrected for autofluorescence.

In Caucasians, roughly half of incident 320–400-nm (UVA) radiation reaches the dermis (1). Furthermore, although only a small fraction of incident radiation of wavelengths less than 300 nm reaches the dermis, it cannot be assumed that these wavelengths exert no direct dermal effects. Delayed erythema induced by 254-nm radiation (Caucasian epidermal transmittance 1%) may involve direct damage to dermal vessels (40). A transient decrease in circulating T lymphocytes is caused by total-body 290–320-nm (UVB) exposure (41), or 320–400-nm (UVA) exposure after ingestion of psoralens (42) at incident exposure doses that are consistent with direct damage to these cells, based upon Caucasian epidermal transmittance and in vitro dose–response studies of lethality or induction of DNA repair in T lymphocytes irradiated in serum-free media (43) (cf. also Chapter 10).

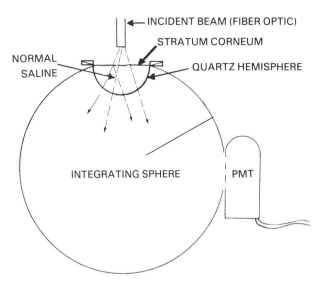

INCIDENT BEAM (FIBER OPTIC)

STRATUM CORNEUM

NORMAL SALINE

QUARTZ HEMISPHERE

INTEGRATING SPHERE

PMT

Fig. 6-8. Apparatus for appropriate measurement of spectral transmission through stratum corneum or epidermis. Because of autofluorescence of the tissue, the photomultiplier detector (PMT) should be of a "solar blind" type (Cs–Te photocathode material) for measurements at wavelengths less than 320 nm. The hemispherical shape of the chamber holding the skin and the presence of saline beneath the sample are necessary to avoid errors due to regular reflectance at the bottom surface of the sample, rendering the measurement, and the sample's environment, analogous to the in vivo situation.

For reference, absorption spectra of major epidermal pigments are given in Fig. 6-10. It can be seen upon careful inspection of these data that epidermal or corneal transmittance spectra are compositely determined by absorption by these (and certainly other) substances. It is largely variations in the concentrations, distributions, or amounts of these chromophores that determine individual and anatomic variations in epidermal spectral trans-mission. One would expect the protein-bound and nucleic acid-bound chromophores to be of rather constant concentration and distribution in normal skin since these chromophores are necessarily inherent to the cellular matrix of the tissue. As such, the magnitude of the 275-nm epidermal absorption maximum varies almost linearly with variations in epidermal or corneal thickness (R. R. Anderson, unpublished observations). For both melanin and urocanic acid, however, their concentrations and distributions are variable, and unlike protein or nucleic acid, UV optical absorption may be their major functional role in human skin.

Melanogenesis is well known to be induced or enhanced by UV radiation exposure with or without photosensitizers, whereas there are conflicting reports on the possible photoinduction of urocanic acid synthesis in the epidermis (44, 45). Thomson (10) showed clearly that racial variations in epidermal melanin content account for a much greater effect on the optical

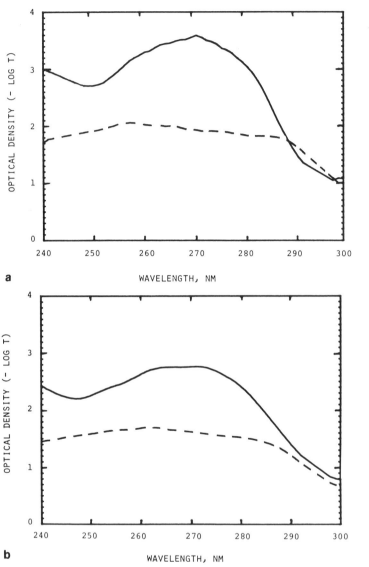

Fig. 6-9. (a) Spectral transmittance, expressed in optical density units, of Caucasian human epidermis sample taken with solar-blind PMT (—) vs. conventional broadband PMT (- - -) in the apparatus shown in Fig. 6-8. Note the large overestimation of transmittance which occurs due to tissue autofluorescence when a broadband detector is used. Sample was obtained from amputated thigh skin, was separated by immersion in 60°C water for 30 sec, and consisted of the entire epidermis minus the basal cell layer. (b) Spectral transmission, expressed in optical density units, of stratum corneum from skin adjacent to that shown in (a), taken with solar-blind PMT (—) vs. conventional broadband PMT (- - -). Sample was separated by 8-hr incubation at 37°C in the presence of 10 mg/ml staphylococcal scalded-skin syndrome epidermolytic toxin in Hepe's buffer with 20% FCS, and consisted of stratum corneum plus stratum granulosum.

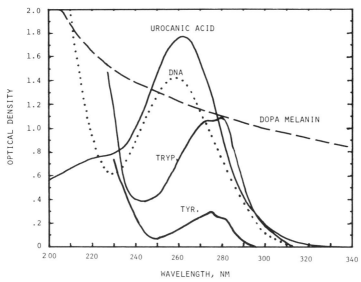

Fig. 6-10. UV absorption spectra of major epidermal chromophores. DOPA-melanin, 1.5 mg%
in H_2O; urocanic acid, 10^{-4} M in H_2O; calf thymus DNA, 10 mg% in H_2O (pH 4.5); tryptophane,
2×10^{-4} M (pH 7); tyrosine, 2×10^{-4} M (pH 7). The broad epidermal absorption band near 275
nm is the result of absorption by protein, urocanic acid, nucleic acids, and other aromatic
chromophores.

near-UV and visible transmittance of the epidermis than do variations in
thickness. Although he used rather crude methods for measuring transmittance, and did not consider that there might be racial differences in the
density of the stratum corneum as has been subsequently suggested (46), his
basic conclusion is beyond dispute. Indeed, it is common experience that
variations in melanin pigmentation have profound effects on the transmittance of solar UVB into and through the human epidermis to cause sunburn.
In the visible portion of the spectrum, melanin is essentially the only pigment
affecting the transmittance of normal human epidermis, giving rise to the wide
range of discernible skin colors from "black" to "white." The 300-nm
transmittance of full-thickness epidermis including the basal cell layer varies
by 2–3 orders of magnitude from fair-skinned to darkly pigmented individuals
(R. R. Anderson, unpublished observations). The relative importance of
melanogenesis vs. epidermal hyperplasia as two UV-inducible mechanisms
for photoprotection against various wavelength regions can be seen from the
absorption spectra given above. For UVC and UVB wavelengths, even mild
hyperplasia alone could exert a highly significant photoprotective effect
because of the absorption by protein and other constitutive epidermal
chromophores. For protection against UVA or visible radiation effects,
however, hyperplasia alone would not offer practically significant photo-

protection compared with the induction of melanogenesis. A thorough test of these simple ideas has yet to be demonstrated in vivo.

Contrary to popular beliefs, melanin is not a "neutral density" filter of the skin. Absorption by melanin increases steadily toward shorter wavelengths over the broad spectrum of 250–1200 nm. In the near-infrared beyond about 1100 nm, the absorbance of melanin is essentially negligible. For wavelengths longer than 1100 nm, both transmittance (12) and remittance (47, 48) are unaffected by melanin pigmentation. Figure 6-11 compares the spectral remittance of dark Negroid and fair Caucasian skin. The prevalence of sunburn, abnormal photosensitivity, skin cancers, and cutaneous "aging" decreases with increasing melanin pigmentation. Despite these apparent inverse correlations between skin sensitivity to UV radiation and melanin content, there remain many fundamental questions about how the distribution and quantity of melanin relate to its photoprotective effects. Although melanin may theoretically protect keratinocytes from some UV-induced damage mechanisms by undergoing oxidation–reduction reactions or acting as a free radical quencher, it is apparent from studies of epidermal transmission that absorption of UV radiation primarily accounts for melanin's photoprotective effects. Furthermore, it is well established that, in normal skin, the majority of the melanin present is located in the basal cell layer, and often appears histologically as "caps" of pigment granules overlying the nuclei of many basal cells (49). The majority of basal cells, which are in a resting state, may derive more photoprotection against nuclear DNA damage

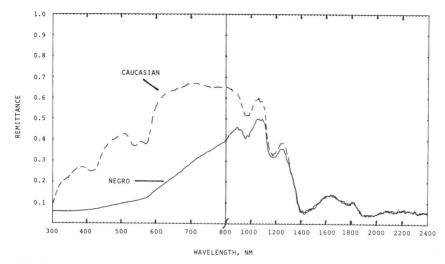

Fig. 6-11. Spectral remittance of dark Negroid and fair Caucasian skin (flexor surface of forearm in each case). The lack of significant absorption by melanin for wavelengths longer than approximately 1100 nm and increased absorption at shorter wavelengths are apparent. Note also that remittance is never less than 5% due to regular reflectance.

by this supranuclear intracellular distribution of melanin than by a random intracellular distribution.

There are no significant racial differences in the numbers of melanocytes per unit area of skin (50) or in the rate of corneocyte loss, although Negroid stratum corneum may have greater physical density (46). Hence, racial differences in melanin content of the skin must be due mainly to differences in the rate at which individual melanocytes produce and transfer melanin to keratinocytes, and to some extent racial differences in melanosome distribution.

Melanin is a remarkably stable protein–polymer complex, the chromophoric backbone of which survives attack by proteases, acids, and bases. Caucasian melanosomes typically contain a greater number of melanin granules, but less total melanin, than Negroid or Mongolian melanosomes, and also appear to suffer greater degradation within keratinocytes (51). The above considerations account for the observation of free "melanin dust" in the Caucasian stratum corneum, whereas Negroid stratum corneum contains numerous intact melanosomes in addition to "melanin dust" (14, 52). The optical effects associated with dispersed "melanin dust" vs. intact melanosomes have not been quantitated, but it is likely that dispersal of melanin pigment in the Caucasian stratum corneum affords somewhat greater protection than would the same quantity of melanin sequestered in intact melanosomes. This is because the pigment presents a greater physical cross section to optical radiation. Interestingly, Caucasian skin sites exposed to UVA after oral administration of photosensitizing psoralens (52) are induced to produce single-granule melanosomes similar to those of Negroid skin.

Given that, across the range of human pigmentation, there are gross differences in the dispersion and concentration of melanin and the stability of melanosomes, and that melanin is preferentially concentrated in the basal cell layer, there exist grossly different distributions of internal optical dosimetry between heavily pigmented skin and lightly pigmented skin. Furthermore, such differences, if quantitatively correlated with variations in thresholds for photobiologic responses, may give clues to the location of tissue layers involved in initiating photobiologic responses. In an attempt to correlate the photoprotection offered by melanin with its quantity and distribution, Kaidbey et al. (53) measured the UVB and UVA spectral transmittance of Caucasian and Negroid stratum corneum and epidermis samples. In addition to spectrophotometric measurements of transmittance, the minimal delayed erythema doses (MEDs) of broadband UVB from fluorescent sunlamps and UVA from a filtered xenon source were determined with and without the skin samples placed over test sites on fair Caucasian subjects. The transmittance of erythemogenic radiation through each skin sample was taken to be the ratio of MED without divided by MED with the sample placed over the subject's skin. Both the UVB and UVA transmittance values measured in these two ways were in general agreement with the UVB and UVA transmittances measured spectrophotometrically. Whereas there was a fivefold average difference in the UVB and UVA transmittance of black vs. white epidermis, the average racial difference in UVB and UVA transmittance of the stratum corneum samples was less than twofold. This study therefore suggests that the large racial differences in sensitivity to UV radiation of 10–30-fold (54, 55) correlate poorly with the small racial differences noted in corneal transmission. However, the minimal erythema dose of black and white subjects has never been directly compared with accurate corneal or epidermal transmittance measurements of skin samples from the same subjects. Such a study might be a rather direct means of determining the tissue layers involved in initiating delayed erythema response.

Urocanic acid is thought to play some role as an "endogenous sunscreen" of the epidermis and stratum corneum (56, 57). Unlike the dermis and most other tissues, the epidermis lacks urocanase (58), the enzyme that oxidatively degrades urocanic acid, while histidine deaminase, the enzyme responsible for urocanic acid synthesis, is present and apparently most active in the latter stages of keratinocyte differentiation at the stratum granulosum (59). There is some evidence that human epidermal urocanic acid levels (44) and histidine deaminase activity in guinea pigs (58) increase for weeks following UV radiation exposure, but these observations may be wholly or in part due to UV-induced epidermal hyperplasia (45).

In those studies that have compared diffuse vs. direct (total transmittance vs. transmittance along an optical path in line with the incident beam) transmittance of epidermis or stratum corneum, the ratio of diffuse/direct transmission does not appear to be wavelength dependent (11, 34, 35) for either UV or visible wavelengths. This broadband independence of wavelength suggests that the diffuse nature of epidermal transmission of UV wavelengths is due more to the irregular refractive surface of skin than to particle scattering within the epidermis. Furthermore, less than 5% of collimated, normally incident radiation in the 280–3000-nm region is remitted by scattering within Caucasian epidermis (21). This observation is consistent with a thin sample in which backscattering (S) is small compared with the reciprocal of sample thickness ($\simeq 100$ cm^{-1}), and/or absorption relative to scattering (K/S) is large. The epidermal transmittance spectra presented above for fair-skinned Caucasians indicate that most of incident near-UV, visible, and near-infrared radiation is transmitted through epidermis. Scattering of visible light within the epidermis is minor enough that, when a layer of oil is applied to diminish refraction at the irregular skin–air interface, one can readily see the capillary tufts of the dermis upon microscopic examination (60). The logical conclusion from the above observations is that whatever backscattering occurs in normal epidermis over this spectral region is for practical purposes weak, and that any strong scattering within epidermis that does occur must be highly forward-directed, i.e., off-axis refraction occurring at the skin surface and large-particle scattering within the tissue.

For wavelengths less than 320 nm, epidermal absorption increases dramatically. Therefore, even though one would expect these shorter wavelengths to experience greater scattering, a concomitant large increase in absorption, and hence K/S, explains why little incident energy in this region is remitted (cf., Fig. 6-7). If one neglects epidermal backscattering over much of the optical spectrum, a greatly simplified analysis of in vivo skin remittance spectra can be obtained, as shall be discussed. However, despite its central role in cutaneous and systemic photoprotection, a precise model of epidermal optics is still lacking.

Optics of the Dermis

Relatively few studies of optical radiation transfer in the dermis or other connective tissue have been reported. Hardy et al. (12) performed goniometric studies (1) of transmission and remission of a collimated incident beam through tangentially sectioned Caucasian and Negroid skin samples of various thicknesses and including both the epidermis and various amounts of dermis. Their findings were that, as greater thicknesses of dermis were included, the transmission decreased with thickness and was more diffuse, suggesting multiple scattering. The Lambert–Beer law was invalid for the visible and near-infrared wavelengths tested as the thickness became greater than 0.5 mm, suggesting that considerable scattering was present in the dermis. In general, longer wavelengths across the visible and near-infrared spectra exhibited both greater and more forward-directed (less diffuse) transmission, which is consistent with scattering by structures with dimensions on the same order as, or greater than, the wavelength of light, most probably bundles of collagen. Of the wavelengths studied, Hardy et al. found 1.23 μm (1230 nm) to be the most penetrating wavelength.

Findlay (61), in an attempt to explain blue skin colors, noted that when the epidermis was removed from a blue nevus of Ota (caused by an abnormal deposition of melanin in the dermis), the dermis was "intensively blue upon direct inspection." He correctly concluded that the epidermis had little to do with blue skin, and went on to measure visible transmittance and remittance spectra of thin sections of pig dermis, or sheets of dura mater (a thin sheet of connective tissue) of newborn humans. Both showed greater transmittance of longer wavelengths, similar to Hardy et al.'s findings, but exhibited greater remittance of shorter wavelengths. Summing Findlay's transmittance and remittance spectra gives values close to 1.0 (100%) across the entire visible spectrum, indicating that very little visible light is absorbed by dura mater or pig dermis in vitro. Visualizing the dermal deposition of melanin pigment in the nevus as being the optical equivalent of providing only a thin layer of dermis for remittance of incident light, Findlay concluded that "subtractive color mixing" accounted for blue skin colors. The only explanation for his spectral transmittance and remittance curves is that light scattering in the dermis must vary inversely with wavelength. Thus, the average dermal pathlength of the scattered light remitted at shorter wavelengths is much less than that of longer wavelengths. Blue light therefore encounters less melanin than red light, and may therefore suffer less absorption. Such scattering is the only means by which a pigment, such as melanin, which absorbs shorter wavelengths more strongly than longer wavelengths, can produce blue colors.

Anderson et al. (21) have presented calculations of spectral scattering (S) and absorption (K) coefficients for human dermis in vitro by application of a modified Kubelka–Munk theory to measurements of transmittance and remittance of thin dermal sections. Measurements were made under conditions appropriate to the assumptions inherent in this model. Measurements of the spectral transmittance and remittance of a typical 200-μm-thick human dermal section, analogous to those of Findlay, are shown in Fig. 6-12. Calculated values for S and K are shown in Fig. 6-13. As expected from Findlay's work, dermal scattering is markedly increased at shorter wavelengths. The absorption coefficient K for bloodless dermis is smaller than S except at the prominent absorption bands of water in the infrared region. Dermal scattering therefore plays a major role in determining the depth to which radiation of various wavelengths penetrates the dermis, and largely accounts for the observations of Hardy et al. (12) and others (31–33, 35) that, in general, longer wavelengths across the UV–visible–near-infrared spectrum penetrate the dermis to a greater extent than do shorter wavelengths.

In vivo, the blood-borne pigments hemoglobin, oxyhemoglobin, beta-carotene, and bilirubin are the major absorbers of visible radiation in the

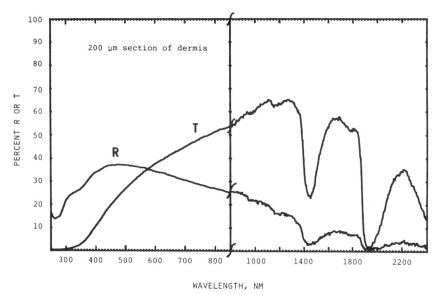

Fig. 6-12. Spectral transmittance and remittance of 200-μm-thickness section of human dermis.

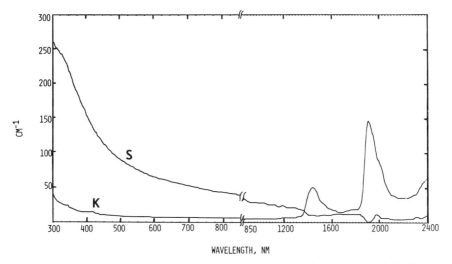

WAVELENGTH, NM

Fig. 6-13. Diffuse scattering (S) and absorption (K) coefficients for human dermis in vitro, calculated from measurements of spectral remittance and transmittance of thin dermal sections under conditions appropriate to application of the Kubelka–Munk theory of radiation transfer (20).

dermis. Absorption spectra for these dermal chromophores and for melanin are shown in Fig. 6-14. In addition, typically less than 1% of the total hemoglobin in blood is methemoglobin, which has an absorption band in the red visible region. The effect of these substances on K is not seen in the in vitro dermal spectra presented above, but can be estimated or inferred from in vivo remittance spectra (21, 62). Estimates of the depth at which various wavelengths are attenuated to $1/e$ (37%) of the (diffuse) incident energy density in fair-skinned Caucasians in vivo are given in Table 6-2 (R. R. Anderson, unpublished calculations). The depth was estimated using Eq. (8), assuming known values for S from in vitro studies of dermis to remain constant in vivo, and calculating K in vivo from measurements of R. Vitiligo skin was studied in order to avoid the influence of melanin, such that the $1/e$ penetration depths given in Table 6-2 represent estimated maximum values.

While all of the various forms of hemoglobin are entirely intravascular pigments, bilirubin occurs in both albumin-bound and free forms, and is therefore both intravascular and extravascular. The fraction of bilirubin that is extravascular may be influenced by both vascular permeability and, in hyperbilirubinemia, saturation of albumin binding sites (63). Beta-carotene is highly lipophilic and is sequestered in subcutaneous fat, dermal lipid, and to some extent stratum corneum. Most other mammals retain relatively little beta-carotene and have white subcutaneous fat as opposed to the yellow fat found in humans. These physical distributions of the dermal pigments have great importance from an optical point of view. First, a pigment's physical cross section is important. For example, absorption by hemoglobin and by

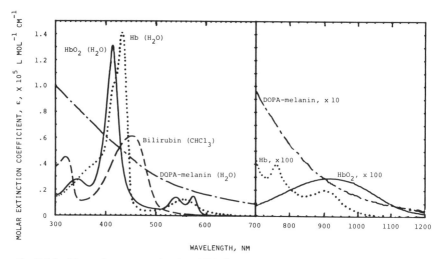

Fig. 6-14. Absorption spectra of major visible-light-absorbing pigments of human skin, HbO₂
(—), Hb (· · ·), bilirubin (- - -), and DOPA-melanin (- · -). Parentheses indicate solvent. The
spectrum shown for DOPA-melanin is the absorbance on a scale of 0 to 1.5 of a 1.5 mg % aqueous
solution. Not shown is beta-carotene, which has a broad absorption band qualitatively similar to
that for bilirubin in the 400–500-nm region, with maxima at 466 and 497 nm in CHCl₃. Note scale
changes in the near-infrared.

oxyhemoglobin is not nearly as great as if these chromophores were uniformly
distributed throughout the dermal tissue. This effect is conceptually similar to
the difference in optical absorption between a sheet of paper with numerous
small dots of ink on it and a similar sheet with the same quantity of ink
uniformly coating the paper. Second, since the penetration of optical
radiation in the tissue is wavelength dependent, stratification of pigments at

Table 6-2. Approximate Depth for Penetration of Optical Radiation in Fair
Caucasian Skin to a Value of 1/e (37%) of the Incident Energy Density

Wavelength, nm	Depth, μm
250	2
280	1.5
300	6
350	60
400	90
450	150
500	230
600	550
700	750
800	1200
1000	1600
1200	2200

different depths influences the spectral distribution of the radiation reaching a given stratum. For example, the blue visible light corresponding to the major absorption band of beta-carotene is essentially absent at the 1–4-mm depths associated with the upper limits of the subcutaneous fat layer. The yellow color of carotenemic individuals can therefore be due only to that beta-carotene in the stratum corneum, epidermis, and superficial dermis. Carotenemic individuals typically exhibit selective yellowing of the palms and soles, sites in which the thick corneum can retain enough carotenoids to noticeably affect skin color. Similarly, the stratification of the cutaneous vascular architecture from tiny capillaries to venules, arterioles, and major vessels at greater depths influences optical absorption by cutaneous blood. Only the superficial vessels—capillaries and the venular plexis—will be exposed to significant blue or UV radiation.

Because of the increased dermal scattering and optical absorption in vivo for wavelengths less than 600 nm, and the high optical absorption of wavelengths longer than about 1300 nm by water, an optical "window" exists in skin and most other soft tissue in the region 600–1300 nm. Another such "window" exists from 1600 to 1850 nm, between two water absorption bands. Whenever it is possible to use some portion of the penetrating 600–1300-nm wavelength region to cause phototoxicity, the volume and depth of tissue affected will be large. This has been taken advantage of in hematoporphyrin-derivative (HPD) photoradiation therapy for cancer, using 630-nm radiation (see Chapter 23). The 600–1300-nm region carries a quantum energy of only 2–0.95 ev, respectively, and hence can only exert photobiologic influences other than heating by affecting very weak bonds. For example, the production of singlet oxygen, the putative intermediate involved in HPD phototoxicity, requires approximately 1 eV. It is possible that other photodynamic photosensitizers exist which can produce singlet oxygen upon absorption of wavelengths even longer than the 630-nm (1.97 eV) radiation used with HPD.

Some weak endogenously occurring bonds are also influenced by 600–1300-nm radiation, and it is therefore possible that these long wavelengths have some effect on metabolic processes in skin and perhaps even on internal organs. CO and O_2 liganded to hemoproteins can often be photodissociated from the heme groups. Carbon monoxide bound to hemoglobin, myoglobin, and some cytochromes has been shown to be photodissociable (64–66), and the action spectrum for photodissociation of human HbCO includes wavelengths as long as 700 nm (67). Despite earlier, largely uncontrolled experiments suggesting an effect of visible light on clearance of CO from animals (68, 69), deliberate exposure to intense radiation in the 400–1000-nm region, even directly upon the lungs, has little effect upon clearance of CO from experimentally CO-poisoned animals (67). It is nonetheless possible that visible and near-infrared wavelengths might influence cutaneous blood gas exchange, oxidative phosphorylation, or other metabolic processes. Preliminary measurements of spectral transmission through the human chest wall and abdomen postmortem indicate that up to 1% (10^{-2}) of 650–850-nm radiation may reach internal organs, whereas the chest wall transmittance of wavelengths less than 550 nm is less than 10^{-6}.

BIOMEDICAL APPLICATIONS INVOLVING CUTANEOUS OPTICS

In Vivo Remittance Spectroscopy

Absorption bands related to each of the major dermal chromophores (cf. Fig. 6-14) can be distinctly seen as minima in the spectral remittance of Caucasian skin in vivo (13, 70–73). Because melanin lacks discrete absorption bands but absorbs more strongly at shorter wavelengths, its effect is to decrease remittance at shorter wavelengths more so than at longer wavelengths (cf. Fig. 6-11). Accurate measurements of skin remittance at carefully chosen wavelengths can in theory be used to quantify or monitor changes in cutaneous pigments. Possibilities for this general technique therefore include determinations of states of vasodilatation (erythema), oxygen saturation of cutaneous blood, bilirubin levels, and melanin pigmentation. Over the past approximately 50 years, all of these measurements have been attempted with varying degrees of success depending mainly upon each author's choice of wavelengths and ability to interpret the data obtained. Therefore, before examining each measurement scheme specifically, a more general model for the remittance of human skin will be presented.

Over the broad spectral region of approximately 350 nm to approximately 1300 nm, the remittance of skin can be qualitatively and to a large extent quantitatively modeled by considering the thin epidermis to be an optically absorbing element with negligible scattering, overlying the thick dermis, which acts as a diffuse reflector (21). Normally, epidermal transmittance can be assumed to depend only upon melanin content and distribution. Remittance of the dermal element depends upon both scattering, mainly by collagen, and absorption, mainly by the dermal pigments of interest. The dermal remittance component must pass back through the epidermis and eventually through the skin surface to the outside world, to be measured as remittance in vivo.

The justification for neglecting any remittance due to scattering within the epidermis is apparent in Fig. 6-15, which compares the spectral remittance of full-thickness Caucasian skin in vitro with the spectral remittance of the heat-separated epidermis alone placed in optical contact with a black glass background (21). Over the entire 350–1300-nm region, the epidermal remittance is essentially only that due to regular reflectance at the skin surface. The much higher values for full-thickness skin remittance must therefore be due to radiation that has passed through the epidermis, been backscattered within the dermis, and passed through the epidermis once again to be measured.

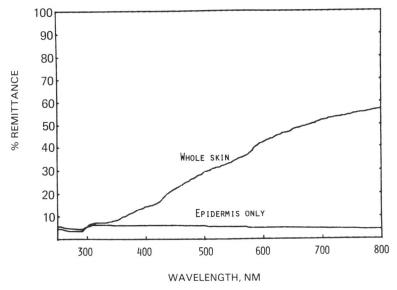

Fig. 6-15. Spectral remittance of full-thickness Caucasian skin (abdominal) in vitro, compared with spectral remittance of the isolated epidermis alone, from the same tissue. The remittance of the epidermis is essentially only that due to regular reflectance. The higher values for full-thickness skin remittance at wavelengths greater than 350 nm are therefore due to radiation that traverses the epidermis, is backscattered from the dermis, and returns through the epidermis once more.

Since this simple model of skin remittance neglects scattering within the epidermis, the effective pathlength of the diffuse radiation returning from the dermis on its second pass through the epidermis is roughly twice that of the epidermis (23, 24). Let us neglect regular reflectance at the skin surface for the moment, and let T_e represent epidermal transmittance for a collimated, normally incident beam, and R_D represent the dermal remittance if the epidermis were not present. The remittance of skin in vivo is then simply $T_e^3 R_D$ (cf. Fig. 6-16). This is derived by inspection as follows: the fraction of the collimated incident flux reaching the dermis is T_e; the dermis then returns a fraction R_D such that the outward-directed diffuse flux at the bottom of the epidermis is $T_e R_D$; finally, this diffuse flux is attenuated by a factor T_e^2 (squared because the effective pathlength is twice as great for the now diffuse radiation) in passing through the epidermis, such that the skin's remittance is $T_e^3 R_D$. To complete this oversimplified model, the effects of regular reflectance occurring at the skin–air interface must be included, both for the incident beam ($R_{reg} = 5$–7% for a collimated, normally incident beam) and for the diffuse flux encountering the same surface from within the tissue. When one then considers the effects of regular reflection occurring at the skin–air interface, the expression for remittance is complicated by an infinite series of terms representing multiple passes of radiation through the epidermis (21), but T_e and R_D are still treatable as separate parameters (21). An improvement in this simple model would be to model both the epidermis and dermis as discrete layers using the Kubelka-Munk or similar theory.

The main advantage of this model is its simplicity. By separating epidermal and dermal elements, the effect of dermal chromophores upon the dermal remittance parameter R_D might be treated using the Kubelka–Munk or similar radiation transfer theories. The dermal scattering coefficient S should not be greatly affected by changes in states of vasodilatation in the papillary dermis, because (1) S is determined largely by scattering by collagen; (2) blood vessels occupy a relatively small volume fraction of the dermis; and (3) the analogous scattering coefficient for whole human blood is only slightly less than that determined for bloodless dermis in vitro (R. R. Anderson; unpublished observations). The effects of edema on S may be more drastic, but are unknown at present. Treating S as a constant, then, one might use variations in R_D caused by dermal chromophores to calculate K, the effective dermal absorption coefficient corresponding to "concentrations" of dermal chromophores.

For the model to be useful practically, one must be able to somehow measure the melanin-dependent epidermal transmittance term T_e independently of the effects of dermal chromophores. Fortunately, there are two widely separated spectral regions in which melanin absorbs, but none of the normal dermal chromophores exerts a major influence on in vivo remittance. One such region is 650–700 nm, where blood shows very little absorption, the other is 330–400 nm, where melanin exhibits high absorption but other epidermal chromophores do not (Fig. 6-10), absorption by hemoglobin or oxyhemoglobin is relatively weak (Fig. 6-14), and the dermal penetration depth is superficial (Table 6-2) such that only the small volume of blood present in superficial capillaries can significantly affect the remittance.

Remittance measurements in these two spectral regions have been used for monitoring melanin pigmentation, with the choice of wavelength based largely upon empirical observations rather than on an optical model for in vivo spectral remittance. Numerous authors simply have used a single measurement of skin remittance in the red visible region for this purpose (13, 71, 74, 75). The technique is adequate for measuring gross pigmentation differences across the wide "spectrum" from Caucasians to blacks, but is not especially sensitive for detecting small differences in melanin pigmentation of lightly pigmented skin, because melanin's absorbance is not particularly high in the red visible region. In contrast, remittance in the spectral region around 350 nm is quite sensitive to small differences in the pigmentation of fair-skinned individuals. Consequently, UVA (320–400 nm) photography of skin (76) or the visible autofluorescence of skin excited by UVA (77) can be used to visualize small variations in melanin pigmentation.

The measurement of erythema has most often been accomplished by comparing remittance in the 540–575-nm (green) region with remittance in the 630–700-nm (red) region (74, 75, 78, 79). Neither absorption by melanin nor the dermal scattering coefficient varies extremely between these two nearby wavelength regions, but absorption by oxyhemoglobin is several orders of magnitude higher in the wavelength region from 540 to 575 nm than from 640 to 700 nm. Most authors have chosen to arithmetically subtract the green remittance from the red remittance to provide a scale for monitoring vasodilatation. Despite the arbitrary nature of such analysis, this simple approach does offer a more objective means than visual inspection for monitoring vasodilatation. However, in view of the basic model presented above, arithmetic subtraction of the remittance leads at best to an arbitrary, nonlinear scale for vasodilatation which is also somewhat dependent upon melanin pigmentation.

Expressing the spectral remittance of skin in optical density units ($OD_R = -\log R$) and in essence subtracting these values at the green wavelengths associated with HbO_2 absorption from those in the red region gives better results. Here, one must be aware that OD_R is an *apparent* optical density unit, and will be proportional to K only as a first approximation, over narrow spectral regions where S can be treated as wavelength independent. This approach was taken by Feather et al. (80), who used spectral comparisons of OD_R between UV-exposed and adjacent unexposed sites to establish scales for melanin pigmentation and erythema. Melanin pigmentation was measured by determining the slope for differences in OD_R between exposed and unexposed sites over the region 645–705 nm, based on the rationale that melanin is the major cutaneous pigment affecting remittance in this region, and that melanin's absorption spectrum climbs gradually toward the shorter wavelengths. An index of vasodilatation was defined by taking the area under the OD_R curve corresponding to the 542-nm and 577-nm absorption bands of oxyhemoglobin, i.e., in the range 510–610 nm. These scales for erythema and pigmentation experimentally proved not to be entirely independent, and the authors derived a linear correction coefficient, which, when applied to the OD_R measurement scale for melanin, rendered their vasodilatation scale relatively independent of melanin pigmentation.

This study offers significant improvement over previous methods, because optical density units are used to derive measures of melanin pigmentation and vasodilatation; the measures for pigments should therefore show greater linearity with actual changes in melanin "concentration" or blood volume. However, the effect of variations in absorption coefficients (pigments) upon the effective pathlength and depth being sampled was not included in the analysis. Furthermore, the analysis is comparative between sites and it is not clear whether absolute states of vasodilatation or pigmentation can be assessed in this manner.

Application of more rigorous radiation-transfer models for the purpose of measuring melanin pigmentation or vasodilatation remains to be accomplished. In theory, it should be possible to estimate absolute states of vasodilatation and melanin pigmentation from remittance spectra by calculation of a dermal and epidermal absorption coefficient at wavelengths of strong and weak absorption by blood, respectively. To do this, one must be able to treat dermal scattering (S) as a known parameter, to measure T_e separately from R_D as discussed above, and correct for or eliminate regular reflections occurring at the skin–air interface. This seemingly more complex approach offers the potential advantage of arriving at measurements of cutaneous chromophores that relate directly to their effects upon optical radiation transfer in the skin. Second because the average dermal pathlength involved varies inversely as a function of wavelength, determined by S and K, it is also theoretically feasible to at least monitor changes in vasodilatation as a function of depth within the dermis (21). This may be possible in practice because hemoglobin and oxyhemoglobin have discrete, widely spaced absorption bands over the 400–1000-nm region. Dermal penetration of radiation over this wavelength region varies by more than an order of magnitude (cf. Table 6-2). Therefore, the influence of blood on in vivo remittance at the HbO_2 Soret absorption band near 420 nm corresponds only to blood in superficial vesels (i.e., <100 μm dermal depth). The influence at longer wavelength bands corresponds to blood in vessels at successively greater depths, up to several millimeters in the near-infrared region.

Several studies have shown that in vivo remittance spectra in the 400–510-nm region can be used to noninvasively estimate serum bilirubin levels. Ballowitz and Avery (81) showed that the depression of neonatal skin remittance over the absorption band of bilirubin centered near 460 nm ($\epsilon \simeq 60,000$ mol^{-1} cm^{-1}) apparently correlated with serum bilirubin levels in jaundiced infants. Subsequently, Bruce (82) developed an instrument and data analysis for estimation of serum bilirubin levels which gave 95% confidence limits as low as ±2.2 mg/100 ml for Caucasian neonates not receiving phototherapy. For infants receiving phototherapy, the correlation was poor, presumably due to induction of melanin pigmentation and transients in the distributions of free vs. albumin-bound bilirubin, which have different absorption spectra. The author suggests that maintaining an unexposed test patch during phototherapy might reduce these errors. Data analysis was accomplished by fitting coefficients to a linear summation of remittances at 424, 465, 511, 556, and 629 nm to obtain the best correlation between this function and measured serum bilirubin. Using a similar estimation technique, Hannemann et al. (83) also correlated skin remittance at five wavelengths with bilirubin levels in 56 Caucasian neonates, with ±2 mg/100 ml 95% confidence limits. These authors, using somewhat different wavelengths (425, 460, 525, 535, and 545 nm) found in addition that a polynomial nonlinear regression analysis gave a slightly better correlation with measured serum bilirubin that did multiple linear regression such as used by Bruce.

Photography is in essence a recording of remittance in which the image is preserved. By placing spectral filters over the camera lens, one can record images of skin remittance of wavelengths of choice across the UV, visible, and near-infrared spectral regions. Judicious choice of wavelength can therefore allow one to enhance the appearance of various pigments or structures. Applications of this technique include UVA photography for visualizing epidermal melanin (76) and near-infrared photography (around 900 nm) for visualization of the deeper cutaneous vessels, even in blacks (84). It has been suggested that near-infrared photographs of pigmented lesions can be used to screen for malignant melanomas, which appear to have less remittance in this region than benign pigmented lesions (85). Whether this effect is due to some difference in the absorption spectrum of melanin produced by malignant melanoma cells or differences in the vascularization or distribution of melanin between benign and malignant lesions is unknown. The recent advent of computerized spectral image-processing systems may some day offer an analogous but sophisticated and diagnostically more powerful tool for visualization of cutaneous pathologies. These devices can enhance and display real-time images based upon computerized analysis of spectral images. To our knowledge, such systems have yet to be applied in any detail for cutaneous analyses.

In Vivo Fluorescence of Skin: Wood's Lamp

In 1908, R. W. Wood (86) placed a UVA-transmitting, visible-absorbing filter over a mercury discharge lamp, and noted that the device caused visible luminescence of many objects, including skin. Dermatologists have since used "Wood's lamps" to diagnose tinea capitis, erythrasma, and some *Pseudomonas* infections, and the appearance of porphyrins in hair, skin, or urine (87). Another application of Wood's lamp is that of visualizing subtle changes in epidermal melanin pigmentation and assessing whether pigmented lesions are due to epidermal vs. dermal deposition of pigment (77). Variations in epidermal pigmentation are much more apparent under Wood's lamp than under visible light. In contrast, lesions due to dermal melanin pigmentation, which often have a blue hue as discussed above, are either less apparent or vanish entirely when viewed under Wood's lamp.

If one sections fresh, lightly pigmented Caucasian skin in vitro and observes the intensity of visible autofluorescence under a Wood's lamp, it is apparent that the dermis fluoresces brightly, while epidermal autofluorescence is comparatively much less. Furthermore, if the entire epidermis including basal layer is separated from the dermis by suction, the separated epidermis alone shows little fluorescence under Wood's lamp, but when placed back over the dermis, the fluorescence increases and is subjectively similar to that for the full-thickness tissue before separation and for in vivo skin (R. R. Anderson, unpublished observations). These observations strongly suggest that fluorescence seen under Wood's lamp is largely due to dermal autofluorescence, caused by UVA penetrating the epidermis, and of course viewed through the epidermis. The fact that variations in epidermal pigmentation are more apparent under Wood's lamp than under visible light is therefore most likely due to the greater absorption by melanin in the UVA vs. the visible spectrum. When the melanin is dermal, however, a very different effect is obtained. UVA penetrates the dermis only superficially compared with visible light, largely because of dermal scattering (cf. Table 6-2). Thus, most of the dermal autofluorescence seen under Wood's lamp is limited to the superficial dermis, and melanin pigment occurring beyond some shallow depth (on the order of 50 μm) within the dermis will cause little or no reduction in this autofluorescence. The effect is conceptually similar to that discussed above for blue skin colors when dermally deposited melanin is present, but is more pronounced under Wood's lamp because UVA is of even shorter wavelength than blue light. The fluorophores or phosphores responsible for visible autofluorescence of the dermis are unknown.

PHOTOMEDICAL TREATMENTS AND CUTANEOUS OPTICS

Knowledge of cutaneous optics is helpful both in explaining certain photobiologic phenomena and in designing new forms of phototherapy or photochemotherapy. In the absence of spectrally dependent tissue optics, biologic action spectra parallel absorption or excitation spectra for the chromophores initiating a biologic response pathway. In skin, however, action spectra will only resemble absorption spectra for a putative chromophore if one corrects for the spectral attenuation of incident radiation by the tissue before reaching the chromophore. As such, the optical properties of the tissue overlying the chromophore and the depth of the chromophore become very important in determining the relative effectiveness of incident radiation as a function of wavelength.

For example, the distinct minimum near 280 nm in delayed erythema action spectra of human skin is largely if not entirely due to absorption of incident radiation of the stratum corneum and epidermis (88). It recently has been shown that the action spectrum for phototherapy of psoriasis vulgaris is similar to that for delayed erythema in normal skin, except for wavelengths less than approximately 295 nm, which are comparatively ineffective (89) (cf. Chapter 17). Wavelengths of 295 nm are on the edge of the strong absorption band for stratum corneum centered near 275 nm. Therefore, the most direct explanation for this important observation is that transmission of wavelengths less than 295 nm through the thick stratum corneum of psoriatic plaques is much less than that for normal skin, resulting in a gross difference in the phototoxicity between psoriatic and normal skin induced by these wavelengths. The 275-nm apparent absorbance ($-\log T$) or normal, fair-skinned Caucasian stratum corneum is typically 1.5–2. The psoriatic stratum corneum, being several times thicker, may have an absorbance of 4–6 at this wavelength. The net result would be several orders of magnitude difference in the incident dose at 275 nm necessary to cause phototoxic effects in viable keratinocytes of psoriatic vs. normal skin. At the longer UV wavelengths outside this broad absorption band, i.e., greater than or equal to approximately 300 nm, the effect of the increased corneal thickness in plaques would be much less dramatic. Other explanations, such as different mechanisms initiated by different chromophores at different sites being involved in delayed erythema of normal skin vs. regression of psoriatic plaques, are also possible.

The depth to which optical radiation penetrates cutaneous tissues varies by several orders of magnitude over the 250–1300-nm spectral region. Because many phototoxic drugs exhibit wide action spectra, it is possible in theory to control the depth of photochemotherapeutic treatments of skin by simply varying the wavelength. For example, if the phototoxic action spectrum includes most of the visible spectrum, the depth of treatment can be controlled to either maximize or avoid exposure of blood cells. It is likely that the depth of photochemotherapeutic treatments with HPD or other phototoxic drugs can be controlled in this manner not only for skin, but also for other connective tissues or organs accessible by optical fiber endoscopes.

MANIPULATING THE OPTICS OF SKIN

Decreasing Photobiologic Sensitivity

The sensitivity of skin to UV radiation can be decreased or increased by topical applications. If a UV-absorbing or -scattering compound is applied to the skin in the form of a "sunscreen," sensitivity to radiation in the spectral regions involved will decrease. Numerous sunscreen formulations exist, with different absorption spectra, water solubilities, and other characteristics (cf Chapter 15).

The relative decrease in sensitivity as measured by increases in the minimal delayed erythema dose (MED) at specified wavelengths is proportional to the relative decrease in transmittance of the stratum corneum after application of the sunscreen (90). Calculations of protection offered by any given sunscreen on the basis of assuming a uniform-thickness layer of the sunscreen with a known absorption coefficient as measured in solution give falsely high estimates of protection (91). The skin surface is far from planar and one would not expect to obtain a uniform-thickness layer of the applied material. Furthermore, many sunscreening compounds crystalize on the skin surface after evaporation of the solvent. Both of these mechanisms would act to create a distinctly nonuniform distribution of sunscreen, and result in significantly greater transmission of radiation than would be obtained for a uniform layer. Other possible losses of protection result from either the washing or rubbing off of the sunscreen, or diffusion of the sunscreening compound through the stratum corneum and into interstitial and/or intracellular fluids of the epidermis (92).

Increasing Photobiologic Sensitivity

Prolonged application of water or aqueous media to normal Caucasian skin results in the extraction of UV-absorbing compounds from the skin both in vivo and in vitro. This results in a corresponding increase in transmittance of the stratum corneum as appropriately measured in vitro, and an increase in sensitivity to UVC and UVB radiation, as measured by decreases in MEDs of fair-skinned subjects (93, 94). In contrast, lipophilic substances such as mineral oil neither extract significant amounts of UV-absorbing material from normal skin nor affect the MED to UVB radiation when applied in vivo. The broad absorbance maximum of the cutaneous materials extracted into topically applied water occurs between 265 and 275 nm and correlates both spectrally and quantitatively with the decrease in optical density of human stratum corneum measured in vitro after application and removal of water. The kinetics for extraction of the UV-absorbing compounds into water are such that application times of $\frac{1}{2}$ hr or more are necessary to observe decreases in the MED to UVB radiation from FS40 lamps of 20% or more. The maximum decrease in MED to UVB radiation obtained was a 40–50% decrease after 4 hr of continuous application of water (94). Application of aqueous 5% lactic acid appears to act similarly to water application.

These observations show that extraction of water-soluble, i.e., relatively polar, freely diffusable, UV-absorbing compounds from skin accounts for the increased sensitivity of skin to UVB radiation after soaking the skin for prolonged periods. Chromatographic analysis of the extracted materials indicated that, while most of the material extracted was lipid or protein, a small fraction (about 0.2%) of the material was urocanic acid. Because of its high extinction coefficient ($18,800 \, mol^{-1} cm^{-1}$ at 277 nm, pH 7.4), however, this small quantity of urocanic acid accounts for approximately 75% of the optical absorbance of the extracted materials. As has been suggested (56, 57), urocanic acid appears to play some role as an "endogenous sunscreen" in human skin. In addition to its epidermal synthesis, urocanic acid is also present in human sweat (56), and is deposited on the skin surface after profuse sweating. Because extensive exposure to sunlight is often associated with sweating, it is possible that sweating may serve to some extent as a thermally induced photoprotective mechanism.

Normal skin has a single, continuous, though somewhat irregular air-tissue interface, in which the refractive index (n_D) changes from that of air, 1.0, to that of stratum corneum, 1.55 (20). As discussed above, this causes a regular reflectance of 5–7% across the UV, visible, and near-infrared spectra. Adding a layer of some clear, lipophilic liquid such as mineral oil, which readily spreads over the surface of skin and has a refractive index ($n_D = 1.48$) between that of air and stratum corneum, does little to reduce regular reflectance occurring at the optical interface with air. However, if there are multiple air–tissue interfaces along the path of incident radiation as it enters the stratum corneum, regular reflectance occurs at each such interface, and the total regular reflectance is considerably greater than for a single air–tissue interface. When mineral oil is applied to the scaly plaques typical of psoriasis vulgaris, it apparently fills air spaces between superficial flakes of corneo-cytes. In this case, the regular reflectance of the plaque is decreased after application of the oil because the oil provides a much better match of refractive index *between* the flakes of corneocytes than does air. Reducing regular reflectance in this manner must necessarily increase the fraction of incident light transmitted into the tissue.

Typical spectral remittance of psoriatic and normal Caucasian skin before and after application of mineral oil is shown in Fig. 6-16 (95). The significant, broad-spectrum decrease in remittance of plaques occurs within seconds after application of oils. Other optically transparent oils produce essentially the same results, but application of water requires up to several minutes to produce a similar effect. The extremely broad spectral character of the decrease in remittance, and the fact that it occurs immediately after application of oils, are entirely consistent with the refractive index-matching mechanism proposed above. Water does not spread readily on the skin surface compared with less polar liquids, which may explain why a longer application time is required for water to cause a similar effect as oils.

The decrease in regular reflectance of psoriasis vulgaris plaques after treatment with oils is typically 10–15%, but varies from as low as 5% decrease to as much as 25% decrease. The expected increase in the fraction of incident radiation transmitted into the psoriatic stratum corneum is essentially the same, 10–15%. However, the increase in that fraction of relatively collimated incident radiation reaching viable keratinocytes is probably considerably greater than 10–15%, perhaps by several times. This may occur because the oil will also drastically reduce off-axis refraction of the incident radiation as it traverses the air–tissue interfaces, resulting in a shorter average pathlength within the stratum corneum, and hence less absorption. Measurements of increased transmittance through psoriatic stratum corneum as a result of application of oils are yet to be accomplished.

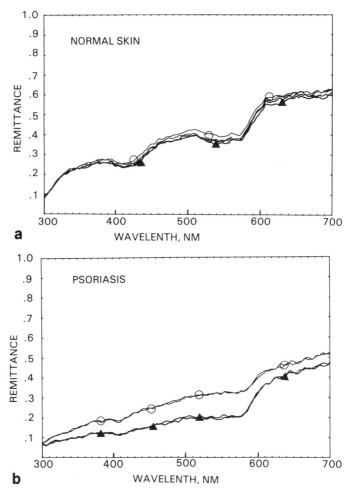

a

b

Fig. 6-16. (a) Spectral remittance of normal Caucasian skin before (O) and after (▲) application of mineral oil. (b) Spectral remittance of typical psoriasis vulgaris plaque before (O) and after (▲) application of mineral oil. The immediate, broad-spectrum decrease in remittance is consistent with a reduction of regular reflectance occurring at the surface(s) of the plaque.

Because the optics of normal skin is not significantly affected by application of oils, one can easily maximize transmission of UVB or UVA radiation into psoriatic plaques during phototherapy without affecting the responses of normal skin, which is generally the limiting factor in the aggressiveness of therapy. Oily lubricants, such as petrolatum, when applied before UVB treatment of psoriasis, significantly enhance phototherapeutic effectiveness (96). Some or all of this effect must be related to the optical changes discussed above. For FS40-lamp UVB phototherapy, the addition of tar compounds to an oily base may be no more effective than the base alone

(96). Because of the very wide spectral character of the reduction in regular reflectance of plaques, use of oily lubricants should be of some benefit for all wavebands used in phototherapy or photochemotherapy of psoriasis. It is probable, however, that the added therapeutic benefit will be somewhat greater for relatively collimated incident radiation sources at wavelengths less than or equal to approximately 300 nm, which are more strongly absorbed by stratum corneum.

LASER-INDUCED SELECTIVE THERMAL DESTRUCTION OF PIGMENTED STRUCTURES

Lasers are sources of optical radiation with the special characteristics of essentially absolute monochromaticity, spatial and temporal coherence, and, for many lasers, high power. The coherence of lasers allows their output beam to be focused to very small diameters, on the order of the wavelength of the radiation emitted. Thus, it is possible to achieve extremely high optical energy densities over areas small enough to destroy, for example, only a small fragment of a single chromosome (97). Pulsed lasers often exhibit extremely short pulse times, as short as 10^{-12} sec or less, and as long as tens of milliseconds, and peak power outputs as high as 10^{10} W or greater. These characteristics of pulsed lasers have made it possible to study very fast processes, such as time-resolved spectroscopy of the transient excited states involved in photochemical reactions. Continuous (CW or nonpulsed) lasers are also available. The many different common types of lasers emit radiation over the spectrum from the vacuum-UV through far-infrared, usually only in one or more discrete spectral lines for each type of laser. Pulsed or continuous tunable organic dye lasers are also available, in which the output wavelength can be tuned over the near-UV through near-infrared spectral regions. In addition, special crystals for the nonlinear generation of optical harmonic frequencies can be used with pulsed lasers to shift the output wavelength to precisely one-half or one-third of the fundamental wavelength.

Medically, lasers have in general, but not exclusively, been used for surgical applications. The vast majority of optical energy at any wavelength absorbed in tissues is rapidly converted to heat by nonradiative processes. The high focal power of lasers can therefore cause confined heating and thermal destruction of tissue, depending upon the wavelength, power, and beam size of the laser, and the optical absorption and scattering properties of the tissue. The main advantage of using a laser instead of a surgical scalpel is that blood vessels are thermally coagulated, reducing or eliminating blood loss. Also, if the power and exposure duration of the laser are carefully controlled, the depth of the incision and photocoagulation can be controlled with some precision. The most common "surgical knife" laser is the continuous CO_2

laser, operating at a wavelength of 10.6 m (10,600 nm). Water absorbs very strongly at this wavelength, and therefore the CO_2 laser generally causes relatively equal thermal destruction of many different soft tissues for a given set of exposure conditions. In contrast, the thermal damage and volume or depth of tissue or structures affected by lasers operating over the near-UV, visible, and near-infrared spectral regions vary greatly depending upon the optical properties of the specific tissue exposed.

The laser most commonly used for dermatologic treatments of port-wine stains, hemangiomas, and tattoos is the argon-ion laser, a continuous laser emitting 1–20 W total power in emission lines at 476, 488, and 514 nm. Pulsed ruby lasers, emitting pulses of a few milliseconds' duration at 694 nm, have also been used for treatment of tattoos and pigmented lesions (98). Choice of lasers and exposure parameters has in general been based upon clinical comparison of results with various lasers rather than an understanding of the mechanisms for treatment, the optical and thermal properties of the tissue, and a rational theoretical approach to maximize the therapeutic benefits and minimize adverse reactions such as scarring. Still, argon laser treatment of port-wine stains and other cutaneous hemangiomas or telangiectases has been developed to the extent that it is often the treatment of choice.

Both grossly and histologically, argon-laser treatments of port-wine stains as currently performed cause extensive thermal necrosis of the entire epidermis and the first 1–2 nm of dermis (99). The lesion is blanched immediately, and a superficial crust of thermally denatured tissue is formed. Over 3–6 months following treatment, fibrosis and reepithelialization occur. The characteristic numerous ectactic vessels responsible for the pink or red color of port-wine stains are replaced by smaller vessels, and a more normal skin color results. Patients under the age of approximately 30 tend to exhibit pink-colored lesions in which the ectatic vessels are of smaller diameter than in older patients, whose lesions tend to be red or violaceous. The pink lesions associated with younger patients generally respond poorly to treatment (100). Often, superficial or, occasionally, extensive scarring results, and because the epidermis is destroyed, there is some risk of infection and loss of normal epidermal pigmentation. Some denaturation of collagen and fibrosis may in fact be necessary for the formation of smaller vessels after treatment, but it is unlikely that extensive fibrosis or epidermal necrosis is necessary for successful treatment.

Through appropriate theoretical consideration of the optical and thermal transfer processes involved in causing thermal damage, it has been possible to select laser wavelengths, exposure times, and incident energy densities which cause highly selective thermal damage to vessels without significant damage to other dermal structures or epidermis (R. R. Anderson and J. A. Parrish, unpublished observations). The general theoretical approach used is applicable to any situation in which one wishes to selectively damage a particular pigmented structure in skin or other organs, and may therefore find application for many other treatments as well.

If the overall goal is to selectively heat a certain pigmented structure such as vessels, the wavelength chosen should correspond to high absorption by the targeted structure relative to other optically absorbing structures. Choice of wavelength also determines the depth to which the optical radiation will penetrate with sufficient optical energy density to cause thermal effects. For vessels, oxyhemoglobin is the logical target chromophore, because it is entirely intravascular and is the dominant hemoglobin species. The wavelengths suitable for consideration are the HbO_2 Soret absorption band at 418 nm and the α and β absorption bands at 542 and 577 nm. Despite the higher extinction coefficient of the Soret band, this wavelength can be rejected on the grounds that penetration into the dermis (cf. Table 6-2) is insufficient for exposure of vessels at depths greater than approximately 0.1 mm. Furthermore, absorption by epidermal melanin is higher at shorter wavelengths such that if one can take advantage of the longer wavelength HbO_2 absorption bands, less heating of the epidermis will occur, and a greater fraction of the incident energy will be transmitted to the dermis. Given that the extinction coefficients of HbO_2 at the 542- and 577-nm absorption bands are comparable, it is logical to choose the 577-nm wavelength. The wavelengths currently used with the argon laser (488 and 514 nm) are fortuitously located in a region between absorption bands of HbO_2 and within the absorption bands for bilirubin, which is both intravascular and extravascular.

The size of the targeted structures should be commensurate with absorption of a significant fraction of the radiation incident upon it. The ectatic vessels associated with the red lesions of older patients are typically 50–100 μm in diameter (100). At 577 nm, the absorbed fraction of radiation incident on such vessels can be estimated to be 30–50%, based on an effective hemoglobin concentration of 2×10^{-3} M and molar extinction coefficient of 1.52×10^4 at 577 nm. For vessels of 20–50 μm diameter, typical of younger patients, the estimated absorbed fractions are 16–30%, respectively.

Exposure duration determines the degree of selective heating of tissue immediately surrounding the absorbing chromophores, as compared with the heating of large tissue volumes heated to temperatures sufficient to cause thermal damage. If the exposure duration is long compared with the time required for diffusion of a significant quantity of heat to structures, such as the epidermis, which are some distance away from the target chromophore, then thermal damage will be extensive and nonspecific regardless of how carefully one has chosen a wavelength for heating of the target structure. This is because the absorbed energy will be invested almost uniformly in heating of the tissue during exposure, despite its origin in the target structure. However, if the incident energy is delivered within the time corresponding to retention of heat within the target structure, a maximum, transient temperature differential

Table 6-3. Estimated Times for Vessel Temperature to Drop to $1/e$ (37%) of Initial Temperature As a Function of Vessel Diameter, Assuming No Blood Flow (101)

Vessel diameter, μm	Estimated thermal relaxation time, msec
5	0.01
10	0.05
20	0.2
30	0.4
50	1.2
70	2.4
100	4.8
150	11.0

between the target structure and its surroundings will be achieved. When the incident energy ceases, this localized heat in the target structure will then diffuse to surrounding structures, and in the process be dissipated over a greater volume such that the macroscopic temperature rise of the tissue will be much less than that achieved briefly in the target structure. The time associated with retention of heat within a target structure depends solely upon the size and thermal properties of the structure and its surroundings. For blood vessels, removal of heat by blood flow must also be considered.

Assuming that blood, blood vessels, and the dermis have approximately the same thermal properties as stagnant water, and modeling vessels as infinite cylinders, one can apply thermal diffusion theory to estimate the time for retention of heat in a vessel that is instantaneously heated to some temperature greater than that of the surrounding tissue. Table 6-3 shows estimated times for the vessel temperature to drop to $1/e$ (37%) of its initial temperature as a function of vessel diameter, assuming no blood flow (101). For the range of ectatic vessel diameters encountered in port-wine lesions the estimated thermal relaxation times range from about 0.5 to about 15 msec. Assuming a blood flow velocity of $0.5 \, \text{cm sec}^{-1}$ or less, the blood will move, at most, a few tens of micrometers during the longest thermal relaxation times. Given that the length of the vessel exposed to significant laser radiation is much larger than this distance, one can, for the purposes of estimation, neglect the influence that axial removal of heat by blood flow may have upon the thermal relaxation time. Therefore, if the exposure duration of the laser is kept to approximately 1 msec or less, maximum differential heating of blood vessels should occur.

Finally, one can estimate the transient microscopic (target structure) and macroscopic temperature rises produced as a function of incident energy density if the optical and thermal properties of the tissue are known. Based on the optical data and models given above for normal fair-skinned Caucasians, it is reasonable to expect that the average energy density at 577 nm within the first 200 μm of the dermis is roughly 50% of the incident energy density. If the exposure duration is less than 1 msec, the peak vessel temperature rise will be simply the energy absorbed per unit vessel length divided by the product of vessel cross-sectional area and the heat capacity of blood. For a 50-μm-diameter vessel and an initial ambient skin temperature of 33° C, the estimated peak vessel temperature is 58° C for an incident energy density of 2.5 J cm^{-2}, 80° C for 5 J cm^{-2}, and 130° C (vaporization) for 10 J cm^{-2}. The estimated peak temperatures for vessels of 20 and 100 μm diameter are similar. Thermal denaturation of proteins typically occurs over the 60–100° C temperature range, such that one would expect an incident energy density on the order of 5 J cm^{-2} to produce significant thermal damage to vessels, while incident energy densities greater than or equal to approximately 10 J cm^{-2} might cause vaporization of blood within the vessel.

Preliminary investigations in normal Caucasian skin (102) using a pulsed organic dye laser operating at 577 nm with a pulse duration of 0.3 μsec, which is much less than the calculated thermal relaxation times for even the smallest vessels, support the above theoretical estimates. In normal fair-skinned Caucasians, exposures of 3–5 J cm^{-2} incident energy density from this laser immediately cause purpura, with no signs of gross damage to the epidermis. Histologically, sites exposed to 3–5 J cm^{-2} incident energy density show marked vasculitis, and some hemorrhaging when biopsied immediately after exposure, and subsequently a polymorphonuclear cell infiltrate. Histologically, the epidermis appeared normal. For incident energy densities of 10 J cm^{-2} or greater, purpura and occasionally epidermal perforation occurred. Histologically, a subepidermal blister and/or rupture of the epidermis were apparent for incident doses of 10 J cm^{-2} or greater. These observations are consistent with vaporization damage. When the laser output was tuned to 600 nm, which is not strongly absorbed by either blood or melanin, no effects were noted up to an incident energy density of 20 J cm^{-2}; higher exposure doses were not possible at this wavelength.

Whether organic dye lasers operating at 577 nm offer a better treatment for port-wine stains is unknown as of the printing of this chapter. However, the theoretical considerations given above have been substantiated, and a conceptually similar approach to predicting laser-induced selective thermal damage might be applied for other medical applications of lasers.

SUMMARY

The optics of human skin is dynamic and variable, and depends upon many different chromophores and scattering structures. Nonetheless, a general and quantitative approach to modeling cutaneous optics is possible, which aids in understanding photobiologic phenomena, in making useful optical measurements of cutaneous and systemic conditions and responses, and in improving and devising new photomedical treatments. By deliberately changing the optical properties of skin and selecting appropriate wavelengths lying within action spectra for photosensitized responses, one can often maximize therapeutic effectiveness, minimize risks to normal skin, and determine the depth of tissues treated by photochemically induced mechanisms. For thermally induced mechanisms, one can similarly choose optimal wavelengths and exposure durations for achieving selective thermal damage to pigmented target structures. There remain many questions regarding the optics of human skin and other organs accessible to optical radiation, and probably a greater number of undiscovered photomedical applications which await this knowledge.

ACKNOWLEDGMENTS. This work was supported by NIH Grant #AM 25395-02 and by funds from the Arthur O. and Gullan M. Wellman Foundation.

REFERENCES

1. Parrish, J. A., Anderson, R. R., Urbach, F., et al. (1978): *UV-A: Biologic Effects of Ultraviolet Radiation With Emphasis on Human Responses to Longwave Ultraviolet.* Plenum Press, New York.
2. Magnus, I. A. (1976): *Dermatological Photobiology*, pp. 11–22. Blackwell Scientific, Oxford.
3. Treagar, R. T. (1966): *Physical Functions of the Skin*, pp. 96–107. Academic Press, New York.
4. Parrish, J. A. (1975): *Dermatology and Skin Care.* McGraw-Hill, New York.
5. Montagna, W., and Parakkal, P. F. (1974): *The Structure and Function of Skin*, 3rd ed. Academic Press, New York.
6. Montagna, W., and Lobitz, W. (1964): *The Epidermis.* Academic Press, New York.
7. Fitzpatrick, T. B., Arndt, K. A., Clark, W. H., Jr., et al. (Eds.) (1971): *Dermatology in General Medicine.* McGraw-Hill, New York.
8. Malpighi, M. (1665): *De Externo Tactus Organo Anatomica Observario.* Naples.
9. Pechlin, J. (1677): *De Habitu et Colore Aethiopum.* Koln.
10. Thomson, M. L. (1955): The relative efficiency of pigment and horny layer thickness in protecting the skin of Europeans and Africans against solar ultraviolet radiation. *J. Physiol. (Lond.)* 127:236–246.
11. Everett, M. A., Yeargers, E., Sayre, R. M., et al (1966): Penetration of epidermis by ultraviolet rays. *Photochem. Photobiol.* 5:533–542.
12. Hardy, J. D., Hammell, H. T., and Murgatroyd D. (1956): Spectral transmittance and reflectance of excised human skin. *J. Appl. Physiol.* 9:257–264.
13. Edwards, E. A., and Duntley, S. Q. (1939): The pigments and color of human skin. *Am. J. Anat.* 65:1–33.
14. Kligman, A. (1969): Comments on the stratum corneum. In: *The Biologic Effects of Ultraviolet Radiation (with Emphasis on the Skin)*, edited by F. Urbach, pp. 165–167. Pergamon Press, Oxford.
15. Baden, H. P., and Pearlman, C. (1964): The effects of ultraviolet light on protein and nucleic acid synthesis in the epidermis. *J. Invest. Dermatol.* 48:71–75.

16. Epstein, J. H., Fukuyama, K., and Fye, K. (1970): Effects of ultraviolet radiation on the mitotic cycle and DNA, RNA and protein synthesis in mammalian epidermis *in vivo. Photochem. Photobiol.* 12:57-65.

17. Parrish, J. A., Zaynoun, S., and Anderson, R. R. (1981): Cumulative effects of repeated subthreshold doses of ultraviolet radiation. *J. Invest. Dermatol.* 76:352-355.

18. Langner, A., and Kligman, A. (1972): Tanning without sunburn with aminobenzoic acid type sunscreen. *Arch. Dermatol.* 106:338-343.

19. Kaidbey, K. H., and Kligman, A. M. (1978): Sunburn protection by longwave ultraviolet radiation-induced pigmentation. *Arch. Dermatol.* 114:46-48.

20. Scheuplein, R. J. (1964): A survey of some fundamental aspects of the absorption and reflection of light by tissue. *J. Soc. Cosmet. Chem.* 15:111-122.

21. Anderson, R. R., Hu, J. H., and Parrish, J. A. (1980): Optical radiation transfer in the human skin and application in *in vivo* remittance spectroscopy. In: *Proceedings of the Symposium on Bioengineering and the Skin, Cardiff, Wales, July 19-21, 1979.* MTP Press, London.

22. Jagger, J. (1967): *Introduction to Research in Ultraviolet Photobiology.* Prentice-Hall, Englewood Cliffs, N.J.

23. Kortüm, G. (1969): *Reflectance Spectroscopy.* Springer-Verlag, New York.

24. Kubelka, P., and Munk, F. (1931): Ein Beitrag zür Optik der Farbanstriche. *Z. technichse Physik* 12:593-601.

25. Kubelka, P. (1948): New contributions to the optics of intensely light-scattering materials. I. *J. Opt. Soc. Am.* 38:448-457.

26. Kubelka, P. (1954): New contributions to the optics of intensely light-scattering materials. II: Nonhomogeneous layers. *J. Opt. Soc. Am.* 44:330-335.

27. Schuster, A. (1905): Radiation through a foggy atmosphere. *Astrophys. J.* 21:1.

28. Wendlandt, W. W., and Hecht, H. G. (1966): *Reflectance Spectroscopy.* Interscience, New York.

29. Atkins, J. T. (1969): Optical properties of turbid materials. In: *The Biologic Effects of Ultraviolet Radiation (with Emphasis on the Skin),* edited by F. Urbach, pp. 141-150. Pergamon Press, Oxford.

30. Hasselbalch, K. A. (1911): Quantitative Untersuchungen uber die Absorption der menschlichen Haut von ultravioletten Strahlen. *Skand. Arch. Physiol.* 25:5-68.

31. Bachem, A. (1929): The ultraviolet transparency of the various layers of human skin. *Am. J. Physiol.* 91:58-64.

32. Macht, D. I., Anderson, W. T., and Bell, F. K. (1928): The penetration of ultraviolet rays into live animal tissues. *JAMA* 90:161-165.

33. Bachem, A., and Reed, C. I. (1930): The penetration of ultraviolet light through the human skin. *Arch. Phys. Ther.* 11:49-56.

34. Kirby-Smith, J. S., Blum, H. F., and Grady, H. G. (1942): Penetration of ultraviolet radiation into skin as a factor in carcinogenesis. *J. Natl. Canc. Inst.* 2:403-412.

35. Bachem. A., and Reed, C. I. (1929): The transparency of live and dead animal tissue to ultraviolet light. *Am. J. Physiol.* 90:600-606.

36. Lucas, N. S. (1930): The permeability of human epidermis to ultraviolet radiation. *Biochem. J.* 25:57-70.

37. Pathak, M. A. (1967): Photobiology of melanogenesis: biophysical aspects. In: *Advances in Biology of the Skin, Vol. VIII, The Pigmentary System,* edited by W. Montagna and F. Hu, pp. 397-420. Pergamon Press, Oxford.

38. Konev, S. V. (1967): *Fluorescence and Phosphorescence of Proteins and Nucleic Acids.* Plenum Press, New York.

39. Fellner, M. J. (1976): Green autofluorescence of human epidermal cells. *Arch. Dermatol.* 112:667-670.

40. van der Leun, J. C. (1966): Ultraviolet erythema: a study on diffusion processes in human skin. Thesis, Utrecht, The Netherlands.

192   R. R. Anderson and J. A. Parrish

41. Morison, W. L., Parrish, J. A., Bloch, K. J., et al. (1979): *In vivo* effect of UVB on lymphocyte function. *Br. J. Dermatol.* **101**:513–519.
42. Ortonne, J.-P., Claudy, A., Alario, A., et al. (1978): Impairment of thymus derived rosette forming cells during photochemotherapy (psoralen-UVA). *Arch. Dermatol. Res.* **262**: 143–151.
43. Morison, W. L., Parrish, J. A., Anderson, R. R., et al. (1979): Sensitivity of mononuclear cells to UV radiation. *Photochem. Photobiol.* **29**:1045–1047.
44. Hais, I. M., and Strych, A. (1969): Increase in urocanic acid concentration in human epidermis following insolation. *Coll. Czech. Chem. Comm.* **34**:649–655.
45. Baden, H. P., and Pathak, M. A. (1967): The metabolism and function of urocanic acid in skin. *J. Invest. Dermatol.* **48**:11–17.
46. Weigand, D. A., Haygood, C., and Gaylor, J. R. (1974): Cell layers and density of Negro and Caucasian stratum corneum. *J. Invest. Dermatol.* **62**:563–568.
47. Jacquez, J. A., Huss, J., McKeehan, W., et al (1956): Spectral reflectance of human skin in the region 0.7–2.6 μ. *J. Appl. Physiol.* **8**:297–299.
48. Kuppenheim, H., and Heer, R. R., Jr. (1952): Spectral reflectance of white and Negro skin between 400 and 1000 mμ. *J. Appl. Physiol.* **4**:800–806.
49. Gates, R. R., and Zimmerman, A. A. (1953): Comparison of skin color with melanin content. *J. Invest. Dermatol.* **21**:339–348.
50. Szabo, G., Gerald, A. B., Pathak, M. A., et al. (1972): The ultrastructure of racial color differences in man. In: *Pigmentation: Its Genesis and Control*, edited by V. Riley, p. 23. Appleton-Century-Crofts, New York.
51. Quevedo, W. C., Jr., Fitzpatrick, T. B., Pathak, M. A., et al. (1974): Light and skin color. In: *Sunlight and Man: Normal and Abnormal Photobiologic Responses*, edited by M. A. Pathak, L. C. Harber, M. Seiji, et al. (T. B. Fitzpatrick, consulting ed.), pp. 165–194. Univ. of Tokyo Press, Tokyo.
52. Toda, K., Pathak, M. A., Parrish, J. A., et al. (1972): Alteration of racial differences in melanosome distribution in human epidermis after exposure to ultraviolet light. *Nature* [*New Biol.*] **236**:143–145.
53. Kaidbey, K. H., Poh-Agin, P., Sayre, R. R., et al. (1979): Photoprotection by melanin—a comparison of black and Caucasian skin. *J. Am. Acad. Dermatol.* **1**:249–260.
54. Olson, R. L., Gaylor, J., and Everett, M. A. (1973): Skin color, melanin, and erythema. *Arch. Dermatol.* **108**:541–544.
55. Hausser, K. W., and Vahle, W. (1969): Sunburn and suntanning. In: *The Biologic Effects of Ultraviolet Radiation (with Emphasis on the Skin)*, edited by F. Urbach, pp. 3–21. Pergamon Press, Oxford.
56. Zenisek, A., and Krahl, J. A. (1953): The occurrence of urocanic acid in sweat. *Biochim. Biophys. Acta* **12**:479–484.
57. Everett, M. A., Anglin, J. H., and Bever, A. T. (1961): Ultraviolet-induced biochemical alterations in skin. *Arch. Dermatol.* **84**:717–724.
58. Anglin, J. H., Jones, D. H., Bever, A. T., et al. (1966): The effect of ultraviolet light and thiol compounds on guinea pig skin histidase. *J. Invest. Dermatol.* **46**:34–39.
59. Cox, A. J., and Reaven, E. P. (1967): Histidine and keratohyalin granules. *J. Invest. Dermatol.* **49**:31–34.
60. Davis, E., and Landau, J. (1966): *Clinical Capillary Microscopy.* C C Thomas, Springfield, Ill.
61. Findlay, G. H. (1970): Blue skin. *Br. J. Dermatol.* **83**:127–134.
62. Hanley, E. J., and DeWitt, D. P. (1978): A physical model for detection of neonatal jaundice by multispectral skin reflectance analysis. In: *Proceedings of the 6th New England Bioengineering Conference*, edited by D. Jaron, pp. 346–349. Pergamon Press, New York.
63. Odell, G., Schaffer, R., and Simopoulos, A. (Eds.) (1974): *Phototherapy in the Newborn, an Overview*, National Academy of Sciences, Washington, D.C.

64. Noble, R. W., Brunori, M., Wyman, J., et al. (1967): Studies on the quantum yields of the photodissociation of carbon monoxide from hemoglobin and myoglobin. *Biochemistry* 6:1216.

65. Spartalian, K., Lang, G., and Yonetani, T. (1976): Low temperature photodissociation studies of ferrous hemoglobin and myoglobin complexes by Mossbauer spectroscopy. *Biochim. Biophys. Acta* 428:281–285.

66. Yoshida, S., and Orii, Y. (1977): Can hemo–CO complexes always be photodissociated? *FEBS Lett.* 79:129–132.

67. Anderson, R. R., Flicker, W., Roberts, J., et al. (1980): *In vitro* and *in vivo* photodissociation of carboxyhemoglobin in whole blood (abstract). In: *Program and Abstracts, 8th Annual Meeting of the American Society for Photobiology, Colorado Springs, February 1980*, p. 138.

68. Macht, D. I., Blackmann, S. S., and Kelley, E. B. (1923): An experimental contribution to the treatment of carbon monoxide poisoning. *Proc. Soc. Exp. Biol. Med.* 21:289–290.

69. Linder, E., Sakai, Y., and Paton, B. C. (1963): Experimental treatment of carbon monoxide poisoning by extracorporeal irradiation. *Surg. Forum* 14:277–278.

70. Jacquez, J. A., Kuppenheim, H. F., Dimitroff, J. M., et al. (1956): Spectral reflectance of human skin in the region 235–700 mμ. *J. Appl. Physiol.* 8:212–214.

71. Goldzieher, J. W., Roberts, I. S., Rawls, W. B., et al. (1951): "Chemical" analysis of the intact skin by reflectance spectrophotometry. *Arch. Dermatol. Syphilol.* 64:533–548.

72. Edwards, E. A., Finkelstein, N. A., and Duntley, S. Q. (1951): Spectrophotometry of living human skin in ultraviolet range. *J. Invest. Dermatol.* 16:311–321.

73. Sheard, C., and Brown, E. (1926): The spectrophotometric analysis of the color of the skin. *Arch. Intern. Med.* 38:816–831.

74. Daniels, F., and Imbrie, J. D. (1958): Comparison between visual grading and reflectance measurements of erythema produced by sunlight. *J. Invest. Dermatol.* 30:295–301.

75. Breit, R., and Kligman, A. M. (1969): Measurement of erythemal and pigmentary responses to ultraviolet radiation of different spectral qualities. In: *The Biologic Effects of Ultraviolet Radiation (with Emphasis on the Skin)*, edited by F. Urbach, pp. 267–275. Pergamon Press, Oxford.

76. Mustakallio, K. K., and Korhonen, P. (1966): Monochromatic ultraviolet-photography in dermatology. *J. Invest. Dermatol.* 47:351–356.

77. Gilchrest, B. A., Fitzpatrick, T. B., Anderson, R. R., et al. (1977): Localization of melanin pigmentation with Wood's lamp. *Br. J. Dermatol.* 96:245–248.

78. Frank, L., Rapp, Y., and Bergman, L. V. (1962): An instrument for the objective measurement of erythema. *J. Invest. Dermatol.* 38:21–24.

79. Tronnier, H. (1969) Evaluation and measurement of ultraviolet erythema. In: *The Biologic Effects of Ultraviolet Radiation (with Emphasis on the Skin)*, edited by F. Urbach, pp. 255–265. Pergamon Press, Oxford.

80. Feather, J. W., Dawson, J. B., Barker, D. J., et al. (1980): A theoretical and experimental study of the optical properties of skin *in vivo*. In: *Proceedings of the Symposium on Bioengineering and the Skin*. MTP Press, International Medical Publishers, Cardiff.

81. Ballowitz, L., and Avery, M. E. (1970): Spectral reflectance of the skin. *Biol. Neonate* 15:348–360.

82. Bruce, R. A. (1978): Noninvasive estimation of bilirubin and hemoglobin oxygen saturation in the skin by reflection spectrophotometry. Ph.D. Thesis, Duke University, Durham, North Carolina.

83. Hannemann, R. E., DeWitt, D. P., and Weichel, J. F. (1978): Neonatal serum bilirubin from skin reflectance. *Pediatr. Res.* 12:207–210.

84. Salthouse, T. N. (1958): Photography of the Negro skin. *Med. Biol. Illus.* 8:150.

85. Marshall, R. J. (1976): Infrared and ultraviolet photography in a study of the selective absorption of radiation by pigmented lesions of skin. *Med. Biol. Illus.* 26:71–84.

86. Wood, R. W. (1919): Secret communications concerning light rays. *J. Physiol. (Paris) 5e Serie* **IX** (March 1919).

87. Caplan, R. M. (1967): Medical uses of the Wood's lamp. *JAMA* **202**:1035–1038.

88. Mitchell, J. S. (1938): The origin of the erythema curve and the pharmacological action of ultraviolet radiation. *Proc. R. Soc. Lond. [Biol.]* **126**:241–246.

89. Parrish, J. A. (1980): Action spectrum of phototherapy of psoriasis (abstract). *J. Invest. Dermatol.* **74**:251.

90. Groves, G. A., Poh-Agin, P., and Sayre, R. M. (1979): *In vitro* and *in vivo* methods to define sunscreen protection, *Australas J. Dermatol.* **20**:112–119.

91. Sayre, R. M., Poh-Agin, P., LeVee, G. J., et al. (1979): A comparison of *in vivo* and *in vitro* testing of sunscreen formulas. *Photochem. Photobiol.* **29**:559–566.

92. Blank, I. H., Ornellas, L., Anderson, R. R., et al. (1979): Observations on the substantivity of sunscreens (abstract). In: *Program and Abstracts, 7th Annual Meeting of the American Society for Photobiology, Pacific Grove, California, June 1979*, p. 127.

93. White, H. A. D., Anderson, R. R., Blank, I. H., et al. (1978): Enhancement of transmission of optical radiation through human epidermis by topical applications (abstract). In: *Program and Abstracts, 6th Annual Meeting of the American Society for Photobiology, Burlington, Vermont, June 1978*, p. 68.

94. Anderson, R. R., Blank, I. H., and Parrish, J. A. (1979): Mechanisms of increased ultraviolet transmittance through human skin after topical applications (abstract). In: *Program and Abstracts, 7th Annual Meeting of the American Society for Photobiology, Pacific Grove, California, June 1979*, p. 141.

95. Anderson, R. R., LeVine, M. J., and Parrish, J. A. (1980): Selective modification of the optical properties of psoriatic vs. normal skin. In: *Book of Abstracts, 8th International Photobiology Congress, Strasbourg, France, July 1980*, p. 152.

96. LeVine, M. J., White, H. A. D., and Parrish, J. A. (1979): Components of the Goeckerman regimen. *J. Invest. Dermatol.* **73**:170–173.

97. Berns, M. W. (1974): *Biological Microirradiation—Classical and Laser Sources.* Prentice-Hall, Englewood Cliffs, N.J.

98. Goldman, L. (1973): Effects of new laser systems on the skin. *Arch. Dermatol.* **108**:385–390.

99. Rosen, S., Noe, J. M., Kamat, B., et al. (1980): Healing of portwine stain after argon laser therapy. *Arch. Dermatol.*, in press.

100. Noe, J. M., Barsky, S. H., Geer, D. E., et al. (1980): Portwine stains and the response to argon laser therapy: Successful treatment and the predictive role of color, age, and biopsy. *Plast. Reconstr. Surg.* **65**:130–136.

101. Rohsenow, W. M., and Hartnett, J. P. (1973): *Handbook of Heat Transfer*, pp. 3–59. McGraw-Hill, New York.

102. Greenwald, J., Rosen, S., Anderson, R. R., et al. (1981): Comparative histological studies of the tunable dye (at 577 nm) laser and argon laser: the specific vascular effects of the dye laser. *J. Invest. Dermatol.*, **77**:305–310.

7

The Photochemistry and Photobiology of Vitamin D₃

M. F. Holick, J. A. MacLaughlin, J. A. Parrish, and R. R. Anderson

SUNLIGHT AND ITS CURATIVE EFFECTS ON RICKETS

Some historians state that the disease rickets was reported to occur in humans as early as the second century A.D. (1, 2), but the disease was not considered a significant health problem until people began to congregate in the cities of Northern Europe during the Renaissance (1–4). In the mid-17th century, Whistler, DeBoot, and Glisson each independently recognized many of the major diagnostic signs of this disease and established rickets as a clinical entity. They noted that it was associated with deformities of the skeleton, particularly enlargement of the epiphyses at the joints of the long bones and the rib cage (rachitic rosary), enlargement of the head, bending of the spine, curvature of the thighs, and flabby and toneless legs that were usually unable to sustain the weight of the body (1, 3, 4). The incidence of this debilitating bone disease increased dramatically during the industrial revolution, especially in Northern Europe and North America, and, by the latter part of the

M. F. Holick and J. A. MacLaughlin • Department of Medicine, Harvard Medical School, Vitamin D Laboratory and Endocrine Unit, Massachusetts General Hospital, Boston, Massachusetts 02114, and Department of Nutrition and Food Sciences, Massachusetts Institute of Technology, Cambridge, Massachusetts 02139. *J. A. Parrish and R. R. Anderson* • Department of Dermatology, Harvard Medical School, Massachusetts General Hospital, Boston, Massachusetts 02114.

19th century, autopsy studies suggested that approximately 90% of the children raised in the crowded cities of these areas had the disease.

As early as 1822, the Polish physician Sniadecki realized the importance of sun exposure for the prevention and cure of rickets (5). He advocated, "If the parents' financial status permits, it is best to take the children out into the country and keep them as much as possible in the dry, open and pure air. If not, at least they should be carried out in the open air, especially in the sun, the direct action of which on our bodies must be regarded as one of the most efficient methods for the prevention and cure of this disease . . . . Thus strong and obvious is the influence of the sun on the cure of the English disease [i.e., rickets], and the frequent occurrence of the disease in densely populated towns, where the streets are narrow and the dwellings of the working-class people low and very poorly lit." However, little attention was focused on the environment as a cause for this disease until 1889 when an investigative committee of the British Medical Association reported that rickets was unknown in the rural districts of the British Islands but that it was prevalent in the large industrialized towns (6). A year later, Palm (7) collated clinical observations from a number of physicians throughout the British empire and the Orient and reported that, in Great Britain, one of the wealthiest nations in the world, rickets abounded, whereas in India and the Orient, where the people were the poorest and lived in squalor, the disease was rare. In conclusion, he urged the following: "(a) The establishment of a sunshine recorder in the heart of the city to record the chemical activity of the sun's rays rather than its heat, (b) the removal of rachitic children as early as possible from large towns to a locality where sunshine abounds and the air is dry and bracing, (c) the systematic use of sun-baths as a preventive and therapeutic measure in rickets and other diseases, and (d) the education of the public to the appreciation of sunshine as a means of health" (7). These insightful observations and comments set the stage for the birth of modern photo-medicine.

In 1905, Buchholz (8) exposed 16 rachitic children to a carbon-arc light source and suggested that there was a favorable response. In 1919, Huldschin-sky (9) demonstrated unequivocally for the first time that phototherapy alone was curative. He reported four patients with severe rickets who were cured (based on x-ray examination) after being treated with exposures to a mercury-vapor quartz lamp. He also showed that the effect of phototherapy was not local, inasmuch as exposure of one arm had equal and dramatic curative effects on both arms. Two years later, Hess and Unger (10) exposed seven rachitic children in New York to varying periods of sunshine and reported that x-ray examination showed marked improvement in the rickets of each child as evidenced by calcification of the epiphyses. Thus, 32 years after Palm first suggested the systematic use of sunbaths to cure this disease, it was finally shown that sunlight alone had a curative effect on rickets.

ROLE OF DIETARY ADDITIVES AND THEIR CURATIVE
EFFECTS ON RICKETS

By the beginning of the 20th century, rickets was a major health problem in the industrialized cities of Europe and North America. Numerous investigators from almost every field of science began a major effort to define the cause and to find a cure for this dreaded bone disease. The five most popular theories of etiology were: (1) lack of sunshine, (2) a heritable disorder, (3) an infectious disease, (4) a nutritional deficiency, and (5) lack of physical activity. In 1918, Mellanby (11, 12) announced the successful production of rickets in puppies as a result of feeding them a diet that lacked a fat-soluble nutritional factor that would later be known as the antirachitic factor. This observation was the impetus for extensive investigations into food substances that could prevent and cure rickets. Although initially Mellanby noted that the antirachitic factor was similar to, if not identical to, vitamin A, subsequent observations led him to the incorrect conclusion that the antirachitic factor was vitamin A (12).

In 1921, McCollum and colleagues (13) reported the profound influence of dietary phosphorus on the calcification of cartilage and ossification of bone in growing rats. They demonstrated that rats given a diet deficient in phosphorus and the antirachitic factor developed rickets, whereas rats given a diet adequate in calcium and phosphorus but deficient in the antirachitic factor developed osteoporosis but not rickets. With this experimental rachitic model, they reexamined the question of whether the antirachitic factor in cod-liver oil was identical with or distinct from vitamin A. In 1922 these workers (14) oxidized cod-liver oil according to the procedure of Hopkins (15), destroying all of the vitamin A activity, and showed that the oxidized oil retained its antirachitic properties. Thus it became clear that the antirachitic factor present in cod-liver oil was not vitamin A but a new vitamin later to be called vitamin D.

The great confusion over whether rickets was cured by ultraviolet (UV) irradiation or by a dietary factor was resolved when Powers et al. (16) reported that radiation from a mercury-vapor quartz lamp had similar, if not identical, healing effects in rachitic rats when compared with those brought about by administration of cod-liver oil. At first it was believed that the UV radiation effects on the body resulted in the mobilization of the fat-soluble antirachitic factor from the tissue stores rather than in a direct photosynthesis of the vitamin in the body (17). Steenbock and Black (18, 19) used rachitic rats that had been fed livers from other rachitic rats exposed to UV radiation or kept in the dark, and showed that livers from nonirradiated rats were less effective than livers from irradiated rats in promoting growth. These workers also found that exposure of rat liver and muscle to UV radiation imparted growth and bone calcification properties when the tissue was subsequently fed to rachitic rats. Furthermore, they found that UV irradiation of the diet also imparted antirachitic properties. Simultaneously it was reported (20) that UV irradiation of olive, cotton, and linseed oils, milk cream, human serum, growing wheat, and green lettuce leaves endowed each with antirachitic properties.

These observations demonstrating the production of the antirachitic factor in vitro outside the living organism bridged a gap in understanding the nutritional antirachitic factor and the antirachitic properties of direct exposure to either sunlight or UV radiation and paved the way for the isolation and structural characterization of the antirachitic vitamin a decade later.

ISOLATION AND STRUCTURAL CHARACTERIZATION OF VITAMIN D

Once it was established that the antirachitic factor could be produced in vitro by the UV irradiation of plant and animal tissues, many investigators concluded that the substance that was activated by UV radiation was cholesterol (21) in animals and phytosterol in vegetable foods. However, cholesterol lost the property of becoming antirachitic when it was purified by chemical means (22). Furthermore, bromination and oxidation of cholesterol rendered it inert to UV radiation and eliminated its UV absorption band at 280 nm. It was concluded that the precursor of vitamin D (called provitamin D) was not cholesterol itself but a substance associated with it (23). The findings that ergosterol, a yeast sterol, had an intense UV absorption band at 280 nm (which was similar to the UV absorption maximum for the cholesterol-like sterol) and that this yeast sterol could be rendered antirachitic by exposure to UV radiation suggested that the parent substance of vitamin D was either ergosterol or a highly unsaturated sterol similar to ergosterol.

Numerous investigators irradiated ergosterol in an attempt to photo-synthesize enough vitamin D to determine its structure. Reerink and van Wijk (24) and Askew et al. (25) purified vitamin D and reported almost identical UV absorption spectra with λ_{max} at 265 and 262 nm, respectively. Initial characterization of vitamin D established that the structure retained the secondary hydroxy group of the parent ergosterol, that ring B was opened at the C_9—C_{10} position (Fig. 7-1), and that three double bonds existed in the ring system. [For an excellent review of the complex chemical derivations and structural analyses by numerous investigators, see Fieser and Fieser (26)]. Finally, in 1948 (27), by x-ray crystal analysis of a heavy-atom derivative of vitamin D_2, the spatial orientation of the vitamin D molecule was determined as outlined in Fig. 7-1.

At first, the vitamin D that was isolated by the irradiation of ergosterol

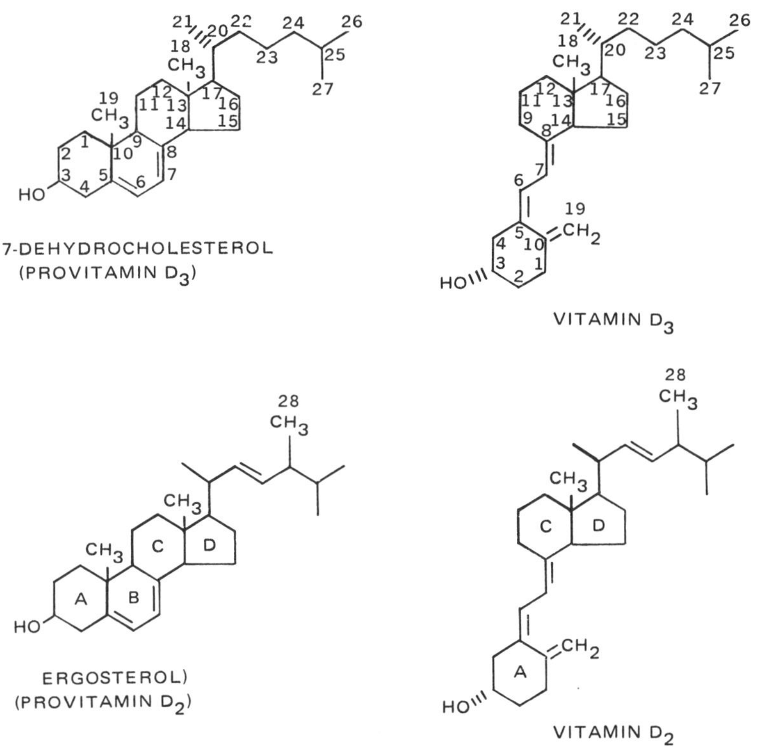

Fig. 7-1. Structures for 7-dehydrocholesterol, ergosterol, vitamin D_3, and vitamin D_2.

was designated vitamin D_1. However, it was quickly realized that the product obtained was an impure mixture, and the term was dropped. Final purification of the vitamin D from its parent ergosterol was achieved and was named ergocalciferol (vitamin D_2) (24–26, 28, 29). Initially, it was believed that vitamin D_2 was identical to the vitamin D that was present in fish-liver oils and was produced in the skin by sunlight exposure. However, a number of investigators (30–32) presented biologic evidence that vitamin D_2 (isolated from irradiated ergosterol solutions) was not the same compound that was isolated from UV-irradiated solutions of cholesterol (which was contaminated with 7-dehydrocholesterol). They based their conclusion on studies that showed that UV-irradiated solutions of cholesterol had marked biologic activity in chickens, whereas irradiated solutions of ergosterol possessed minimum antirachitic activity in this species. At the same time Windaus et al. (33) reported the synthesis of a new vitamin D that was made by exposing 7-dehydrocholesterol (Fig. 7-1) to UV radiation. This new vitamin D, called cholecalciferol (vitamin D_3), was shown to have equal antirachitic activity in the chick and the rat and to be identical in structure to the vitamin D isolated from fish-liver oils and skin (34). Therefore it was concluded that 7-dehydrocholesterol rather than ergosterol was the parent compound present in skin and the photoproduct that resulted was vitamin D_3.

PHOTOCHEMISTRY OF VITAMIN D

In the 1930s, it was established that the parent structure, or the provitamin of vitamin D_2 and vitamin D_3, was composed of a four-member ring steroid structure with a side chain (ergosterol or 7-dehydrocholesterol) and two conjugated double bonds at C_5 and C_7 ($\Delta^{5,7}$-diene) in the B ring (Fig. 7-1). Furthermore, it became evident that vitamin D (the designation of vitamin D without a subscript means vitamin D_3 and/or vitamin D_2 interchangeably) is not the only compound that results from UV irradiation of the parent $\Delta^{5,7}$-diene sterol. Reerink and van Wijk (24) reported that the photochemical reaction of ergosterol is dependent on the wavelength as well as the time of exposure. Windaus and co-workers conducted numerous experiments to elucidate the sequence of photochemical reactions that leads to vitamin D. They concluded that during UV irradiation the following sequence of reactions occurs: ergosterol $\rightarrow$ lumisterol$_2$ $\rightarrow$ tachysterol$_2$ $\rightarrow$ vitamin D_2. However in 1949, Velluz et al. (35) made the startling observation that vitamin D_2 is not a photoproduct of ergosterol. Irradiation of ergosterol at temperatures below $10°C$ resulted in a compound that these workers isolated, characterized, and called previtamin D_2. They also demonstrated that previtamin D_2 was thermally labile and underwent a thermally induced isomerization of the triene system to form vitamin D_2 (35). This reaction was later characterized as an intramolecular [1—7] hydrogen shift from $(CH_3)_{19}$ to $(CH)_9$ (36), followed by a rearrangement of the 6,7-cis-triene to the 5,6-cis-triene for vitamin D_2 (Fig. 7-2).

During the past 30 years, principally through the efforts of Havinga and collaborators, the principal sequence of photochemical and thermal events leading to the formation of vitamin D is now well documented. Upon UV irradiation, the $\Delta^{5,7}$-diene sterol (such as 7-dehydrocholesterol) absorbs a quantum of radiation energy, transforming the ground state to an excited singlet state that may undergo ring opening at C_9—C_{10} to yield a 6,7-cis-hexatriene derivative, previtamin D. Previtamin D then undergoes a non-photochemical, temperature-dependent isomerization to the more thermo-dynamically stable 5,6-cis isomer, vitamin D, in an equilibrium reaction. Previtamin D can also absorb UV radiation and undergo either (1) ring closure, to form the parent compound (7-dehydrocholesterol), or its stereo-isomer, lumisterol; or (2) isomerization of its triene chromaphore to form tachysterol. Upon continued irradiation, a "quasi" photoequilibrium state is reached, as illustrated in Figure 7-2 (37).

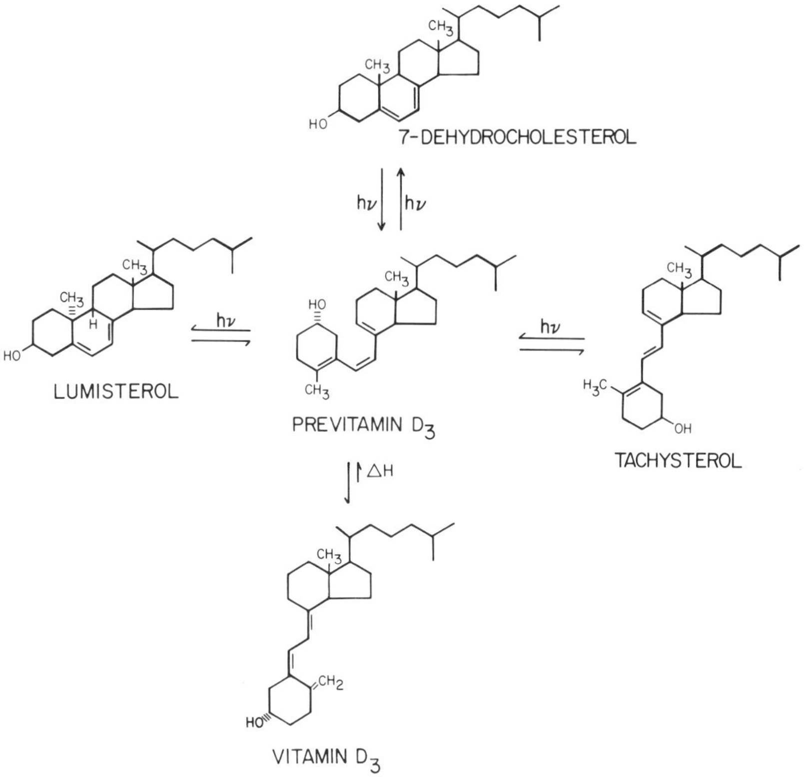

Fig. 7-2. In vitro photoconversion of 7-dehydrocholesterol to previtamin D₃, lumisterol₃, and tachysterol₃. Previtamin D₃ is converted to vitamin D₃ by thermal energy. [Reproduced from Holick et al. (47) with permission.]

It was noted in 1929 that when ergosterol was exposed to UV irradiation for prolonged periods, the resultant reaction mixture was devoid of biologic activity (24). There are a remarkable number of additional photoproducts of previtamin D and tachysterol, called toxisterols (38)—at least 13 have been reported so far—and, under continued irradiation, vitamin D isomerizes to photoproducts called suprasterols (37), of which six major representatives are known (Fig. 7-3). Both groups of photoisomers are believed to be devoid of biologic activity.

THE EFFECT OF WAVELENGTH ON THE PHOTOCHEMICAL REACTIONS OF Δ⁵,⁷-DIENE STEROLS

The recognition that UV radiation from either artificial sources or sunlight was an important therapeutic agent prompted many investigators to

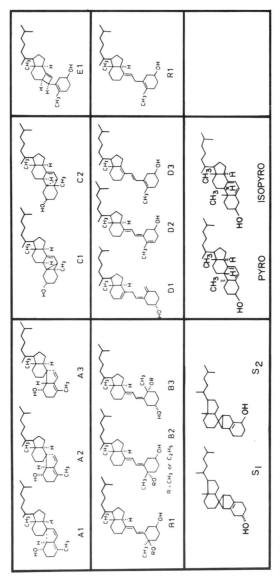

Fig. 7-3. Structures for toxisterols (A_1, A_2, A_3, B_1, B_2, B_3, C_1, C_2, D_1, D_2, D_3, E_1, R_1), suprasterols (S_1, S_2), and isopyrovitamin D_3 (isopyro) and pyrovitamin D_3 (pyro).

examine the effectiveness of specific wavelengths in the cure and prevention of rickets. In 1922, Hess et al. (39) noted that when rachitic rats were placed in a box containing flint-glass windows, the sun's rays lost their antirachitic activity. They interposed various filters in front of a mercury-quartz lamp and exposed rachitic rats to the filtered radiation. No antirachitic activity was noted in rats exposed to radiation filtered through window glass that transmits wavelengths of 334 nm and longer, whereas rats exposed to filtered wavelengths 313 nm and shorter demonstrated marked healing of rickets. It was concluded that wavelengths effective in producing antirachitic activity lie in the UV spectral region of wavelengths shorter than 313 nm. At first it was believed that the quantity of radiant energy necessary to form vitamin D by irradiation of ergosterol with monochromatic radiation was constant for wavelengths between 256 and 293 nm (40). However, in 1929, Reerink and van Wijk (24) reported that when a solution of ergosterol was exposed to wavelengths longer than 275 nm, a series of products was obtained that differed from those obtained when an ergosterol solution was irradiated with monochromatic radiation at 254 nm. Bunker and Harris (41) exposed depilitated rats to monochromatic radiation and determined the amount of energy required at various wavelengths to produce an antirachitic response. Their data demonstrated that 297 nm was the most efficient wavelength to cure rickets. A year later, Knudson and Benford (42) conducted similar experiments and concluded that wavelengths 265, 280, 289, 297, 302, and 312 nm were effective in curing rickets, but that monochromatic radiation at 280 nm was the most effective wavelength. In 1940, Bunker et al. (43) reported the relative antirachitic activity of solutions of 7-dehydrocholesterol exposed to equal quanta of various wavelengths of UV radiation. The products from the irradiation of 7-dehydrocholesterol were fed to rachitic rats, and the antirachitic response was then measured. They concluded that the photo-chemical activation of 7-dehydrocholesterol by monochromatic radiation at 248, 253, 265, 280, and 302 nm was substantially uniform per quantum of energy applied. However, the activation at 297 nm was significantly greater than at other wavelengths examined, and there was no antirachitic activity in the solutions irradiated at 313 nm.

The development of chromatographic systems that permit the separation of the various photoproducts from their parent sterol has permitted a detailed analysis of the effect of wavelength on the component photoproducts produced. Kobayashi and Yasumura (44) irradiated a solution of ergosterol (1 mg/ml ethanol) with monochromatic radiation at wavelengths between 230 and 400 nm. Immediately after irradiation, the reaction mixture was derivatized to the corresponding trimethylsilyl ether derivatives and then separated by gas–liquid chromatography. However, because previtamin D and vitamin D pyrolyze at temperatures above 200°C to form two products, pyrovitamin D and isopyrovitamin D (45) (see Fig. 7-3 for structures), these

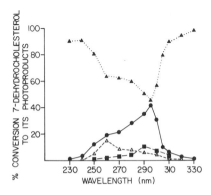

Fig. 7-4. Percent conversion of 7-dehydrocho-
lesterol ($\cdots \blacktriangle \cdots$) to previtamin D₃ (-●-),
tachysterol (- -△- -), and lumisterol (-■-) as a
function of wavelength. 7-Dehydrocholesterol
was dissolved in tetrahydrofuran ($10 \ \mu g \ ml^{-1}$)
and exposed to UV radiation ($0.2 \ J \ cm^{-2}$) at
various wavelengths with a 10-nm half-band-
width. This radiation was obtained from a 2.5-
kW xenon–mercury arc lamp coupled to a
holographic grating monochromator (HL-300,
Jobin Yvon).

experimenters notes that they could determine only the amount of isopyrovitamin D₂ and pyrovitamin D₂ in the gas–liquid chromatograms, and called
the sum of the two products "potential vitamin D₂." Using these techniques,
they concluded that vitamin D₂ could be formed when ergosterol was exposed
to monochromatic radiation at wavelengths as short as 230 nm and as long as
330 nm, but that 295 nm gave the highest yields per quantum of energy
applied. Furthermore, the maximum yield of "potential vitamin D₂" that was
obtained when ergosterol was exposed to 295-nm radiation was about 33%
and further increases in exposure had the effect of decreasing the yield.

Using high-pressure liquid chromatography at room temperature, Holick
et al. (46, 47) developed a method of separating the individual photoproducts
without altering their structures by either chemical derivatization or heat-
induced pyrolization. Solutions of 7-dehydrocholesterol (either 10 μg/ml or 1
mg/ml of tetrahydrofuran) were exposed to the same energy of monochromatic radiation at 10-nm intervals between 240 and 330 nm. Previtamin
D₃ was formed over the entire range, with 295 nm being the most efficient
waveband (Fig. 7-4). Lumisterol₃ and tachysterol₃ were also formed over this
range of radiation, but they were less in amount and had different action
spectra. Maximum tachysterol₃ formation occurs at about 260 nm, whereas
maximum lumisterol formation was most favored at 310 nm (Fig. 7-4).

PHOTOBIOLOGY OF VITAMIN D₃ IN SKIN

Soon after Huldschinsky (9) clearly established that exposure of skin to
the radiation from a mercury-vapor quartz lamp had a therapeutic effect that
could cure rickets and that this benefit was not a local effect, Hess (48)
reported that rats fed UV-radiated cadaver or surgically obtained skin
samples were protected from developing rickets. There was considerable
debate regarding the origin of 7-dehydrocholesterol from which vitamin D₃
was synthesized during exposure of skin to UV radiation. At first it was

believed that 7-dehydrocholesterol was deposited on the surface of the skin in sebum and, when exposed to sunlight, partially converted to vitamin D_3. Once formed on the skin, it was thought that it was absorbed through the skin or licked off and ingested (49). However, Reinertson and Wheatly (50) demonstrated that the highest concentration of 7-dehydrocholesterol was found in the malpighian layer of the epidermis, with only trace amounts in the stratum corneum, and thereby established that the major source of the provitamin was within the epidermis rather than on the surface.

However, because of the multitude of neutral and nonsaponifiable lipids in the skin, little information has been available regarding the mechanism by which vitamin D_3 is made in skin during exposure to the sun. In 1969, Rauschkolb et al. (51) reported the isolation and identification of vitamin D_3 from human cadaver skin. Abdominal skin was separated from subcutaneous fat tissue, saponified, and extracted. Gas–liquid chromatographic analysis demonstrated the two pyrolyzed products of vitamin D_3. Okano et al. (52) and Esvelt et al. (53) saponified rat skin that had been exposed to UV radiation, made lipid extracts, and, after several chromatographic procedures, demonstrated the presence of vitamin D_3. Because saponification was used for purification, any thermally labile intermediate photoproducts such as previtamin D_3 were isomerized.

Petrova et al. (54) reported the first evidence that previtamin D_3 is synthesized in vivo. These workers injected $[22,23\text{-}^3\text{H}]$7-dehydrocholesterol intravenously in previously shaved rats, which, 1.5 hr later, were exposed to UV radiation. Chromatographic analyses of lipid extracts from the whole skin demonstrated the presence of radiolabeled previtamin D_3. However, it was unclear whether the $[22,23\text{-}^3\text{H}]$7-dehydrocholesterol was in the epidermis or present only in the dermal capillary bed. Holick et al. (55–57) synthesized $[3\alpha\text{-}^3\text{H}]$7-dehydrocholesterol (Fig. 7-5) and topically applied this isotope to previously shaven vitamin D-deficient rats. Twenty-four hours after application, groups of animals were exposed to 0.2 J cm^{-2} of UV radiation (F40-T12 Westinghouse sunlamp, broadband 253–400 nm, maximum at 315 nm) and

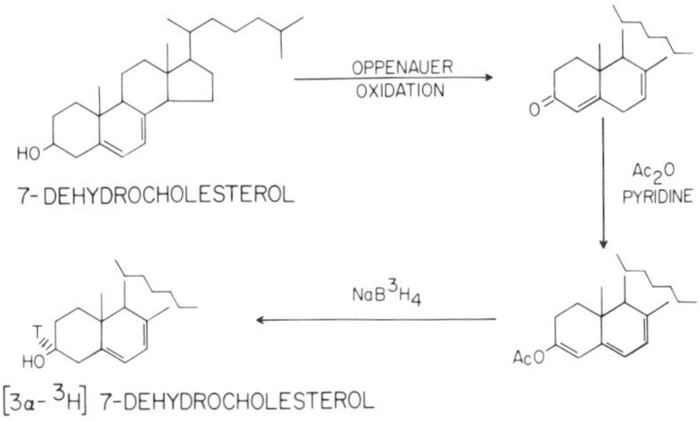

Fig. 7-5. Chemical synthesis of $[3\alpha\text{-}^3\text{H}]$ 7-DEHYDROCHOLESTEROL
$[3\alpha\text{-}^3\text{H}]$ 7-dehydrocholesterol.

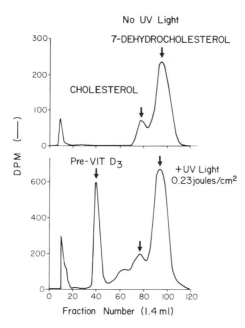

Fig. 7-6. Neodox 1518 Sephadex column (1×60 cm packed in 19:1 n-hexane: chloroform) profiles of skin lipid extracts from animals treated with topical application of 2 μCi [3α-^{3}H] 7-dehydrocholesterol and then killed 24 hr later (top) or irradiated with 0.23 J cm^{-2} and then killed (bottom). [Reproduced from Holick et al. (56) with permission.]

the irradiated skin was excised, extracted, and chromatographed. Lipid extracts from the skin of control (unirradiated) animals contained 7-dehydrocholesterol and its reduction product, cholesterol (Fig. 7-6, top). Skin from exposed animals exhibited radiolabeled 7-dehydrocholesterol, cholesterol, and an additional major compound identified as previtamin D$_3$ (Fig. 7-6, bottom). To be certain that this observation was not due only to the photoconversion of radiolabeled 7-dehydrocholesterol on the stratum corneum surface but also occurred intraepidermally, 40 vitamin D-deficient rats were exposed to 0.2 J cm^{-2} of UV irradiation, and the whole skin was immediately excised and extracted in organic solvents. All the purification steps were carried out at 4° C to ensure that any thermally labile photoproduct would not be altered during the extraction and chromatography procedures. After numerous chromatographic procedures, previtamin D$_3$ was isolated in pure form and identified based upon its (a) UV absorption spectrum, λ_{max} 260 and λ_{min} 230 nm, which is characteristic for the 6,7-cis-triene chromophore of the previtamin D, (b) mass spectrum, m/e 384 (M$^+$), 271 (M$^+$ − side chain), 253 (271 − H$_2$O), 136 [ring A + (HC)$_6$, (HC)$_7$, and (H$_2$C)$_{19}$], and 118 (136 − H$_2$O), and (c) subsequent thermally controlled conversion to vitamin D$_3$, as demonstrated by spectral shift in its UV absorption from λ_{max} 260 nm to λ_{max} 265 nm and an almost doubling of its extinction coefficient (Fig. 7-7). To determine whether any vitamin D$_3$ was formed in the skin simultaneously with previtamin D$_3$ during exposure to UV radiation, tracer quantities of [3α-^{3}H]-vitamin D$_3$ were added to the same rat-skin extract (kept at 4° C), and the lipid

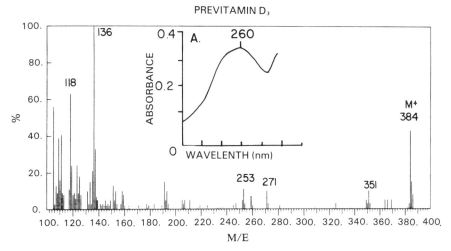

Fig. 7-7. Mass spectrum of previtamin D₃ isolated from rat skin after it was thermally converted to vitamin D₃. Ultraviolet absorption spectrum of previtamin D₃ isolated from rat skin (inset). [Reproduced from Holick et al. (57) with permission.]

fraction that comigrated with the $[3\alpha\text{-}^{3}H]$vitamin D₃ was exhaustively purified. There was no detectable vitamin D₃ present in the skin. Furthermore, a careful analysis of the rat-skin lipid extract did not demonstrate significant quantities of either lumisterol₃ or tachysterol₃ (57). In human skin exposed to UV radiation, the principal photoproduct is also previtamin D₃ (46, 47).

PHYSIOLOGY OF VITAMIN D₃ SYNTHESIS IN THE SKIN

The thermal isomerization of previtamin D₃ to vitamin D₃ has been studied in vitro to determine the time course of this thermal equilibrium reaction at various temperatures, including those that approximate the temperature of the epidermis (46, 47). At 25°C, previtamin D₃ slowly equilibrates to vitamin D₃, with 50% conversion occurring in approximately 48 hr and equilibrium reached in approximately 14 days, with 83% of previtamin D₃ converting to vitamin D₃ (Fig. 7-8). In comparison, at 37°C, 50% conversion occurs by 28 hr and equilibrium is reached after 4 days, whereas at −20°C less than 2% of the previtamin is converted to vitamin D₃ even after 7 days' incubation (Fig. 7-8). These analyses of the temperature and time dependence of this conversion process suggest that, at physiologic temperature, vitamin D₃ synthesis can occur over several days, even in the absence of further exposure to UV radiation (46, 47).

Holick et al. (46, 47, 58) investigated the possibility that there was a transport system that would preferentially remove vitamin D₃ from the skin as

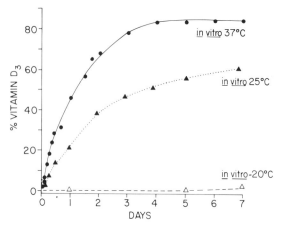

Fig. 7-8. Thermal conversion of previtamin D₃ to vitamin D₃ as a function of time at 37° C (-●-), 25° C (· · ·▲· · ·), and −20° C (- -△- -). [Reproduced from Holick et al. (47) with permission.]

it was being made, leaving behind previtamin D_3 to continue its thermal isomerization to vitamin D_3. The binding affinity of the plasma vitamin D binding protein (an α_1-globulin that is believed to be important for the transport of vitamin D_3 and its metabolites in the circulation) for previtamin D_3, lumisterol₃, tachysterol₃, and vitamin D_3 was determined. This protein has essentially no affinity for previtamin D_3 compared with its affinity for vitamin D_3 (Fig. 7-9) (46, 47, 58). The physiologic advantage of the formation of previtamin D_3 in the skin during exposure to the sun and the role of the vitamin D binding protein in the processing of the thermal product of the previtamin are illustrated schematically in Fig. 7-10. During exposure to sunlight, the UVB (290–310 nm) portion of the solar spectrum produces the photochemical conversion of epidermal 7-dehydrocholesterol to previtamin D_3. As soon as previtamin D_3 is made in the skin, it begins to isomerize to vitamin D_3, the rate of the reaction being controlled by the temperature of the

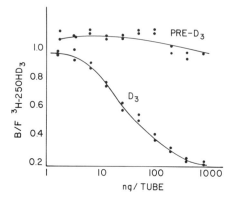

Fig. 7-9. Displacement of ³H-25-hydroxy-vitamin D₃ (³H-25-OH-D₃) from rat vitamin D binding protein by vitamin D₃ (D₃) and previtamin D₃ (pre-D₃). [Reproduced from Holick et al. (47) with permission.]

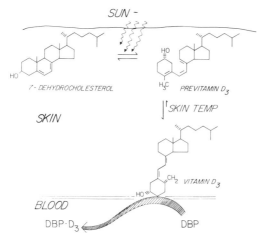

Fig. 7-10. Diagrammatic representation of the formation of previtamin D₃ in the skin during sun exposure and its subsequent thermal conversion to vitamin D₃, which in turn binds to the plasma vitamin D binding protein for transport into the circulation. [Reproduced from Holick et al. (47) with permission.]

skin. Once vitamin D₃ is formed from its precursor, it is preferentially bound to the vitamin D binding protein in the capillaries and transported into the circulation. Thus the skin is the site for the synthesis of provitamin D₃, a reservoir for the storage of the primary photoproduct, previtamin D₃, and the site for the slow thermal conversion to vitamin D₃. The slow thermal conversion to vitamin D₃ and the selective removal of vitamin D₃ by the vitamin D binding protein permit the efficient use of small quantities of previtamin D₃ that are generated in the skin during sun exposure.

Reinertson and Wheatley (50) suggested that the malpighian layer of the epidermis is the major site for vitamin D₃ synthesis; however, there have been no experimental data available to precisely locate where vitamin D₃ synthesis occurs in the epidermis and dermis. Using techniques that separate layers of epidermis without altering the stratum corneum barrier or disrupting the integrity of the cells, Holick et al. (47, 58) recently examined this issue. To determine whether previtamin D₃ could be synthesized in the layers of epidermis below the stratum corneum and stratum granulosum, surgically obtained Caucasian skin was incubated with staphylococcal exfoliatin, a substance produced by phage-infected staphylococci. Exfoliatin causes the skin to separate between the stratum granulosum and stratum malpighii without any known alterations in structure or function of the cells and is one cause of toxic epidermal necrolysis (59). After incubation, the skin was either exposed to 1.0 J cm⁻² of UVB or kept in the dark. Immediately after UVB exposure, the top layer (stratum corneum plus stratum granulosum) was removed as a single sheet. Separate lipid extracts of the upper layer and

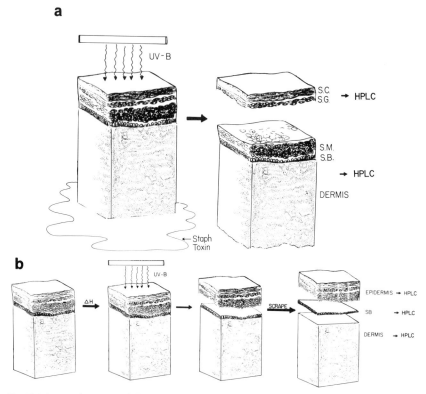

Fig. 7-11. (a) Diagrammatic illustration of the separation of the stratum corneum and stratum granulosum from the rest of the epidermis and dermis by toxin treatment. (b) Diagrammatic illustration of the separation of the skin into the epidermis minus stratum basalis, and stratum basalis plus dermis, by a heat separation technique.

bottom layer (malpighian layer plus dermis) were obtained and chromato-graphed on a high-pressure liquid chromatograph (Fig. 7-11a). Other surgically obtained human-skin samples were immersed in water at 60° C for 45 sec, according to the procedure of Scheuplein (60), blotted dry, and subsequently exposed to UVB or kept in the dark. The hot water immersion makes it possible to later separate skin samples into two sections: the top (entire epidermis minus basal layer) and bottom (entire dermis plus basal layer). The basal layer was mechanically scraped from the bottom section, and the three isolated layers were extracted and chromatographed on a high-pressure liquid chromatograph (Fig. 7-11b). The chromatograms demon-strate that although previtamin D_3 synthesis occurs throughout the entire epidermis, the basal layer and the malpighian layer had the highest concentration of previtamin D_3 (47, 58). Furthermore, there is also a small amount of previtamin D_3 produced in the dermis.

THE INFLUENCE OF SUNLIGHT ON THE SYNTHESIS AND METABOLISM OF VITAMIN D_3

There are several excellent reviews of new developments regarding the metabolism of vitamin D, to which the reader is referred (61–64). During the past decade, investigations into vitamin D metabolism have led to the conclusion that vitamin D (the designation of vitamin D metabolites without a subscript means vitamin D_2 and/or vitamin D_3 metabolites interchangeably) is a hormone and not a vitamin (because this secosteroid requires activation in two separate organs before it is transported to its target tissues to induce a biologic response). Once vitamin D_3 is made in the skin or ingested in the diet, it, along with dietary vitamin D_2, enters the circulation and both are transported on the vitamin D binding protein to the liver, where they are hydroxylated on C_{25} to form 25-hydroxyvitamin D (25-OH-D). Then 25-OH-D is subsequently transported to the kidney, where hydroxylation on either C_{24} or C_1 (Fig. 7-12) occurs. It is generally believed that when there is a demand for an increase in the absorption of intestinal calcium, the secretion of parathyroid hormone increases. This peptide hormone, in addition to acting on mineral metabolism in the bone and kidney, also acts physiologically as a trophic hormone to increase the renal metabolism of 25-OH-D to the more metabolically active $1\alpha,25$-dihydroxyvitamin D [$1\alpha,25$-(OH)₂-D]. The $1\alpha,25$-(OH)₂-D is transported to the small intestine, where it stimulates absorption of intestinal calcium, and to the bone, where, in conjunction with parathyroid hormone, it mobilizes bone calcium. When there is less demand for intestinal calcium absorption, 25-OH-D is metabolized to 24,25-dihydroxyvitamin D [24,25-(OH)₂-D]. At present, little is known about the physiologic role of this metabolite, but recent evidence suggests that it may be important for fetal bone growth and development (61).

At the turn of this century, rickets was recognized as a seasonal disease, with the number of cases peaking in early spring and diminishing in early summer. Hess and Lundagen (65) correlated these observations to plasma phosphate levels and noted that they were at their lowest in March and then gradually increased to peak levels in June. It became evident that these occurrences were a result of the seasonal variation in the intensity of the sun's spectrum combined with the area of uncovered skin exposed to sunshine, thus allowing the consequent synthesis of vitamin D_3.

Bekemeier and Pfennigsdorf (66) estimated that 1 cm² of human skin can produce up to 18 IU (1 International Unit = 0.025 μg) of vitamin D_3 bioactivity during 1.5–3 hr of exposure to UV radiation. There is, however, little information on the blood levels of vitamin D_3 as a result of exposure to the sun. Because 25-OH-D₃ is the major circulating metabolite of vitamin D_3 and the concentrations of this metabolite correlate with dietary intake of vitamin D_3, many investigators have measured the circulating levels of this

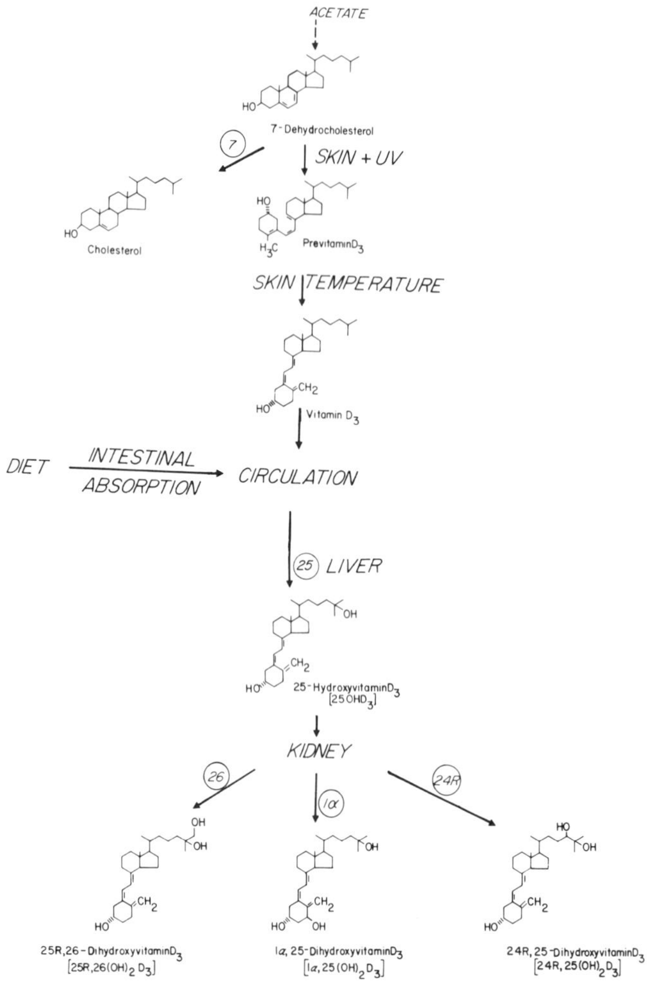

Fig. 7-12. The photochemical, thermal, and metabolic pathways for vitamin D₃. Circled letters and numbers denote specific enzymes: 7 = 7-dehydrocholesterol reductase; 25 = vitamin-D-25-hydroxylase; 1α = 25-OH-D-1α-hydroxylase; 24R = 25-OH-D-24R-hydroxylase; 26 = 25-OH-D-26-hydroxylase.

metabolite during a variety of environmental conditions and demonstrated that serum 25-OH-D₃ levels reflect directly upon the cutaneous synthesis of vitamin D₃. Preece et al. (67) and Fairney et al. (68) reported a marked lowering of serum 25-OH-D levels in submariners and in one antarctic explorer during prolonged periods of lack of sunshine, whereas Haddad and Chyu (69) observed that lifeguards on the beach have almost a doubling in their serum 25-OH-D levels (normal range is 5–80 ng ml^{-1}). There is now strong evidence in both children and adults that serum 25-OH-D levels vary with the season, with the peak levels occurring in the summer, when exposure to the sun and the intensity of UV radiation are maximized, and the lowest levels occurring in the middle of winter, when exposure to the sun and the intensity of UV radiation are minimized. The contribution of cutaneous production of vitamin D_3 in preventing osteomalacia and rickets relative to the dietary intake of either vitamin D_2 or vitamin D_3 has been the subject of much examination. In the British Isles, where vitamin D supplementation of foods is not practiced, the cutaneous photosynthesis of previtamin D_3 is quite important. In the United States, however, dietary supplementation is widely practiced, and the role of cutaneous previtamin D_3 synthesis for maintenance of calcium homeostasis is less significant. Neer et al. (70) compared serum 25-OH-D levels in groups of adult males who either worked primarily indoors (telephone switchmen and office workers) or primarily outdoors (telephone linemen and installers) in six cities across the United States at intervals of 6 weeks after the summer and winter solstices, and soon after the vernal and autumnal equinoxes. Although all of the serum levels of 25-OH-D were within the normal range of between 15 and 80 ng ml^{-1}, at every season, the blood 25-OH-D levels were 10–15 ng ml^{-1} lower in the indoor workers. The conclusion from this study was that the significant determinants of blood 25-OH-D levels in normal adult men are: geography $>$ individual variation $>$ occupational exposure to sun $>$ season of the year.

Unlike serum 25-OH-D and 24,25-$(OH)_2$-D levels, which vary according to environmental exposure to the sun, serum 1,25-$(OH)_2$-D levels do not appear to change significantly with a change in season, probably because the synthesis of this metabolite is tightly regulated by many ionic and hormonal factors (61–64).

THE ROLE OF SKIN PIGMENTATION IN THE CUTANEOUS PRODUCTION OF VITAMIN D₃

In the early 1920s, Hess (71) suggested that one of the factors that would influence the antirachitic potency of sunlight is the amount of skin pigment (melanin). He subjected six white and six black rats to a minimal protective dose of UV radiation and noted that only the black rats developed rickets. These observations correlated with the clinical observations that black infants were more susceptible to rickets than white infants from the same socio-economic environment. Kramer et al. (72) and Levinsohn (73) disputed this concept. They treated black and white rachitic children with equal doses of UV radiation and concluded that pigmentation did not retard the antirachitic effect of UV radiation. However, as noted by these investigators, they used more than the minimum effective dose of UV radiation and thus they could not discriminate between small differences.

In 1967, Loomis (74) popularized the thesis that skin depigmentation evolved for the purpose of increasing the cutaneous photosynthesis of vitamin D_3 as humans migrated successively north and south of the equator. He suggested that in the southern latitudes, hypopigmentation of the skin allows maximum penetration of UV radiation for maximum vitamin D_3 synthesis, whereas near and at the equator, heavily pigmented skin allows minimum penetration of UV radiation through the stratum corneum and thus controls vitamin D_3 photosynthesis and prevents an overproduction of vitamin D_3 that would lead to vitamin D_3 toxicity. Beadle (75) agreed that, theoretically, production of vitamin D_3 in heavily pigmented skin is diminished when compared with nonpigmented skin, but calculated that the difference is about 60% rather than 90–95%, as suggested by Loomis.

Our new understanding of the cutaneous photochemical events regarding vitamin D_3 production reveals that additional variables are involved in such calculations and that they probably invalidate many of the conclusions reached by these two authors. When human skin is exposed to a simulated UVB sun spectrum of 0.01–0.05 J cm^{-2}, approximately 1–10% of the epidermal 7-dehydrocholesterol converts primarily to previtamin D_3. When the exposure dose is increased to above 0.5 J cm^{-2} of UVB irradiation, the previtamin D_3 that is initially formed absorbs UVB radiation and photo-isomerizes to lumisterol$_3$ and tachysterol$_3$, which are biologically inert. Furthermore, because previtamin D_3 needs up to 4 days to reach thermal equilibrium with vitamin D_3, only small quantities of vitamin D_3 are released into the circulation at any one time, making it less likely that very high levels of vitamin D_3 can be achieved in the serum at any one time. Probably the most important factor that would prevent vitamin D_3 toxicity (if, in fact, excessive production of vitamin D_3 in the skin can be achieved) is cascading metabolic events that are required before vitamin D becomes biologically active. Although the hepatic 25-hydroxylation is not well controlled, the subsequent renal 1α-hydroxylation is tightly regulated.

SUMMARY

The concept that exposure to sunlight causes the formation of vitamin D_3 in the skin is well established. Until recently, however, very little was known about the sequential events involved in the photoproduction of vitamin D_3 in the skin and, once it is made, how it is transferred from the skin into the circulation. When skin is exposed to UV radiation, the 7-dehydrocholesterol stores in the epidermis (mainly in the malpighian layer) undergo a photochemical reaction and convert to previtamin D_3. Once formed, the previtamin in the skin undergoes a nonphotochemical temperature-dependent isomerization to vitamin D_3. At physiologic temperatures (in warm-blooded animals and humans), this thermal equilibrium reaction requires several days before ~80% of the previtamin D₃ is converted to vitamin D₃. Vitamin D₃ is then preferentially transported from the epidermis into the circulation by the plasma vitamin D binding protein.

The development of new extraction procedures, skin-layer separation methods, and chromatographic techniques that permit the direct analysis of skin lipid extracts for 7-dehydrocholesterol and its photoproducts should be helpful in the future in determining (1) the in vivo production rates for previtamin D₃, (2) what role, if any, melanin has on previtamin D₃ formation, and (3) what factors other than melanin limit the cutaneous synthesis of vitamin D₃.

REFERENCES

1. Mettler, C. C. (1947): *History of Medicine*, pp. 720–723. Blakiston, Philadelphia.
2. Foote, J. A. (1927): Evidence of rickets prior to 1650. *Am. J. Dis. Child.* **34**:443–452.
3. Griffenhagen, G. (1952): A brief history of nutritional diseases. II. Rickets. *Bull. Natl. Inst. Nutr.* **2**(9):1–2.
4. Guthrie, D. (1946): In: *A History of Medicine*, p. 69. Lippincott, Philadelphia.
5. Sniadecki, J. (1840). [Cited by W. Mozolowski: Jedrzej Sniadecki (1768–1883) on the cure of rickets. *Nature* **143**:121 (1939).]
6. Owen, I. (1889): Geographical distribution of rickets, acute and subacute rheumatism, chorea, cancer and urinary calculus in the British Islands. *Br. Med. J.* **1**:113–116.
7. Palm, T. A. (1890): The geographic distribution and etiology of rickets. *Practitioner* **45**:270–279, 321–342.
8. Park, E. A. (1923): The etiology of rickets. *Physiol. Rev.* **3**:106–159.
9. Huldschinsky, K. (1919): Heilung von Rachitis durch künstliche Höhensonne. *Detsch. Med. Wochenschr.* **14**:712–713.
10. Hess A. F., and Unger, L. J. (1921): Cure of infantile rickets by sunlight. *J. A.M.A.* **77**:39.
11. Mellanby, E. (1918): The part played by an "accessory factor" in the production of experimental rickets. *J. Physiol.* **52**:11–14.
12. Mellanby, E. (1919): An experimental investigation on rickets. *Lancet* **1**:407–412.
13. McCollum, E. V., Simmonds, N., Shipley, P. G., et al. (1921): Studies on experimental rickets. The production of rickets by diets low in phosphorus and fat-soluble A. *J. Biol. Chem.* **47**:507–527.
14. McCollum, E. V., Simmonds, N., Becker, J. E., et al. (1922): Studies on experimental rickets. An experimental demonstration of the existence of a vitamin which promotes calcium deposition. *J. Biol. Chem.* **53**:293–312.
15. Hopkins, F. G. (1920): The effects of heat and aeration upon the fat-soluble vitamin. *Biochem. J.* **14**:725–730.
16. Powers, G. F., Park, E. A., Shipley, P. G., et al. (1921): The prevention of rickets in the rat by means of radiation with the mercury vapor quartz lamp. *Proc. Soc. Exp. Biol. Med.* **19**:120–121.
17. Goldblatt, H., and Soames, K. M. (1923): Studies on the fat soluble growth-promoting factor. *Biochem. J.* **17**:446–453.
18. Steenbock, H. (1924): The induction of growth promoting and calcifying properties in a ration exposed to light. *Science* **60**:224–225.

19. Steenbock, H., and Black, A. (1924): The reduction of growth-promoting and calcifying properties in a ration by exposure to ultraviolet light. *J. Biol. Chem.* **61**:408–422.

20. Hess, A. F., Weinstock, M. (1924): Antirachitic properties imparted to inert fluids and green vegetables by ultraviolet irradiation. *J. Biol. Chem.* **62**:301–313.

21. Hess, A. F., Weinstock, M., and Helman, D. F. (1925): The antirachitic value of irradiated phytosterol and cholesterol. *J. Biol. Chem.* **63**:305–308.

22. Rosenheim, O., and Webster, T. A. (1926): The anti-rachitic properties of irradiated sterols. *Biochem. J.* **20**:537–544.

23. Rosenheim, O., and Webster, T. A. (1927): On the nature of the parent substance of vitamin D. *Lancet* **1**:306–307.

24. Reerink, E. H., and van Wijk, A. (1929): The photochemical reactions of ergosterol. *Biochem. J.* **23**:1294–1307.

25. Askew, F. A., Bourdillon, R. B., Bruce, H. M., et al. (1931): The distillation of vitamin D. *Proc. R. Soc. Lond. [Biol.]* **107**:76–90.

26. Fieser, L. D., and Fieser, M. (1959): Vitamin D. In: *Steroids*, pp. 90–168. Reinhold, New York.

27. Crawfoot, D., and Dunitz, J. D. (1948): Structure of calciferol. *Nature* **162**:608–610.

28. Windaus, A., Lüttringhaus, A., and Deppe, M. (1931): Über das krystallisierte Vitamin D. *Justus Liebig's Ann. Chem.* **489**:252–269.

29. Windaus, A., Linsert, O., Lüttringhaus, A., et al. (1932): Über das krystallisierte Vitamin D₂. *Justus Liebig's Ann. Chem.* **492**:226–241.

30. Massengale, O. N., and Nussmeier, M. (1930): The action of activated ergosterol in the chicken. *J. Biol. Chem.* **87**:423–425.

31. Steenbock, H., and Kletzien, S. W. F. (1932): The reaction of the chicken to irradiated ergosterol and irradiated yeast as contrasted with the natural vitamin D in fish liver oil. *J. Biol. Chem.* **97**:249–264.

32. Waddell, J. (1934): The provitamin D of cholesterol. I. The antirachitic efficacy of irradiated cholesterol. *J. Biol. Chem.* **105**:711–739.

33. Windaus, A., Schenck, Fr., and von Werder, F. (1936): Über das antirachitisch wirksame Bestrahlungsprodukt aus 7-dehydrocholesterin. *Z. Physiol.* **241**:100–103.

34. Brockmann, H. (1936): Die Isolierung des antirachitischen Vitamins aus Tunfischleberol. *Hoppe Seylers Z. Physiol. Chem.* **241**:104–113.

35. Velluz, L., Amiard, G., and Petit, A. (1949): Le precalciferol—ses relations d'équilibre avec le calciferol. *Bull. Soc. Chim. Fr.* **16**:501–508.

36. Schlatmann, J. L. M., Pot, J., and Havinga, E. (1964): An investigation into the interconversion of precalciferol and calciferol and analogous compounds. *Recl. Trav. Chim. Pays-Bas* **83**:1173–1184.

37. Havinga, E. (1973): Vitamin D, example and challenge. *Experientia* **29**:1181–1193.

38. Jacobs, H. J. C., Boamsma, F., Havinga, E., et al. (1977): The photochemistry of previtamin D and tachysterol. *Recl. Trav. Chim. Pays-Bas Belg.* **96**:113–117.

39. Hess, A., Pappenheimer, A. M., and Weinstock, M. (1922): A study of light waves in relation to their protective action in rickets. *Proc. Soc. Exp. Biol. Med.* **20**:14–16.

40. Kon, S. K., Daniels, F., and Steenbock, H. (1928): The quantitative study of the photochemical activation of sterols in the cure of rickets. *J. Am. Chem. Soc.* **50**:2573–2581.

41. Bunker, J. W. M., and Harris, R. S. (1937): Precise evaluation of ultraviolet therapy in experimental rickets. *N. Engl. J. Med.* **216**:165–169.

42. Knudson, A., and Benford, F. (1938): Quantitative studies of the effectiveness of ultraviolet radiation of various wavelengths on rickets. *J. Biol. Chem.* **124**:287–299.

43. Bunker, J. W. M., Harris, R. S., and Mosher, M. L. (1940): Relative efficiency of active wavelengths of ultraviolet light in activation of 7-dehydrocholesterol. *J. Am. Chem. Soc.* **62**:508–511.

44. Kobayashi, T., and Yasumura, M. (1973): Studies on the ultraviolet irradiation of provitamin

D and its related compounds. Effect of wavelength on the formation of potential vitamin D_2 in the irradiation of ergosterol by monochromatic ultraviolet rays. *J. Nutr. Sci. Vitaminol.* (*Tokyo*) **19**:123–128.

45. Ziffer, H., Vanden Heuvel, W. J. A., Haahti, E. O. A., et al. (1960): Gas chromatographic behavior of vitamin D_2 and D_3. *J. Am. Chem. Soc.* **82**:6411–6415.

46. Holick, M. F., Holick, S. A., McNeill, S. C., et al. (1979): The photobiochemistry of vitamin D_3 *in vivo* in the skin. In: *Vitamin D: Basic Research and Its Clinical Application* (Proceedings of the Fourth Workshop on Vitamin D, Berlin, West Germany, February 1979), edited by A. W. Norman, K. Schaefer, D. v. Herrath, et al. pp. 173–176. Walter de Gruyter, Berlin/New York.

47. Holick, M. F., McNeill, S. C., MacLaughlin, J. A., et al. (1979): The physiologic implications of the formation of previtamin D_3 in skin. *Trans. Assoc. Am. Physicians* **XCII**:54–63.

48. Hess, A. F. (1925): The antirachitic activation of foods and of cholesterol by ultraviolet radiation. *J. Am. Med. Soc.* **84**:1910–1913.

49. Hou, H. (1931): Relation of preen gland of birds to rickets III. Site of activation during irradiation. *Chin. J. Physiol.* **5**:11–18.

50. Reinertson, R. P., and Wheatly, V. R. (1959): Studies on the chemical composition of human epidermal lipids. *J. Invest. Dermatol.* **32**:49–59.

51. Rauschkolb, E. W., Winston, D. Fenimore, D. C., Black, H. S., and Fabre, L. F. (1969): Identification of vitamin D_3 in human skin. *J. Invest. Dermatol.* **53**:289–293.

52. Okano, T., Yasumura, M., Mizuno, K., and Kobayashi, T. (1977): Photochemical conversion of 7-dehydrocholesterol into vitamin D_3 in rat skins. *J. Nutr. Sci. Vitaminol.* (*Tokyo*) **23**:165–168.

53. Esvelt, R. P., Schnoes, H. K., and DeLuca, H. F. (1978): Vitamin D_3 from rat skins irradiated *in vitro* with ultraviolet light. *Arch. Biochem. Biophys.* **188**:282–286.

54. Petrova, E. A., Nikulicheva, S. I., and Lazareva, N. P. (1976): Obrazovanie prekholekal'-tsiferola in vivo. *Vopr. Pitan.,* **5**:50–52.

55. Holick, M. F., Frommer, J., McNeill, S., Richtand, N., Henley, J., and Potts, J. T., Jr. (1977): Conversion of 7-dehydrocholesterol to vitamin D_3 in vivo: Isolation and identification of previtamin D_3 from skin. In: *Vitamin D: Biochemical, Chemical and Clinical Aspects Related to Calcium Metabolism* (Proceedings of the Third Workshop on Vitamin D, Asilomar, California, January 1977), edited by A. W. Norman, K. Schaefer, J. W. Coburn, H. F. DeLuca, D. Fraser, H. G. Grigoleit, and D. v. Herrath, pp. 135–137. Walter de Gruyter, Berlin/New York.

56. Holick, M. F., Frommer, J. E., McNeill, S. C., Richtand, N. M., Henley, J. F., and Potts, J. T., Jr. (1977): Photometabolism of 7-dehydrocholesterol to previtamin D_3 in skin. *Biochem. Biophys. Res. Commun.* **76**:107–114.

57. Holick, M. F., Richtand, N. M., McNeill, S. C., Holick, S. A., Frommer, J. E., Henley, J. W., and Potts, J. T., Jr. (1979): Isolation and identification of previtamin D_3 from the skin of rats exposed to ultraviolet irradiation. *Biochemistry* **18**:1003–1008.

58. Holick, M. F., McNeill, S. C., MacLaughlin, J., Clark, M. B., Holick, S. A., and Potts, J. T., Jr. (1979): The epidermis: A unique organ responsible for the photo-biosynthesis of vitamin D_3. In: *Endrocrinology '79*, pp. 301–307, Elsevier/North-Holland Biomedical Press, Amsterdam.

59. Elias, P. M., Fritsch, P., and Epstein, E. H. (1977): Staphylococcal scalded-skin syndrome. Clinical features, pathogenesis, and recent microbiological and biochemical developments. *Arch. Dermatol.* **113**:207–211.

60. Scheuplein, R. J. (1965): Mechanism of percutaneous absorption. Routes of penetration and the influence of solubility. *J. Invest. Dermatol.* **45**:334–346.

61. Holick, M. F., and Potts, J. T., Jr. (1980): Vitamin D. In: *Harrison's Princples of Internal Medicine*, 9th ed., edited by K. J. Isselbacher, R. D. Adams, E. Braunwald, R. G. Petersdorf, and J. D. Wilson, pp. 1843–1849. McGraw-Hill, New York.

62. Haussler, M. R., and McCain, T. A. (1977): Basic and clincal concepts related to vitamin D metabolism and action. *N. Engl. J. Med.* **297**:974–983, 1041–1050.
63. DeLuca, H. F., and Schnoes, H. K. (1976): Metabolism and mechanism of action of vitamin D. *Annu. Rev. Biochem.* **45**:631–642.
64. Norman, A. W., and Henry, H. (1974): 1,25-Dihydroxycholecalciferol—a hormonally active form of vitamin D₃. *Recent Prog. Horm. Res.* **30**:431–480.
65. Hess, A. F., and Lundagen, M. A. (1922): A seasonal tide of blood phosphate in infants. *J. AMA* **79**:2210–2212.
66. Bekemeier, H., and Pfennigsdorf, G. (1959): Versuche zur erschopfanden UV-Aktiverung des Provitamin D in Schweineschwarte. *Hoppe Seylers Z. Physiol. Chem.* **314**:120–124.
67. Preece, M. A., Tomlinson, S., Ribot, C. A., Pietrek, J., Korn, H. T., Davies, D. M., Ford, J. A., Dunnigan, M. G., and O'Riordan, J. L. H. (1975): Studies of vitamin D deficiency in man. *Q. J. Med.* **44**:575–589.
68. Fairney, A., Fry, J., and Lipscomb, A. (1979): The effect of darkness on vitamin D in adults. *Postgrad. Med. J.* **55**:248–250.
69. Haddad, J. G. and Chyu, K. J. (1971): Competitive protein binding radioassay for 25-hydroxycholecalciferol. *J. Clin. Endocrinol. Metab.* **33**:992–996.
70. Neer, R., Clark, M., Friedman, V., Belsey, R., Sweeney, M., Buonchristiani, J., and Potts, J., Jr. (1977): Environmental and nutritional influences on plasma 25-hydroxyvitamin D concentration and calcium metabolism in man. In: *Vitamin D: Biochemical, Chemical and Clinical Aspects Related to Calcium Metabolism* (Proceedings of the Third Workshop on Vitamin D), edited by A. W. Norman, K. Schaefer, J. W. Coburn, H. F. DeLuca, D. Fraser, H. G. Grigoleit, and D. v. Herrath, pp. 595–606. Walter de Gruyter, Berlin/New York.
71. Hess. A. F. (1922): New aspects of the rickets problem. *J. A.M.A.* **78**:1177–1183.
72. Kramer, B., Casparis, H., and Howland, J. (1923): Ultraviolet radiation in rickets: Effect on the calcium and inorganic phosphorus concentration of the serum. *Am. J. Dis. Child.* **24**:20–26.
73. Levinsohn, S. (1927): Rickets in the Negro: Effect of treatment with ultraviolet rays. *Am. J. Dis. Child.* **34**:955–966.
74. Loomis, F. (1967): Skin-pigment regulation of vitamin D biosynthesis in man. *Science* **157**:501–506.
75. Beadle, P. C. (1977): The epidermal biosynthesis of cholecalciferol (vitamin D₃). *Photochem. Photobiol.* **25**:519–527.

8

Responses of Normal Skin to Ultraviolet Radiation

J. L. M. Hawk and J. A. Parrish

The skin of humans is frequently exposed to ultraviolet (UV) radiation from the sun, either during everyday activity or during intentional exposure to achieve tanning. Exposure may also occur from any of a number of artificial sources which emit UV radiation. These include the increasingly popular commercial sunlamps and solaria used in an attempt to produce year-round tanning, the therapeutic UVB and UVA lamps used in the treatment of psoriasis and other skin ailments, welding arcs, gas discharge arc lamps, fluorescent lamps, and lasers used in industry or research. Physiologic mechanisms exist to deal with the absorbed energy, but they are not totally efficient. Sufficient damage at tissue, cellular, subcellular, and molecular levels invokes an inflammatory response, repair processes, and an increase in the function of protective processes. If no further exposure occurs, these processes run a short course and then cease to act. If multiple exposures occur, the processes continue and intensify. Since neither repair nor protective process is perfect, continuing exposure leads to long-term damage as discussed in Chapter 9. In this chapter, unless otherwise stated, only the effects of single, short UV exposures sufficient to produce a discernible response will be considered.

When UV radiation strikes the skin, photons may be reflected from the skin surface or pass across the air–skin interface into the skin, where they are *scattered* or *absorbed*, or both (see Chapter 6). Following scattering, photons may pass back out of the skin, pass through the skin, or be absorbed by any

J. L. M. Hawk • Department of Photobiology, Institute of Dermatology, St. John's Hospital for Diseases of Skin, London, England. *J. A. Parrish* • Department of Dermatology, Harvard Medical School, Massachusetts General Hospital, Boston, Massachusetts 02114.

molecule in their path capable of accepting their exact photon energy. Only those photons that are absorbed contribute to the clinical response, and the absorbing molecule is termed a *chromophore*. In general, only unsaturated organic compounds are good UV radiation chromophores at wavelengths longer than about 220 nm. These compounds usually contain alternating single and double bonds and are frequently cyclic or polycyclic. Important substances in the skin capable of absorbing UV radiation are the purine and pyrimidine bases of nucleic acids, which absorb maximally at about 260 nm; the amino acids of proteins (especially the aromatic tryptophan, tyrosine, and phenylalanine and the nonaromatic cystine and cysteine), which absorb maximally at about 280 nm (1); melanin; and hemoglobin (2). Less important are urocanic acid (3), the porphyrins, riboflavin, steroids, nicotinamide adenine dinucleotide, isoprenoid quinones (such as vitamin K), beta-carotene (1), and bilirubin. Many of the major biomolecules in vitro absorb optimally in the UVC region, which is outside the range of terrestrial sunlight, but they also absorb, if less efficiently, in the UVB range and are thus susceptible to sunlight-induced damage (4).

Following absorption of a photon, the electrically excited absorbing molecule rapidly returns to a more stable energy state (a) by relaxation through vibrational or rotational energy levels resulting in production of heat; (b) by reemission of a photon with lower energy in the form of fluorescence or phosphorescence; (c) by undergoing a permanent structural change; or (d) by reacting with an appropriate nearby molecule. After the initial photochemical reaction, so-called "dark" thermal chemical reactions may cause direct tissue damage or release of mediators and result in the observable clinical response. Exact details of the photochemical and subsequent thermal chemical reactions associated with given clinical responses are not known in most cases, although there is some information concerning the products of the latter reactions.

The response of normal skin to UV irradiation is in part an example of *inflammation*, a nonspecific response to a damaging agent (in this case UV photons). This reaction comprises a series of changes in the microcirculation and in tissue, tending to remove the injurious agent and to repair the damage. Inflammation may result from any injury and the degree of the response increases with the severity of the insult. The well-known symptoms and signs originally described by Celsus in about A.D. 178 are present, namely redness or erythema as a result of increased vasodilatation, heat from increased blood flow, swelling because of increased exudation of plasma and cells from the blood, and pain, probably due to the action of chemical mediators on tissue nerve endings. In skin, the inflammatory reaction is often followed by a pigmentary response, most marked after UV injury and hyperplastic changes, both of which tend to protect against further damage. After UV irradiation in normal skin, there also occur many molecular events which may well have little or no role in the inflammatory response. For example, induction of enzymes such as ornithine decarboxylase takes place and there is damage to nuclear DNA.

The clinical responses of skin to a single UV exposure sufficient to produce observable changes are:

1. *Erythema*, often called *sunburn*, which is the most visible and best-known component of UV inflammation, but is only one of many consequences of in vivo UV injury. Marked erythema is often accompanied by edema.

2. *Tanning*, which consists of two types: (a) *immediate tanning* (IT), otherwise known as *immediate pigment darkening* (IPD) or *immediate pigmentation*; and (b) *delayed tanning* (DT), otherwise known as *delayed pigmentation* or *true melanogenesis.*

3. *Thickening*, which results from a hyperplastic response of the skin.

These events will now be considered in detail.

ERYTHEMA

Mechanism of Production of UV Inflammation

General. UV erythema (redness) is caused by vasodilatation and consequent increased blood content in the dermis. Such erythema is often called sunburn, but to avoid confusion, this term is better reserved for the sun-induced erythema. Otherwise *UV erythema* should be used, the spectral composition of the inducing radiation being specified if necessary. UV inflammation may be induced by a single adequate dose of UV radiation of wavelengths longer than about 230 nm. There may be a biphasic response, particularly marked in some laboratory animals, consisting of a transient immediate reaction, beginning in seconds and lasting a few minutes, followed about ½–8 hr later by a prolonged delayed reaction. The biphasic nature of the reaction applies to only some of the events in UV inflammation, the division thus being largely artificial and likely to be discarded as more becomes known about cellular and molecular details. In humans, the immediate inflammatory responses are usually not clinically apparent.

The Immediate Phase of UV Inflammation. In humans, following UVB or UVC irradiation, immediate erythema has been described only occasionally (5–7). Following UVA irradiation of sufficient dose, however, it is a common observation (8, 9). In guinea pigs irradiated with a predominantly UVB source, immediate erythema is usual, fading quickly within 1–15 min (10, 11). The reaction probably affects arterioles, capillaries, and venules. Vasopermeability has been studied only in laboratory animals, occurring in guinea pigs about 1 min after irradiation as the erythema is fading, reaching a maximum in 10 min, and returning to normal permeability within 5 more min

(7, 10). It also occurs in rats, but not hairless mice (7). The affected vessels are venules (7, 12). These immediate vascular responses may result from direct vascular damage by photons or from the effects of chemical mediators or both. Direct irradiation of dermal arterial blood vessels in the dog, rabbit, and humans with about 3–5 MEDs (minimal erythema doses) of UVB or UVC produces immediate arteriolar vasodilatation which recovers rapidly when irradiation ceases (13). These are high exposure doses and equivalent to higher doses in vivo where intact epidermis attenuates the radiation, and thus this direct effect in vivo may be minimal.

Histamine, a substance stored in mast cells, may play some role in the immediate phase of UV inflammation, although evidence in humans is sparse. However, there is a suggestion in animals that mast cells are degranulated by UV irradiation (14, 15). Further, histamine produces erythema and edema on intradermal injection in humans (16) and injection of histamine in rats produces endothelial gaps similar to those of acute inflammation (17). Also, the specific antihistamine triprolidine virtually suppresses the early vasopermeability following UV irradiation in guinea pigs (10, 18). In humans, histamine has been looked for unsuccessfully in the immediate phase after UV irradiation using tissue perfusion (19) and suction blister techniques (20), but on one occasion bioassay of venous blood draining UVB-irradiated skin showed an immediate minimal and transient rise of histamine to about 2.5 μg ml^{-1} in two out of five subjects.* Serotonin, a substance also present in mast cells, is found in the skin of rats (21) and has been isolated from the urine of humans (22) following UV irradiation, but its exact role in the immediate phase of UV inflammation in humans is not certain. Prostaglandins (PGs) also are released in human skin in vitro, possibly from membrane receptor sites, immediately following high-dose UVB irradiation (23), but the in vivo significance of this observation is not known.

The Delayed Phase of UV Inflammation. Following the immediate phase of the inflammatory response, there is a period of clinical quiescence before onset of the delayed phase. Tissue elements contributing to this phase of UV inflammation are the blood vessels, the blood contents (cells and plasma), and the cells of the skin. The temporal responses of these various tissue elements have been elucidated by histologic, histochemical, and pharmacologic studies, but in all cases the exact pathophysiologic mechanisms remain uncertain.

Delayed vasodilatation or erythema after UVB irradiation appears in ½–8 hr, reaches a maximum at about 12–24 hr, and fades in a further few hours to several days (5, 24–29). Very small doses may produce reactions lasting for a total of a few hours only. Increasing doses progressively shorten the time before the appearance of the delayed erythema, lengthen its persistence, and increase its intensity. UVC irradiation tends to produce an

---

*Hawk, J. L. M., Black, A. K., and Greaves, M. W. (1979): Unpublished observations.

earlier and shorter delayed erythema than UVB, the redness peaking at about 5–8 hr and fading within a few hours up to about 72 hr after exposure, depending on exposure dose (5, 25). UVA irradiation commonly leads to an immediate erythema persisting into a delayed phase lasting hours to days (8, 9). The site of delayed vasodilatation has been debated, but arterioles, capillaries, and venules all seem to be affected (6, 30–32).

In guinea pigs, rats, and hairless mice (7, 10), delayed vasopermeability begins within about 4–6 hr of irradiation, reaches a maximum after the erythema peak (10) between 12 and 24 hr, and subsides within the next 48 hr. The sites of the delayed vasopermeability in rats, guinea pigs, and hairless mice appear to be the venules and capillary bed (7, 12). The increased vasopermeability is sufficient to permit passage of leukocytes and plasma into the exposed sites (7, 12). Neutrophil migration from blood to tissues occurs in guinea pigs within ½ hr of irradiation and reaches a peak at about 8 hr, coinciding with or just preceding the erythema peak (10, 33). These tissue neutrophil levels return virtually to normal by 48 hr after irradiation. Monocytes in guinea pigs begin migration after UV irradiation simultaneously with the neutrophils, also reach a peak at 8 hr, but persist in large numbers at 48 hr (33).

As in the immediate phase, it is possible that direct vascular injury contributes to the delayed phase of UV inflammation. Repeated UV irradiation of isolated blood vessels with high doses of UVB and UVC causes prolonged vasodilatation (13). It also seems unlikely that inflammatory mediators alone can lead to necrosis of blood vessels which has been seen following UV injury (34, 35). Direct vascular insult by photons may play a more prominent role at larger exposure doses and is most likely wavelength dependent.

Possible chemical mediators of delayed UV inflammation are many. PGs appear to have an important role. These compounds are cyclic oxygenated 20-carbon fatty acids which induce vasodilatation and enhance the vasopermeability effects of other mediators, particularly histamine and bradykinin (36). They were first noted to be elevated following UV irradiation in human dermal perfusates after about 24–48 hr (19). Their presence was later confirmed in delayed UV inflammation in human (37), rat (37), and guinea pig (11) skin. The increased levels occur in both epidermis and dermis (37). Recently, PGE_2 and $PGF_{2\alpha}$ have been recovered in human suction blister fluid from both UVB (38, 39) and UVC (40) irradiation sites. After UVB irradiation PGD_2 has also been found (39). Their occurrence in UVA erythema has not yet been reported. Values have been elevated at 1–6 hr after irradiation, reaching a peak at 18–24 hr, and falling virtually to normal by 48 hr (11, 38–40). This closely parallels the time course of delayed UVC erythema, but delayed UVB erythema persists well beyond the return of the PG levels to normal. Attempts to abolish the changes of delayed UVB- and UVC-induced inflammation by means of the cyclo-oxygenase inhibitor indomethacin, used topically or orally, have met with only partial success. Pain and erythema are merely reduced but not abolished (41–44) even though elevation of PGE_2 and $PGF_{2\alpha}$ levels in human suction blister fluid from UVB- and UVC-irradiated sites is totally suppressed (45). After UVA irradiation, topical indomethacin caused no visible reduction in erythema in one study (44). PGs thus appear to have an important but only a partial role in the production of UV erythema. The exact site of origin of the PGs during UV inflammation is not known, although in non-UV studies PG formation has been shown within epidermis (46), neutrophils (47), monocytes (48), platelets (49), and vascular endothelium (50).

Mast cell histamine may also be a mediator in delayed UV inflammation. Its importance, however, is uncertain. It may be released in non-UV delayed inflammation by activation of complement (51) and by the action of cationic proteins from neutrophil lysosomes (52). Elevated histamine has recently been isolated from human suction blister fluid 3–4 hr after UVB irradiation, just before the appearance of erythema, but not at any other time in the 24-hr period studied (20). An earlier human study, however, showed histamine elevation after UVB irradiation in six of 17 subjects at 24 and 48 hr (19).

Mediators may also be formed in the tissues from the plasma exudate during cutaneous inflammation. These include the kinin polypeptides, the best known of which is bradykinin (53). They all cause pain, vasodilatation, increased vascular permeability, and increased leukocyte migration (53, 54). Formation is complex, nonspecific injury activating the plasma protein prekallikrein (55, 56), leading to kinin production in a variety of ways (57, 58). After UVB irradiation in humans, kinins have been detected by a dermal perfusion technique within a few minutes, and possibly as late as $6\frac{1}{2}$ hr, usually well before the appearance of delayed erythema (59). On the other hand, in a similar UVB study, kinin was detected only at 24 and 48 hr after irradiation in about one-third of both irradiated and control subjects (19). Thus, as in some other types of inflammation (60, 61), it appears that kinins probably have only a variable and minor role in delayed UV inflammation, although this role may be increased by the potentiating effect of PGs (36). Another plasma-derived mediator in some types of inflammation is the complement system, activation of which may lead to increased vasodilatation, vasopermeability, and neutrophil chemotaxis (51, 62), but there are as yet no data concerning its role in UV inflammation.

Neutrophil leukocytes are possibly causally related to delayed UV inflammatory changes in skin. The peak neutrophil concentration in guinea pig dermis coincides with or just precedes the peaks of delayed erythema (10, 33) and vasopermeability (10). Further, neutropenia in guinea pigs reduces the intensity and duration of delayed UVB erythema (although possibly not of UVC erythema) (18, 33). It has been shown, although not yet following UV irradiation, that neutrophils are attracted to sites of injury by tissue damage (63–65). They may then break down and release their own granule (lysosome) contents (66), the latter increasing erythema (36, 67) and vasopermeability (36, 52, 67–71), and enabling further chemoattraction of neutrophils (62, 66). Monocytes, too, are attracted by neutrophil breakdown products (72) and may help mediate the later stages of delayed cutaneous inflammation (33, 73), although such participation in UV inflammation has net yet been demonstrated.

Absorption of UV radiation at various sites in the epidermis and dermis may result in damage to cells and organelles and consequent release of proinflammatory substances. After UV irradiation, lysosomal rupture in epidermal cells has been detected electron microscopically at about 2 hr in guinea pigs (74) and histochemically at about 4 hr in humans (75), and the damage is UV radiation dose-related (76). Therefore it has been suggested that UV radiation-induced lysosomal breakdown may play an important part in the delayed phase of UV inflammation (3, 77, 78). However, electron microscopic evidence of cell damage is apparent before lysosomal damage occurs and even lethally damaged cells may contain completely normal lysosomes (74). Further, no products of lysosomal breakdown are detectable in epidermal suction blister fluid until at least 11 hr after irradiation (79) and maximal levels do not occur until 4–7 days (80). Thus, released epidermal lysosomal contents may not initiate UV inflammation but may accentuate it, especially in the later stages of the delayed phase. It has also been shown that nucleosides, nucleotides, and RNA cause a moderate increase in vasopermeability and chemotaxis of neutrophils and monocytes (81, 82). Hence, damage to nucleic acids (83, 84) and cell death (34, 35, 85), both of which may follow UV irradiation, may conceivably enhance the delayed phase of UV inflammation, although this has not yet been demonstrated.

The chromophores responsible for initial absorption of UV radiation and the associated photochemical reactions leading to delayed UV inflammation are unknown. Nucleic acids (86) and proteins (87) have been suggested as targets. Absorption of UV radiation by nucleic acids leads to formation of pyrimidine dimers (83, 84), and other products (88). Sufficient damage may lead to cell death. Proteins can also absorb UV radiation, and absorption by membrane lipoproteins may lead through lipid peroxidation to membrane breakdown (89). Absorption of UV radiation by any skin chromophore may lead to formation of unstable reactive free radicals and free radical ions (90, 91). Any of these reactions could initiate inflammation, but the exact photochemistry is not yet understood.

The relative effectiveness of various wavelengths of the UV spectrum is measured by plotting the reciprocal of the lowest exposure dose that results in erythema (minimal erythema dose, MED) against wavelength. This is called the *erythema action spectrum*. In general, decreasing erythemal effectiveness

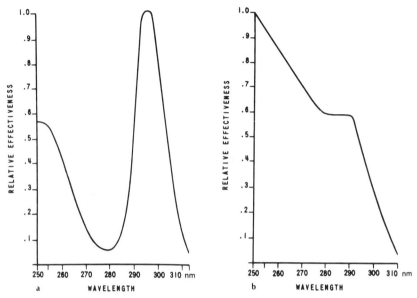

Fig. 8-1.   (a) Standard erythema action spectrum [modified from (24)]. (b) More recent research indicates maximum effectiveness at 250 nm with gradual decreasing effectiveness at longer wavelengths [from (27)].

has been found up to about 320 nm from a broad peak at about 300 nm (92). In one case no 300-nm peak was found, but there was a flat shoulder at about 280–290 nm (27). Two examples of the resulting curves are shown in Fig. 8-1 (24, 27). Calculations from early literature have shown that the erythemal effectiveness probably falls gradually from 100% at 300 nm to slightly below 1% at 320 nm, about 0.1% at 365 nm, and 0.05% at 400 nm (93). All the action spectra described are probably equivalent if differences in time of observation of the erythema, site of irradiation, and definition of the MED are taken into account (94). It is thus claimed that the action spectrum obtained by each different set of investigators depicts the same unknown epidermal events (94).

By comparing the time courses of erythema induced by 250-nm and 300-nm radiation, skin temperature changes, and migration of the border of irradiated sites, van der Leun (93, 95) postulated that:

1.   There is a broad peak of erythemal effectiveness around 250 nm, caused by direct action of UV radiation on or at the level of the blood vessels, this effectiveness probably diminishing gradually with increasing wavelength up to about 400 nm.

2.   Superimposed on this curve, there is also a sharp peak of erythemal effectiveness at about 300 nm caused by action on the dermal blood vessels of a diffusing substance released just below the stratum corneum at the time of irradiation.

The nature of the diffusing substance is unknown, but by his calculation even nonmacromolecular substances could have a diffusion time long enough to explain the delay in appearance of the erythema.

Minimal Erythema Dose (MED). This useful and easily measured response enables semiquantitative evaluation of skin reactions to UV irradiation and has been widely used and studied. However, it has a number of disadvantages:

1. It is only one component of a complicated cascade of events induced in skin by exposure to UV radiation.

2. Different definitions are used by different workers. Perhaps the MED is most commonly defined as the least UV-radiation dose giving a distinct erythema with sharp margins 7–24 hr after irradiation (96). However, many workers probably use the dose producing minimal perceptible erythema (MPE) or other personally convenient response for routine assessments of the threshold dose. The MED is a dose, not a time or a visual grading, and is expressed preferably in $J\ m^{-2}$, although $mJ\ cm^{-2}$ or equivalent units are still used. If grading of erythema and not dose is required, the convention outlined in Table 8-1 may be used. Such a practice of visual grading has proved convenient and fairly repeatable and compares well with existing quantitative methods (97).

3. The MED (and the dose required to produce other erythematous responses) varies according to the circumstances relating to the irradiation. The variables are summarized in Table 8-2 and some are listed below:

a. *Wavelength.* In Caucasian subjects, various workers have found slightly differing ranges of MED values at each of the wavelengths studied. The results from all the studies are presented in Table 8-3. It can be seen that MED values differing by a factor of about 2–3 may be within normal limits.

b. *Season.* The MED on the exposed skin of the back increases in spring and summer and decreases in autumn and winter (99, 100).

c. *Position of subject.* MED assessments should always be made with the subject in the same position, to prevent MED variations presumably induced by alterations in blood flow.

Table 8-1. Convention for Grading of Skin Erythema

Symbol	Abbreviation	Definition
0	NR	No reaction; identical to surrounding nonirradiated skin
±	MPE	Minimal perceptible erythema; blotchy areas of faint erythema confined to the irradiated site; borders indefinite
+	1+	Minimal erythema with four sharp borders
++	2+	More pronounced erythema without edema
+++	3+	Marked erythema with edema
++++	4+	Violaceous erythema with vesiculation

Table 8-2. Variables Affecting the Assessment of Minimal Erythema Dose Following UV Radiation Exposure

Conditions related to the optical source
  Spectral distribution of emitted radiation
  Radiant power of source
  Constancy of power output
  Size of exit slit of source
  Degree of collimation of emitted radiation
Conditions related to irradiation of subject
  Distance of subject from exit slit of source
  Irradiance at skin of subject
  Duration of irradiation
  Angle of incidence of radiation
  Field size of irradiated area
  Possible shadow effects at margins of irradiated area
  Ambient conditions (temperature, humidity, wind)
  Ability of subject to remain still
Conditions related to the skin
  Color (skin type or pigmentation)
  Previous exposure to radiation at same site
  Season of year
  Age of subject
  Anatomic site of irradiation on subject
  Presence of a dermatosis on irradiation site
  Presence of an abnormal reaction to UV radiation (i.e., a photodermatosis)
  Presence of topical or systemic agent which changes radiation absorption or effect (e.g., water, sebum, beta-carotene)
Conditions related to assessment of erythema
  Definition of MED
  Amount of time elapsed after irradiation before MED reading
  Radiation doses and increments given
  Position of subject during reading
  Ambient lighting (color, intensity, and angle) during reading

d. *Size of irradiation site.* Small irradiation sites less than about 1 cm in diameter or width increase the MED. This effect is not marked until the field size becomes less than 1 mm (101).

e. *Age of subject.* The MED of children below 6 years of age and adults over about 70 years of age may be lower, and that of people between about 7–20 years of age may be higher, than at other ages (100, 102).

f. *Sex of subject.* There is no difference in MED values between sexes (100, 103).

g. *Irradiation site.* For UVB radiation, the MED is the same for both sides of the body (102). At 297 nm on the face, neck, and trunk it is 2–4 times

Table 8-3. Values of MED for Selected Wavelengths and Selected Wavebands
Compiled from the Findings of Several Studies (8, 9, 28, 98)

	MED range, mJ cm^{-2}	MED rounded value, mJ cm^{-2}
UVC (254 nm) (28)	6.9–12.0	10
UVB (300 nm) (28, 98)	11.6–25.2	20
UVB (310 nm) (28, 98)	205.0–238.0	200
UVB (broadband) (9)	18.3–47.8	30
	MED range, J/cm^{-2}	MED rounded value J cm^{-2}
UVA (337.1 nm) (8)		
Immediate	12.7–21.2	15
at 24 hr	14.8–27.5	20
UVA (broadband) (9)		
Immediate	5–30	13
Persisting 4–6 hr	14–60	30
Persisting 24 hr	25–80	50

lower (20–25 mJ cm^{-2}) than on the limbs (40–85 mJ cm^{-2}), the most distal areas having the highest MED (28). The upper back is more sensitive than the lumbar region (102).

h. *Pigmentation.* Caucasians have UVB MED values 3–5 times less than moderately pigmented races and up to about 30 times less than very pigmented races (25, 34, 104). For solar-simulating radiation, fair-skinned races have MEDs about five times lower than pigmented peoples (105). Facultative tanning in the absence of stratum corneum thickening increases the MED in Caucasians by a factor of only 2–3 (106).

The "color" of skin responses varies with the UV waveband. The erythema of UVC is pink, whereas that of UVB is red. UVA erythema is usually deep red. Increasing dose intensifies the erythema and tends to minimize the color differences between wavebands.

The dose–response curve is also a function of wavelength (Fig. 8-2). The UVC dose–response curve is very flat, particularly at shorter wavelengths, the intensity of the erythema increasing very gradually with increasing dose (24, 25). Fifty MEDs of 254-nm radiation usually produces marked erythema and later desquamation, but epidermal vesiculation or evidence of tissue necrosis does not normally occur. The UVB dose–response curve is relatively steep (24, 25) and 5–10 MEDs produce severe erythema, pain, vesiculation, and peeling in fair-skinned subjects. The UVA dose-response curve appears to be at least as steep as that for UVB.*

Erythemal Response in Differing Atmospheric Conditions. Wind (107),

*Parrish, J. A., and Hawk, J. L. M. (1980): Unpublished observations.

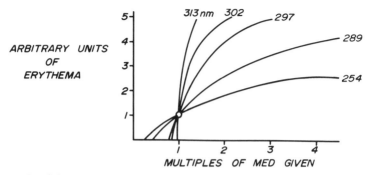

Fig. 8-2. UV erythema dose–response according to wavelength [from (24)].

humidity (108), and heat (109) increase the degree of UVB erythema in mice. Human data are not available.

The Law of Reciprocity in Relation to UV Erythema. The Bunsen–Roscoe law of reciprocity for a photochemical reaction states that the intensity of radiation is inversely related to the time of exposure to produce a given effect. That is, the effect is directly proportional to the total dose whether that dose be achieved with high irradiance for a short time or low irradiance for a long time. This may break down with very high intensities if two-photon absorption occurs, or with very low intensities if biologic repair occurs during the exposure. Temperature effects and effects of intermediate photoproducts may also cause deviation from reciprocity. It has been shown, however, that the reciprocity law holds for UV-induced delayed erythema over seven orders of magnitude of irradiance (110) and, in a recent preliminary study using lasers, over ten orders of magnitude of irradiance (111). It has been said that the law is valid only approximately for polychromatic radiation (112) but unless the spectral characteristics of the radiation change with varying intensity (as with sunlight), reciprocity seems to hold.

Solar Erythemal Effectiveness. The effectiveness spectrum for production of UV erythema in sunlight (i.e., solar erythemal effectiveness) is not the same as the classical erythema action spectrum, as the sun's intensity is not constant from wavelength to wavelength. Its spectral irradiance, which is zero below about 286 nm at low latitudes and about 300 nm in the temperate zones, rises rapidly to a peak at about 550 nm, thereafter falling off gradually through the longer visible and infrared wavelengths. The UVB irradiance at the solar zenith in midsummer in Davos, Switzerland, can be calculated to be about 150 μW cm^{-2}, or about 3% of the UVA irradiance of about 3.5 m W cm^{-2} (113). At all other times the greater atmospheric attenuation of UVB reduces its relative irradiance still further. By convoluting the curves for solar spectral irradiance and erythema action spectrum, the relative erythemal effectiveness at each solar wavelength can be calculated (Fig. 8-3). The action spectrum for UVA erythema is not known, but if there is assumed to be

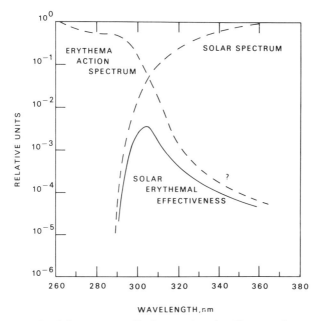

Fig. 8-3. Erythemal effectiveness of sunlight [from (114)].

a gradual falloff in erythemal efficiency with increasing wavelength (93); it can be seen from Fig. 8-3 that UVA contributes significantly to solar erythema at the solar zenith [10–15% has been suggested (114)] and more at other times. The most erythemogenic wavelength in sunlight at the solar zenith is about 306–309 nm (115) rather than about 300 nm, as in the erythema action spectrum.

Photorecovery, Photoaddition, and Photoaugmentation. Photorecovery, a phenomenon previously noted in single-cell systems (116), was later suspected in animals (117) and finally in humans (118) following the discovery that the MED for UVB and UVC was increased by 15–25% if irradiation was followed by exposure to window glass-filtered sunlight (UVA). If the glass-filtered sun exposure preceded the UVB or UVC irradiation, erythema equivalent to addition of the UVB or UVC to the UVA solar radiation doses apparently occurred. Such *photoaddition* of two UV wavebands had previously been suggested as a likely phenomenon (29, 119). More recently, workers combining UVB and UVA described yet another response, an erythema apparently more marked than that expected with photoaddition, and called this phenomenon *photoaugmentation* (120). A debate has ensued, both photoaddition (121, 122) and *photoaugmentation* (123) having since been reported. One recent study described approximate photoaddition if UVB- and UVC-irradiated sites were pre- or postirradiated with UVA, but called it photoaugmentation (124). The matter remains unresolved.

Histology

Early studies on the histology of UV inflammation were carried out by Miescher (34, 35, 85), who irradiated guinea pigs and human subjects with UVB. Since then other studies have been undertaken using different wavebands and different doses of UVB, UVC, and UVA irradiation in both animals and human subjects (125–127).

The early histologic features of UV inflammation of all wavebands in guinea pigs include a dermal inflammatory infiltrate of neutrophils most marked at about 8 hr, much reduced by 24 hr, and minimal by 48 hr (10, 33). A round cell or mononuclear infiltrate begins with the neutrophils but then persists at a fairly constant level from 24 hr onward, the number of these cells always being somewhat more numerous than that of the neutrophils and markedly so from 24 hr onward (33). Exactly similar early studies have not been carried out in humans. However, in a recent investigation of the cutaneous effects of UVB irradiation in four Caucasian subjects, only a few dermal neutrophils were seen at 4 and 24 hr (128). No information is available concerning the intervening period. The mononuclear infiltrate in humans peaks at 48–72 hr and still persists to a lesser degree at 7 days. It is most marked with UVA and may involve most of the dermis, whereas UVB and UVC produce less marked infiltrates, tending to affect mostly the upper dermis. All infiltrates are most noticeable at 48 and 72 hr, their density being inversely proportional to their dermal depth (127).

Vascular effects after UVB and UVC irradiation in animals include an immediate increase in venular permeability as manifested by exudation of trypan blue and deposition in the venular walls of colloidal carbon. A similar increase in capillary permeability follows within a few hours (7, 12). Endothelial swelling, nuclear dust, and extravasation of red blood cells are visible to a mild degree in humans within 24 hr with all wavebands. These changes disappear within 7 days with UVB and UVC but persist slightly with UVA (127). Vascular damage is most marked with UVA, and vascular necrosis has been noted (35). UVA may also cause edema of the papillary dermis and perivenular space (127). Thus, in all aspects studied, UVA is the waveband most affecting the dermis.

In contrast, the epidermis appears most affected by UVC and UVB and little by UVA. Increasing number of dyskeratotic cells (so-called sunburn cells) (75, 129–132) are seen following UVC and UVB during the first 24 hr after irradiation in humans and animals, appearing initially within 2-1/2 hr in mice (131) and within 8 hr in rabbits (132), and after high doses in humans coalescing into a band of necrotic tissue persisting at 7 days (127). Only very few sunburn cells occur after UVA, from 72 hr onward (127). Sunburn cells have homogeneous eosinophilic cytoplasm and pyknotic nuclei and are usually scattered singly among normal epidermal cells. Their increased susceptibility to UV irradiation may result from inadequate ability to repair DNA (133) or possibly from lysosomal breakdown and damage related in some way to an increased cellular melanin content (134). However, sunburn cells may contain intact lysosomes and thus the latter explanation has been disputed (74). The cells are characteristic but not pathognomonic of UV erythema, similar cells appearing in other tissues and processes. Epidermal spongiosis is also most marked with UVB and UVC, appearing in 24 hr, peaking at 48 hr, and persisting moderately at 7 days, whereas UVA produces only mild spongiosis at 48 and 72 hr, and is still present at 7 days (127). Nuclear diameter is increased by a factor of three within 7 days of UVB and UVC irradiation, returning to normal by about 6 weeks (135). The nucleolar size of keratinocytes is affected mostly by UVB and UVC, being increased at 48 and 72 hr, whereas UVA has only a minimal effect at 7 days (127, 136). Hyperkeratosis, parakeratosis, and acanthosis are induced particularly by UVC and moderately by UVB but not by UVA, the change not being present until 72 hr after irradiation (127). There is patchy loss of the granular layer at 24 and 48 hr with UVB and UVC (127) and patchy increase with all wavebands by 72 hr, which is still present at 7 days (127, 137). Scattered intracellular edema is present with UVA, UVB, and UVC at all times up to 7 days (127). Epidermal mitoses are infrequent (127). These changes are summarized in Table 8-4.

Ultrastructural studies have been carried out following irradiation with UVB (74, 136–139), UVA (6), and solar-simulating radiation (6). Immediately after 10–20 MEDs of UVB radiation, scattered superficial epidermal cells show nuclear and perinuclear edema and perinuclear vacuoles, apparently of distended endoplasmic reticulum (74). Mild immediate lysosomal disruption may also be present, but no more than in control skin, and many cells show no lysosomal damage, even the few exhibiting immediate cytolysis (74). Later, also after lower doses of UVB radiation, groups of cells containing vacuoles or diffuse clear cytoplasm seem to migrate from the basal layer to the granular layer, mostly during the 1–72-hr period after irradiation (74, 137, 138). Over the same time period a similar movement of cells containing ovoid dense bodies about 0.5 μm in length seems to occur. These structures, possibly of glycolipid or glycoprotein, and normally present in small numbers in the basal cells of unirradiated epidermis, seem to pass into the stratum corneum, appearing first as oval lacunae by 72 hr, and later as multiple dark structures by 7 days (74, 137–139). The exact nature of the vacuolated and clear cells and of the ovoid dense bodies remains uncertain. Epidermal changes following UVA irradiation seem mild at 48 hr, consisting of intracellular vacuolation and lipid droplets along with widening of the intercellular spaces (6). Similar but more marked changes follow solar-simulating radiation (6). Dermal ultrastructural changes following UVA irradiation at 48 hr apparently consist of widely opened endothelial gaps in blood vessels of all types in the papillary and reticular dermis, platelet aggregation, leukocyte degranulation, and extravasation of blood cells (6). There are also signs of mast cell degranu-

Table 8-4. Comparison of Histologic Changes Induced by Equally Erythemogenic Single Doses of UVA, UVB, and UVC Radiation to Produce 2+ Erythema, Noted at 24, 48, and 72 hr and at 7 Days (127)[a]

Abnormality		24 hr	48 hr	72 hr	7 Days
Dyskeratotic ("sunburn") cells (0–4)	UVA	0	0	1	1
	UVB	2	3	4	4
	UVC	2	3	4	4
Spongiosis	UVA	0	1	1	1
	UVB	1	2	1	1
	UVC	1	2	1	1
Nucleolar size	UVA	0	0	0	1
	UVB	0	1	2	0
	UVC	0	1	2	0
Hyperkeratosis	UVA	0	0	0	0
Parakeratosis	UVB	0	0	1	1
Acanthosis	UVC	0	0	2	2
Patchy loss of granular layer	UVA	0	0	0	0
	UVB	1	1	0	0
	UVC	1	1	0	0
Patchy increase in granular layer	UVA	0	0	1	1
	UVB	0	0	1	1
	UVC	0	0	1	1
Scattered intracellular edema	UVA	2	2	2	2
	UVB	2	2	2	2
	UVC	2	2	2	2
Mononuclear infiltrate	UVA	2	3	3	2
	UVB	1	2	2	1
	UVC	1	2	2	1
Direct vessel damage (endothelial swelling,	UVA	1	1	2	1
extravasation of cells, nuclear dust)	UVB	1	1	1	0
	UVC	1	1	1	0
Perivenular and papillary dermal edema	UVA	0	0	1	1
	UVB	0	0	0	0
	UVC	0	0	0	0

[a]All categories graded on scale of 0 to 3, except dyskeratotic cells, graded 0 to 4; 0 = control; 1 = minimal; 2 = moderate; 3 = marked; 4 = very marked.

lation, fibrin deposition, and fibroblast abnormalities consisting of cytoplasmic changes and pyknotic nuclei (6). However, some of these effects may have been due to heat as a result of the very high irradiances used. Dermal changes after UVB irradiation consist of immediate vasodilatation probably affecting vessels of all types, this apparently also occurring with solar-simulating radiation, in addition to mild endothelial gap formation, extravasation of blood cells, and occurrence of lipid droplets in fibroblasts (6).

Thus, the histologic alterations induced by UVB and UVC are mainly in the epidermis and less marked in the dermis, whereas UVA affects mostly the dermis.

Prevention and Treatment of UV Erythema

Prevention of UV Erythema. Prevention of UV erythema is achieved by avoidance of excessive UV exposure, wearing of protective clothing, application of topical sunscreens (see Chapter 15), or (theoretically) medication with photoprotective drugs (see Chapter 11).

Excessive UV exposure may occur from artificial sources and from sunlight. Since solar UV radiation is attenuated by the atmosphere, the burning potential of the sun is greatest at the solar zenith, in the tropical zones, and at high altitudes, where its radiation pathlength through the atmosphere is shortest (Fig. 8-4). The shorter the wavelength, the greater the attenuation, and thus the relatively erythemogenic UVB radiation decreases most rapidly in intensity away from the solar zenith, away from the tropics, and with decreasing altitude. Sunburn is unlikely to occur in susceptible subjects in temperate zones in summer more than 2 hr from the time of the solar zenith.

Ambient conditions may alter the likelihood of sunburn. Any cooling effect such as from wind and water may induce subjects to remain exposed for longer times. In addition, wind possibly leads to a potentiated sunburn (107) and water permits sunburning during swimming by transmitting UV radiation well, by washing off topical sunscreens, and possibly by enhancing UV transmission because of optical changes in the stratum corneum. Atmospheric haze and shade from clouds or objects still allow sunburning from UV radiation transmitted through the haze, reflected from the clouds, or scattered from the blue sky; such UV radiation may sometimes contain up to two-thirds of the total incident solar UVB radiation. Conversely, the early morning and late afternoon sunshine, even if very hot, contains minimal UVB radiation and has minimal sunburning potential.

Sunburn may be reduced by attenuation of UV radiation as a result of atmospheric pollution or screening by buildings, and enhanced by UV reflection from snow (85%), sand (17%), white wall plaster (46%), shiny

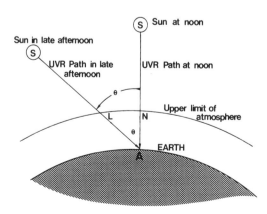

Fig. 8-4. Diagram showing longer path length of sun's rays through earth's atmosphere as sun moves away from its zenith. In the figure, $AL = AN \cos \theta = AN \sec \theta$, and is always greater than or equal to AN.

metals, and to a certain extent by water (5%, or more if ripples permit multiple reflections) (140). City, countryside, seaside, and mountain areas have increasing sunburning potential in the order listed.

Treatment of UV Erythema. To be most effective all treatments need to be commenced during or immediately after exposure, at which time the subject is usually not aware of the need or in reach of the treatment. Once redness and pain begin, treatment can be only symptomatic and partially effective. This is obvious if one considers the diverse mechanisms involved in UV inflammation, including probably direct vessel damage and release of mediators from mast cells, leukocytes, plasma exudate, and epidermal cells. Perhaps multiple therapy might be expected to be more helpful than single agents, but direct vessel damage presumably cannot be cured by drugs and it is also difficult to see how damage to epidermal cells can be prevented by a drug given after irradiation. However, the symptoms and vasodilatation can be partially prevented, improved, or reversed, and certain components of the ongoing inflammatory response may be diminished. Many therapies have been tried, among which are nonsteroidal anti-inflammatory agents, corticosteroids, antihistamines, antioxidants, vitamin A, psoralen photochemotherapy (PUVA), antimalarials, and beta-carotene.

Nonsteroidal Anti-inflammatory Agents. Because of the known association of PGs and UV erythema (see above), antiprostaglandin agents have been tried in therapy, the most commonly used being the cyclo-oxygenase inhibitor, indomethacin (141, 142). UVC erythema might be expected to respond best since its time course correlates closely with the elevation of skin PG levels (40), but although these levels are returned to normal, oral indomethacin only partly inhibits the erythema (45) and intradermal indomethacin seems effective only in high doses and not in all cases (43). Similarly in UVB erythema, although skin PG levels are again returned to normal (45), there is only moderate inhibition and sometimes delay in onset of the erythema, the inhibition lasting for a few hours up to 24 hr in most cases, and perhaps up to 48 hr if therapy is given immediately or repeatedly after irradiation (11, 42, 44, 45, 143–146). The histologic changes in UVB erythema are unaffected by indomethacin (11, 42). UVA erythema in one study was not inhibited by topical, oral, or intradermal indomethacin (44). Further studies have looked at the effect of other nonsteroidal anti-inflammatory agents, such as aspirin (41, 147, 148), fenoprofen (66, 143), flufenamic acid, mefenamic acid (149), naproxen (66, 149), ibuprofen (149), niflumic acid, phenylbutazone, paracetamol (148), and suprofen (150). All these substances have had at least a mild but never a marked effect. Indomethacin appears to be satisfactory as symptomatic therapy and may be applied topically as a 2.5% solution in a vehicle of absolute ethanol:propylene glycol:dimethylacetamide 19:19:2 by volume (41, 44, 45) as soon as possible after exposure, one application seeming moderately effective for up to 24 hr (42) and repeated applications for up to 48 hr (44).

Corticosteroids. Corticosteroids have also been used in UV erythema. They appear to reduce PG synthesis by preventing formation of arachidonic acid in membranes (151) while apparently not affecting synthesis beyond this stage (149, 151, 152) and have been noted mildly to antagonize the erythematous action of intradermal PGE_1 (153). Steroids may also inhibit leukocyte accumulation in inflammation and inhibit lysosomal breakdown (154–156), although the importance of this last factor in UV inflammation is not certain.

Steroids seem to be less effective in UV erythema than nonsteroidal anti-inflammatory agents (41, 146, 150). Systemic steroids in large doses have been said to protect by a factor of two against UV irradiation (157), but in a bilateral comparison study they seemed not to reduce UVB-induced erythema, tenderness, or edema (158). UVB erythema may be moderately reduced by topical and intradermal betamethasone valerate following doses of less than 2 MEDs, and totally abolished following 1 MED (146). It is significantly reduced for more than 24 hr by intradermal triamcinolone acetonide following 2-1/2 MEDs and totally abolished if the drug is given just prior to irradiation (41). The combination of a nonsteroidal anti-inflammatory agent (suprofen as a 5% cream) and a corticosteroid (triamcinolone acetonide as a 0.1% cream) is moderately effective for about 30 hr when topically applied 6 hr, or preferably immediately, after UVB irradiation, suprofen alone being better than triamcinolone alone and the combination being better than either single agent (150).

Other Agents. Antihistamines may theoretically decrease immediate and possibly delayed UV erythema, as histamine release can apparently occur during UV inflammation (see above). A single uncontrolled study of triprolidine supports this (159), although clinical experience strongly suggests otherwise. However, oral antihistamine therapy might give slight additional symptomatic relief.

Antioxidants may act by preventing photooxidation of vulnerable cell structures. Vitamin C, vitamin E, glutathione, and butylated hydroxytoluene (BHT) have been tried (160, 161). Oral BHT has been reported to protect by a factor of about two (160) and topical vitamin E by a factor of about 1.5 (161). Topical vitamin E applied several times from 1 min to 60 hr after UVC irradiation in mice apparently may prevent or reduce ultrastructural damage (162). Oral BHT is not a safe medication, but topical antioxidants may prove to play a role in the prevention of sunburn.

Vitamin A was used orally for many years, but there appears to be no evidence for its efficacy (163). By inducing delayed pigmentation, psoralen photochemotherapy (PUVA) may protect by a factor of about two (164) following a single dose, and by a factor of 4–7 following a short course of treatment (165). UV radiation alone also induces pigmentation, which subsequently raises the threshold for erythema. *Antimalarial drugs* such as chloroquine and quinacrine have not been shown to work (166). $PGF_{2\alpha}$

synthesis can be inhibited by chloroquine, but this PG does not appear to be very active in promoting inflammation (167, 168). *Beta-carotene* does not appear to be effective in prevention or treatment of UV-induced inflammation in normal persons (see Chapters 13 and 14).

Treatment of sunburn is therefore not fully effective. Most cases need only soothing creams or cooling shake lotions (e.g., calamine lotion) and mild analgesics. More severe cases can be treated with a topical preparation of 2.5% indomethacin in ethanol:propylene glycol:dimethylacetamide 19:19:2 by volume applied as soon as possible after irradiation and then every hour or so for 24 hr. Theoretically, a better therapy is topical application of a combined preparation of nonsteroid anti-inflammatory agent, such as 5% suprofen, and corticosteroid, such as 0.1% triamcinolone acetonide, as soon as possible after irradiation and then every few hours. Presumably other combinations of steroid and nonsteroid would do as well.

No other treatment is currently convenient, effective, safe, and available, although the use of antioxidants may eventually prove useful. Topical preparations containing a number of active agents seem likely to be used in the future, but avoidance of sunburn remains the most effective approach. Agents that diminish pain or vascular response but do not affect epidermal and dermal cell injury, mutagenesis, chronic actinic changes, or photocarcinogenesis may lead to an overall increase in UV-induced skin damage if people become unafraid of overexposure.

TANNING

Melanin pigmentation of skin may conveniently be divided into two types:

1. *Constitutive,* or baseline, i.e., the coloring induced by genetic factors only, uninfluenced by external stimuli.
2. *Facultative*, i.e., the reversible increase in tanning in response to external stimuli, particularly UV radiation (169).

Constitutive skin coloring is generally seen on covered areas such as the buttocks and facultative tanning on areas exposed to sunlight. Such coloring is usually related to ethnic background and is also an indication of how readily a facultative tan will develop. Subjects with marked constitutive coloring tend readily to develop a marked facultative tan as well.

Biology of the Melanin Pigmentary System

This subject is discussed fully elsewhere (170). Melanin in humans is of two types: (1) phaeomelanin, responsible for the reddish and yellowish hair and possibly skin pigmentation in subjects of that coloring; and (2) eumelanin, the major chromophore responsible for skin color, for the familiar summer tan in sun-exposed Caucasians, and for the brown-black pigmentation for dark-skinned races. Eumelanin is a high-molecular-weight insoluble substance thought to consist of a complex arrangement of linked indoles. Cuttlefish melanin consists of 5,6-dihydroxyindole and 5,6-dihydroxyindole-2-carboxylic acid units forming an irregular three-dimensional, highly conjugated heteropolymer bonded to protein by cysteine (171). It exists as a stable free radical with indole units in various states of oxidation, a fact supported by electron spin resonance (esr) studies in skin (172). Melanin appears to have the characteristics necessary for directly absorbing UV radiation and energy from excited molecules and for trapping free radicals and electrons formed in skin (91, 173). It then harmlessly dissipates this energy as heat (174). Thus it appears well suited to averting or reducing UV-induced skin damage.

The functions of melanin are possibly multiple, but certainly seem to include photoprotection, although the pigment is far from completely effective in this role (25, 34, 104, 106, 165). Constitutive pigmentation may be more important than facultative pigmentation. The former seems to give about 5–30 times protection against UV radiation (25, 24, 104) whereas the latter, in one study, seemed to protect by a factor of only 2–3 (106). The possibility that these differences in UV tolerance may be due to variations not in pigmentation but in stratum corneum or epidermal thickening has been excluded (106, 175–177). Other functions suggested for melanin are animal camouflage, thermoregulation, regulation of vitamin D synthesis, coloring to emphasize aggressive display behavior patterns (169), and conversion of acoustic to electrical energy (174).

Melanin is formed in the melanocytes of the basal layer of the epidermis. In transverse histologic sections one melanocyte occurs for about every ten basal keratinocytes (178), although if inactive melanocytes are also included one melanocyte for about 4–6 basal keratinocytes has been suggested (179). Three-dimensionally, each melanocyte is related to about 36 living keratinocytes of the basal layer and stratum spinosum (169). These keratinocytes are entangled within the dendrites of the melanocyte to which they are related, and hence they receive melanin, such a melanocyte–keratinocyte complex being known as an epidermal melanin unit (180) (Fig. 8-5). Melanocytes seem to maintain their population by occasional mitotic division (181).

Melanin is formed by a complex series of reactions starting with the action of tyrosinase on tyrosine. The tyrosine probably initially accumulates in the Golgi apparatus and is incorporated into a protein matrix derived from the rough endoplasmic reticulum to form an ovoid cytoplasmic unit of variable size known as a melanosome. Melanosomes are larger in darkly pigmented races and are singly distributed within a membrane-bound vesicle. In fair-skinned races they are smaller and several appear together within one membrane-bound vesicle. Mongoloids may have a mixture of single and

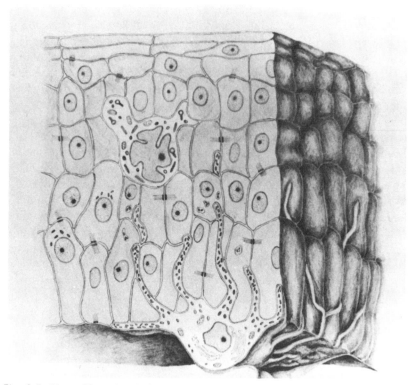

Fig. 8-5. The epidermal melanin unit. Relationship of a basal melanocyte, "high-level" Langerhans cell, and keratinocytes in mammalian epidermis. [From Quevedo (215).]

aggregated melanosome complexes and exposure to UV radiation may increase the number of larger single melanosomes (169, 182). The size at which melanosomes invariably seem to be in single membrane-bound organelles is about 0.7 by 0.3 μm (104). The melanosome matrix is gradually melanized while the melanosome is being passed along the dendrite either singly or clustered with other melanosomes in a membrane-bound lysosome-like organelle. Movement seems to be aided by 100-Å filaments in the dendrites (183). The melanosome is fully melanized before transfer of the membrane-bound structure to the keratinocyte during very close apposition of parts of the donor and receptor cells (184, 185). Degradation of melanosomes occurs within the keratinocyte, with disruption of the melanosomes and dispersal of melanin particles. This degradation is most marked in the stratum corneum. The exact steps in the metabolic pathway of melanin pigmentation are shown in Fig. 8-6.

Photobiology of the Melanin Pigmentary System

Immediate Tanning (IT). This is a transient light brown, dark brown, or occasionally greyish facultative tan and may be induced by UV wavelengths

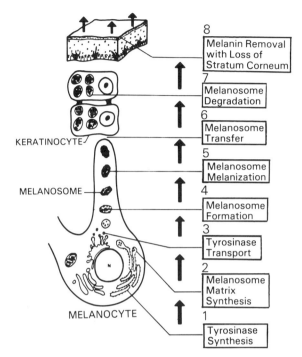

Fig. 8-6. Morpholotic and metabolic pathway of epidermal melanin pigmentation. [Modified from (170).]

from 320 to 700 nm (5, 9, 186–188). The effect seems most marked between about 380 and 500 nm (188). IT may begin immediately and fade within seconds to minutes or may persist with higher doses or longer exposures for 1/2–1 hr, up to 24 hr, or rarely for 36–48 hr after prolonged exposure, at which stage it blends with delayed tanning (DT) (5, 9, 186, 187). A dose of 2–12 J cm^{-2} of UVA appears sufficient to produce IT in Caucasians who tan fairly readily (9).

The function of IT has not yet been demonstrated. Immediate photoprotection would be expected, but UVB and UVC erythema seems not to be reduced by IT (124). However, melanin forms predominantly supranuclear caps in basal cells (34, 189) and as this is the most satisfactory distribution for protection of genetic material in epidermal germinative cells, IT may somehow be useful although erythema reduction may be minimal.

During IT there is a photooxidation of existing melanin. Studies in human skin suggest that parts of the melanin molecule are oxidized to semiquinone-like free radicals (91), this change apparently being responsible for the darkening of melanin and thus of melanosomes and skin. There are also changes in the distribution of epidermal melanosomes. They cease to be arranged predominantly around the melanocytic nucleus and become spread throughout the melanocytic dendrites and surrounding keratinocytes (190), presumably as a result of rapid movement (183). At the same time, the 100-Å filaments which are also normally clustered about the nucleus are seen surrounding the melanosomes in the dendrites, suggesting that they are the motive force for the melanosomes (183). Other changes during IT are an increase in prominence of the melanocytic dendrites, an increase in dopa reactivity of the melanocytes, and an increase in melanocytic nucleolar size. However, there is apparently no change in the number of melanosomes or of melanocytes (183).

   Delayed Tanning (DT). This is the familiar long-lasting facultative tan induced by repeated sun exposure in outdoor workers and vacationers and to a much lesser degree by adequate single exposures. DT may follow UVC, UVB, and UVA irradiation, the time course, degree, and color of tan varying with waveband. UVC-induced DT follows small radiation doses probably greater than 1 MED (25), may become visible by about 24 hr, is faint and light-brown in color, and fades within a few days to a week or two (5). UVB-induced DT follows radiation doses above about 1.5 MEDs (9, 191), i.e., about 40 mJ cm^{-2} (9), may be visible after about 24 hr, becomes obvious by about 3–5 days, is deeper brown in color than after UVC, and may persist for weeks to months (5). UVA-induced DT is more difficult to assess because of IT, which nearly always precedes and blends imperceptibly into DT (5, 8, 9), occasionally with a transient intermediate phase of lighter pigmentation (8). UVA-induced DT seems to become visible by about 36–48 hr (8), is deep brown in color, and may last for weeks up to more than a year (5). The minimal UVA dose for DT has been assessed at 17.8 ± 8.7 J cm^{-2} (range, 5.6–37.1 J cm^{-2}) for monochromatic UVA of 337.1 nm (8), and almost identically at 17.7 ± 8.0 J cm^{-2} (range 8–40 J cm^{-2}) for broadband UVA (9), which is about two-thirds to one-half (8, 9) of the MED read at 24 hr, contrasting with the higher than MED doses necessary for UVC- and UVB-induced DT. Visible light-induced DT apparently resembles that following UVA, its action spectrum extending at least as far as 520 nm (186).

   The stimulus for induction of DT is not known, but is possibly nonspecifically related to UV injury to melanocytes or keratinocytes. Melanocytes are probably always damaged by UV radiation before melanogenesis begins, since ¼ MED or less of solar-simulating radiation can lead to DNA damage in basal cells (165). On the other hand, there is conceivably a specific UV-induced trigger for melanogenesis.

   In that it entails formation of new melanin in response to UV exposure, the main function of DT is likely to be photoprotection. Such protection, however, seems to be no more than moderate, a factor of only 2–3 being achieved against solar-simulating radiation in Caucasians by a dark UVA tan in one study in the absence of horny layer thickening (106), although a factor of 4–7 was obtained against similar radiation in another study by a PUVA-induced tan, probably because of the presence of horny layer thickening (165). Further, DNA damage, albeit reduced, still occurs at all levels in tanned skin

(165). Melanin therefore cannot be considered an extremely effective sunscreen for Caucasians, particularly when compared with the best presently available commercial products.

During DT in humans and animals there is an increase in the number of functioning melanocytes. This has been observed following UVA (192), UVB (179, 193), and UVC (194) irradiation, but, at least for UVA and UVB in humans, only following multiple exposures (182). There has been discussion as to whether increase in number by mitosis or by activation of already present but dormant melanocytes is responsible. Both mechanisms may be important. Repeated UVC irradiation in mice induces a gradual increase in functioning melanocytes throughout the irradiation period with a decrease to normal levels over the next two weeks, the increase at least partly due to activation of previously nonfunctioning melanocytes, although mitotic increase was not ruled out (194). Repeated exposures to UVB radiation cause a 4–6 fold increase in the number of melanocytes in mice within 8–11 days, associated with a higher rate of melanocyte mitosis than in unirradiated control sites. This rate of mitosis as assessed by cumulative thymidine labeling seems high enough to account for the total increase in functioning melanocytes, but activation of already present cells is not definitely excluded. Following cessation of irradiation after 2 weeks, the number of melanocytes gradually drops towards normal over the next few months (193). On nonirradiated sites in mice there seems to be a delayed and slightly smaller increase in melanocyte numbers after 2 weeks' irradiation, a peak being reached in 2–3 months and a slow return to normal occurring in parallel with the population in irradiated sites. The presence of a systemic factor arising from the irradiated site was suggested as responsible for the generalized increase (195). Other studies have also noted an increase in melanocyte population following UVB irradiation (179, 195); one, however, using a histochemical technique, attributed it at least partly to structural and functional activation of already present melanocytes (179). With repeated UVA irradiation in mice over 2 weeks, electron microscopic examination shows a marked increase in functioning melano-cytes, in part due to activation of nonfunctioning melanocytes already present as well as to mitosis (192). After irradiation, mitosis has been seen and the mitotic index is higher (192) than in unirradiated melanocytes (181). Increase in the number of functioning melanocytes after UVA irradiation has also been described in humans (182), but more recently in mice absent or minimal increase was reported, possibly because the UVA dose used was much lower (196). The increase in numbers of melanocytes is probably associated with increased numbers of keratinocytes, thereby maintaining the basic epidermal melanin unit structure (182).

Following UVB or UVA irradiation in humans, increase in melanocyte size and increased branching (arborization) of dendrites occurs within 2–3 days and 7 days, respectively, and melanocyte tyrosinase activity is enhanced, especially after multiple exposures. Multiple exposures also lead to an

Table 8-5. Responses of Human Melanocytes to UV Radiation[a]

		Unirradiated skin	UV-irradiated skin (single exposure)	
			Immediate tanning (IT)	Delayed tanning (DT)
Light microscopy				
DOPA reaction		Weak	No definite change	Markedly increased
Number of melanocytes			No change	Increased, but variable
Perikaryon		Small	Small	Markedly enlarged
Dendrites		Poorly developed	Well developed	Well developed
Electron microscopy	Nucleus shape	Oval, round	Indented	Markedly indented
	Chromatin	Heterochromatin granules in the periphery, sparse euchromatin	Increased heterochromatin granules; no change in euchromatin	Increased euchromatin
	Nucleolus	Few in number, small	No increase in number, but slightly enlarged in size	Increased in number and enlarged in size; occasional segregation of nucleolar components
	Melanosomes (number)	Few	No change; possibly decreased (?)	Markedly increased
	Stages of formation of melanosomes	In pigmented skin, mostly melanized stages, but in light skin, unmelanized stages	Larger proportion of melanized melanosomes (?)	Melanosomes in various stages, particularly in melanized stages
	Distribution pattern	Perinuclear	Dendrites (predominantly)	Perinuclear areas and dendrites

100-Å filaments	Dense, perinuclear aggregation	Dense aggregation in dendrites, and melanosomes interspersed between filaments	Diffusely scattered in perikaryon and dendrites
Golgi apparatus	Poorly developed	Poorly developed	Well developed; marked increase in size and number
Rough endoplasmic reticulum	Poorly developed	Poorly developed	Well developed
Free ribosomes	A few	A few	Abundant
Microtubules	Perinuclear area	Dendrites	Perinuclear area and dendrites
Autophagic vacuole	Absent	Absent	Present
Lipid droplet	Absent	Absent	Present
Basal lamina below melanocyte	Monolayered	Multilayered	Multilayered

[a] After Quevedo et al. (169).

increase in size and number of melanosomes in both melanocytes and keratinocytes as a result of accentuated synthesis and transfer of these organelles (182), although possibly only in number after UVA irradiation in guinea pigs (197). There is also a moderate decrease in the number of melanosomes per melanosome complex and a great increase in the number of melanin granules throughout the epidermis (182).

Thus, in general, a single UVA or UVB irradiation tends to increase the functional activity of the melanocyte only, whereas multiple irradiations stimulate an increase in the number of melanocytes and epidermal melanin units as well. A summary of the light and electron microscopic differences in irradiated and nonirradiated skin with respect to IT and DT, including some features not mentioned in the text, is shown in Table 8-5.

Skin Thickening

In addition to erythema and tanning, UV irradiation of the skin results in skin thickening. After UV injury there is an initial depression in many aspects of cellular activity, a subsequent increase toward normal, and then above-normal cell replication during repair. The increase in activity persists, leading to increased skin thickness until, in the absence of further UV irradiation, there is a gradual reduction to normal replication and thickness. These phases proceed smoothly from one stage to the next and lead to changes in skin tolerance to UV irradiation.

Changes in Epidermal Kinetics

Studies of changes in rate of macromolecular synthesis have been carried out, mostly following single doses of UVB irradiation. There is a biphasic response in the rate of synthesis of DNA, RNA, and proteins in humans and animals (198–204). Semiconservative DNA synthesis, which precedes cell division, normally occurs in about 4–5% of all epidermal cells. It is usually measured by studying the incorporation of tritiated thymidine into the nucleus (199, 203). DNA synthesis is depressed in the first few minutes after irradiation, reaching maximum reduction in between 1 and 6 hr (198, 203) after irradiation. At this time, synthesis is between about 10% and 50% (198, 200) of normal. Maximum stimulation occurs between 2 and 48 hr (199, 203) after irradiation, reaching from about 125–700% (199, 200) of normal. At 7 days, the changes may still persist to a moderate degree or have virtually disappeared (199, 203). One study also shows some stimulation of DNA synthesis at 24 and 48 hr after UVA irradiation (120). Dose–response aspects of this effect are uncertain. One study tended to show that increased dosage increased all the effects up to a point, but continued further increase seemed inexplicably to reverse this trend (203). RNA and protein synthesis are similarly depressed in the first few hours after UVB irradiation and are markedly increased by 72 hr (199). The effect on protein is apparently a direct effect rather than secondary to RNA damage, and the effects are more marked in the upper layers of the epidermis, the basal layer not obviously being affected (204).

The changes are associated with similar changes in mitotic rate of epidermal cells. There is an initial decrease to zero in the number of cells entering mitosis within 1 hr of irradiation, this number increasing to normal by 24 hr and being much increased by 72 hr (199). The increase continues until 7 days after irradiation and gradually drops toward normal by 6 weeks (135). Thus, cells divide more frequently, and the daughter cells also divide sooner than usual, leading to a great increase in epidermal tissue growth rate. This leads to an up to 2–3-fold increase in the number of cells per unit cross-sectional area of epidermis, greater after UVB than after UVC; the maximum occurs at about 14 days after UVB and 11 days after UVC irradiation and still persists somewhat above normal at 6 weeks (135).

Changes in Skin Thickness

The changes in cellular activity described above eventually lead to skin thickening affecting both dermis and epidermis (135, 205). A 2–4-fold increase in epidermal thickness occurs in the mouse ear following a single UVB or UVC irradiation. When irradiated animals are subsequently kept in the dark, increased thickness, becoming evident after about a day, is maximum at about 12 days and persists over 40 days (135). If animals are kept in the light after UV exposure, it appears that photorecovery may decrease the thickening by half (117). The finding of increased thickness is associated with an up to fivefold increase in the number of epidermal cell layers, although the cells are very possibly smaller than normal (206).

Studies of the increase in thickness of human skin following UV irradiation have shown that after single UVB exposures in tanned and untanned Caucasian subjects, the stratum spinosum tends to thicken up to about twofold (85) and the stratum corneum by about 1.5–3-fold (85, 207) within 1–3 weeks. In vitiliginous skin the increase in thickness, at least of stratum corneum, is up to twice as great as in normal Caucasian skin (207). After multiple exposures every 1–2 days for up to 7 weeks, there is only a little thickening of the stratum spinosum, but a marked 3–5-fold thickening of the stratum corneum, possibly slightly more marked in vitiliginous kin (85); this returns to nearly normal within about 4 weeks of ceasing irradiation. The longer the period of repeated exposure, the thicker the skin becomes, one subject after 8 months of regular UVB therapy for cutaneous tuberculosis having a stratum spinosum about 2–3 times thicker and a stratum corneum about 7–10 times thicker than normal, although the possibility of disease effects on the skin is not discussed (85).

Dermal thickening also occurs after single UVB and UVC exposures in the mouse ear, first becoming apparent at about 1 day after irradiation, reaching a maximum of up to four times normal at 9–12 days, and returning toward normal by 6 weeks (135).

Changes in Skin Tolerance to UV Radiation Due to Skin Thickening

Thickening of the skin, especially of the dead horny layer, should theoretically lead to increased UV skin tolerance even in the absence of increased melanin. Vitiliginous skin is less sensitive to UV radiation after repeated UV exposure (208–210); this has been attributed to increased horny layer thickness (210). Repeated UVB irradiation of albino mouse skin produces an approximately twofold reduction in UVB transmission (211). Conversely, stripping of the stratum corneum with tape increases skin sensitivity to UVB (212) and in one study also to UVC (213). Miescher (85) investigated protection factors as assessed by the erythema response to UVB radiation in Caucasian subjects, single irradiation inducing a slight increase in protection. Repeated irradiations every 1–2 days led to an 18-fold increase in UV tolerance after 4 weeks of irradiation, reducing to threefold 1 month after cessation of exposure. In a subject with vitiligo, there was a 15-fold increase in UV tolerance after 7 weeks of daily suberythemogenic doses, and in the patient with cutaneous tuberculosis mentioned above it became impossible to induce UVB erythema following 8 months of almost daily exposure.

Thus thickening of the skin, and probably especially of the horny layer, after UV exposure leads to a significant increase in protection against UV radiation. That this is not so effective as in association with melanin protection has been shown in transmission studies in human skin (211) and is evident from the fact that albino Cuna Indians develop multiple skin carcinomas as compared to their pigmented neighbors (214). However, particularly since the stratum corneum and epidermis are of essentially equal thickness in all races (175–177), it seems likely that pigmentation is the most important means of protection against UV radiation in races of marked constitutive coloring—dark races are 5–30 times better protected than Caucasians (25, 34, 104). On the other hand, skin thickening is probably more important in races of light constitutive coloring, since dark facultative pigmentation without horny layer thickening apparently gives only a mild increase in UV tolerance—tanned Caucasians with an unthickened horny layer are only 2–3 times better protected than similar untanned subjects (106). However, only one study of this type appears to have been carried out (106). It is, of course, possible that protection of vital structures (i.e., nuclear material) and not prevention of erythema is provided by melanin. Nevertheless, it is evident that skin thickening is an important adjunct to melanization in minimizing UV-induced skin damage. Further studies should clarify the relative value of each mechanism.

SUMMARY

UV inflammation is initiated following absorption of UV photons by unknown chromophores, although nucleic acids and proteins may be involved. Free radicals are also formed and damage to other susceptible structures, such as membranes, may also result. The details of these reactions are, however. not known. UV radiation induces inflammation, tanning, and skin thickening in humans. Adequate doses of any combination of UVC, UVB, and UVA irradiation are capable of inducing cutaneous inflammation. This inflammation is an example of the general inflammatory response to a noxious invading agent. There are two phases: (1) an immediate phase, and (2) a delayed phase. In humans, only a few subjects show a clinically discernible immediate phase. The immediate phase consists of transient erythema and vasopermeability beginning within seconds and lasting only a few minutes, and may be mediated to some extent by histamine release following direct action of UV radiation on mast cells. Direct vessel damage may also contribute to some extent in the immediate phase, and continue to have an effect during the delayed phase.

The delayed phase ensues within a few hours and lasts for hours to a few days. Neutrophils are present in delayed UVB and UVC inflammation in guinea pigs and are important in other types of delayed inflammation where they tend to break down, releasing multiple substances from their granules or lysosomes, leading to chemoattraction of more neutrophils, a further or delayed phase of erythema, and a further or delayed phase of vasopermeability. The neutrophil invasion peaks in guinea pigs at about 8 hr after UVB radiation, vasopermeability probably peaking at about the same time, and erythema reaching its height at about 12–24 hr. A role for neutrophils in human UV inflammation, however, has not yet been documented. Tissue neutrophil levels in guinea pigs fall to near normal by 24 hr after irradiation, but monocytes may persist for much longer. Their exact role, if any, in UV inflammation is not known. There is also passage of plasma into the tissues, leading to probable formation of bradykinin. Bradykinin enhances vasopermeability, erythema, and pain, and has been isolated in humans at an early stage following UVB irradiation. After UVB and UVC irradiation skin prostaglandin levels rise within about 6 hr and peak at about 12–24 hr. Prostaglandin enhances erythema and in association with histamine and bradykinin may enhance vasopermeability. Breakdown of epidermal lysosomes and of epidermal and possibly many other cells may contribute to continued elevation of tissue prostaglandin levels. Inhibitors of prostaglandin formation reduce UV erythema, but not the histologic evidence of epidermal cell injury.

It must be stressed that exact or complete data are lacking on many of these points, particularly in humans, and further studies are needed to clarify the situation.

Treatment of UV inflammation is not very effective; prevention of burning by avoidance of excessive exposure and by use of effective sunscreening agents is more useful. However, most likely to be helpful symptomatically is a combination of topical steroid and topical cyclo-oxygenase inhibitor.

In people genetically able to pigment, delayed tanning appears gradually as delayed erythema fades. Previous immediate tanning may be induced within seconds by UVA and visible wavelengths and is due to alteration and redistribution of melanin already present. It persists for one to several hours, or in some cases, a day or two. Delayed tanning results from UV-induced production of new melanin by melanocytes and recruitment of new melanocytes, probably both by mitosis and by activation of already present melanocytes. The pigment is passed up through the epidermis to the stratum corneum, and protects against further UV damage apparently by scattering, reflecting, or absorbing UV radiation, and possibly by taking up free radicals and electrons produced in skin by such radiation.

Skin thickening is a process that follows the initial and virtually immediate reduction of DNA, RNA, and protein synthesis caused by UV irradiation. Initially mitosis also ceases. Within a few hours to a day or so, these processes increase enormously and hyperplasia of the epidermis and dermis ensues, especially after repeated irradiation. The stratum corneum is very much thickened within a week or two and acts in conjunction with melanin in protecting against further UV-radiation damage by absorbing such radiation. During the 1–2 months after cessation of exposure the skin gradually returns toward normal.

REFERENCES

1. Jagger, J. (1967): *Introduction to Research in Ultraviolet Photobiology*, pp. 53–59. Prentice-Hall, Englewood Cliffs, N. J.
2. Parrish, J. A., Anderson, R. R., Urbach, F., et al. (1978): *UV-A: Biological Effects of Ultraviolet Radiation with Emphasis on Human Responses to Longwave Ultraviolet*, p. 76. Plenum Press, New York.
3. Daniels, F., Jr., and Johnson, B. E. (1974): Normal, physiological, and pathologic effects of solar radiation on the skin. In: *Sunlight and Man: Normal and Abnormal Photobiologic Responses*, edited by M. A. Pathak, L. C. Harber, M. Seiji, and A. Kukita (T. B. Fitzpatrick, consulting editor), pp. 117–130. University of Tokyo Press, Tokyo.
4. Johnson, B. E., Magnus, I. A., and White, J. E. (1979): Solar radiation damage and the induction of skin cancer. An International Workshop-Meeting, Lausanne, Switzerland, September 26–29, 1978. *Brit. J. Dermatol.* 100:593–595.
5. Bachem, A. (1955): Time factors of erythema and pigmentation, produced by ultraviolet rays of different wavelengths. *J. Invest. Dermatol.* 25:215–218.
6. Kumakiri, M., Hashimoto, K., and Willis, I. (1977): Biologic changes due to longwave ultraviolet irradiation on human skin: ultrastructural study. *J. Invest. Dermatol.* 69: 392–400.

7. Cotran, R. S., and Pathak, M. A. (1968): The pattern of vascular leakage induced by monochromatic UV irradiation in rats, guinea pigs and hairless mice. *J. Invest. Dermatol.* **51**:155–164.

8. Parrish, J. A., Anderson, R. R., Ying, C. Y., et al. (1976): Cutaneous effects of pulsed nitrogen gas laser irradiation. *J. Invest. Dermatol.* **67**:603–608.

9. Kaidbey, K. H., and Kligman, A. M. (1979): The acute effects of long-wave ultraviolet radiation on human skin. *J. Invest. Dermatol.* **72**:253–256.

10. Logan, G., and Wilhelm, D. L. (1963): Ultra-violet injury as an experimental model of the inflammatory reaction. *Nature* **198**:968–969.

11. Snyder, D. S. (1976): Effect of topical indomethacin on UVR-induced redness and prostaglandin E levels in sunburned guinea pig skin. *Prostaglandins* **11**:631–643.

12. Rea, T. H. (1968): The anatomic site of vascular injury in mouse skin exposed to ultraviolet light. *J. Invest. Dermatol.* **51**:100–107.

13. Sams, W. M., Jr., and Winkelmann, R. K. (1969): The effect of ultraviolet light on isolated cutaneous blood vessels. *J. Invest. Dermatol.* **53**:79–83.

14. Uvnäs, B. (1964): Release processes in mast cells and their activation by injury. *Ann. N. Y. Acad. Sci.* **116**:880–890.

15. Valtonen, E. J., Jänne, J., and Siimes, M. (1964): The effect of the erythemal reaction caused by ultra-violet irradiation on mast cell degranulation in the skin. *Acta Derm. Venereol. (Stockh.)* **44**:269–272.

16. Lewis, T. H. (1927): *The Blood Vessels of the Human Skin and Their Responses*, p. 117–138. Shaw, London.

17. Majno, G., and Palade, G. E. (1961): Studies on inflammation. I. The effect of histamine and serotonin on vascular permeability: an electron microscopic study. *J. Biophys. Biochem. Cytol.* **11**:571–605.

18. Logan, G., and Wilhelm, D. L. (1966): Vascular permeability changes in inflammation: I. The role of endogenous permeability factors in ultraviolet injury. *Br. J. Exp. Pathol.* **47**:300–314.

19. Greaves, M. W., and Sondergaard, J. (1970): Pharmacologic agents released in ultraviolet inflammation studied by continuous skin perfusion. *J. Invest. Dermatol.* **54**:365–367.

20. Gilchrest, B. A., Soter, N. A., and Stoff, J. (1980): A possible role for histamine in the human reaction. In: *Program and Abstracts*, pp. 135–136. 8th Annual Meeting of the American Society for Photobiology.

21. Claesson, S., Wettermark, G., and Juhlin, L. (1959): Action of ultra-violet light on skin: effect of the histamine liberator 48/80 and methotrimeprazine. *Nature* **183**:1451–1452.

22. Veninga, T. S., and de Boer, J. E. (1968): Urinary excretion pattern of serotonin and 5-hydroxyindole acetic acid in ultraviolet induced erythema. *J. Invest. Dermatol.* **50**:1–8.

23. Lord, J. T., and Ziboh, V. A. (1979): Specific binding of prostaglandin E_2 to membrane preparations from human skin: receptor modulation by UVB-irradiation and chemical agents. *J. Invest. Dermatol.* **73**:373–377.

24. Hausser, K. W., and Vahle, W. (1922): Die Abhängigkeit des Lichterythems und der Pigmentbildung von der Schwingungszahl (Wellenlänge) der erregenden Strahlung. *Strahlentherapie* **13**:41–71.

25. Hausser, K. W., and Vahle, W. (1927): Sonnenbrand und Sonnenbräunung. *Wissenschaftliche Veröffnungen des Siemens Konzern* **6**:101–120.

26. Rottier, P. B. (1953): The erythematous action of ultraviolet light on human skin. I. Some measurements of the spectral response with continuous and intermittent light. *J. Clin. Invest.* **32**:681–689.

27. Everett, M. A., Olsen, R. L., and Sayre, R. M. (1965): Ultraviolet erythema. *Arch. Dermatol.* **92**:713–719.

28. Olson, R. L., Sayre, R. M., and Everett, M. A. (1966): Effect of anatomic location and time on ultraviolet erythema. *Arch. Dermatol.* **93**:211–215.

29. Sayre, R. M., Olson, R. L., and Everett, M. A. (1966): Quantitative studies on erythema. *J. Invest. Dermatol.* **46**:240–244.
30. Lewis, T., and Zotterman, Y. (1926): Vascular reactions of the skin to injury. VI. Some effects of ultra-violet light. *Heart* **13**:203–217.
31. Ramsay, C. A., and Cripps, D. J. (1970): Cutaneous arteriolar dilatation elicited by ultraviolet irradiation. *J. Invest. Dermatol.* **54**:332–337.
32. Ramsay, C. A., and Challoner, A. V. J. (1976): Vascular changes in human skin after ultraviolet irradiation. *Br. J. Dermatol.* **94**:487–493.
33. Eaglstein, W. H., Sakai, M., and Mizuno, N. (1979): Ultraviolet radiation-induced inflammation and leukocytes. *J. Invest. Dermatol.* **72**:59–63.
34. Miescher, G. (1932): Untersuchungen über die Bedeutung des Pigments für den UV.-Lichtschutz der Haut. *Strahlentherapie* **45**:201–216.
35. Miescher, G. (1957): Zur Histologie der lichtbedingten Reaktionen. *Dermatologica* **115**:345–357.
36. Johnston, M. G., Hay, J. B., and Movat, H. Z. (1976): The modulation of enhanced vascular permeability by prostaglandins through alterations in blood flow (hyperemia). *Agents Actions* **6**:705–711.
37. Mathur, G. P., and Gandhi, V. M. (1972): Prostaglandin in human and albino rat skin. *J. Invest. Dermatol.* **58**:291–295.
38. Black, A. K., Greaves, M. W., Hensby, C. N., et al. (1978): Increased prostaglandins E_2 and $F_{2\alpha}$ in human skin at 6 and 24 h after ultraviolet B irradiation (290–320 nm). *Br. J. Clin. Pharmacol.* **5**:431–436.
39. Black, A. K., Fincham, N., Greaves, M. W., et al. (1980): Time course changes in levels of arachidonic acid and prostaglandins D_2, E_2, $F_{2\alpha}$ in human skin following ultraviolet B irradiation. *Br. J. Clin. Pharmacol.* **10**:453–457.
40. Camp, R. D., Greaves, M. W., Hensby, C. N., et al. (1978): Irradiation of human skin by short wavelength ultraviolet radiation (100–290 nm) (u.v.C.): increased concentrations of arachidonic acid and prostaglandins E_2 and $F_{2\alpha}$. *Br. J. Clin. Pharmacol.* **6**:145–148.
41. Snyder, D. S., and Eaglstein, W. H. (1974): Topical indomethacin and sunburn. *Br. J. Dermatol.* **90**:91–93.
42. Snyder, D. S. (1975): Cutaneous effects of topical indomethacin, an inhibitor of prostaglandin synthesis, on UV-damaged skin. *J. Invest. Dermatol.* **64**:322–325.
43. Eaglstein, W. H., and Marsico, A. R. (1975): Dichotomy in response to indomethacin in UV-C and UV-B induced ultraviolet light inflammation. *J. Invest. Dermatol.* **65**:238–240.
44. Morison, W. L., Paul B. S., and Parrish, J. A. (1977): The effects of indomethacin on long-wave ultraviolet-induced delayed erythema. *J. Invest. Dermatol.* **68**:130–133.
45. Black, A. K., Greaves, M. W., Hensby, C. N., et al. (1978): The effects of indomethacin on arachidonic acid and prostaglandins E_2 and $F_{2\alpha}$ levels in human skin 24 h after u.v.B and u.v.C. irradiation. *Br. J. Clin. Pharmacol.* **6**:261–266.
46. Ziboh, V. A., Lord, J. T., Uematsu, S., et al. (1978): Activation of phospholipase A_2 and increased release of prostaglandin precursor from skin by ultraviolet irradiation. *J. Invest. Dermatol.* **70**:211.
47. Movat, H. Z., Macmorine, D. R. L., and Takeuchi, Y. (1971): The role of PMN-leukocyte lysosomes in tissue injury, inflammation and hypersensitivity. VIII. Mode of action and properties of vascular permeability factors released by PMN-leukocytes during *in vitro* phagocytosis. *Int. Arch. Allergy Appl. Immunol.* **40**:218–235.
48. Davies, P., and Allison, A. C. (1976): The macrophage as a secretory cell in chronic inflammation. *Agents Actions* **6**:60–74.
49. Smith, J. B., Ingerman, C., Kocsis, J. J., et al. (1973): Formation of prostaglandins during the aggregation of human blood platelets. *J. Clin. Invest.* **52**:965–969.
50. Gimbrone, M. A., Jr., and Alexander, R. W. (1975): Angiotensin II stimulation of prostaglandin production in cultured human vascular endothelium. *Science* **189**:219–220.

51. Johnson, A. R., Hugli, T. E., and Müller-Eberhard, H. J. (1975): Release of histamine from rat mast cells by the complement peptides C3a and C5a. *Immunology* **28:**1067–1080.
52. Ranadive, N. S., and Cochrane, C. G. (1971): Mechanism of histamine release from mast cells by cationic protein (band 2) from neutrophil lysosomes. *J. Immunol.* **106:**506–516.
53. Lewis, G. P. (1964): Plasma kinins and other vasoactive compounds in acute inflammation. *Ann. N. Y. Acad. Sci.* **116:**847–854.
54. Reis, M. L., Okino, L., and Rocha e Silva, M. (1971): Comparative pharmacological actions of bradykinin and related kinins of larger molecular weights. *Biochem. Pharmacol.* **20:**2935–2946.
55. Davies, G. E., Holman, G., and Lowe, J. S. (1967): Role of Hageman factor in the activation of guinea-pig pre-kallikrein. *Br. J. Pharmacol.* **29:**55–62.
56. Kaplan, A. P., and Austen, K. F. (1971): A prealbumin activator of prekallikrein. II. Derivation of activators of prekallikrein from active Hageman factor by digestion with plasmin. *J. Exp. Med.* **133:**696–712.
57. Habal, F. M., Movat, H. Z., and Burrowes, C. E. (1974): Isolation of two functionally different kininogens from human plasma—separation from proteinase inhibitors and interaction with plasma kallikrein. *Biochem. Pharmacol.* **23:**2291–2303.
58. Habal, F. M., Burrowes, C. E., and Movat, H. Z. (1975): Generation of kinin by plasmin. *Fed. Proc.* **34:**859.
59. Epstein, J. H., and Winkelmann, R. K. (1967): Ultraviolet light-induced kinin formation in human skin. *Arch. Dermatol.* **95:**532–536.
60. Willis, A. L. (1969): Release of histamine, kinin and prostaglandins during carrageenon-induced inflammation in the rat, in *Prostaglandins, Peptides and Amines*, edited by P. Mantegazza and W. Horton, pp. 31–38. Academic Press, London.
61. Di Rosa, M., Giroud, J. P., and Willoughby, D. A. (1971): Studies of the mediators of the acute inflammatory response induced in rats in different sites by carrageenan and turpentine. *J. Pathol.* **104:**15–29.
62. Goldstein, I. M., and Weissmann, G. (1974): Generation of C5-derived lysosomal enzyme-releasing activity (C5a) by lysates of leukocyte lysosomes. *J. Immunol.* **113:**1583–1588.
63. Weimar, V. (1957): Polymorphonuclear invasion of wounded corneas. Inhibition by topically applied sodium salicylate and soybean trypsin inhibitor. *J. Exp. Med.* **105:**141–152.
64. Buckley, I. K. (1963): Delayed secondary damage and leucocyte chemotaxis following focal aseptic heat injury *in vivo. Exp. Mol. Pathol.* **2:**402–417.
65. Hurley, J. V. (1963): Incubation of serum with tissue extracts as a cause of chemotaxis of granulocytes. *Nature* **198:**1212–1213.
66. Blackham, A., and Owen, R. T. (1975): Prostaglandin synthetase inhibitors and leucocytic emigration. *J. Pharm. Pharmacol.* **27:**201–203.
67. Franson, R., Patriarca, P., and Elsbach, P. (1974): Phospholipid metabolism by phagocytic cells. Phospholipases A₂ associated with rabbit polymorphonuclear leukocyte granules. *J. Lipid Res.* **15:**380–388.
68. Prokopowicz, J. (1968): Purification of plasminogen from human granulocytes using DEAE–Sephadex column chromatography. *Biochim. Biophys. Acta* **154:**91–95.
69. Greenbaum, L. M., Prakash, A., Semente, G., et al. (1973): The leukokinin system; its role in fluid accumulation in malignancy and inflammation. *Agents Actions* **3:**332–334.
70. Movat, H. Z., Steinberg, S. G., Habal, F. M., et al. (1973): Kinin-forming and kinin-inactivating enzymes in human neutrophil leukocytes. *Agents Actions* **3:**284–291.
71. Movat, H. Z., Minta, J. O., Saya, M. J., et al. (1976): Neutrophil generation of permeability enhancing peptides from plasma substrates. In: *Molecular and Biological Aspects of the Acute Allergic Reactions*, edited by S. O. G. Johansson, K. Strandberg, and B. Uvnäs, pp. 391–416. Plenum Press, New York.
72. Ward, P. A. (1968): Chemotaxis of mononuclear cells. *J. Exp. Med.* **128:**1201–1221.
73. Steinman, R. M., and Cohn, Z. A. (1974): The metabolism and physiology of the

mononuclear phagocytes. In: *The Inflammatory Process,* 2nd ed., edited by B. W. Zweifach, L. Grant, and R. T. McCluskey, pp. 449–510. Academic Press, New York.

74. Hönigsmann, H., Wolff, K., and Konrad, K. (1974): Epidermal lysosomes and ultraviolet light. *J. Invest. Dermatol.* **63**:337–342.

75. Johnson, B. E., and Daniels, F., Jr. (1969): Lysosomes and the reactions of skin to ultraviolet radiation. *J. Invest. Dermatol.* **53**:85–94.

76. Desai, I. D., Sawant, P. L., and Tappel, A. L. (1964): Peroxidative and radiation damage to isolated lysosomes. *Biochim. Biophys. Acta* **86**:277–285.

77. Sams, W. M., Jr. (1974): Inflammatory mediators in ultraviolet erythema. In: *Sunlight and Man: Normal and Abnormal Photobiologic Responses,* edited by M. A. Pathak, L. C. Harber, M. Seiji, et al. (T. B. Fitzpatrick, consulting editor), pp. 143–146. University of Tokyo Press, Tokyo.

78. Allison, A. C., Magnus, I. A., and Young, M. R. (1966): Role of lysosomes and of cell membranes in photosensitization. *Nature* **209**:874–878.

79. Volden, G. (1978): Acid hydrolases in blister fluid. 4. Influence of ultraviolet radiation. *Br. J. Dermatol.* **99**:53–60.

80. Mier, P. D., van den Hurk, J. J. M. A., Bauer, F. W., et al. (1977): Mitotic activity and acid hydrolase levels in human epidermis following a single dose of ultraviolet radiation. *Br. J. Dermatol.* **96**:163–165.

81. Drury, A. N. (1936): The physiological activity of nucleic acid and its derivatives. *Physiol. Rev.* **16**:292–325.

82. Willoughby, D. A., Walters, M. N.-I., and Spector, W. G. (1964): Effect of RNA on vascular permeability in the rat. *Nature* **203**:882.

83. Beukers, R., and Berends, W. (1960): Isolation and identification of the irradiation product of thymine. *Biochim. Biophys. Acta* **41**:550–551.

84. Pathak, M. A., Krämer, D. M., and Gungerich, U. (1972): Formation of thymine dimer 7′5′ in mammalian skin by ultraviolet radiation in vivo. *Photochem. Photobiol.* **15**:177–185.

85. Miescher, G. (1930): Das Problem des Lichtschutzes und der Lichtgewöhnung. *Strahlentherapie* **35**:403–443.

86. Hamperl, H., Henschke, U., and Schulze, R. (1939): Über den Primärvorgang bei der Erythemerzeugung durch ultraviolette Strahlung. *Naturwiss.* **27**:486.

87. Mitchell, J. S. (1938): The origin of the erythema curve and the pharmacological action of ultra-violet radiation. *Proc. R. Soc. Lond. [Biol]* **126**:241–261.

88. Deering, R. A. (1962): Ultraviolet radiation and nucleic acid. The damaging effects of ultraviolet on living things have long been known. Now they are being explained in terms of specific changes in molecules of the genetic material. *Sci. Am.* **207**:135–144.

89. Meffert, H., Dressler, C., and Meffert, B. (1972): UV-provozierte Lipidperoxydation in Epidermis, Korium und Subkutis des Menschen in vitro. *Acta Biol. Med. Germ.* **29**:667–675.

90. Norins, A. L. (1962): Free radical formation in the skin following exposure to ultraviolet light. *J. Invest. Dermatol.* **39**:445–448.

91. Pathak, M. A., and Stratton, K. (1968): Free radicals in human skin before and after exposure to light. *Arch. Biochem. Biophys.* **123**:468–476.

92. Johnson, B. E., Daniels, F., Jr., and Magnus, I. A. (1968): Response of human skin to ultraviolet light. In:*Photophysiology,* Vol. IV, edited by A. C. Giese, pp. 139–202. Academic Press, London.

93. van der Leun, J. C. (1965): Theory of ultraviolet erythema. *Photochem. Photobiol.* **4**:453–458.

94. van der Leun, J. C. (1972): On the action spectrum of ultraviolet erythema. In: *Research Progress in Organic, Biological and Medicinal Chemistry,* Vol. 3, Part II, edited by L. Santamaria and U. Gallo, pp. 711–735. North-Holland, Amsterdam/London.

95. van der Leun, J. C. (1966): Ultraviolet erythema: A study on diffusion processes in human skin. Thesis, Utrecht, The Netherlands.

96. Wucherpfennig, V. (1942): Zur Messung und Bemessung des Ultraviolett. *Klin. Wochenschr.* **21**:926–930.

97. Daniels, F., and Imbrie, J. D. (1958): Comparison between visual grading and reflectance measurements of erythema produced by sunlight. *J. Invest. Dermatol.* **30**:295–304.

98. Cripps, D. J., and Ramsay, C. A. (1970): Ultraviolet action spectrum with a prism-grating monochromator. *Br. J. Dermatol.* **82**:584–592.

99. Brodthagen, H. (1969): Seasonal variations in ultraviolet sensitivity of normal skin. In: *The Biologic Effects of Ultraviolet Radiation (with Emphasis on the Skin),* edited by F. Urbach, pp. 459–467. Pergamon Press, Oxford.

100. Wucherpfennig, V., Ehring, F. J., and Heite, H. J. (1953): Die Beziehungen des UV Erythems zu Konstitution und Umwelt. *Strahlentherapie* **92**:212–218.

101. Olson, R. L., Sayre, R. M., and Everett, M. A. (1965): Effect of field size on ultraviolet minimal erythema dose. *J. Invest. Dermatol.* **45**:516–519.

102. Barth, J., and Jacobi, U. (1979): UV-Erythemschwellenbestimmung mit der Hg-Hochdrucklampe SL 500. II. Einfluss von Alter der Probanden, Lokalisation und Zeitpunkt der Erythemschwellenbestimmung. *Dermatol. Monatsschr.* **165**:220–223.

103. Barth, J. (1979): UV-Erythemschwellenbestimmung mit der Hg-Hochdrucklampe SL 500. I. Einfluss von Geschlecht, Ablesezeitpunkt und Spektralverteilung auf die Schwellenwerter mittlung. *Dermatol. Monatsschr.* **165**:216–219.

104. Olson, R. L., Gaylor, J., and Everett, M. A. (1973): Skin color, melanin, and erythema. *Arch. Dermatol.* **108**:541–544.

105. Kaidbey, K. H., Agin, P. P., Sayre, R. M., et al. (1979): Photoprotection by melanin—a comparison of black and Caucasian skin. *J. Am. Acad. Dermatol.* **1**:249–260.

106. Kaidbey, K. H., and Kligman, A. M. (1978): Sunburn protection by longwave ultraviolet radiation-induced pigmentation. *Arch. Dermatol.* **114**:46–48.

107. Owens, D. W., Knox, J. M., Hudson, H. T., et al. (1974): Influence of wind on ultraviolet injury. *Arch. Dermatol.* **109**:200–201.

108. Owens, D. W., Knox, J. M., Hudson, H. T., et al. (1975): Influence of humidity on ultraviolet injury. *J. Invest. Dermatol.* **64**:250–252.

109. Freeman, R. G., and Knox, J. M. (1964): Influence of temperature on ultraviolet injury. *Arch. Dermatol.* **89**:858–864.

110. Claesson, S., Juhlin, L., and Wettermark, G. (1958): The reciprocity law of UV-irradiation effects. Damage on mouse skin exposed to UV-light varied over a 10^7-fold intensity range. *Acta Derm. Venereol. (Stockh.)* **38**:123–136.

111. Anderson, R. R., and Parrish, J. A. (1980): A survey of the acute effects of UV lasers on human and animal skin. In: *Lasers in Photomedicine and Photobiology,* edited by R. Pratesi and C. A. Sacchi, pp. 109–114. Springer-Verlag, Berlin/Heidelberg.

112. Blum, H. F., and Terus, W. S. (1946): The erythemal threshold for sunburn. *Am. J. Physiol.* **146**:107–117.

113. Bener, P. (1963): The diurnal and annual variations of the spectral intensity of ultraviolet sky and global radiation on cloudless days at Davos, 1950 m.a.s.l., Air Force Contract AF61 (052)-618, Technical Note No. 2, Davos.

114. Parrish, J. A., Anderson, R. R., Urbach, F., et al. (1978): *UV-A: Biological Effects of Ultraviolet Radiation with Emphasis on Human Responses to Longwave Ultraviolet,* pp. 122–123. Plenum Press, New York.

115. Schulze, R., and Gräfe, K. (1969): Consideration of sky ultraviolet radiation in the measurement of solar ultraviolet radiation. In: *The Biologic Effects of Ultraviolet Radiation (with Emphasis on the Skin),* edited by F. Urbach, pp. 359–373. Pergamon Press, Oxford.

116. Kelner, A. (1949): Effect on visible light on the recovery of *Streptomyces griseus* conidia from ultraviolet irradiation injury. *Proc. Natl. Acad. Sci. U.S.A.* **35**:73–79.

117. Rieck, A. F., and Rudich, E. C. (1955): Skin response of albino mouse to ultraviolet radiation and photorecovery. *Fed. Proc.* **15**:151.

118. van der Leun, J. C., and Stoop, T. (1969): Photorecovery of ultraviolet erythema. In: *The*

Biologic Effects of Ultraviolet Radiation (with Emphasis on the Skin), edited by F. Urbach, pp. 251–254. Pergamon Press, Oxford.

119. Adams, E. Q., Barnes, B. T., and Forsythe, W. E. (1933): Über die Erythemwirksamkeit ultravioletten Lichtes. Strahlentherapie 48:235–249.

120. Willis, I., Kligman, A., and Epstein, J. (1972): Effects of long ultraviolet rays on human skin: photoprotective or photoaugmentative? J. Invest. Dermatol. 59:416–420.

121. Ying, C. Y., Parrish, J. A., and Pathak, M. A. (1974): Additive erythemogenic effects of middle- (280–320 nm) and long- (320–400 nm) wave ultraviolet light. J. Invest. Dermatol. 63:273–278.

122. Parrish, J. A., Ying, C. Y., Pathak, M. A., et al. (1974): Erythemogenic properties of long-wave ultraviolet light. In: Sunlight and Man: Normal and Abnormal Photobiologic Responses, edited by M. A. Pathak, L. C. Harber, M. Seiji, et al. T. B. Fitzpatrick, consulting editor, pp. 131–141. University of Tokyo Press, Tokyo.

123. Kaidbey, K. H., and Kligman, A. M. (1975): Further studies of photoaugmentation in humans: phototoxic reactions. J. Invest. Dermatol. 65:472–475.

124. Spiegel, H., Plewig, G., Hofmann, C., et al. (1978): Photoaugmentation. Ein photobiologisches Phanomen. Arch. Dermatol. Res. 261:189–200.

125. Stern, W. K. (1972): Anatomic localization of the response to ultraviolet radiation in human skin. Dermatologica 145:361–370.

126. Willis, I., and Cylus, L. (1977): UVA erythema in skin: is it a sunburn? J. Invest. Dermatol. 68:128–129.

127. Rosario, R., Mark, G. J., Parrish, J. A., et al. (1979): Histological changes produced in skin by equally erythemogenic doses of UV-A, UV-B, UV-C and UV-A with psoralens. Br. J. Dermatol. 101:299–308.

128. Gilchrest, B. A., Soter, N. A., Stoff, J., et al. (1981): Human sunburn reaction: Biochemical and histologic studies. J. Am. Acad. Dermatol., 5:411–422.

129. Daniels, F., Jr., Brophy, D., and Lobitz, W. C. (1961): Histochemical responses of human skin following ultraviolet irradiation. J. Invest. Dermatol. 37:351–357.

130. Wilgram, G. F., Kidd, R. L., Krawczyk, W. S., et al. (1970): Sunburn effect on keratinosomes. A report with special note on ultraviolet-induced dyskeratosis. Arch. Dermatol. 101:505–519.

131. Woodcock, A., and Magnus, I. A. (1976): The sunburn cell in mouse skin: preliminary quantitative studies on its production. Br. J. Dermatol. 95:459–468.

132. Danno, K., and Horio, T. (1980): Histochemical staining of sunburn cells for sulphhydryl and disulphide groups: a time course study. Br. J. Dermatol. 102:535–539.

133. Brenner, W., and Gschnait, F. (1979): Decreased DNA repair activity in sunburn cells. A possible pathogenetic factor of the epidermal sunburn reaction. Arch. Dermatol. Res. 266:11–16.

134. Johnson, B. E., Mandell, G., and Daniels, F., Jr. (1972): Melanin and cellular reactions to ultraviolet radiation. Nature [New Biol.] 235:147–149.

135. Soffen, G. A., and Blum, H. F. (1961): Quantitative measurements of changes in mouse skin following a single dose of ultraviolet light. J. Cell. Comp. Physiol. 58:81–96.

136. Nix, T. E., Jr., Nordquist, R. E., Scott, J. R., et al. (1965): An ultrastructural study of nucleolar enlargement following ultraviolet irradiation of human epidermis. J. Invest. Dermatol. 45:114–118.

137. Nix, T. E., Jr., Nordquist, R. E., and Everett, M. A. (1965): Ultrastructural changes induced by ultraviolet light in human epidermis: granular and transitional cell layers. J. Ultrastruct. Res. 12:547–573.

138. Nix, T. E., Jr., Nordquist, R. E., Scott, J. R., et al. (1965): Ultrastructural changes induced by ultraviolet light in human epidermis: basal and spinous layers. J. Invest. Dermatol. 45:52–64.

139. Nix, T. E., Jr., Nordquist, R. E., Scott, J. R., et al. (1964): Ultrastructural changes in stratum corneum induced by ultraviolet light. J. Invest. Dermatol. 43:301–317.

140. Jagger, J. (1967): *Introduction to Research in Ultraviolet Photobiology,* p. 130. Prentice-Hall, Englewood Cliffs, N.J.

141. Smith, W. L., and Lands, W. E. M. (1971): Stimulation and blockade of prostaglandin biosynthesis. *J. Biol. Chem.* **246:**6700–6702.

142. Vane, J. R. (1971): Inhibition of prostaglandin synthesis as a mechanism of action of aspirin-like drugs. *Nature [New Biol.]* **231:**232–235.

143. Gruber, C. M., Jr., Ridolfo, A. S., Nickander, R., et al. (1972): Delay of erythema of human skin by anti-inflammatory drugs after ultraviolet irradiation. *Clin. Pharmacol. Ther.* **13:**109–113.

144. Greenberg, R. A., Eaglstein, W. H., Turnier, H., et al. (1975): Orally given indomethacin and blood flow response to UVL. *Arch. Dermatol.* **111:**328–330.

145. Snyder, D. S., and Eaglstein, W. H. (1974): Intradermal anti-prostaglandin agents and sunburn. *J. Invest. Dermatol.* **62:**47–50.

146. Kaidbey, K. H., and Kurban, A. K. (1976): The influence of corticosteroids and topical indomethacin on sunburn erythema. *J. Invest. Dermatol.* **66:**153–156.

147. Greaves, M. W., and McDonald-Gibson, W. (1972): Inhibition of prostaglandin biosynthesis by corticosteroids. *Br. Med. J.* **2:**83–84.

148. Flower, R., Gryglewski, R., Herbaczyńska-Cedro, K., et al. (1972): Effects of anti-inflammatory drugs on prostaglandin biosynthesis. *Nature [New Biol.]* **238:**104–106.

149. Greaves, M. W., Kingston, W. P., and Pretty, K. (1975): Action of a series of non-steroid and steroid anti-inflammatory drugs on prostaglandin synthesis by the microsomal fraction of rat skin. *Br. J. Pharmacol.* **53:**47OP.

150. Eaglstein, W. H., Ginsberg, L. D., and Mertz, P. M. (1979): Ultraviolet irradiation-induced inflammation. Effects of steroid and nonsteroid anti-inflammatory agents. *Arch. Dermatol.* **115:**1421–1423.

151. Hong, S. L., and Levine, L. (1976): Inhibition of arachidonic acid release from cells as the biochemical action of anti-inflammatory corticosteroids. *Proc. Natl. Acad. Sci. U.S.A.* **73:**1730–1734.

152. Lewis, G. P., and Piper, P. J. (1975): Inhibition of release of prostaglandins as an explanation of some of the actions of anti-inflammatory corticosteroids. *Nature* **254:**308–311.

153. Michaëlsson, G. (1970): Effects of antihistamines, acetylsalicylic acid and prednisone on cutaneous reactions to kallikrein and prostaglandin E_1. *Acta Derm. Venereol. (Stockh.)* **50:**31–36.

154. Weissmann, G., and Fell, H. B. (1962): The effect of hydrocortisone on the response of fetal rat skin in culture to ultraviolet irradiation. *J. Exp. Med.* **116:**365–380.

155. Weissmann, G., and Dingle, J. (1962): Release of lysosomal protease by ultraviolet irradiation and inhibition by hydrocortisone. *Exp. Cell Res.* **25:**207–210.

156. Vogt, W., Meyer, U., Kunze, H., et al. (1969): Entstehung von SRS-C in der durchströmten Meerschweinchenlunge durch Phospholipase A. Identifizierung mit prostaglandin. *Naunyn Schmiedebergs Arch. Pharmacol. Exp. Pathol.* **262:**124–134.

157. Järvinen, K. A. J. (1951): Effect of cortisone on reaction of skin to ultra-violet light. *Br. Med. J.* **2:**1377–1378.

158. Greenwald, J. S., Parrish, J. A., Jaenicke, K. F., et al. (1981): Failure of systemically administered corticosteroids to suppress UVB-induced delayed erythema. *J. Am. Acad. Dermatol.,* **5:**197–202.

159. Loewenthal, L. J. A. (1963): Triprolidine hydrochloride in the prevention of some solar dermatoses. *Br. J. Dermatol.* **75:**254–256.

160. De Rios, G., Chan, J. T., Black, H. S., et al. (1978): Systemic protection by antioxidants against UVL-induced erythema. *J. Invest. Dermatol.* **70:**123–125.

161. Roshchupkin, D. I., Pistsov, M. Y., and Potapenko, A. Y. (1979): Inhibition of ultraviolet light-induced erythema by antioxidants. *Arch. Dermatol. Res.* **266:**91–94.

162. Watabiki, T., and Ogawa, K. (1975): Electron microscopic studies of effects of vitamin

E on changes in the mouse skin following ultraviolet irradiation. *Vitamins (Japan)* **49**:121–142.

163. Findlay, G. H., and van der Merwe, L. W. (1965): Epidermal vitamin A and sunburn in man. *Br. J. Dermatol.* **77**:622–626.

164. Imbrie, J. D., Daniels, F., Jr., Bergeron, L., et al. (1959): Increased erythema threshold six weeks after a single exposure to sunlight plus oral methoxsalen. *J. Invest. Dermatol.* **32**:331–337.

165. Gschnait, F., Brenner, W., and Wolff, K. (1978): Photoprotective effect of a psoralen-UVA-induced tan. *Arch. Dermatol. Res.* **263**:181–188.

166. Findlay, G. H. (1969): Oral interceptives that do not work. In: *The Biologic Effects of Ultraviolet Radiation (with Emphasis on the Skin)*, edited by F. Urbach, pp. 693–695. Pergamon Press, Oxford.

167. Greaves, M. W., and McDonald-Gibson, W. (1973): Effect of nonsteroid anti-inflammatory and antipyretic drugs on prostaglandin biosynthesis by human skin. *J. Invest. Dermatol.* **61**:127–129.

168. Crunkhorn, P., and Willis, A. L. (1971): Cutaneous reactions to intradermal prostaglandins. *Br. J. Pharmacol.* **41**:49–56.

169. Quevedo, W. C., Jr., Fitzpatrick, T. B., Pathak, M. A., et al. (1974): Light and skin color. In: *Sunlight and Man: Normal and Abnormal Photobiologic Responses*, edited by M. A. Pathak, L. C. Harber, M. Seiji, et al. (T. B. Fitzpatrick, consulting editor), pp. 165–194. University of Tokyo Press, Tokyo.

170. Fitzpatrick, T. B., Szabó, G., Seiji, M., et al. (1979): Biology of the melanin pigmentary system. In: *Dermatology in General Medicine*, 2nd ed., edited by T. B. Fitzpatrick, A. Z. Eisen, K. Wolff, et al., pp. 131–163. McGraw-Hill, New York.

171. Nicolaus, R. A., and Piatelli, M. (1965): Progress in the chemistry of natural black pigments. *Rend. Acc. Sci. Fis. Mat.* **32**:1–17.

172. Blois, M. S., Zahlan, A. B., and Maling, J. E. (1964): Electron spin resonance studies on melanin. *Biophys. J.* **4**:471–490.

173. Commoner, B., Townsend, J., and Pake, G. E. (1954): Free radicals in biological materials. *Nature* **174**:689–691.

174. McGinness, J., and Proctor, P. (1973): The importance of the fact that melanin is black. *J. Theor. Biol.* **39**:677–678.

175. Thomson, M. L. (1955): Relative efficiency of pigment and horny layer thickness in protecting the skin of Europeans and Africans against solar ultraviolet radiation. *J. Physiol.* **127**:236–246.

176. Weigand, D. A., Haygood, C., and Gaylor, J. R. (1974): Cell layers and density of Negro and Caucasian stratum corneum. *J. Invest. Dermatol.* **62**:563–568.

177. Freeman, R. G., Cockerell, E. G., Armstrong, J., et al. (1962): Sunlight as a factor influencing the thickness of epidermis. *J. Invest. Dermatol.* **39**:295–298.

178. Cochran, A. J. (1970): The incidence of melanocytes in normal human skin. *J. Invest. Dermatol.* **55**:65–70.

179. Mishima, Y., and Widlan, S. (1967): Enzymically active and inactive melanocyte populations and ultraviolet irradiation: combined DOPA-premelanin reaction and electron microscopy. *J. Invest. Dermatol.* **49**:273–281.

180. Fitzpatrick, T. B., and Breathnach, A. S. (1963): Das epidermale Melanin-Einheit-System. *Dermatol. Wochenschr.* **147**:481–489.

181. Jimbow, K., Roth, S. I., Fitzpatrick, T. B., et al. (1975): Mitotic activity in non-neoplastic melanocytes in vivo as determined by histochemical, autoradiographic and electron microscope studies. *J. Cell. Biol.* **66**:663–671.

182. Pathak, M. A., Jimbow, K., Parrish, J. A., et al (1976): Effect of UV-A, UV-B, and psoralen on *in vivo* human melanin pigmentation. Cellular and subcellular characterization on delayed tanning reaction induced by single or multiple exposures to UV-A, UV-B or UV-A

plus 8-methoxypsoralen. In: *Pigment Cell*, Vol. 3, edited by V. Riley, pp. 291–298. S. Karger, Basel.

183. Jimbow, K., Davison, P. F., Pathak, M. A., et al. (1975): Cytoplasmic filaments in melanocytes. Their nature and role in melanin pigmentation. In: *Pigment Cell*, Vol. 3, edited by V. Riley, pp. 13–32. S. Karger, Basel.

184. Szabo, G., Garcia, R. I., and Fletcher, C. (1977): Effects of ultraviolet light on melanogenesis and melanocyte-keratinocyte interactions. *J. Cell Biol.* **75**:48a.

185. Seiji, M., Toda, K., Okazaki, K., et al. (1975): Melanocyte–keratinocyte interaction in pigment transfer. A film presented at the IX International Pigment Cell Conference, Houston, Texas.

186. Pathak, M. A., Riley, F. C., and Fitzpatrick, T. B. (1962): Melanogenesis in human skin following exposure to long-wave ultraviolet and visible light. *J. Invest. Dermatol.* **39**:435–443.

187. Hausser, I. (1938): Über spezifische Wirkungen des langwelligen ultravioletten Lichts auf die menschliche Haut. *Strahlentherapie* **62**:315–322.

188. Henschke, U., and Schulze, R. (1939): Untersuchungen zum Problem der Ultraviolett-Dosimetrie. 3. Über Pigmentierung durch langwelliges Ultraviolett. *Strahlentherapie* **64**:14–42.

189. Gates, R. R., and Zimmerman, A. A. (1953): Comparison of skin color with melanin content. *J. Invest. Dermatol.* **21**:339–348.

190. Jimbow, K., Pathak, M. A., Szabo, G., et al. (1974): Ultrastructural changes in human melanocytes after ultraviolet radiation. In: *Sunlight and Man: Normal and Abnormal Photobiologic Responses*, edited by M. A. Pathak, L. C. Harber, M. Seiji, et al. (T. B. Fitzpatrick, consulting editor), pp. 195–215. University of Tokyo Press, Tokyo.

191. Langen, D. (1938): Experimentelle Studien über die Erythembildung der Sonnen- und Himmelsstrahlung. *Strahlentherapie* **63**:142–170.

192. Uesugi, T., Katoh, M., Horikoshi, T., et al. (1979): Mode of activation and differentiation of dormant melanocytes after UV exposure on mouse skin. Autoradiographic, histochemical, and cytochemical studies of melanogenesis. In: *Pigment Cell*, Vol. 4, edited by V. Riley, pp. 337–344. S. Karger, Basel.

193. Rosdahl, I. K., and Szabo, G. (1978): Mitotic activity of epidermal melanocytes in UV-irradiated mouse skin. *J. Invest. Dermatol.* **70**:143–148.

194. Miyazaki, H., Kawada, A., Takaki, Y., et al. (1974): Effects of ultraviolet light on epidermal dendritic cells of hairless mice. In: *Sunlight and Man: Normal and Abnormal Photobiologic Responses*, edited by M. A. Pathak, L. C. Harber, M. Seiji, et al. (T. B. Fitzpatrick, consulting editor), pp. 217–229. University of Tokyo Press, Tokyo.

195. Rosdahl, I. K. (1979): Local and systemic effects on the epidermal melanocyte population in UV-irradiated mouse skin. *J. Invest. Dermatol.* **73**:306–309.

196. Blog, F. B., and Szabó, G. (1979): The effects of psoralen and UVA (PUVA) on epidermal melanocytes of the tail in C57BL mice. *J. Invest. Dermatol.* **73**:533–537.

197. Toda, K., and Shono, S. (1979): Effect of UVA irradiation on the epidermal pigment darkening. In: *Pigment Cell*, Vol. 4, edited by V. Riley, pp. 318–322. S. Karger, Basel.

198. Epstein, J. H., Fukuyama, K., and Epstein, W. L. (1968): UVL induced stimulation of DNA synthesis in hairless mouse epidermis. *J. Invest. Dermatol.* **51**:445–453.

199. Epstein, J. H., Fukuyama, K., and Fye, K. (1970): Effects of ultraviolet radiation on the mitotic cycle and DNA, RNA and protein synthesis in mammalian epidermis *in vivo*. *Photochem. Photobiol.* **12**:57–65.

200. Epstein, W. L., Fukuyama, K., and Epstein, J. H. (1969): Early effects of ultraviolet light on DNA synthesis in human skin in vivo. *Arch. Dermatol.* **100**:84–89.

201. Baden, H. P., and Pearlman, C. (1964): The effect of ultraviolet light on protein and nucleic acid synthesis in the epidermis. *J. Invest. Dermatol.* **43**:71–75.

202. Krämer, D. M., Pathak, M. A., Kornhauser, A., et al. (1974): Effect of ultraviolet

irradiation on biosynthesis on DNA in guinea-pig skin *in vivo. J. Invest. Dermatol.* **62**:388–393.

203. Pullmann, H., Galosi, A., Jakobeit, C., et al. (1980): Effects of selective ultraviolet phototherapy (SUP) and local PUVA treatment on DNA synthesis in guinea pig skin. *Arch. Dermatol. Res.* **267**:37–45.

204. Fukuyama, K., Epstein, W. L., and Epstein, J. H. (1967): Effect of ultraviolet light on RNA and protein synthesis in differentiated epidermal cells. *Nature* **216**:1031–1032.

205. Blum, H. F. (1969): Hyperplasia induced by ultraviolet light: possible relationship to cancer induction. In: *The Biologic Effects of Ultraviolet Radiation (with Emphasis on the Skin),* edited by F. Urbach, pp. 83–89. Pergamon Press, Oxford.

206. Blum, H. F., Butler, E. G., Dailey, T. H., et al. (1959): Irradiation of mouse skin with single doses of ultraviolet light. *J. Natl. Cancer Inst.* **22**:979–993.

207. Everett, M. A. (1961): Protection from sunlight in vitiligo. *Arch. Dermatol.* **84**:997–998.

208. With, C. (1920): Studies on the effect of light on vitiligo. *Br. J. Dermatol. Syphilol* **32**:145–155.

209. Meyer, P. S. (1924): Gewöhnung vitiliginöser Hautstellen an ultravioletten Licht und andere Reize. *Arch. Dermatol. Syphilol. (Berlin)* **147**:238–241.

210. Guillaume, A.-C. (1926): Le pigment épidermique, la pénétration des rayons U.V. et le mécanisme de protection de l'organisme vis-à-vis de ces radiations. *Bull. Mém. Soc. Med. Hôpitaux de Paris* **50**:1133–1135.

211. Kirby-Smith, J. S., Blum, H. F., and Grady, H. G. (1942): Penetration of ultraviolet radiation into skin, as a factor in carcinogenesis. *J. Natl. Cancer Inst.* **2**:403–412.

212. Rottier, P. B., and Mullink, J. A. M. (1952): Localization of erythemal processes caused by ultra-violet light in human skin. *Nature* **170**:574–575.

213. Claesson, S., Juhlin, L., and Wettermark, G. (1959): The action of ultraviolet light on skin with and without horny layer. The effect of 48/80 and methotrimeprazine. *Acta Derm. Venereol. (Stockh.)* **39**:3–11.

214. McFadden, A. W. (1961): Skin disease in the Cuna Indians. Dermatology and geography of the San Blas coast of Panama. *Arch. Dermatol.* **84**:1013–1023.

215. Quevado, Jr., W. C. (1969): The control of the color in mammals. *Am. Zool.* **9**:531–540.

9

Photocarcinogenesis

F. Urbach

There has been a recent reawakening of interest in the field of photobiology. This has been largely due to rapid advances in photochemistry, particularly due to a much better understanding of photobiologic phenomena occurring on the molecular level, and a recent concern about potential alteration of the ozone layer. Furthermore, the great improvement in design, versatility, and intensity of modern light sources and the development of accurate measuring devices capable of determining the intensity of very narrow bands of light even in the ultraviolet (UV) region of the electromagnetic spectrum have made more elegant studies possible.

That sunlight can cause demonstrable acute and chronic changes in apparently normal skin certainly has been known since antiquity: "I am dark, because the sun has scorched me" (*Song of Solomon* 1:6). Charcot (1) determined that UV radiation caused acute erythema and Unna (2) proved that pigmentation can be induced by UV radiation. It soon became apparent that the capability of the skin to react to light by pigmenting was most variable, and that this variability pertained not only to different races, but also to individuals of apparently similar ancestry. Hausser and Vahle (3) showed that the longer UV wavelengths were more effective in producing pigmentation than the more erythemogenic shorter wavelengths. Bloch carried out his classical experiments on the mechanism of melanin formation in human skin, discovered dopaoxidase, and laid the groundwork for the development of skin histochemistry (4).

The dominant inheritance of freckling was noted by Ehrman (5) and by Hammer (6), an observation that decades later was correlated with predisposition to skin carcinogenesis.

F. Urbach • Department of Dermatology, Skin and Cancer Hospital, Temple University School of Medicine, Philadelphia, Pennsylvania 19140.

Changes in the stratum corneum, epidermis, and dermis due to chronic light exposure were first associated with UV radiation by Unna (2), who noted thickening and brownish discoloration of the stratum corneum of light-exposed skin areas and hyperplasia of the epidermis. Thickening of the stratum corneum provided some measure of protection against further UV radiation injury, as first noted by With (7), and later documented in detail by Guillaume (8) and then Miescher (9). Eventually a peculiar degeneration of the elastica and collagen of the skin develops, virtually only on the most exposed areas of very heavily sun-exposed persons (9).

It is an ancient observation that the face and hands, in addition to their more marked pigmentation, usually show a more warm-red coloration. This persistent erythema is primarily due to UV radiation, as shown originally by Finsen (10). He also noted that skin, intensively irradiated with UV, continued to react to minor mechanical or thermal irritation many months after both the early erythema and pigmentation had disappeared. In other words, a single dose of UV radiation was sufficient to cause permanent blood vessel damage. Chronic insolation caused permanent vasodilatation, e.g., the "dermatose du triangle sternoclaviculaire" of Brocq—occurring in the V of the neck area of women.

The first suggestion that skin cancer may be due to prolonged and repeated exposure to light came almost simultaneously from two directions. Unna (2) noted severe degeneration skin changes on exposed areas of the skin of sailors and associated these with the development of skin cancer which was seen with great regularity in his clinic in Hamburg, an old Hanseatic seaport town. Dubreuilh (11), studying skin diseases in the Bordeaux region of France, noted the frequent occurrence of keratoses and skin cancer in vineyard workers while the nearby city dwellers showed few such lesions. The observations were soon confirmed by Shield (12), Hyde (13), Paul (14), and others, who noted a high incidence of skin cancer in rural areas of the United States and Australia, where sun exposure was much more intense than in central Europe. It is interesting (and almost prophetic) that Bruusgard (15) considered the sailor's skin cancer as being due to a combination of sunlight and coal tar (to which sailors were heavily exposed in those days).

Following the clinical observation of a relationship of chronic sunlight exposure to skin cancer, there was much discussion among dermatologists as to whether this association applied to all white-skinned people or, as Haxthausen and Hausmann (16) had proposed, really occurred only in those carrying a forme fruste trait of xeroderma pigmentosum. This view began to change when Findlay (17) showed that daily irradiation of mice with UV from a mercury arc caused the induction of skin cancers. Incidentally, Findlay also noted that when mice were tarred prior to UV radiation exposure, the period necessary for the induction of skin cancer was reduced. His findings were soon reproduced by Putschar and Holtz (18). Sarcomas of the eyes of rats were produced with UV radiation by Huldschinsky in 1933 (19).

The individual most responsible for calling attention to the causal relationship of solar and artificial UV radiation to skin cancer in humans and in experimental animals was Roffo (20, 21). In a series of studies between 1930 and 1936, Roffo showed that skin cancer could be induced in rats with natural sunlight as well as with mercury-arc radiation, and carried out the first real epidemiologic study of human skin cancer. As had Dubreuilh, he pointed out that the same skin areas most likely to develop skin cancer also showed a great tendency to develop hyperkeratoses, and considered these keratoses as premalignant lesions. Finally, Roffo (22) carried out the first action spectrum studies of skin photocarcinogenesis: he showed that clear window glass was sufficient to stop skin cancer production by both natural sunlight and mercury-arc radiation, thus setting an approximate limit for the effective UV radiation of shorter than 320 nm.

That light and certain chemical compounds can exert a biologic effect together which neither possesses alone was first shown by Raab (23), and subsequently was elegantly documented by Tappeiner (24), Jodlbauer (25), Busk (26), Haxthausen and Hausmann (16), and many others. The first group of photoactive agents was found to be halogenated derivatives of fluorescein, anthracene, and anthracene analogs (acridines, phenothiazines, etc.). They were found to profoundly affect protozoa, bacteria, fungi, cells in tissue culture, and, if injected, whole animals (including humans) if light of an appropriate wavelength was administered and reached the photodynamic compound.

In the early 1930s, chemically pure phenanthrene compounds which were able to produce skin cancer in rodents had been isolated. As previously noted, Findlay (17) had already reported that application of coal tar followed by UV radiation increased the probability of skin carcinogenesis and shortened the development time of the tumors. In 1935, Lewis (27) made a prophetic observation: "When certain cancer-producing hydrocarbons were added to cultures of chick embryo tissue, the cells developed photosensitivity to the electric light used for the study of cells in tissue cultures. The photodynamic action caused definite changes in the state of the cell protoplasm, which were often accompanied by inhibited cell division. This brought about a later occurrence of abnormalities of mitosis that duplicated many of the types of abnormal mitosis characteristic of malignant growth."

By the end of the third decade of this century, the groundwork had been laid for the detailed studies of various aspects of photocarcinogenesis that were to follow.

PHOTOCARCINOGENESIS—EXPERIMENTAL ASPECTS

The skin, especially of rodents, has been used as one of the primary sites for study of carcinogenic stimuli. As a result, a vast catalog of agents, ranging from aromatic hydrocarbons to viruses and rare metals, have proven to be tumorigenic. However, only a very few of these have been found as yet to be related to the development of human skin cancer neoplasms. Of such stimuli, light energy is by far the most important and most extensively studied.

From 1940 to 1944 Blum, Kirby-Smith, and Grady (28) carried out a comprehensive series of experiments on UV radiation carcinogenesis in mice at the National Cancer Institute. Taking advantage of a stable photoelectric cell developed by Rentschler of Westinghouse and an integrating meter devised by Kuper, Brochett, and Eichen at the National Institutes of Health, Blum and his associates were able to expose albino mice repeatedly to UV radiation with confidence in the reproducibility of the dosage from day to day and with the ultimate satisfaction of obtaining higher reproducible cancer incidence in the populations of exposed mice. Variability was reduced by using one sex only (male), by using a genetically homogeneous strain of mice (Strain A), and by limiting the quantitative observations to only one part of the body (the ear). For details of these elegant experiments, Blum's classic work, *Carcinogenesis by Ultraviolet Light* (29), should be consulted.

Blum reported several important observations on tumor induction:

1. A single dose of UV radiation did not cause development of tumors in the lifetime of the animals.

2. A useful measure for tumor induction was the "development time," i.e., the time elapsed between the first UV radiation dose and the appearance of a tumor of a certain volume. This was found to be distributed, within an identically treated population of mice, in a consistently regular fashion

3. Differences in dose, intensity, or interval between doses did not alter the shape or the slope of the dose–response relationships, but only moved their relative postion along with dose axis.

4. Reciprocity held until the dose became too small to produce tumors in the lifetime of the animal.

Reciprocity and Time–Dose Rate Relationships

The second law of photochemistry (law of Bunsen and Roscoe) states that photochemical action depends only on the product of light intensity and the duration of exposure. This law, however, holds only for primary photochemical action, and cannot be applied to secondary reactions (30). Since the biologic end points that can be observed, such as erythema, pigmentation, skin cancer production, etc., are certainly indirect effects, and since we still know little about the primary photochemical reactions that underlie them, it is not surprising that "reciprocity" holds only for some of the effects studied.

Blum (31), in the first quantitative photocarcinogenesis experiments ever performed, found that, within relatively narrow limits (approximate factors of five), differences in dose, intensity, or interval between doses did not alter the shape or slope of tumor incidence curves, but only their positions on the log time axis. Blum, however, was careful to point out that this was true only so long as the experimental conditions remained the same until the time the tumors appeared.

With the accumulated data, Blum surmised that UV-induced cancer formation is a continuous process that begins with the initial exposure. The appearance of tumors within a lifetime of the animal depends on sufficient acceleration of the growth process. In support of the concept that growth acceleration is an important component of carcinogenesis, Rogers (32) produced adenomas in mouse lung with a single UV-radiation exposure, and later Epstein and Roth (33) reported the production of squamous cell carcinomas in hairless mouse skin with one exposure when croton oil was utilized to promote carcinogenesis. Pound (34) has subsequently confirmed the findings of Epstein and Roth.

More recently, skin tumors in hairless mice were produced within 6–16 weeks after a single dose of UV radiation with no further light of chemical treatment. The tumors appeared only in those mice that had received sufficient UV irradiation to cause severe acute burns (necrosis, desquamation, crust formation, scar formation), and the tumors (primarily papillomas) arose only at the edge of severely damaged tissue (35). It is possible that this phenomenon is nonspecific and related to epidermal hyperplasia secondary to severe skin damage, and thus has little direct bearing on human skin carcinogenesis, which is apparently related to multiple, lesser exposures to UV radiation.

In the majority of photocarcinogenesis studies performed to date, fixed doses of UV radiation were given at a fixed dose rate, and the interval between doses was altered, but in increments of at least 24 hr. Such experiments, while very valuable, are far removed from the conditions found in nature to which human skin is exposed. Humans are exposed to relatively low UV-radiation flux, which varies with time of day, season, and environmental conditions such as cloud cover, but generally rises and falls *during* the exposure period (Fig. 9-1). Figure 9-2 uses squares and rectangles to model the flux–time relationships for radiation doses usually assumed in animal experiments (top three figures); other geometric figures probably come closer to real conditions: lamp warmup time, sunrise and sunset, etc. (bottom three figures). In each case, the total dose delivered (i.e., the shaded area) is equal.

Figure 9-3 shows several ways in which the total dose can be delivered. Thus experiments utilizing such doses as outlined in Fig. 9-3 would give some insight into the limits of reciprocity for photocarcinogenesis. Some studies of this type have been begun by Forbes and Urbach (36), utilizing the Skh hairless-1 mice.

Two experiments were designed to test the relative effect of protraction vs. that of fractionation. In the first experiment, groups of hairless mice were

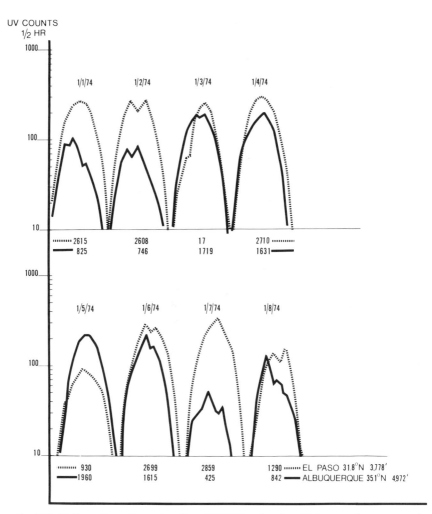

Fig. 9-1. Half-hourly readings of erythemal UV light taken from Robertson–Berger meters in Albuquerque, New Mexico and El Paso, Texas in January 1974. Note the marked effect of cloud cover at Albuquerque compared with the almost daily clear weather at El Paso (101).

exposed to suberythemal doses of UV radiation from a bank of fluorescent "sun" (FS) lamps known to produce skin cancer in these animals. The design used to test the protraction effect is shown in Fig. 9-4. Equal doses of UV radiation were delivered in 5, 50, or 500 min. Thus, while the doses (given five times weekly) were the same, the flux varied by a factor of 10 or 100. A striking difference in both tumor development time and tumor yield was noted. The animals given the total UV-radiation dose in 5 min developed tumors later, and in smaller number, than did those given the same total dose in 50 or 500 min.

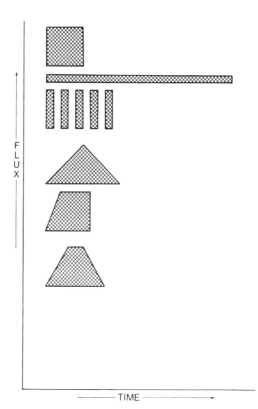

Fig. 9-2. Geometric model of dose (area) as a function of flux (ordinate) and time (abscissa). Shaded areas (doses) are equal in all cases. The top three figures represent relationships usually assumed in animal experiments; the bottom three figures probably come closer to actual exposure conditions (gradual warm-up of lamp, sunrise and sunset, etc.).

Thus, protracting the UV radiation dose over longer time periods resulted in a striking increase in the carcinogenic effect of the radiation.

In the second experiment, the total UV-radiation dose was delivered either in a single 5- min period or in five 1-min periods, 1 hr apart, each day the mice were exposed (Fig. 9-5). The rationale was to separate the possible effect of flux from that of delivery time. The result was not clear-cut: the longer delivery time yielded a somewhat steeper tumor accumulation rate, but with a longer "latent" period.

Another approach to the question of reciprocity involves comparing the following two experiments. In the first, two groups of mice were exposed daily (Monday through Friday) to either 600 or 300 J m^{-2} of erythema effective energy (EEE) from banks of FS fluorescent sunlamps. As had Blum et al. previously (28), we found that the lower daily dose resulted in delayed onset of first tumors, without significantly changing the shape of the response curve (Fig. 9-6). The second of this pair of experiments included two groups of mice, both exposed daily to 600 J m^{-2} but for either 36 weeks (group I) or 10 weeks (group II). Here, the initiation of tumors was apparently not influenced, but the subsequent shape of the response curve was altered (Fig. 9-7), and

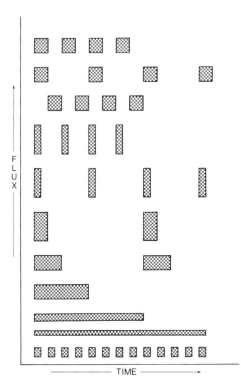

Fig. 9-3. Geometric model of dose accumulation under several different conditions of flux, time, and fractionation. Each horizontal line of figures totals the same dose. The figures could represent varying "rest" intervals, day-night cycles, and number of exposures, as well as differences in flux and total exposure time.

individual tumor growth and development was different. Tumors first appeared in both groups at 13 weeks after the first exposure. At 18 weeks, the two groups were virtually indistinguishable in terms of tumor size and gross tumor morphology. Half the survivors in each group had at least one tumor (prevalence = 0.5), and there was an average of one tumor per survivor (tumor yield = 1.0). Subsequently, the growth of these tumors was more rapid and invasive in group I than in group II. At 27 weeks, the prevalence was 0.7 (group II) or 1.0 (group I); tumor yields were 3.0 (group II) and 6.5 (group I). Continued exposure not only increased prevalence of affected individuals and tumor yield, but also resulted in the development of larger and more aggressive growths (37).

These experiments are only a first attempt at designing studies relating flux, dose fractionation, and total dose to animal skin carcinogenesis. Such studies are greatly needed so that better models for human skin carcinogenesis can be developed. However, these preliminary experiments strongly suggest that the *rate* of UV exposure is of great and fundamental influence for the development of photocarcinogenesis.

Despite these and numerous other biologic and biochemical studies, the pathogenic mechanism of UV carcinogenesis on the cellular level remains

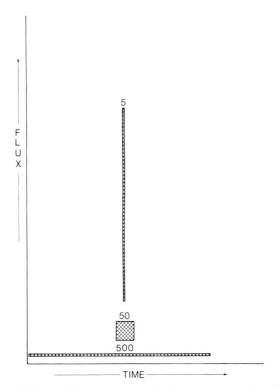

Fig. 9-4. Scheme of doses used in an experiment designed to test the effect of protraction on photocarcinogenesis. The shaded areas represent daily dose and are equal in all three arrangements, with the dose being delivered in 5, 50, or 500 min.

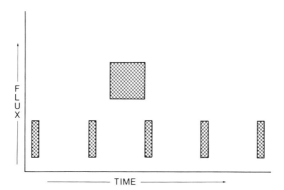

Fig. 9-5. Scheme of doses used in an experiment designed to test the effect of fractionation of doses on photocarcinogenesis. The shaded areas represent daily dose and are equal in both arrangements.

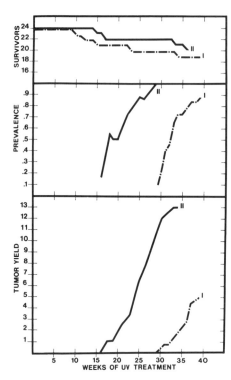

Fig. 9-6. Effects of exposing mice to 300 (I) or 600 (II) J m^{-2} of UV radiation (erythema effective energy: EEE) per day (Monday to Friday) for 40 weeks.

obscure. Basic data about the molecular effect of UV radiation on DNA had not helped either until recently, when pyrimidine dimer formation, excision, and repair by unscheduled DNA replication were demonstrated in mammalian cells in vitro (38) and in vivo (39) and in cultured cells from skin of cancer-prone patients (xeroderma pigmentosum) (40). This last observation resulted in a flurry of research activity because the possible implication of unrepaired DNA damage in cancer production hit a responsive chord—a "Zeitgeist" phenomenon. However, xeroderma pigmentosum variants were soon discovered in which excision repair systems were apparently normal, although the patients were as exquisitely cancer-prone as those showing little or no DNA repair (41).

Excision repair is now known to occur after damage in the skin of humans and mice (42), rat liver and kidney, rabbit brain, UV-induced squamous cell carcinoma of hairless mouse skin (43), and human tumor cell suspensions (44) produced by both carcinogenic and noncarcinogenic agents (45). It is thus clear that a great variety of mammalian cells and at least some malignant cells have excision repair capacity.

In addition to the well-documented capability of UV radiation to induce cancer of the skin in humans and mice, Setlow and Hart have to show that fish liver cells UV-irradiated in vitro and reinjected into isogenic recipients give

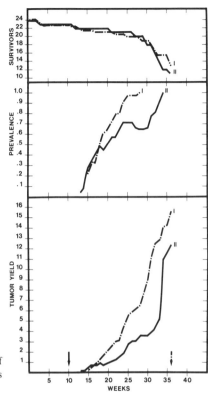

Fig. 9-7. Effects of exposing mice to 600 J m⁻² of UV radiation per day for 36 weeks (I) or 10 weeks (II).

rise to tumors (46). The tumor induction is UV dose dependent, and illumination of the irradiated cells with visible light before injection markedly reduces tumor production. Since fish cells possess the photoreactivating enzyme, these data may support the concept that pyrimidine dimers induced in cellular DNA by UV irradiation are related to the development of the tumors.

The available evidence suggests that injury to DNA is somehow related to carcinogenesis. In view of the evidence that DNA damage is related to mutagenesis in cells, this is a tenable assumption. However, in mouse skin and in most cancer patients, the DNA repair systems seem to be capable of repairing UV-radiation damage; thus absence of DNA repair cannot be the basis of most skin cancers. An elegant experiment of Zajdela and Latarjet (47) suggests a possible reason. They painted a solution of caffeine, a potent inhibitor of postreplication DNA repair, on the skin of mice during UV irradiation. The caffeine-treated skin developed fewer skin cancers than an unpainted control area on the same animal. Epstein et al. (42) and Zajdela and Latarjet (47) suggest that the production of skin cancer by UV radiation is initiated by repair of DNA, allowing the cell to survive, yet leaving in place or even favoring subsequent errors in DNA replication, resulting in a greater likelihood of malignant change.

The recent discovery of additional error-prone DNA repair mechanisms such as recombination repair and the complicated system repairing inter-strand links, together with the increasing evidence for the association of error-prone DNA repair systems with mutagenesis, make these hypotheses progressively more attractive.

The explanation for the significantly greater carcinogenic effect of protracted UVB doses may also rest in mechanisms of DNA repair. It is known that DNA repair is initiated immediately after injury and progresses rapidly. Thus, long continued injury may lead to either overloading of the repair systems or injury so close to the onset of cell division that repair has to occur post replication. In contrast, in high-flux, short-duration doses, more injury may occur in a shorter period of time, but time for repair is very much longer, and so the more efficient excision repair systems may predominate.

In any case, the door has now been opened for more detailed studies of the mechanisms of photocarcinogenesis and, knowing where to look, much progress can be expected in the near future.

The Action Spectrum for Photocarcinogenesis

The various studies described above and those to follow have been carried out with light sources delivering various mixtures of UV radiation, particularly UV radiation of wavelengths below 320 nm. The restriction to that waveband was based on the early observations of Roffo (21) that sunlight filtered through window glass was not effective for skin photocarcinogenesis. However, the precise shape of the photocarcinogenesis action spectrum is not known. Determinations of action spectra are beset with problems, both practical and theoretical. The relative effectiveness of different wavelengths often differs by orders of magnitude; experimental and equipment limitations usually dictate that their effects be studied at greatly different intensitites, a procedure fraught with hazards, as suggested by the protraction experiments described above.

Most attempts to define an action spectrum for skin photocarcinogenesis were performed with reasonably monochromatic radiation at or near the mercury resonance lines of 297 (300) nm, 303 nm, and 310 (313) nm. The most detailed of these studies are those of Freeman and co-workers (49–51) and Wetzel (52). These authors found that, within the limits of such an experiment, the wavelengths' effectiveness roughly paralleled that expected based on the human skin erythema action spectrum.

It is certainly not self-evident that the action spectrum for human skin erythema and mouse skin photocarcinogenesis should be similar, unless a common chromophore or action mechanism were involved. Setlow (53) has proposed that the common denominator is the action spectrum for affecting DNA. He has shown that making some assumption for skin transmission of

UV radiation, the shapes of the DNA, erythema, and (perhaps) skin cancer action spectra are similar, and can be made to coincide. A recent report of Forbes et al. (54) suggest that wavelengths shorter than 290 nm are more efficient in producing skin cancer in mice than erythema, thus suggesting that the action spectra for skin erythema and skin photocarcinogenesis indeed differ.

Much more work on the details of photocarcinogenesis action spectra is needed, most of which will have to await the development of more potent and sophisticated light sources.

Immunologic Effects on Photocarcinogenesis

Several lines of evidence indicate that the immune status of the host and carcinogenesis are potentially interactive processes. Increased cancer risk in humans under prolonged immunosuppression following organ transplant-ation has been reported. Some investigators believe that chemical carcinogens depress the immune system of the host. Kripke and Fisher (55, 56) have shown that UV-induced skin tumors, induced in C_3Hf mice, are highly antigenic, and are usually immunologically rejected when transplanted to normal, non-irradiated syngeneic recipients. This raised the question of why these tumors are able to grow progressively in their primary hosts. In an extensive series of experiments, Kripke found that preirradiation of mice for periods of time too short to induce skin tumors in the lifetime of the animals made them susceptible to challenge with UV-induced tumors. This effect was not specific, i.e., tumors did take and grow on areas not directly irradiated (such as the abdomen). This indicates that UV-irradiated mice are systemically altered in a way that prevents immunologic rejection of highly antigenic tumors, and that UV radiation can alter the host response against a tumor in addition to initiating the neoplastic transformation. It appears that UVB irradiation induces specific suppressor lymphoid cells that prevent the development of an immune response to UV-induced skin tumor antigens (57).

Another pertinent finding relates to the effects of immunosuppressive drugs on photocarcinogenesis (58). Several lines of evidence indicate that immunity and carcinogenesis can be interactive processes. Immunosup-pressed patients appear to be at increased risk for several types of tumors, and some laboratory studies show enhancement of tumor initiation or growth in animals receiving immunosuppressive drugs. However, such other data show no such relationship, and a number of questions about the direction and extent of immunosuppressive drug influence on carcinogenesis remain unanswered.

Photomodified Chemical Carcinogenesis

The interrelationship among light, chemicals, and skin carcinogenesis, first noted by Findlay in 1928, is of increasing interest and significance. Since all early studies of chemically induced skin carcinogenesis were performed using coal tar as the inducing agent, attention was drawn to the observation of Lewin (59) that coal tars exhibited photodynamic action. In 1930 Fleischhauer (60) showed that the action spectrum of coal tar for skin erythema was primarily located in the long-UV (UVA 340–390 nm) region. Soon after the purification of the first phenanthrene carcinogens by Kennaway, Lewis (27) noted that 20-methylcholanthrene, 7,12-dimethylbenzanthracene, and benzpyrene showed evidence of photodynamic action in tissue culture, and Doniach and Mottram (61) showed that most skin carcinogens then known were photodynamically active, and that in all these the activating wavelengths were found in the UVA band.

Reports on the effects of combined UV and visible radiation and polycyclic hydrocarbon treatment of animal skin have presented conflicting results. Acceleration of tumorigenesis was reported by Findlay (17) and others in the 1930s, and more recently, Clark (62) showed that UVA irradiation immediately after 20-methylcholanthrene painting accelerated papilloma formation without affecting incidence of carcinomas. This effect was, up to a point, dose related, but prolonged or intense irradiation had an inhibiting effect on tumor formation. Stenbäck (63) found that pretreatment of mouse skin with UVB caused a marked increase of 7,12-dimethylbenzanthracene-induced skin tumors, while irradiation *after* application of the carcinogen significantly decreased tumor induction.

In contrast were the findings of Doniach and Mottram (61), Morton et al. (64), Kohn-Speyer (65), and Seelig and Cooper (66), who found either no effect or a decrease in skin tumor production, although most observers noted development of acute skin phototoxicity.

Santamaria (67), in extensive in vitro and in vivo experiments, concluded that benzpyrene-induced carcinogenicity can be influenced by UV or daylight irradiation causing either acceleration *or* inhibition of tumorigenesis. He concluded that acceleration of tumor production was due to a benzpyrene-dependent photodynamic reaction compatible with cellular life, and inhibition due to severe photodynamic damage to cells and extracellular components rather than the alteration of the carcinogen by photooxidation.

On the other hand, Schonberg et al. (68) had already suggested that light might destroy externally applied carcinogens: their suggested mechanism was photodimerization, known to occur in some anthracene-type compounds. Cook and Martin (69) had shown that a number of substituted benzanthracenes (many of which are carcinogenic) undergo photooxidation when exposed to light. Despite these observations, few investigators have seriously considered in situ photochemical changes as factors in the combined effects of carcinogens and light, except in the sense of photoactivation of an inactive precursor or of localized energy transduction.

The studies of Davies et al. (70–73) showed that, under clearly defined conditions, the potency of a well-known carcinogen, 7,12-dimethylbenz(a)anthracene (DMBA), is reduced by light in accord with the demonstrable photochemical activity of the compound. There is also evidence that an additional time-dependent factor can influence this effect. However, given appropriate conditions, the carcinogen can also produce a phototoxic response, with resulting increase in tumor yield.

Thus, the reason for the conflicting results of so many competent investigators has now become clear: depending on the wavelengths of the UV radiation used, the carcinogen can be photodegraded to a less carcinogenic compound or cause phototoxicity, which may augment carcinogenesis, or cause such severe local phototoxic reaction that epithelial skin cells are mostly destroyed. Thus, either enhancement or inhibition of skin carcinogenesis may occur, depending on the carcinogen and the wavelength and dose of radiation used.

Chemically Enhanced Photocarcinogenesis

An equally significant problem concerns photoinduced carcinogenesis following application of agents to the skin which are phototoxic, but not in themselves carcinogenic. The literature is brief: Büngeler (74) reported that subcutaneous injection of eosin, hematoporphyrin, and a tar solution enhanced the ability of light to produce skin tumors. His experiments are difficult to interpret, since the mortality in each of the experimental groups was very high, occurring long before tumors appeared.

Miescher (75) did not succeed in producing tumors in mice exposed five times weekly to a clinically phototoxic combination of UVA and anthracene. He concluded that there were no reasons for viewing photodynamic action as "a new, specific carcinogenic agent." Heller (76), in an attempt to reproduce Miescher's results, produced necrotizing phototoxic skin changes with UVA and anthracene in mice, which developed neoplasia at the borders of the phototoxically produced skin ulcerations. Heller's conclusion was diametrically opposed to that of Miescher—he concluded, in fact, that photodynamic reactions "should be recognized as a new carcinogenic principle."

The introduction of 8-methoxypsoralen (8-MOP) as a therapeutic agent for certain human skin diseases was followed by reports that it could enhance photocarcinogenesis in mice (77, 78). These demonstrations had the experimental advantage of newer and more convenient lamps which produced less stress on the animals, limited skin ulceration, and improved animal survival. Evidence indicated that carcinogenesis could result from the interacting effects of a compound and irradiation with a particular waveband of radiation, neither of these agents being a primary carcinogen.

A portion of the sunlight spectrum is carcinogenic even in the absence of an exogenous photosensitizer. At the current rate of introduction of new compounds into the environment, it has become increasingly important to determine whether a readily demonstrable property such as phototoxicity can be used to predict compounds or treatment regimes that could enhance photocarcinogenesis.

Forbes et al. (79) investigated the relative enhancing effect of two widely recognized photoactive compounds (8-MOP and anthracene) on photocarcinogenesis. These were selected because they were available in 99% pure form, leaving no doubt as to the identity of the active ingredient, they

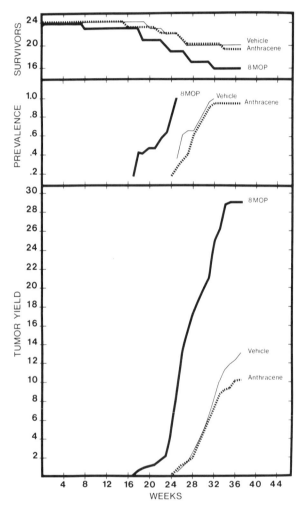

Fig. 9-8. Effects of pretreatment with 8-MOP, anthracene, or the vehicle, on the survival, the proportion of mice with tumors at any given time, and the average number of tumors/survivor in groups of irradiated mice.

represented different classes of chemicals inducing similar but not identical physiologic responses, and neither was a chemical carcinogen.

The results of the study are pertinent to the opposing conclusions of Miescher and Heller. The development of more appropriate light sources (solar simulators), animals (hairless mice), and test procedures (subacute phototoxicity) has, in fact, made possible a type of study envisaged by Miescher.

The experiments utilized genetically hairless mice pretreated three times weekly with application of 40 μl of a 0.1 g l^{-1} solution of either 8-MOP or anthracene dissolved in reagent-grade methanol. This volume covers about 20 cm^2 of skin on the back of a mouse. Approximately 1/2 hr later, the animals were exposed to a dose of simulated sunlight containing 300 J m^{-2} UVB (equivalent to about 1 human MED) from a xenon-arc solar simulator. Chemical and UV treatment continued for 38 weeks.

Compared with the vehicle alone, the 8-MOP solution, but not the anthracene solution, markedly enhanced photocarcinogenesis (Fig. 9-8). The times to 50% prevalence for the vehicle-treated and anthracene groups were 27 and 28 weeks, respectively. These values were not significantly different, but the time to 50% prevalence for the 8-MOP group differed significantly from each of the other two groups ($P < 0.01$). Similarily, tumor prevalence was significantly ($P < 0.05$) greater in the 8-MOP group. Beginning with week 18, tumor yield was significantly greater in the 8-MOP group than in either of the other groups ($P < 0.01$).

Under the conditions of the experiment, both test compounds were phototoxic, but only 8-MOP enhanced photocarcinogenesis.

Recent studies of Fry et al. (80) confirmed that photosensitization of the skin of hairless mice with 8-MOP increases the tumorigenic effect of UV radiation. Their studies suggest that photoadducts to DNA induced by this treatment are related to tumorigenesis. However, there was no quantitative relationship in several mouse strains between DNA cross-links and tumor production. This apparent lack of relationship appears to be due to a difference between strains of mice in the *expression*, not the *initiation* events. Thus it appears that *tumor promotion* is strain dependent.

Chemical Promotion of Photocarcinogenesis

Chemical promotion of photocarcinogenesis in the skin of hairless mice was shown, using croton oil as the promoter, by Epstein et al. (39) and Pound (34). Stenbäck (81) was able to show some promotion in a classic two-stage experiment, using UV radiation as the initiator.

Several other chemical agents have been studied for their potential promoting activity of photocarcinogenesis. Most important of these are *all-trans*-retinoic acid (RA) and BCNU, a nitrosourea chemotherapeutic agent.

Epstein (82) reported that topical application of 0.3% RA in a cream base, preceded by UV radiation exposures, enhanced photocarcinogenesis. In a later experiment, using lower concentrations of RA, he could not substantiate these findings. Forbes et al. (83) showed a marked effect of potentiation of photocarcinogenesis using a solar simulator as the radiation source and 0.01% or 0.001% RA in methanol topically. Subsequent experiments by Forbes strongly suggest that this potentiating effect of RA is due to promotion of UV-induced photocarcinogenesis.

Epstein (82), using a system similar to the RA experiments, reported that BCNU in low concentration also promoted UV-induced skin carcinogenesis.

THE IMPACT OF MOLECULAR BIOLOGY ON THE UNDERSTANDING OF MECHANISMS OF PHOTOCARCINOGENESIS

The spectacular advances in the field of molecular biology and, in particular, studies of alteration of DNA molecules and their repair have led to fascinating and biologically important observations on the characteristics of photoreactions of psoralens with biologic molecules.

It has been shown that the commonly investigated photodynamic agents, such as fluoresceine derivative dyes and porphyrins, carry out photosensitized oxidation reactions dependent on the presence of O_2. In contrast, the photosensitizing effect of psoralens is not oxygen dependent. Some psoralens form cycloadducts with pyrimidine bases, which are attached to only a single strand of the DNA molecule. Even more important, the photosensitizing psoralens which are linearly annulated are capable of intercalating between two base pairs of DNA and give interstrand cross-linkages upon irradiation (84).

Thus it appears that the damage caused to biologic systems may occur at the DNA level. Since single-strand covalent linkages to DNA can be more easily repaired by relatively error-free excision repair systems, the ability of the strongly photosensitizing 5- and 8–methoxypsoralens to form interstrand linkages may be of great importance for development of photocarcinogenesis. This is particularly likely, since cross-links remaining in cellular DNA should block separation of the strands during semiconservative replication and, if left unrepaired, might prevent normal cell division. There is evidence that DNA containing interstrand cross-links can be repaired. As can be seen in the scheme proposed by Cole and Sinden (85), the postulated repair mechanism is complicated, requires strand exchanges and repair synthesis, and is thus likely to be error-prone. The present thinking of scientists in the field of molecular biology (48) suggests strongly that mutagenesis and carcinogenesis are a consequence of errors in DNA repair. Thus it is a reasonable suggestion that some psoralens (because of their DNA cross-linking capability) will be photocarcinogenic, while most photodynamic compounds, including anthracene, causing either photooxidation or covalent DNA single-strand adducts, have less likelihood of serious DNA change and thus should be relatively less photocarcinogenic.

Blackburn and Taussig (86) have reported that UVA irradiation of mammalian epithelial cell cultures after treatment with anthracene produces covalent binding of anthracene to DNA. Their suggestion that this constitutes a potentially carcinogenic lesion is not borne out by the animal studies of Forbes et al. (79).

The problem of attempting to predict the relative potential of photoactive agents for neoplastic transformation is further complicated by the observations of Fry et al. (80). They demonstrated an action spectrum for formation of cross-links in DNA in the presence of 8-MOP, in the sense that irradiation with relatively narrowband 365-nm photons was one-fourth to one-fifth as efficient in forming DNA cross-links as was the 320–400-nm wideband radiation. Moreover, 365-nm radiation was much less effective for carcinogenesis in 8-MOP treated, irradiated mice even when UV doses were made equivalent for in vitro cross-linking effect. Their data demonstrate a spectral dependence of oncogenic effects, which must relate in part to the formation of some psoralen photoproduct, since the exposure to wavelengths of 320–400 nm is normally carcinogenic only in photosensitized skin. Thus, their experiments tentatively suggest that it is unlikely that the photoproduct involved is the bifunctional adduct. Time, much more experimentation, and further studies on the action spectrum of both UVB-induced and chemically augmented photocarcinogenesis will solve this riddle.

HUMAN PHOTOCARCINOGENESIS

Human Skin Cancer Production by UV Radiation

Examination of the sun's role in the production of human skin cancers does not lend itself to direct experimentation. However, extensive astute observations have strongly suggested the etiologic significance of radiation energy in the induction of these tumors. Skin cancers in Caucasians, in general, are most prevalent in geographical areas with the greatest insolation and among people who receive the most exposure, i.e., individuals who work outdoors. They are rare in blacks and other deeply pigmented individuals, who have the greatest protection against UV radiation injury. Further, the lightest complexioned individuals, such as those of Scottish and Irish descent, appear to be most susceptible to skin cancer when they live in geographic areas of high UV exposure. When skin cancers do occur in the darkly pigmented races, they are not distributed primarily in the sun-exposed areas as they are in light-skinned people. The tumors in these pigmented individuals are more commonly stimulated by other forms of trauma, such as chronic leg ulcers, irritation due to not wearing shoes, the use of a Kangri (an earthenware pot that is filled with burning charcoal and strapped to the abdomen for warmth), the wearing of a Dhoti (loin cloth), and so on. In contrast, the distribution of skin cancer in the Bantu albino and in patients with xeroderma pigmentosum follows sun exposure patterns.

Blum (31), Urbach et al. (87, 88), and Emmett (89) have reviewed the evidence supporting the role of sunlight in human skin cancer development. Briefly, the main arguments are:

1. It is clearly established that superficial skin cancers occur most frequently on the head, neck, arms, and hands—parts of the body habitually exposed to sunlight.

2. Pigmented races, who sunburn much less rapidly than people with white skin, have very much less skin cancer, and when it does occur, it most frequently affects areas not exposed to sunlight.

3. Among Caucasians there appears to be much greater incidence of skin cancer in those who spend more time outdoors than in those who work predominantly indoors.

4. Skin cancer is more common in white-skinned people living in areas where insolation is greater.

5. Genetic diseases resulting in greater sensitivity of skin to the effect of solar UV radiation are associated with marked increases in skin cancer and premature skin cancer development (albinism, xeroderma pigmentosum).

6. Superficial skin cancers, particularly squamous cell carcinoma of the skin, occur predominantly on the areas receiving the maximum amounts of solar UV radiation and where histologic changes of chronic UV-radiation damage are most severe.

7. Skin cancer can be produced readily on the skin of mice and rats with repeated doses of UV radiation, and the upper wavelength limit of the most effective cancer-producing radiation is about 320 nm, that is, the same spectral range that produces erythema solare in human skin.

Though these arguments do not consitute absolute proof, there is excellent epidmiologic evidence supporting the role of sunlight in three types of skin cancers: basal cell carcinomas, squamous cell carcinomas, and malignant melanomas.

Together, the first two types of skin cancer add up to the most frequently detected cancer in humans and have had an increased incidence over the past decade. They are also the most easily and most successfully treated human cancers. The quantitative extent to which agents other than UV exposure cause nonmelanoma skin cancer in the white population has not been established. It is, however, believed to be small. Some nonmelanoma skin cancer is caused by exposure to arsenic, pitch, and x-rays, often in the course of work, sometimes following treatment of skin disorders. This latter group of tumors is found among patients of all degrees of skin pigmentation who happen to be exposed to these agents. In some less developed countries, most nonmelanomas seem to arise in neglected wounds.

Nonmelanoma skin cancer is at present a serious problem because of disfigurement and the significant economic burden associated with its treatment, particularly in the United States, Europe, and Australia, and to emigrants from these regions to other parts of the world.

Incidence of Skin Cancer in Humans

Surveys of the incidence of skin cancer have been performed with varying success in the recent past. The major surveys have been those performed by the U.S. National Cancer Institute in 1947–1948 ("Ten City Survey") (90), the recent Third National Cancer Survey (1971–1972) (91), and the M. D. Anderson Institute, Texas Survey (1962–1972) (92). Data are also available from Iowa (93), Minnesota (94), and several prevalence studies carried out in Australia (95, 96).

The enumeration of skin cancer incidence in a population is made very difficult by the relative benignity of the disease, which allows for curative treatment in physicians' offices rather than in hospitals. Surveying *all* inhabitants in any one area is difficult and expensive, so that most skin cancer incidence studies have seriously underestimated actual conditions.

Probably the most accurate surveys have been those of Scotto et al. (91) (Third National Cancer Survey, National Cancer Institute, 1971–1972) and of MacDonald and Heinze (92). In both those surveys and in data from other studies, an inverse relationship with latitude is apparent.

The Third National Cancer Survey shows that the annual incidence rates for skin cancer (excluding malignant melanoma) vary from 379 per 100,000 in Dallas-Fort Worth to 124 per 100,000 in Iowa.

Nonmelanoma skin cancer, like most other forms of cancer, is a disease that occurs more frequently in older age groups. However, unlike other types of cancer, the rates for skin cancer are significantly higher even in the middle age groups, i.e., 35–54-year-old persons.

Comparing the older and more recent studies, there is a strong suggestion that skin cancer has increased in the past several decades. For instance, for Minnesota, comparing the metropolitan areas, an apparent twofold increase has occurred since 1963, perhaps a reflection of the recent trend for many people to expose themselves more, and more of themselves, to the sun's rays as lifestyles, clothing, and leisure time changed.

The best estimate for present annual incidence of nonmelanoma skin cancer in the United States (in Caucasians) is 165 per 100,000 population. This means that at present about 300,000 cases of nonmelanoma skin cancer develop in the United States each year, or about one-third to one-half of all cancers of all sites arise in the skin. It is indeed fortunate that the cure rate for nonmelanoma skin cancer exceeds 95%.

Sunlight and the Etiology of Malignant Melanoma

The influence of latitude of residence on the incidence of and mortality from melanoma is the original and strongest evidence of the importance of exposure to sunlight by white people as a cause of malignant melanoma. The gradient with latitude of death rate from malignant melanoma is not as great as for the other skin cancers, but it is substantial. Both the incidence and the mortality rates from malignant melanoma are rising rapidly in all countries in which they have been studied. Mortality rates are rising by around 3–9% per year, so that the rates have doubled in about the last 15 years (97). In some countries, e.g., Canada, the rate of increase is greater than that of any other tumor except male lung cancer. The changes have been shown to be independent of improved diagnosis or certification. There is some indication that incidence rates have risen more rapidly, showing that improved diagnosis and treatment have reduced case fataility, but not to a great extent. All these relationships are most unlikely to be due to chance. Where exposure of particular sites is different between the sexes because of conventional dresss and hair styles (ears and neck in males; lower limbs in females), the exposed site has higher incidence and mortality rates than the unexposed site in the opposite sex. While no substantial study of the influence of occupation has apparently yet been made, patients with malignant melanoma had higher numbers of hours of exposure and were less pigmented than controls. (98).

In spite of this evidence, the importance of sunlight as an etiologic factor in malignant melanoma has been recognized only in recent years and tends to be minimized in the older literature. Malignant melanomas are not common tumors and, until the sixth revision of the International Statistical Classi- fication of Diseases (World Health Organization, 1948), were not separated from other skin tumors. This effectively prevented recognition of their variation from population to population. However, a more important factor was the lack of concentration cf malignant melanomas on the face and neck, in obvious contrast to squamous cell and basal cell carcinomas.

It is of interest that there is a close relationship between the death rate from squamous cell carcinoma and malignant melanoma in the United States and Canadian provinces, suggesting that a common environmental factor operates (98).

The paradox of the strong relationship of malignant melanomas to exposure–latitude, differential exposure between the sexes, occupation, and the lack of strong concentration of melanomas on exposed sites has been most clearly presented in Australian clinical studies. Not only is there a broad similarity between the anatomical distribution of the malignant melanomas reported from white populations with widely differing incidences of the disease, but direct questioning of Australian patients with malignant melanoma fails to elicit a history of particular exposure on the site of the primary lesion. Furthermore, malignant melanoma appears to affect professionals and skilled workers more than poorer classes. The present best thinking suggests that while nonmelanoma skin cancer is due to accumulated UV radiation dose, malignant melanoma is more likely related to intermittent overdoses of UV radiation (99) (Table 9-1).

The incidence and death rate from malignant melanoma are rising rapidly in many developed societies. This is in spite of the improvements in treatment in the last generation. As a result, the death rate from all forms of skin cancer combined has, surprisingly, shown no decline in recent years. The increase in death rates from malignant melanoma in the younger age groups has balanced the improvements in the death rates from squamous cell carcinomas in the elderly. This rise is a generation effect, and we can expect the general population death rate to rise, even without a further rise in the death rates in the young.

There seems no reasonable doubt that, as industrial societies develop, the exposure of the population to sunlight becomes greater since hours of work become less, vacations become longer, the opportunities for vacation travel become greater, and clothing becomes lighter. There is, at present, no reason to associate the increasing melanoma rates with anything but this. The proportion of rural workers declines as societies industrialize, but this may not make much difference, since, in general, white people living a tradiational country life, whether as peasant farmers in Europe or as cattle herders in the American west, tend to be fairly shy of the sun and dress accordingly. Society clearly cannot go back on these changes, but it does have a responsibility to

Table 9-1. Percentage Distribution by Anatomical Site
of Malignant Melanoma of the Skin
and Other Skin Cancers[a]

	Head and Neck	Trunk	Upper limb	Lower limb	Multiple sites	Total
Malignant melanoma:						
Male	32	25	9	22	12	100
Female	24	19	14	33	10	100
Other skin cancers:						
Male	81	7	4	6	2	100
Female	78	7	8	4	3	100

[a]Denmark, 1943–1957. Data Based on 511 male and 693 female patients with melanoma; 7316 male and 5071 female patients with other skin cancers. Source: Clemmenson (103).

protect those in danger. Only a rather specific identification of people particularly likely to develop a malignant melanoma would be of practical use, as the disease has an incidence of only 2–10 per 100,000 per year.

Under contemporary conditions, basal cell and squamous cell carcinomas are practically unable to start off from white skin except under the prolonged direct effect of exposure to sunlight. In contrast, the relative sensitivity of melanocytes to sunlight is apparently much less, and malignant melanomas can develop at any point on the body surface. Malignant melanomas have a predilection for exposed sites, but it is not as definite as it is for the malignancies derived from other skin cells.

A simple hypothesis to account for this would be that malignant melanomas have two origins—one independent of sunlight and occurring wherever there are melanocytes to undergo malignant change (perhaps related to preexsiting nevi) and the other related to exposure (98).

ESTIMATE OF EFFECT OF OZONE REDUCTION IN THE STRATOSPHERE ON THE INCIDENCE OF SKIN CANCER

As has been pointed out in the preceding sections, there exists extensive evidence that skin cancer, at least of the nonmelanoma type, is caused by cumulative exposure to UVB. This is primarily true of skin unprotected by significant amounts of melanin, and thus mainly applicable to the white races, or about one-third of the world's population.

The weight of the evidence is consistent with the concept that UV-induced photodamage to skin is the main causative factor in skin cancer, and that there is not threshold effect. Thus a relationship should exist between skin cancer incidence and accumulative dose using a sensitivity function. In mice, the quantitative relationship between UV-radiation dose and the production of skin cancer has been thoroughly explored: tumor incidence in this experimental model is proportional to the square of the number of UV-radiation doses, their size, and the interval between doses (31).

Accumulative dosage or exposure is a function of the amount of ozone in the stratosphere, atmospheric conditions (cloudiness, aerosol, etc.), latitude, and lifestyle (which includes time and type of outdoor activity). Of these, the thickness of the stratospheric ozone layer is the major determinant of the amount of spectral distribution of effective UV radiation that can reach any point on earth.

An example of the importance of lifestyle and diurnal exposure has been assembled by Scotto et al. (100). Utilizing integrated erythemal UV measurements, obtained with Robertson–Berger meters at nine locations in the United States (101), the striking variation with season and time of day of such presumably carcinogenic radiation was documented (100) (Fig. 9-9). As

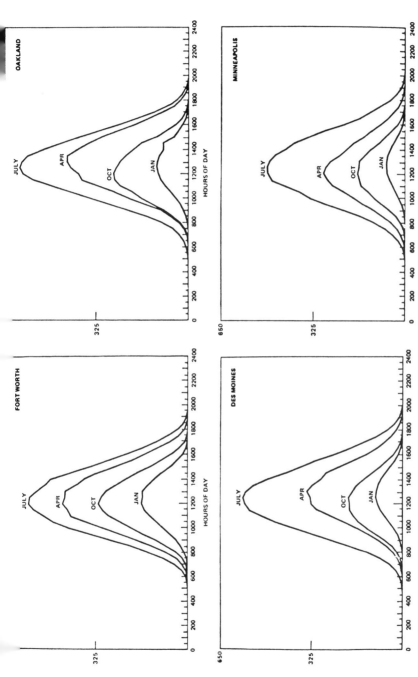

Fig. 9-9. Average half-hourly UV count by time of day for January, April, July, and October. Measurements of solar UVB irradiance obtained with Robertson–Berger meters in four areas of the United States over a 20° latitude span. Note the striking variation of UVB reaching the ground with season, time of day, and latitude (100).

expected, greater amounts of radiation were found at locations that are closer to the equator (low latitude), closer to the sun (high altitude), and with clearer skies. As reported long ago by Schulze, approximately 60% of the day's total erythemogenic radiation is received between the hours of 10 a.m. and 2 p.m. The relative effect of avoiding sunlight during noontime is significantly large. Even for an office worker, whose small exposure occurs primarily on weekends and vacations, the reduction is over 25% by avoiding just 1 hr from 12 noon to 1 p.m. By avoiding two noontime hours, all occupations can achieve reductions in UV exposure of the order of 35–50%. Thus, independent of location, by using a simple plan to avoiding sunlight during noontime period, an individual can reduce exposure substantially without major changes in living habits.

Relationship of Ozone Thickness to UV Radiation

A quantitative relatioship between ozone thickness and UV radiation erythemogenic for untanned white skin has been calculated by a number of investigators. The average increase in UVB effectiveness for a 5% decrease in ozone becomes 9.25% (or a multiplication factor of 1.85). Comparisons of UVB meter readings at Hilo, Hawaii and Bismarck, North Dakota with Dobson meter measurements at these stations showed multiplication factors of 2.15 and 2.0, respectively (101).

Effect on Skin Cancer

Utilizing the figures for incidence of skin cancer in the United States obtained by the Third National Cancer Survey and a variety of assumptions on the relationship of UV radiation and skin cancer, several models for the potential effect of reduction of the stratospheric ozone layer have been proposed.

Underlying all of these models are several assumptions:

1. A decrease in stratospheric ozone will result in an increase in UV radiation shorter than approximately 320 nm.

2. An increase in UV radiation shorter than approximately 320 nm will result in an increase in skin cancer in a susceptible human population.

3. The observed increase in skin cancer with decreasing latitude is due to several interacting factors, of which ozone thickness is one, and a variety of differences in local atmospheric conditions, genetic background of the population, type, length, and kind of outdoor exposure, and other not yet specified conditions make up the rest.

The various models attempting to relate decrease in atmospheric ozone to a possible increase in skin cancer result in the following "amplification" factors:

1. Increase in UVB due to reduction in ozone concentration in the stratosphere: "amplification" factor 2 (range 1.4–2.5).
2. Increase in skin cancer incidence due to increase in UVB radiation at ground level: "Amplification" factor 2 (range 0.5–4).
3. Increase in skin cancer incidence due to reduction in ozone concentration in the stratosphere: Amplification" factor 4 (range 0.5–4).

Utilizing the skin cancer incidence figures of the Third National Cancer Survey as baseline and an overall "amplification" factor of 4 (99), a 5% reduction in ozone concentration could result in an increase of 74 per 100,000 cases of skin cancer per year at the latitude of Dallas–Fort Worth, Texas, and an increase of 25 per 100,000 cases of skin cancer per year at the latitude of Iowa. On the assumption that the incidence of nonmelanoma skin cancer in the United States is approximately 165 per 100,000, a 5% decrease in stratospheric ozone concentration could result in an average increase in the United States of 23 per 100,000 cases of skin cancer (or + 20%).

It cannot be pointed out too strongly that all the calculations by all authors who have attempted to provide such estimates are subject to great, and at this time not measurable, uncertainty, much of which is inherent in the uncertainity of growth of cell populations in cancer. For this reason, until much better data are available, at least on the effects of shifts in spectral distribution of UV radiation, effects of irradiance, time–dose relationships, and on–off (seasonal) cycles of irradiation, as well as relible information on the true incidence of skin cancer, all the numerical estimates must be treated as very preliminary and open to significant corrections as new information accumulates.

SUMMARY

The skin cancers discussed in the above section are principally basal cell and squamous cell carcinomas. Melanomas have been included. The incidence of malignant melanoma, although low, also shows a marked latitude gradient, and the death rates from the two broad groups of primary neoplasms of skin are highly correlated in the United States and the provinces of Canada. The importance of malignant melanomas lies in the high proportion of the patients who die of that tumor (with current methods about 40%, comparable with breast cancer). It can be assumed that the extra deaths from squamous cell carcinomas produced by an environmental change will be associated with an approximately equal number of deaths from malignant melanomas. If the present clinical features of the tumors are unaltered, these melanoma deaths will occur in much younger people than the deaths from other skin cancer.

Furthermore, the preceding observations on the relationship between exposure to sunlight and the incidence of skin cancers and melanomas has largely referred to a static situation. There have been hints that the incidence of skin tumors of all types is rising, but there remains the difficulty of being certain that improving methods of ascertainment have not been largely responsible for this rise. Mortality rates from skin tumors are approximately stable in both the U.S. white population and in Canada. However, investigation of these rates in both countries shows that the mortality from melanomas is rising rapidly, while that from other skin cancers is declining. Further, the death rates are rising in the younger age groups and declining in the elderly. The reasonable explanation of these changes is that improvements in medical care (earlier diagnosis, better surgery, and radiotherapy) are reducing the mortality from the squamous cell carcinomas (better certification may also play a part), while the improvements in treatment are failing to keep pace with the rising incidence of melanomas. The changes in the age distribution of the deaths support this, as the average melanoma patient is much younger than the patient with a squamous cell tumor (98, 99).

Thus, if we are to make projections into the future, we should make estimates of the incidence of human skin tumors in terms of the likely levels that will have been reached by the continuation of present trends, most likely related to changes in human behavior.

Finally, it must be clearly pointed out that all estimates concerning effects of stratospheric ozone depletion on the incidence of skin cancer in humans represent the conditions that could be expected to exist after a *new steady state* of both UV radiation and skin cancer incidence have been reached. Since it is assumed that the development of skin cancer is related to accumulated lifetime UV radiation dose, a new steady state in skin cancer incidence for a population will not be reached until the time when all members of that population have been exposed to the new levels of increased UV radiation over a considerable part of their lifetime. Cutchis (102) has estimated the manner in which skin cancer incidence may be expected to build up from an initial to a new equilibrium rate. Assuming a sudden increase in UVB irradiance, Cutchis shows that one-fourth of the expected increase in skin cancer incidence would develop about 10 years after such an event and that, if the UVB irradiance were returned to its original level at that time, it would take of the order of 15 years for the skin cancer incidence to return to its baseline level. Since UVB-irradiance changes are not likely to occur suddenly, there will be time in which to carry out pertinent experiments which should allow considerably more accurate estimates of potential risks to humans to be performed.

REFERENCES

1. Charcot, P. (1858): Erythème produit par l'action de la lumière électrique. *C. R. Soc. Biol.* (*Paris*) **5**(Ser. 2):63–65.

2. Unna, P. (1894): *Histopathologie der Hautkrankheiten.* August Hirschwald, Berlin.
3. Hausser, K. W., and Vahle, W. (1927): Sonnenbrand und Sonnenbraunung. *Wiss. Veroff. Siemens-Konzern* **6**:101–120.
4. Bloch, B. (1917): Das Problem der Pigmentbildung in der Haut. *Arch. Dermatol. Syphilol. (Berlin)* **124**:129–208.
5. Ehrman, S. (1905): *Mracek's Handbuch,* Vol. 2, pp. 789. Vienna.
6. Hammer, F. (1891): *Uber den Einfluss des Lichtes.* Ferdinand Enke, Stuttgart.
7. With, C. (1920): Studies on the effect of light on vitiligo. *Br. J. Dermatol.* **32**:145–155.
8. Guillaume, A. C. (1926): Le pigment épidermique, la penetration des rayons ultraviolets et le mécanisme de protection de l'organisme vis-à-vis de ces radiations. *Bull. Soc. Med. Hop. (Paris)* **42**:1133–1135.
9. Miescher, G. (1930): Das Problem der Lichtgewöhnung. *Strahlentherapie* **36**:434.
10. Finsen, N. R. (1900): Neue Untersuchungen über die Einwirkung des Lichtes auf die Haut. *Mit. Finsen Institut* **1**:8.
11. Dubreuilh, W. (1896): Des hyperkeratoses circonscriptes. *Ann. Dermatol. Syphiligr. (Paris)* **7**(Ser. 3): 1158–1204.
12. Shield, A. M. (1899): A remarkable case of multiple growths of the skin caused by exposure to the sun. *Lancet* **1**:22–23.
13. Hyde, J. (1906): On the influence of light in the production of cancer of the skin. *Am. J. Med. Sci.* **31**:1–22.
14. Paul, C. N. (1918): *The Influence of Sunlight in the Production of Cancer of the Skin.* H. K. Lewis, London.
15. Bruusgaard, cited in Rasch, C. (1926): Some historical and clinical remarks on the effect of light on the skin and skin diseases. *Proc. R. Soc. Med.* **20**:11–20.
16. Haxthausen, H., and Hausmann, W. (1929): *Die Lichterkrankungen der Haut.* Urban und Schwarzenberg, Vienna.
17. Findlay, G. M. (1928): Ultraviolet light and skin cancer. *Lancet* **2**:1070–1073.
18. Putschar, W., and Holtz, F. (1930): Erzeugung von Hautkrebsen bie Ratten durch langedaurende Ultraviolet Bestrahlung. *Z. Krebsforsch.* **33**:219–260.
19. Huldschinsky, K. (1933): Augensarkom bei Ratten hervorgerufen durch abnorm lange Ultraviolet Bestrahlung. *Dtsch. Med. Wochenschr.* **59**:530–531.
20. Roffo, A. H. (1933): Cancer y sol. *Bol. Inst. Med. Exp. Estud. Trata Cancer* **10**:417–439.
21. Roffo, A. H. (1934): Cancer et soleil. Carcinomes et sarcomes provoques par l'action du soleil in toto. *Bull. Cancer (Paris)* **23**:590–616. 1934.
22. Roffo, A. H. (1939): Uber die physikalische Aetiologie der Krebskrankheit. *Strahlentherapie* **66**:328–350.
23. Raab, O. (1899): Untersuchungen über die Wirkung fluoreszierender Stoffe. *Z. Biol.* **38**:16.
24. Tappeiner, H. V., and Jodlbauer, A. (1907): *Die sensibilisierende Wirkung fluoreszierender Substanzen.* Verlag FCW Vogel. Leipzig.
25. Jodlbauer, A. (1905): Die Beteilung des Sauerstoffes bei der Wirkung fluoreszierenden Stoffe. *Arch. Klin. Med.* **82**:520–546.
26. Busck, G., and Tappeiner, H. (1906): Über Lichtbehandlung blut-parasitärer Krankheiten. *Arch. Klin. Med.* **87**:98–110.
27. Lewis, M. R. (1935): The photosensitivity of chick embryo cells growing in media containing certain carcinogenic substances. *Am. J. Cancer* **25**:305–309.
28. Blum, H. F., Kirby-Smith, S., and Grady, H. G. (1941): Quantitative induction of tumors in mice with ultraviolet radiation. *J. Natl. Cancer Inst.* **2**:259–268.
29. Blum, H. F. (1959): *Carcinogenesis by Ultraviolet Light.* Princeton Univ. Press, Princeton.
30. LeGrand, Y. (1970): *Introduction to Photobiology.* American Elsevier Press, New York.
31. Blum, H. F. (1950): On the mechanism of cancer induction by ultraviolet radiation. *J. Natl. Cancer Inst.* **11**:463–495.
32. Rogers, S. (1955): In vitro initiation of pulmonary adenomas in fetal mouse lung by single exposure ultraviolet irradiation of wavelength 2,537 Å. *J. Natl. Cancer Inst.* **15**:1001–1004.

33. Epstein, J. H., and Roth, H. L. (1968): Experimental ultraviolet light carcinogenesis. *J. Invest. Dermatol.* **50**:387–389.

34. Pound, A. W. (1970): Induced cell proliferation and the initiation of skin tumor formation in mice by ultraviolet light. *Pathology* **2**:269–273.

35. Hsu, T., Forbes, P. D., Harber, L. C., et al. (1975): Induction of skin tumors in hairless mice following single exposure to ultraviolet radiation. *Photochem. Photobiol.* **21**:185–188.

36. Forbes, P. D., and Urbach, F. (1975): Experimental modification of photocarcinogenesis. III. Simulation of exposure to sunlight and fluroescent whitening agents. *Food Cosmet. Toxicol.* **131**:343–345.

37. Forbes, P. D. (1974): Influence of continued exposure to ultraviolet light (UVL) on UVL induced tumors. In: *Abstracts of the 2nd Annual Meeting, American Society for Photobiology, Vancouver, 1974,* p. 102.

38. Evans, R. G., and Norman, A. (1968): Unscheduled incorporation of thymidine in UV irradiated human lymphocytes. *Radiat. Res.* **36**:287–298.

39. Epstein, J. H. Fukuyama, K., and Epstein, W. L. (1968): Ultraviolet light induced stimulation of DNA synthesis in hairless mouse epidermis. *J. Invest. Dermatol.* **51**:445–453.

40. Cleaver, J. E. (1968): Defective repair replication of DNA in xeroderma pigmentosum. *Nature* **218**:652–656.

41. Cleaver, J. E., and Carter, P. M. (1973): Xeroderma pigmentosum: influence of temperature on DNA repair. *J. Invest. Dermatol.* **60**:29–32.

42. Epstein, W. L., Fukuyama, K., and Epstein, J. H. (1971): Ultraviolet light, DNA repair and skin carcinogenesis in man. *Fed. Proc.* **30**:1766–1771.

43. Lieberman, M. W., and Forbes, P. D. (1973): Demonstration of DNA repair in normal and neoplastic tissues after treatment with proximate chemical carcinogens and UV radiation. *Nature [New Biol.]* **241**:199–201.

44. Norman, H., Ottoman, R. E., Chou, P., et al. (1972): Unscheduled DNA synthesis. *Mutat. Res.* **15**:358–360.

45. Roberts, J. J. (1972): In: Molecular and Cellular Repair Processes, edited by R. F. Beers, R. F. Beers, R. M. Herriott, and R. Tilghman. *Johns Hopkins Med. j. Suppl.* **1**:226–238.

46. Setlow, R. B., and Hart, R. W. (1974): Direct evidence that damaged DNA results in neoplastic transformation: a fish story. *Radiat. Res.* **59**:73–74.

47. Zajdela, F., and Latarjet, R. (1973): The inhibiting effect of caffeine on the induction of skin cancer by ultraviolet light in the mouse. *C. R. Acad. Sci.* [*D*] (*Paris*) **277**:1073–1076.

48. Hanawalt, P. C., and Setlow, R. B. (Eds.) (1975): *Molecular Mechanisms for Repair of DNA,* Parts A and B. Plenum Press, New York/London.

49. Freeman, R. G., Hudson, H. T., and Carnes, R. (1970): Ultraviolet wavelength factor in solar radiation and skin cancer. *Int. J. Dermatol.* **9**:232–235.

50. Freeman, R. G. (1975): Data on the action spectrum for ultraviolet carcinogenesis. *J. Natl. Cancer Inst.* **55**:1119–1122.

51. Freeman, R. G. (1978): Action spectrum for ultraviolet carcinogenesis. *Natl. Cancer Inst. Monogr.* **50**:27–30.

52. Wetzel, V. R. (1959): Zum Wirkungsspektrum der cancerogener Eigenschaften des ultravioletten Lichtes. *Arch. Geschwulstforsch.* **14**:120–131; **15**:227–237.

53. Setlow, R. B. (1974): The wavelength in sunlight effective in producing skin cancer: a theoretical analysis. *Proc. Natl. Acad. Sci. U.S.A.* **71**:3363–3366.

54. Forbes, P. D., Davies, R. E., and Urbach, F. (1978): Experimental ultraviolet carcinogenesis: wavelength interaction and time–dose relationships. *Natl. Cancer Inst. Monogr.* **50**:31–38.

55. Kripke, M. L., and Fisher, M. S. (1976): Immunologic parameters of ultraviolet carcinogenesis. *J. Natl. Cancer Inst.* **57**:211–215.

56. Kripke, M. L., and Fisher, M. S. (1978): Immunologic aspects of tumor induction by ultraviolet radiation. *Natl. Cancer Inst. Monogr.* **50**:179–183.

57. Fisher, M. S. (1978): A systemic effect of ultraviolet irradiation and its relationship to tumor immunity. *Natl. Cancer Inst. Monogr.* **50**:185–188.

58. Nathanson, R. B., Forbes, P. D., and Urbach, F. (1976): Modification of photocarcinogenesis by two immunosuppressive agents. *Cancer Letters* **1**:243–247.

59. Lewin, L. (1913): Uber photodynamische Wirkungen von Inhaltsstoffen des Steinkohlenteer Pech's am Menschen. *Munch. Med. Wochenschr.* **60**:1529–1530.

60. Fleischhauer, L. (1930): Über die sensibilisierende Wirkung des Teer präparates Liantral. *Strahlentherapie* **36**:144–160.

61. Doniach, I., and Mottram, J. C. (1940): On the effect of light upon the incidence of tumors in painted mice. *Am. J. Cancer* **39**:234–240.

62. Clark, J. H. (1964): The effect of longwave ultraviolet radiation on the development of tumors induced by 20-methylcholanthrene. *Cancer Res.* **24**:207–211.

63. Stenbäck, F. (1975): Studies on the modifying effect of ultraviolet radiation on chemical skin carcinogenesis. *J. Invest. Dermatol.* **64**:253–257.

64. Morton, J. J., Luce-Clausen, E. M., and Mahoney, E. B. (1942): Visible light and skin tumors induced with benzpyrene in mice. *Cancer Res.* **2**:256–260.

65. Kohn-Speyer, A. C. (1929): Effect on ultraviolet radiation on the incidence of tar cancer in mice. *Lancet* **1**:1305–1306.

66. Seelig, M. G., and Cooper, Z. K. (1933): Light and tar cancer. *Surg. Gynecol. Obstet.* **56**:752–761.

67. Santamaria, L. (1960): Photodynamic action and carcinogenicity. In: *Recent Contributions to Cancer Research in Italy*, Vol. I, edited by P. Bucalossi and U. Veronesi, pp. 107. Rome.

68. Schonberg, A., Mustafa, A., Barakat, M. Z., et al. (1948): Photochemical reactions. XIII. (a) Photochemical reactions to ethylenes with phenanthraquinone and with 1,2,3-triketones. (b) Dimerisation reactions in sunlight. *J. Chem. Soc. (London)* **428**:2126–2129.

69. Cook, J. H., and Martin, R. H. (1940): Polycyclic aromatic hydrocarbons. XXIV. *J. Chem. Soc. (London)* **1940**(Part 2):1125–1127.

70. Davies, R. E., Dodge, H. A., and Austin, W. A. (1972): Carcinogenicity of DMBA under various light sources. In: *Proceedings of the VIth International Congress of Photobiology, Bochum, 1972,* Abstract 347.

71. Davies, R. E., Dodge, H. A., and DeShields, L. H. (1972): Alteration of the carcinogenic activity of DMBA by light (abstract). *Proc. Am. Assoc. Cancer Res.* **13**:14.

72. Davies, R. E., and Dodge, H. A. (1973): Modification of chemical carcinogenesis by phototoxicity and photochemical decomposition of carcinogen. In: *Proceedings of the 1st Annual Meeting of the American Society for Photobiology, Sarasota, 1972,* p. 138.

73. Davies, R. E. (1978): Interaction of light on chemicals in carcinogenesis. *Natl. Cancer Inst. Monogr.* **50**:45–50.

74. Büngeler, W. (1937): Über den Einfluss photosensibilisierender Substanzen auf die Enstehung von Hautgeschwülsten. *Z. Krebsforsch.* **46**:130–167.

75. Miescher, G. (1942): Experimentelle Untersuchungen uber Krebserzeugung durch Photosensibilisierung. *Schweiz. Med. Wochenschr.* **23**:1082–1084.

76. Heller, W. (1950): Experimentelle Untersuchungen über den Lichtkrebs. *Strahlentherapie* **81**:529–548.

77. Griffin, A. C., Hakim, R. E., and Knox, J. (1958): The wavelength effect upon erythemal and carcinogenic response in psoralen treated mice. *J. Invest. Dermatol.* **31**:289–295.

78. Urbach, F. (1959): Modification of ultraviolet carcinogenesis by photoactive agents. *J. Invest. Dermatol.* **32**:373–378.

79. Forbes, P. D., Davies, R. E., and Urbach, F. (1976): Phototoxicity and photocarcinogenesis: comparative effects of anthracene and 8-methoxypsoralen in the skin of mice. *Food Cosmet. Toxicol.* **14**:303–306.

80. Fry, R. J. M., Ley, R. D., and Grube, D. D. (1978): Photosensitized reactions and carcinogenesis. *Natl. Cancer Inst. Monogr.* **50**:39–43.

81. Stenbäck, F. (1975): Ultraviolet light irradiation as initiating agent in skin tumor formation by the two-stage method. *Eur. J. Cancer* **11**:241–246.

82. Epstein, J. H. (1978): Photocarcinogenesis: a review. *Natl. Cancer Inst. Monogr.* **50**:13–25.

83. Forbes, P. D., Urbach, F., and Davies, R. E. (1979): Enhancement of experimental photocarcinogenesis by topical retinoic acid. *Cancer Letters* **7**:85–90.
84. Pathak, M. A., Kramer, D. M., and Fitzpatric, T. B. (1974): Photobiology and photochemistry of furocoumarins (psoralens). In: *Sunlight and Man: Normal and Abmormal Photobiologic Responses,* edited by M. A. Pathak, L. C. Harber, M. Seiji, et al., pp. 335–368. Univ. of Tokyo Press, Tokyo.
85. Cole, R. S., and Sinden, R. R. (1975): Repair of crosslinked DNA in *Escherichia coli.* In: *Molecular Mechanisms for Repair of DNA,* edited by P. C. Hanawalt and R. B. Setlow, pp. 487–495. Plenum Press, New York.
86. Blackburn, M. G., and Taussig, P. E. (1975): The photocarcinogenicity of anthracene: photochemical binding to deoxyribonucleic acid in tissue culture. *Biochem. J.* **149**:289–291.
87. Urbach, F., Rose, D. B., and Bonnem, M. (1972): Genetic and environmental interactions in skin carcinogenesis. In: *Environment and Cancer* (M. D. Anderson Hospital Conference Proceedings), pp. 356–371. Williams & Wilkins, Baltimore.
88. Urbach, F., Epstein, J. H., and Forbes, P. D. (1974): Ultraviolet carcinogenesis: experimental, global, and genetic aspects. In: *Sunlight and Man: Normal and Abnormal Photobiologic Responses,* edited by M. A. Pathak, L. C. Harber, M. Seiji, et al., pp. 259–283. Univ. of Tokyo Press, Tokyo.
89. Emmett, E. A. (1973): Ultraviolet radiation as a cause of skin tumors. *CRC Crit. Rev. Toxicol.* **2**:211–255.
90. Dorn, H. F. (1944): Illness from cancer in the United States. *Public Health Rep.* **59**:33, 65, 77.
91. Scotto, J., Kopf, A. W., and Urbach, F. (1974): Nonmelanoma skin cancer among Caucasians in four areas of the United States. *Cancer* **34**:1333–1138.
92. MacDonald, E. J., and Heinze, E. B. (1978): *Epidemiology of Cancer in Texas.* Raven Press, New York.
93. Haenszel, W., Marcus, S. C., and Zimmeren, E. G. (1956): Cancer morbidity in urban and rural areas. *Public Health Service Publication #462.* U.S. Government Printing Office, Washington, D.C.
94. Lynch, F. W., Seidman, H., and Hammond, E. C. (1970): Incidence of cutaneous cancer in Minnesota. *Cancer* **25**:83–91.
95. Silverstone, H., and Gordon, D. (1966): Regional studies in skin cancer. Second report: Wet tropical and subtropical coast of Queensland. *Med. J. Aust.* **2**:733–740.
96. Gordon, D., Silverstone, H., and Smithhurst, B. A. (1972): The epidemiology of skin cancer in Australia. In: *Melanoma and Skin Cancer,* edited by W. H. McCarthy. New South Wales Government Printer, Sydney.
97. Magnus, K. (1977): Incidence of malignant melanoma of the skin in five Nordic countries. *Int. J. Cancer* **20**:477–485.
98. Lee, J. A. H. (1973): The trend of mortality from primary malignant tumors of the skin. *J. Invest. Dermatol.* **59**:445–448.
99. National Academy of Sciences: *Protection Aganist Depletion of Stratospheric Ozone by Chlorofluorocarbons,* pp. 74–105. Washington, D.C.
100. Scotto, J., Fears, T. R., and Gori, G. A. (1975): *Measurements of Ultraviolet Radiation in the United States and Comparison with Skin Cancer Data.* U.S. Government Printing Office, Washington, D.C.
101. Berger, D., Robertson, D. F., and Davies, R. E. (1975): *Field Measurements of Biologically Effective UV Radiation.* CIAP Monograph 5, Part I, Appendix D, pp. 2–233.
102. Cutchis, P. (1975): Estimates of increase in skin cancer incidence with time following a decrease in stratospheric ozone. In: *CIAP Reports,* Vol. 5, Appendix D to Chapter 7, pp. 7–141. National Technical Information Service, Springfield, Virginia.
103. Clemmeson, J. (1965): *Statistical Studies of the Etiology of Malignant Neoplasms.* Munksgaard, Copenhagen.

10

Photoimmunology

W. L. Morison and J. A. Parrish

Photoimmunology is the study of the interaction between nonionizing radiation and the immune system, a meeting point of the sciences of photobiology and immunology. It is only within the last decade that the potential importance of interactions between nonionizing radiation and the immune system has begun to be appreciated. Most studies prior to that time were conducted by biologists who examined the effects of in vitro exposure to UVC (254 nm) radiation on components of the immune system. It was demonstrated that exposure to such radiation could influence the function of antibodies, decrease the viability and alter the function of lymphocytes, and increase the antigenicity of DNA. At the same time, dermatologists and other physicians were making clinical observations related to photoimmunology— for example, photosensitivity in systemic lupus erythematosus (SLE)—and were mostly interested in longer and more penetrating wavelengths of ultraviolet (UV) radiation. The relationships between the in vitro observations of biologists and in vivo clinical studies were often not fully appreciated. However, recent studies have shown that the biologic effects of UVC and of longer wavelengths of UV radiation are often similar; therefore, the early in vitro observations can be important in our understanding of the effects of nonionizing radiation on the immune system in vivo.

Recent interest in photoimmunology has arisen from three main developments. First is the observation that UVB (290–320 nm) radiation can alter immune responses in the intact host. Exposure to such radiation can, for example, induce the proliferation of clones of lymphocytes that specifically suppress the rejection of UVB-induced skin tumors in mice. Second, studies of

W. L. Morison • National Cancer Institute, Frederick Cancer Research Facility, Frederick, Maryland 21701 J. A. Parrish • Department of Dermatology, Harvard Medical School, Massachusetts General Hospital, Boston, Massachusetts 02114.

the interaction of UV radiation and DNA have resulted in the demonstration of antibodies to UV-altered DNA (UV-DNA) in humans and the production of antinuclear antibodies (ANAs) as a result of UV-radiation exposure in animals. These studies will possibly lead to a better understanding of the pathogenesis of SLE. Finally, the recent findings that phototherapy and photochemotherapy are useful in the treatment of a number of skin disorders with pathogeneses in which the immune system is thought to play a prominent role suggests that these therapies may act via an effect on the immune system. If exposure to nonionizing radiation in humans can affect abnormal immune responses, the question is raised: What is the effect of such radiation on normal immune function?

PHOTOIMMUNOLOGY AND THE IMMUNE SYSTEM

The immune system is a complex organization designed to react to substances, termed antigens, that are recognized as foreign to the host organism. The immune response stimulated by contact with a particular antigen is specific for that antigen or closely related molecules. Although immune responses are very complex, involving interactions between a variety of cells and the generation of numerous effector molecules and mediators, for the purpose of simplicity they are usually divided into two components: cell-mediated and humoral. The cell-mediated component of an immune response involves the sensitization, activation, and proliferation of lymphocytes specifically sensitized to the particular antigen. The humoral component is directed toward the production of antibodies, which are proteins capable of interacting with the antigen that triggered the response. Early studies of immunity identified defense of the body against invasion by infectious organisms to be an important function of the immune system. More recently, it has also been demonstrated that the immune system plays an important role in preventing the development of neoplasia and that abnormal immune responses are involved in the pathogenesis of many diseases.

The skin interfaces with the environment and its chief function is protection; it is therefore not surprising that the immune system is well represented in the skin. Lymphocytes, antibodies, and other serum components are found in dermal blood vessels, the lymphatics, and the tissues of the dermis. Mast cells, effector cells for immediate hypersensitivity, are also found in the dermis. The epidermis is also involved in immune responses. The dendritic Langerhans cells form a network in the epidermis. These cells have surface membrane receptors for immunoglobulins and complement and probably belong to the monocyte–macrophage series; they appear to be concerned with antigen recognition, transport of antigens to the dermis or regional lymph nodes, and presentation of antigens to other cells. Recent evidence suggests that lymphocytes, the cells central to most immune responses, also enter the epidermis; epidermal lymphocytes presumably belong to the body's circulating pool of lymphocytes.

The immune system is represented in almost all tissues of the body and functions as a unified organ regardless of the boundaries of other organ systems. This is achieved through a very efficient communications network of mediators produced and released by lymphocytes, the lymphocytes themselves, and circulating antibodies. Furthermore, mediators released by other tissues can influence immune responses. Therefore, a stimulus applied to one area of the body is readily transmitted to all portions of the immune system. This concept is important in photoimmunology because exposure to nonionizing radiation is not systemic, as with a drug, but is local and confined to the depth of skin penetrated by the radiation. However, a local insult to components of the immune system may result in secondary and distant alterations in immune function.

The influence of nonionizing radiation on various components of the immune system and on immune responses in health and disease will be discussed separately, but of course some overlap is inevitable.

Antigens

Exposure to nonionizing radiation can result in photochemical changes in molecules such that the photoproducts are antigenic or demonstrate increased antigenicity (capacity to stimulate an immune response) as compared to the parent compound. The molecules may be normal body constituents (for example, DNA), abnormal body constituents (as in some cases of solar urticaria), or exogenous substances (as, for example, in photoallergy). There is also some evidence that, in addition to antigen formation, exposure to UV radiation can result in the masking or deletion of normal tissue antigens so that they can no longer be detected using appropriate antisera; this subject will be considered under the section on photocarcinogenesis.

Native DNA is a weak antigen; however, Levine et al. (1) reported that exposure of DNA to UVC radiation produced an alteration of the molecule so that it became strongly antigenic. Immunofluorescence studies confirmed this work and extended it to show that the antiserum to UV–DNA was specific in that it reacted with the nuclei of irradiated tissue, but did not react with nonirradiated tissue (2). The antigenic determinants in UV-DNA are thymine photoproducts, and prior absorption of the antiserum with polydeoxythymidylic acid or irradiated thymine oligonucleotides abolishes the antigen–antibody reaction (1, 3). Cytosine photoproducts do not have this effect. Thymine photoproducts that react with antisera to UV-DNA are produced in vivo in humans and animals following exposure to UV radiation and can be identified in the nuclei of both the dermis and epidermis (4, 5). There is also indirect evidence that the photoproducts are released into the blood (6). The action spectrum for the production of UV-DNA in vivo extends at least from 254 to 320 nm (7), although wavelengths longer than 300 nm are much less active than the shorter wavelengths. One study failed to demonstrate this effect with a radiation source that had an emission spectrum from 290 to 400 nm (8), but the UVA spectrum has not been further investigated. The overall conclusion reached from these studies is that the photoproducts of thymine responsible for the antigenicity of UV-DNA are thymine dimers, but that has not been definitely established.

Not only is UV-DNA produced in vivo, but it can also stimulate an immune response in the host. Exposure of mice to UVC radiation, daily for six weeks, resulted in the development of ANAs; these antibodies appeared earlier and in higher titer in animals kept under dark conditions when not undergoing UV exposure (9). This finding suggests that a photoreactivating enzyme was important in reducing the antigen load in animals housed under ambient light conditions. An unexpected finding of the study was that the ANAs reacted with both irradiated and nonirradiated tissue substrates in the immunofluorescence test. While these observations remain to be confirmed, they do raise the possibility that environmental or therapeutic exposure to UV radiation in humans, resulting in a similar antigenic alteration of cellular DNA, could lead to the production of an ANA.

Systemic lupus erythematosus (SLE) is a disease characterized by the spontaneous appearance of ANAs, often with multiple specificities; these abnormal antibodies are thought to be important in the pathogenesis of the disorder. Nonionizing radiation plays a role in this disease, as photosensitivity is a clinical feature in some patients with SLE and sun exposure can precipitate and aggravate the disease. Antibodies with specificity for UV-DNA have been detected in the sera of some patients with SLE (2). The histologic and immunofluorescence findings in the skin of patients with SLE have been reproduced in mice immunized with UV-DNA and then exposed to UVC radiation (10). The mouse skin showed a deposit of immunoglobulin and complement at the dermal–epidermal junction and an intense poly-morphonuclear cell infiltrate. A possibly theory for the pathogenesis of SLE is that thymine dimers are released from skin cells as a result of exposure to radiation, complex with circulating antibody, and are then deposited locally in the skin, and possibly elsewhere, resulting in disease manifestations. A study of patients with SLE failed to find any correlation between the presence of an ANA specific for UV-DNA and a clinical history of photosensitivity (11). However, photosensitivity was not defined and it is possible that the question has not been fully explored.

Psoralen compounds intercalate into DNA, and subsequent exposure to UVA radiation (referred to by the acronym PUVA) results in the formation of photoadducts. Recently, a specific antiserum to psoralen–DNA photoprod-ucts was produced in rabbits, demonstrating that the products of the action of PUVA on DNA can be antigenic (12). This finding raises the question of whether precipitation of SLE could be an adverse effect of PUVA therapy. The use of PUVA therapy for psoriasis has been associated with the development of SLE in one patient (13) and an SLE-like syndrome in another patient (14). However, many thousands of patients are at present being treated with PUVA therapy and the association may be fortuitous, particularly since SLE is not a rare condition. A preliminary study (15) in 34 patients with psoriasis treated with PUVA therapy has reported a rise in the incidence of a positive test for ANAs as compared with pretreatment results. However, the titers were low and assays for DNA antibodies were negative. A 2-year followup of 1300 patients being treated with PUVA did not reveal an increased incidence of positive tests for ANAs (16). In these studies a standard ANA test was performed and it is quite possible that determination of ANAs using substrates that have been irradiated with UV with and without the addition of psoralen would yield different results. With our present knowledge, all prospective patients for PUVA therapy and UVB phototherapy should be screened for connective tissue disease.

Evidence that the antigenicity of other molecules can be altered by exposure to nonionizing radiation is less direct. Pemphigus and pemphigoid are blistering skin disorders thought to have autoimmune pathogeneses. The main evidence for this theory is that antibodies to the intercellular epidermal matrix in patients with pemphigus, and to epidermal basement membrane in pemphigoid patients, appear to be involved in the development of lesions. In both conditions, exposure to erythemogenic doses of UV radiation results in the development of new lesions and the deposition of immunoglobulin (IgG) and complement (C3) (17–19). One possible explanation for this effect is that UV radiation induces the formation of an abnormal antigen locally in the skin and this altered molecule then reacts with circulating-specific antibody. However, a recent study found that sera from patients with pemphigus could induce acantholysis in normal skin in organ culture (20); exposure to UV radiation did not increase that effect (21). An effect of radiation on skin blood flow or the permeability of the dermal–epidermal barrier may be an alternative explanation for the UV-induced exacerbation of pemphigus in vivo.

Antigen–antibody reactions appear to be responsible for some cases of solar urticaria, as evidenced by passive transfer reactions with sera from these patients. The exact nature of these antigens is unknown, but since exposure to nonionizing radiation is necessary before the reaction can occur, it is reasonable to hypothesize that the antigens are photoproducts. Two classes of antigens have been recognized for this reaction. One type of antigen results from a photochemical alteration of a normal body constituent. The other type can be produced only in the patient and therefore presumably is the result of photochemical alteration of an abnormal body constituent. This subject will be covered in greater detail below.

Contact allergy provides another example of the induction of new antigens by exposure to nonionizing radiation. The most carefully studied examples are the photoreactions of tetrachlorosalicylanilide (TCSA) and related compounds. TCSA, which is a small molecule, is not immunogenic, but instead behaves as a hapten.* Exposure of TCSA to UVA radiation in the presence of a suitable carrier protein results in the formation of a complete antigen capable of stimulating a photoallergic reaction. In vitro, epidermal proteins (22) and human serum albumin (23) can act as carrier proteins, but the nature of the carrier proteins(s) in vivo is unknown. A recent study (24) of TCSA photoallergy found that noncovalent binding of TCSA to the carrier protein was the first step in the formation of the antigen, and this was followed by covalent bonding upon exposure to UVA radiation. An interesting observation in that study was that the carrier protein used, namely albumin, was photochemically altered by exposure to radiation. TCSA mediated the photooxidation of the histidine in albumin, giving rise to an altered molecule. The possibility is raised that this new molecule could itself be antigenic and give rise to a persistent light reaction; this possibility will be discussed further in Chapter 12.

Photocarcinogenesis probably involves the formation of tumor-specific antigens and the masking or deletion of normal tissue antigens. This work will be discussed below.

Antibodies

Exposure to nonionizing radiation could affect the production or function of antibodies. Antibodies are produced by B (bursa-derived) lymphocytes and plasma cells in response to antigenic stimulation; the production is modulated by the influence of suppressor and helper T (thymus-derived) lymphocytes. The surface properties of B and T lymphocytes in humans are altered by exposure to PUVA (25) and the viability of these cells is decreased by exposure to UV radiation in vitro (26). However, the effect of nonionizing radiation on antibody production by B cells has not been studied.

Various functions of antibodies have been defined by in vitro tests; these include cell lysis, complement fixation, agglutination, and the precipitin reaction. Exposure of antisera to UVC radiation in vitro can abolish these reactions (27, 28). The exposure doses required to produce this effect were very high (up to 12 hr of exposure to a low-pressure Hg lamp), so the relevance of the findings to the in vivo situation is questionable. The mechanism by which radiation produces this effect is not clear, although one study (29) demonstrated the formation of complexes between immunoglobulins and albumin, presumably resulting in the masking of antigen-binding sites.

---

*Hapten: A protein-free substance which can react with a specific antibody but cannot stimulate the production of antibodies. A hapten must first combine with a carrier protein to form a complete antigen.

Further studies of the effect of radiation on antibody production, structure, and function are required.

Lymphocytes

Lymphocytes are mononuclear leukocytes found in large numbers in blood, all lymphoid organs, and the bone marrow. As a circulating pool of cells, they are found also in most tissues of the body. Lymphocytes are the central component in the maintenance of normal immune function and are involved in both cell-mediated and humoral immune responses. Not surprisingly, the effect of nonionizing radiation on these cells has attracted more interest than any other facet of photoimmunology. Lymphocytes are altered by exposure to nonionizing radiation, both in vivo and in vitro. How this alteration affects immune function in health and disease is now being studied. To date, most observations have been at a cellular level, and there is relatively little information on how radiation affects the structure and function of these cells on a molecular basis.

Pappenheimer in 1917 (30) first observed that exposure of lymphocytes to sunlight in the presence of hematoporphyrin decreased the ability of the cells to exclude trypan blue dye. Since then a number of studies have explored the sensitivity of lymphocytes to exposure to UV radiation in vitro. Trypan blue dye exclusion by lymphocytes is diminished following exposure to UV radiation; this alteration of cell function is dependent on both the dose of radiation and the wavelength (31). UVC radiation is more active than broadband UVB, which in turn is more active than broadband UVA, in an approximate ratio of UVC:UVC:UVA = $1:10^{-1}:10^{-5}$.

Other functions of lymphocytes are also affected by in vitro exposure to UV radiation. The response to mitogens, such as phytohemagglutinin (PHA), is decreased and the extent of the reduction is dependent on both the dose and wavelength of the radiation; UVC is more toxic than UVB, which in turn is more toxic than UVA (32). Lymphocyte subpopulations and their functional activity vary in their susceptibility to nonionizing radiation. In two studies (33, 34) T lymphocytes were found to be more sensitive than B lymphocytes to exposure to UVC radiation in vitro, but the sensitivities of these two subpopulations to UVB radiation were similar (35). The proliferative response of lymphocytes following antigenic stimulation is more sensitive to UVC (33) or visible radiation in the presence of bromo-2-deoxyuridine (36) than is their ability to produce macrophage inhibitory factor. Activation of lymphocytes by exposure to an antigen also changes their sensitivity to radiation. Lymphocytes are sensitive to small doses of UVC radiation at the time of first exposure to an antigen but relatively resistant once they have been activated (37–39).

The introduction of oral psoralen photochemotherapy for psoriasis and other skin diseases has led to an expansion of research in various fields of photobiology, and photoimmunology is no exception. Exposure of human lymphocytes to UVA radiation in vitro in the presence of 8-methoxypsoralen resulted in a decrease in the viability of the cells as measured by trypan blue dye exclusion (40, 41), and a decreased incorporation of [^{3}H]thymidine into the DNA of the cells following stimulation by PHA (40–44) as well as other mitogens (40, 45). These effects were dependent on the dose of both radiation and psoralen, but whereas the effects tended to be linear for increases in the dose of radiation, this did not apply to increases in the dose of psoralens (41). Individual lymphocyte functions vary in their sensitivity to PUVA just as they do in their sensitivity to UVC radiation. Exposure to PUVA abolished T-cell replication at a dose that did not affect the helper function of these cells in B-lymphocyte antibody production (46).

The mechanism of the effect of radiation on lymphocytes is not clear. There is evidence for two sites of damage in lymphocytes as a result of exposure to UV radiation: DNA and the cell membrane. DNA damage, as reflected by increased levels of unscheduled DNA synthesis (UDS), occurs in lymphocytes as a result of exposure to UVC radiation; this repair synthesis was reported to be essentially complete after 6 hr (47). Broadband UVB and UVA radiation, as well as exposure to PUVA in vitro, similarly produce a rise in UDS (unpublished observations). The distribution of UDS within the nucleus was found to be nonuniform, being mainly adjacent to the nuclear membrane (48); that observation applied to both resting and mitogen-stimulated lymphocytes. The sensitivity of lymphocytes to PUVA has been found to be dependent on their location in the cell cycle (42); cells in the S phase were more sensitive than cells in other parts of the cycle. An alteration in the cell membrane, in terms of its capacity to bind a fluorescent dye, has been observed following exposure of lymphocytes to UVC radiation and it was suggested that this may be responsible for the decreased viability of the cells resulting from such exposure (49). Evidence of membrane damage was also revealed by scanning electron microscopic examination of lymphocytes 3 days after exposure to PUVA in vitro (50).

These studies of the mechanism of radiation effects on lymphocytes are at best preliminary and point to the need for more detailed investigations. It is likely that the effects of radiation are complex, involving multiple sites of damage and secondary interactions between cell functions. Furthermore, it is possible that the targets within the lymphocyte differ with the wavelength of radiation.

An experimental model using in vitro exposure of cells to radiation is useful because it permits precise dosimetry and an examination of the individual functions of the cells. However, it is a model, and does not necessarily reflect the situation in vivo, which is much more complex due to the influences of skin optics and interactions between cells.

Several early studies of the effect of acute and chronic exposure to UV radiation in humans and animals suggested that the total lymphocyte count increased following such exposure. These studies have been reviewed (51). Later studies by Spode in the albino rabbit found that exposure to UVC radiation had no effect on the circulating number of lymphocytes (52), while UVB radiation usually produced an increased number (53). A recent study (54) in humans found that, in normal individuals, a whole-body exposure to an erythemogenic dose of UVB radiation did not produce any alteration of the total lymphocyte count in the peripheral blood; however, the distribution of subpopulations of lymphocytes was altered, there being a decrease in the proportion of T lymphocytes and an increase in the proportion of null cells. These changes appeared within 2 hr of exposure, reached a maximum at 8–12 hr, and reverted to normal by 48 hr. The function of lymphocytes was also changed, with a marked depression of the response of the cells following stimulation by PHA, and this alteration followed the same time course. A dose of UVB radiation which resulted in only a trace erythema produced similar changes that were less marked. Therefore, the type of erythemal response commonly acquired from excessive sun exposure, a fashionable indulgence in Western society, can be associated with striking short-term alterations in the distribution and function of circulating lymphocytes.

The influence of PUVA on lymphocytes in vivo has been examined in a number of studies, with varied results. In most of these studies, patients with psoriasis or other diseases have been examined during a course of PUVA therapy aimed at clearing their disease. PUVA is reported to produce a decrease (55–57), an increase (58), or no change (59, 60) in the proportion of T lymphocytes. Measurements of the response of lymphocytes following stimulation by mitogens have also varied; the response was unchanged in two studies (58, 61) and showed a transient impairment during the first few weeks of PUVA therapy in another study (59). These differing results are probably due to the influence of the disease state, variations in time of blood collection relative to the last PUVA exposure, and differences in the methodology employed. Psoriasis alone tends to be associated with a decrease in the proportion of circulating T lymphocytes and the extent of the decrease is proportional to the activity of the disease. In one study (56), it was found that circulating T lymphocytes decreased during PUVA therapy in patients with inactive disease but progressively increased in patients with active disease who started with low levels. In normal subjects, a single whole-body exposure to an erythemogenic dose of PUVA produced no change in the total lymphocyte count or of response of lymphocytes to PHA. However, that exposure did produce a decrease in the proportions of circulating T and B lymphocytes and a corresponding increase in the proportion of null lymphocytes (25). These changes appeared soon after exposure, reached a maximum at 12–16 hr, and returned to normal levels by 48–72 hr postirradiation. A dose of PUVA that resulted in a trace or no erythema produced similar but less marked changes. Therefore exposures to PUVA and UVB radiation are similar in their effects on the total number of circulating lymphocytes and the proportion of T lymphocytes within that population of cells. However, they differ in that PUVA alters the proportion of circulating B lymphocytes and does not affect mitogen responsiveness, while UVB radiation has the reverse effects.

Some other aspects of lymphocyte function have been examined after exposure to PUVA in vivo. Synthesis of DNA was decreased immediately following individual exposures (62). Although PUVA in vitro produced an increase in sister chromatid exchanges (63, 64), such an effect was not observed after in vivo exposure to PUVA (65).

All these studies indicate that UV radiation, with and without the addition of photosensitizers, does affect lymphocytes in vivo, but it is too early to judge the exact significance of the findings. Both T and B lymphocytes are identified by surface markers, and the failure to identify these cells after irradiation only points directly to an alteration of the cell membrane. The cells may still be present in the circulation as part of the null cell population, or alternatively, they may have lost their viability and been cleared from the circulation. However, since most lymphocytes are long-lived cells, the finding of a normal distribution of their subpopulations after up to 33 months of PUVA treatment (60) points strongly away from cell death as a consequence of exposure to PUVA. The possibility remains that exposure to oral psoralen photochemotherapy may be altering the function of abnormal lymphocytes involved in the pathogenesis of diseases such as mycosis fungoides and that this may be the mechanism of the therapy.

In vivo studies of the effects of radiation on lymphocytes have always been directed toward circulating peripheral blood lymphocytes. This approach has three disadvantages. First, observations reflect only what is happening at the time blood is drawn and this may not represent a true picture of changes that have occurred. For example, the observation that a single exposure to PUVA does not alter the response of lymphocytes to PHA stimulation (25) may be misleading, because it is possible that cells with an impaired response to the mitogen as a result of exposure to PUVA are rapidly removed from the circulation and therefore not collected by venipuncture. Second, it is possible to perform only a limited number of assays of lymphocyte function at one time, and since it is likely that the various functions will vary in their sensitivity to radiation, an effect may easily be missed. Third, peripheral blood lymphocytes may not be the correct population for study since they are only transiently exposed to radiation as they pass through dermal capillaries. In contrast, lymphocytes slowly migrating through the tissue spaces of the dermis receive a much higher radiant exposure dose and presumably sustain more damage. At present there are technical limitations to the study of tissue lymphocytes.

Finally, how does radiation affect lymphocytes in vivo—directly or indirectly? There is no information available on this question. Calculations that take into account the circulation time, exposure dose, and transmission of radiation to the level of the dermis indicate that circulating lymphocytes are exposed to doses of PUVA and UVB radiation that produce alterations in lymphocytes in vitro. Therefore, a direct effect is possible. Alternatively, lymphocytes could be secondarily affected by mediators released from skin as a result of exposure to nonionizing radiation.

Mast Cells

The mast cell is found in the dermis and is a target cell for IgE-mediated, immediate-hypersensitivity reactions. The mast cell granules contain substances such as histamine, serotonin, and chemotactic factors involved in inflammation and the repair of injured tissues. These cells are altered by exposure to nonionizing radiation, but in the few studies on the subject the nature of the alterations has not been clearly defined.

In vitro exposure of rat peritoneal mast cells to sunlight in the presence of hematoporphyrin resulted in a loss of basophilia and the release of a vasodilating substance which was not thought to be histamine (66). Exposure of the cells to UVB and UVA radiation resulted in disruption of the cells and liberation of the mast cell granules (67). The radiant exposure doses required to produce this effect were small and possibly indicate a selective susceptibility of the cell to radiation. Exposure of mouse skin in vivo to UVC radiation (68) resulted in partial degranulation, cytoplasmic edema, and hypertrophy of the endoplasmic reticulum of mast cells. These changes paralleled the time course of delayed erythema. A more detailed study compared the acute and chronic effects of exposure to UVC, UVB, and UVA radiation in vivo on the number of mast cells in mouse ear skin (69). The cells were identified by their staining reaction with toluidine blue. Exposure to UVC radiation in erythemogenic doses initially produced a decrease in the number of identifiable mast cells, but continued exposure was associated with an increase above control values by the fourth day. This increase continued for the full 32 days of exposure, when the number of cells reached 250% above control values. Exposure to UVB radiation, also in erythemogenic doses given by continuous exposure, was associated with a minimal increase in the number of mast cells, while UVA radiation, in minimally erythemogenic doses, resulted in no significant changes in the number of stained cells. These findings are difficult to interpret because this staining reaction of mast cell granules is not a certain guide to the actual presence or absence of mast cells. More recently, another study of skin morphology found that mast cell degranulation occurs in human skin following exposure to erythemogenic doses of PUVA (70).

Cell-Mediated Immune Responses

Exposure to UV radiation inhibits the development and expression of several cell-mediated immune responses in the intact host. Exposure to UVB radiation was found to decrease, but not abolish, the resonse to a challenge dose of dinitrochlorobenzene (DNCB) in guinea pigs sensitized to that contact allergen (71). In that study only a trace of erythema was produced over half of the back of the animals as a result of the exposure to UVB radiation. No evidence of systemic suppression of contact allergy was observed and the results were not influenced by whether the exposures were given before, during, or after sensitization. Reactivity to DNCB was also depressed in mice following chronic exposure to UVB radiation, but this depression was transient and reactivity returned to baseline levels while exposures were still continued (72). This effect appeared to be due to a block in the afferent limb of the immune response at the level of antigen processing or presentation. In another study, UVC radiation decreased the response to an intradermal injection of streptokinase/streptodurnase antigen in a single human subject who was sensitive to the antigen (33).

We have recently conducted a number of studies aimed at comparing the effects of exposure to UVB radiation and PUVA on cell-mediated immune responses in guinea pigs and rabbits. Exposure of less than half of the back of guinea pigs to doses of either radiation that was sufficient to produce a marked erythema almost totally suppressed delayed-hypersensitivity reactions in animals that had been immunized with the antigen in complete Freund's adjuvant. This effect of radiation was both local and systemic and although it was most marked when the exposure to radiation was commenced one week prior to immunization of the animals, suppression was still observed when irradiation was given after immunization and continued until elicitation a week later. Contact allergy to DNCB in the guinea pig has also been studied. Both PUVA and UVB radiation, again in erythemogenic doses, also suppressed this response. However, even at maximal tolerated doses, the response was not totally abolished. Radiation affected DNCB allergy in two ways: local inhibition occurred after exposure of a small area, provided the site of elicitation of contact allergy was included in the field of exposure; systemic inhibition of the allergic response was seen if large area (most of the back) of the animal was exposed, and in that circumstance the site of elicitation did not have to be exposed. It is possible that the local effect is due to an influence of radiation on Langerhans cell function, while the systemic effect may be due to lymphocytotoxicity. There is no evidence for either of these two suggestions and there are other possible mechanisms. Finally, the influence of radiation on skin-graft rejection was studied using a rabbit-ear model. Exposure of both the donor and recipient sites to erythemogenic doses of UVB radiation did not produce a prolongation of graft survival. Exposure to PUVA radiation, also in erythemogenic doses, produced only a minimal prolongation of survival. More work is required to elicit the mechanisms underlying these observations of the effects of nonionizing radiation on immune responses in vivo, as they clearly open up some very interesting possibilities.

Nonspecific Immune Responses

Nonionizing radiation has been used in the treatment of infections and is reported to have beneficial results. The 1903 Nobel Prize for Medicine was awarded to Finsen for his work demonstrating the beneficial effect of UV radiation therapy in cutaneous tuberculosis. In the early part of this century, erysipelas and other bacterial infections of the skin were treated with heliotherapy or with artificial UV radiation sources. A scientific rationale for these treatments arose when it was discovered that microorganisms were killed by in vitro exposure to UV radiation. However, nonspecific and specific immune mechanisms for these treatments have also been considered.

The management of pertussis and prevention of upper respiratory tract infections are two other areas that attracted early interest in phototherapy. The methodology of some of these studies was not ideal, but in others, control groups were included and favorable results reported. Weekly whole-body exposures to mildly erythemogenic doses of UVB radiation produced a 40% reduction in the incidence of respiratory tract infections in young male adults as compared with the incidence in a control, untreated group (73). However, a group of children given alternate-day exposures of a similar radiation had an incidence of respiratory tract infections similar to that in the control group of children (74). Studies of this type have not attracted any recent interest except in the USSR, where there is considerable enthusiasm for the beneficial effects of UV radiation in health and disease (75). Regular exposure of several thousand children to UV radiation was claimed to have an advantageous effect on their health, mediated via the immune system. Carefully controlled studies aimed at neutralizing any placebo effect would be necessary to establish these observations and some objective tests of immune function would be required to demonstrate the immunologic basis of any positive observation.

PHOTOIMMUNOLOGY AND DISEASE

Photobiology and immunology appear to be linked in the pathogenesis and treatment of a number of diseases, all of which affect the skin. The photobiologic aspects of some of these conditions have been explored in depth, but the immunologic features have received less attention.

Photocarcinogenesis

There is a large amount of epidemiologic and experimental evidence that chronic exposure to UV radiation is the main factor in the etiology of nonmelanoma skin cancer, in particular basal cell carcinoma (BCC) and squamous cell carcinoma (SCC). Recently it has been demonstrated that, at least in animals, an interaction between UV radiation and immune responses precedes the expression of neoplasia.

Tumors, usually of a spindle-cell type and less commonly SCCs, induced by exposure to UVB radiation in mice are highly antigenic. If these tumors are transplanted to syngeneic recipients, the presence of tumor-specific antigens causes an immunologic response in the recipient and the tumor is rejected or does not grow (76). In this respect, UV-induced tumors differ from tumors induced by chemical carcinogens, which grow quite readily in syngeneic recipients. The fact that rejection of the transplanted UV-induced tumors is immunologically mediated is suggested by the observation that the transplants will grow progressively in immunosuppressed mice (76). Several observations indicate that specific immunologic response directed against the transplanted tumors can be detected in normal recipients: splenic lymphocytes are cytotoxic for tumor cells (77); macrophage-activating factor is produced by lymphocytes and renders macrophages cytotoxic for the tumor cells (78); and the tumors are infiltrated by T lymphocytes that show cytotoxicity toward tumor cells in an in vitro assay (79). The rejection mechanism is specific for the transplanted tumor and there is little cross-reactivity toward other UV-induced tumors.

These observations raise the question as to why a primary tumor is able to grow in its host. The answer appears to be that chronic exposure of mice to UVB radiation produces a specific systemic alteration of immune function so that animals are then unable to reject a UVB-induced tumor (80, 81). This tolerance appears long before the animals themselves develop tumors and is not associated with evidence of general systemic immunosuppression (82). The tolerance has been found to be mediated by suppressor cells, probably T lymphocytes (83, 84), that influence the induction of a tumor rejection response. The generation of suppressor lymphocytes is probably initiated by a photoproduct produced in the skin by exposure to UVB radiation (85). The evidence for this is that full-thickness skin from exposed animals, when grafted onto nonexposed animals, can confer tolerance to UVB-induced tumors. The nature of the photoproduct is unknown. Kripke has hypothesized that mice have an immune mechanism aimed at preventing the development of UV-induced tumors and that exposure to UVB radiation can suppress this mechanism and permit the initiation and growth of highly antigenic tumors. According to this hypothesis, photocarcinogenesis is a two-stage process, with a UV-induced alteration in immune function being essential for the expression of UV-induced neoplasia. The action spectrum for the tumor-specific alteration in immune function has not been defined, but it may not be restricted to UVB radiation. A recent study found that mice exposed to UVA radiation after topical application of psoralen were unable to reject UVB-induced tumors (86). However, in that system, the specificity of the defect and the involvement of suppressor T lymphocytes were not established.

It has not been established in humans that nonmelanoma skin cancers are antigenic. Circulating antibodies to cytoplasmic and membrane tumor-associated antigens were found in some patients with SCC of the skin (87). The possibility that the antigens were normal tissue antigens was not entirely eliminated. In another study (88), circulating antibodies to BCCs were not detected, but the sensitivity of the system may not have been adequate. Both BCCs and SCCs have been found to be relatively devoid of intercellular substance (89) and basement membrane (90) in studies using antisera directed against antigens normally present at these sites. These findings have been confirmed in mice (91) and, in addition, two polypeptides normally present in rodent epidermis disappear with the progression of UV-induced hyperplasia to neoplasia (92). Antigen deletion, or perhaps masking of epidermal antigens, has been postulated to explain the results of these studies (89–92). However, an equally plausible explanation would be that anaplastic cells, by failing to differentiate, might not reach a stage of development at which these protein antigens are formed.

Evidence for an immune response specific for human nonmelanoma skin cancer is not very strong. Serum cytotoxicity toward cultures of the patient's own tumor cells was demonstrated in three of nine patients with SCC and this was partially complement dependent (87). Six of these nine patients also had evidence of lymphocyte-mediated cytotoxicity, again partially complement dependent. These are interesting results worthy of further study. Lymphocytic infiltration of the tumors in patients with SCCs and BCCs and the number of circulating T lymphocytes in such patients have been studied (93). Small tumors were associated with a marked infiltrate and a T-lymphocyte count just below normal, while large tumors, particularly those with lymph node involvement, were characterized by minimal lymphocytic infiltrate of the tumors and much lower levels of circulating T lymphocytes. Of course, whether the lymphocyte response influenced the size of the tumor or vice versa is unknown.

Although there is little positive evidence that an immune response directed against nonmelanoma skin cancers does occur in humans, there is some evidence that compromised immune responses may lead to increased tumorogenesis. The incidence of skin cancer is increased in immunosuppressed patients. This has been reported in renal transplant recipients receiving immunosuppressive agents on a long-term basis (94–98) and in patients with lymphomas (99). In addition, not only is the incidence of nonmelanoma skin cancer increased in these patients, but multiple lesions are especially common, and SCCs usually outnumber BCCs; the reverse is true in otherwise normal subjects. Most of these lesions occurred on sun-exposed sites in subjects predisposed to skin cancer; this suggests that UV radiation exposure was still the initiating factor and that the absence of normal immune responses played a facilitating role. This concept is supported by animal studies in which it was shown that administration of antilymphocyte serum

(100) or azothioprine (101), plus exposure to UVB radiation, resulted in the development of skin cancers earlier and in greater numbers than in control animals only exposed to radiation. Similar indirect evidence for involvement of the immune system in UV-induced neoplasia was provided by the observation that patients with xeroderma pigmentosum, a disorder characterized by defects in the DNA repair system, had a defect of cell-mediated immunity (102, 103) as manifested by impaired delayed hypersensitivity skin tests, a failure of DNCB sensitization, and a low response of lymphocytes to stimulation by mitogens. A serum factor appeared to be responsible for the decreased response to mitogens. These observations provide evidence for another defect in patients with xeroderma pigmentosum; further studies are necessary to establish a possible link between the immune defect and the known propensity of such patients for the development of UV-induced neoplasia.

Solar Urticaria

Solar urticaria is a disease characterized by the development of urticarial lesions on exposed skin within minutes of exposure to sunlight or artificial sources of radiation that include the action spectrum for the condition. The disease is usually classified on the basis of the action spectra (104), and using that classification two of the six varieties have features that suggest an immunologic pathogenesis. The main evidence for this suggestion is that urticarial reactions occur following injection of the patient's serum into normal subjects and subsequent irradiation of the injection site (a positive passive transfer reaction). However, there are differences in the pathogenic mechanisms mediating these two types of urticaria.

In the so-called Type I solar urticaria (action spectrum 280–320 nm), passive transfer of serum gives a positive reaction, even if exposure to radiation precedes the injection (a positive reversed passive transfer reaction). This observation eliminates the possibility of the reaction being due to a phototoxic substance in the serum and strengthens the immunologic theory of the pathogenesis. Presumably, the serum factor is an antibody that reacts with an antigen produced by the photochemical alteration of a normal constituent of skin. The nature of the antibody in serum has been studied and it has some features of a reagenic antibody (105). The origin and nature of the antigen are unknown.

Type IV solar urticaria (action spectrum 400–500 nm) is also characterized by positive passive transfer reactions, but sera from these patients give a negative reversed passive transfer reaction. An explanation for this has recently been found (106). When serum from a patient was irradiated in vitro and then injected into the patient, an urticarial reaction occurred. However, when the same irradiated patient's serum was injected into normal subjects, no reaction occurred. The investigators concluded that all the antibody in the patient's serum had reacted with antigen that was produced by the exposure of the serum to radiation; however, sufficient antigen remained in the serum to react with antibody in the patient's skin. Injection of irradiated normal serum did not produce a reaction in the patient. These findings indicate that the antigen in this type of solar urticaria is a photoproduct formed from an abnormal constituent in the patient's serum.

The mediator responsible for producing the urticarial skin response in solar urticaria has attracted much interest and speculation. Two recent studies have found that mast cells were activated in solar urticaria and that mediators were released from these cells, specifically histamine (107, 108) and chemotactic factors (108). The relative importance of these or other products of the mast cell in the initiation of lesions in urticaria remains to be determined.

A successful therapy for solar urticaria has been developed using a depletion process; repeated exposures to radiation, including the action spectrum of the individual patient's eruption, resulted in a loss of reactivity and this was maintained by regular exposures to radiation (109). The mechanism underlying this therapy may be a depletion of antigen, antibody, or mast cell mediators. The latter would appear to be most likely since the therapy appears to be effective in all types of solar urticaria. The response to treatment may simply be due to a toxic effect of radiation on mast cells, in which case an adequate dose of radiation, whether or not it included the action spectrum of the eruption in a particular patient, would probably be effective.

Polymorphic Light Eruption

Polymorphic light eruption (PMLE) may be defined as a delayed abnormal response to nonionizing radiation that appears hours to days after exposure, lasts for days or weeks, and is not associated with other cutaneous disorders likely to be responsible for the delayed response. Using this definition, it is quite possible that more than one condition is included under the label and this may explain why separate investigations of the pathogenesis of the condition have yielded different results. For example, we do not include sun-exacerbated atopic eczema under a diagnosis of PMLE; others do, and therefore report a high incidence of atopy among patients. Lack of a uniform definition undoubtedly leads to some confusion.

Several features of PMLE suggest an immunologic pathogenesis: the reaction time for appearance of the eruption is delayed; a perivascular lymphocytic infiltrate is a constant feature of the histology; the rash can develop at nonexposed but previously involved sites following sun exposure; and, in some patients, solar urticaria and PMLE occur in association. Duke, in 1926 (110), first directed attention to the possibility that PMLE might represent an "allergic" reaction to sun exposure while discussing three patients who possibly had the combination of PMLE and solar urticaria. He suggested that a substance formed in the skin under the influence of sun exposure was responsible for their subsequent allergic reaction to nonionizing radiation. Epstein (111) carried this concept further by reporting a positive passive transfer reaction in one patient which took the form of a papular reaction on the ninth day after injection of serum and exposure to radiation. He developed a theory that an antigen–antibody reaction was involved in the pathogenesis of PMLE (112). However, a subsequent study of 13 cases of PMLE found negative passive transfer reactions in all cases (113). Furthermore, the condition could not be transferred using peripheral blood leukocytes, although the details of the technique were not given (114). Probably the most intriguing study of the etiology of PMLE in the early literature is that of Mühlmann and Akobjan in 1930 (115). They found that injection of serum obtained from a patient with PMLE into rats, followed by exposure to UV radiation, produced agitation, edema, conjuctivitis, and even death. This study does not appear to have been repeated.

The possibility of an autoimmune process has been explored. It has been suggested that PMLE belongs to the same clinical spectrum as SLE, and, using indirect immunofluorescence with tumor imprints as a substrate, a third of the patients had a positive ANA (116). In another study (117) using two different subtrates (human leukocytes and rat liver), the ANA test was consistently negative in 35 patients. Furthermore, LE cell tests gave negative results (116, 118) and examination of skin biopsy specimens by direct immunofluorescence did not disclose deposits of immunoglobulins or complement at the basement membrane zone (116, 117, 119).

Lymphocyte function in patients with PMLE has also attracted some interest. Following exposure to UV radiation in vitro, lymphocytes from patients with PMLE were reported to differ from control lymphocytes by having a higher level of S-phase DNA synthesis and RNA synthesis, a low level of UDS, and a greater response following stimulation by PHA (120, 121). No statistical evaluation of the results was provided in these somewhat confusing studies. Furthermore, similar studies failed to support those findings (122, 123). Leukocytes from patients with PMLE have also been reported to be unresponsive to stimulation by homogenates of patients' irradited and nonirradiated skin in an in vitro assay (124).

It appears that in the study of the alleged immune pathogenesis of PMLE every positive observation has been countered by one or more negative studies, leaving the original clinical and histologic observations as the sole supporting evidence. However, bearing in mind those observations and the absence of a more attractive hypothesis, it is quite possible that, as Duke postulated, PMLE is an allergic reaction to nonionizing radiation. A clearer definition of the diagnostic criteria of PMLE, plus the application of modern immunologic techniques to the investigation of the disease, might provide an answer.

Photoallergy

The pathogenesis of photoallergy, as the name implies, is generally considered to be immunologic in nature. While this is true by definition, the term is overused, because the immunologic nature of the reaction is usually not established. The photobiologic, clinical, and histologic aspects of photoallergy have attracted much interest, but the "allergic" element has been studied by only a few workers. Evidence that allergy underlies contact photoallergy is much stronger than in the case of systemic photosensitivity that is classified as photoallergic, and therefore these two conditions will be considered separately.

The clinical and histologic features of contact photoallergy are similar to those of allergic contact dermatitis, and it is presumed that it involves similar immune mechanisms. Eczema is the most common clinical manifestation, although urticarial reactions have been reported, and a dense perivascular lymphocytic infiltrate in the dermis is the characteristic histologic finding. A number of investigations have pointed toward a cell-mediated immune pathogenesis. Photopatch testing gives positive delayed responses that have been interpreted as being allergic, and not toxic, on the basis of the lower concentration of chemical used for their induction, the clinical appearance of eczema and not just erythema, and histology showing spongiosis and infiltration by lymphocytes. Caution must be exercised in placing too much emphasis on positive photopatch tests as evidence of allergy, because a phototoxic reaction can be very similar. Contact photoallergy has been induced in guinea pigs (125–127) and in humans (128, 129) and in some cases this has been associated with simple contact allergy (128). Passive transfer of contact photoallergy has been achieved in guinea pigs using mononuclear cells from peritoneal exudates (127). Sensitivity of mononuclear cells to protein-bound photoproducts of two photoallergens has been detected in two types of in vitro correlates of cell-mediated immunity: migration inhibition (23) and lymphocyte transformation (130). The methodology in some of these studies has attracted reasonable criticism (131) and further investigations are necessary before a cell-mediated immune pathogenesis for contact photo-allergy can be fully accepted.

The role of nonionizing radiation in the induction of contact photoallergy is not clear, but there are several possibilities. Radiation may alter the photoallergen, which is usually a simple chemical, converting it from a prohapten to a hapten which can then combine with a carrier protein. A second possibility is that the formation of a bond between the photoallergen and the carrier protein requires exposure to radiation. Finally, the carrier protein may be photochemically altered, thus permitting it to then react with the photoallergen. Probably each of these mechanisms, and perhaps others, applies in different cases.

Systemic photoallergy, a photoallergic reaction following systemic administration of a chemical agent, is a very confused topic. A variety of drugs and chemicals have been reported to cause this type of reaction, but the evidence for involvement of the immune system has been restricted to clinical and histologic criteria of an allergic reaction. A clinical picture of eczema and the presence of lymphocytes in the dermis cannot be considered as strong evidence of allergy, as has been suggested in some case reports of systemic photoallergy. Occasionally, positive photopatch tests have also been cited as such evidence, but quite possibly that is better support for a systemic phototoxic reaction. Phototoxicity may well explain many reported examples of systemic "photoallergy." Furthermore, systemic photoallergy has not been produced in an experimental animal model. Although it would seem very likely that systemic photoallergy does exist, there is no conclusive evidence to indicate that a systemically administered chemical has ever caused photosensitivity by way of an immunologic mechanism.

Photoallergic reactions are sometimes followed by a long-lasting sensitivity to nonionizing radiation, the so-called persistent light reaction. Such a state of altered reactivity could well have an immunologic pathogenesis, and although this frequently has been suggested, it remains a theoretical possibility without supporting evidence. Most interest has been directed toward identifying the antigen responsible for the reaction. Theories that have been advanced are: persistence of small amounts of antigen in the skin (132), a somewhat unlikely possibility, as the reaction persists for years, if not for life; continued exposure to the antigen or related compounds from unrecognized sources (133); and alteration of the antigenicity of a normal body constituent (134). This latter concept would appear most likely, and recently some evidence has been presented to support it with the demonstration that TCSA can sensitize the photooxidation of histidine in albumin (24). Two features of note regarding the persistent light reaction are that only some contact photoallergens are prone to induce it, and only some patients with contact photoallergy go on to develop the reaction. It can be hypothesized that only some chemicals are capable of inducing a photochemical alteration of the antigenicity of a normal body constituent and that once that happens only some patients develop an allergic reaction to that antigen. Investigation of the photochemical reactions of photoallergens that do cause persistent light reactions and of the immunologic makeup of the affected patients might be fruitful.

Phototherapy and Photochemotherapy

A resurgence of interest in UVB phototherapy and the introduction of successful psoralen photochemotherapy have been two very significant advances in photomedicine over recent years. Most reports have been concerned with defining the therapeutic range of these two treatments, but there has also been work aimed at determining the mechanism of the therapeutic effect. UVB phototherapy is beneficial in psoriasis, a disorder characterized by epidermal cell proliferation. The depression of epidermal S-phase DNA synthesis induced by exposure to UVB radiation (135) and consequent inhibition of cell proliferation has been accepted as its mode of action. PUVA therapy first achieved prominence when it was found to be beneficial in psoriasis and, since exposure to PUVA also depressed epidermal DNA synthesis (136), this action, with the consequent decrease in cell turnover, was presumed to be the mechanism of its therapeutic effect.

However, PUVA therapy is also beneficial in many other disorders— vitiligo, mycosis fungoides, atopic eczema, lichen planus, PMLE, persistent light reactions, and actinic reticuloid. In these diverse diseases, a problem arises in invoking the original theory of how PUVA works, namely repression of DNA synthesis and decreased epidermal cell proliferation, because none of them is characterized by increased epidermal cell turnover. However, an examination of the suggested pathogenic mechanisms of these diseases reveals a common thread, namely that each is considered to involve either an abnormal immune mechanism or infiltration of the skin by cells of the lymphoid series. It is therefore quite possible that PUVA therapy acts by an effect on normal or abnormal immune function in some diseases and by a direct toxic effect on lymphocytes in skin infiltrates in other conditions. This hypothesis can be extended further to provide an alternative theory as to why PUVA therapy, and perhaps UVB therapy, is effective in psoriasis. This disease has long been regarded as involving only the epidermis, but there is increasing evidence, recently summarized (137), that the underlying abnormality may be immunologic. Therefore, photoimmunology may be involved in the beneficial effects of phototherapy and photochemotherapy.

Just as PUVA and UVB phototherapy may produce beneficial effects via the immune system, it is also necessary to consider whether harmful effects may be produced via the same pathway. The possibility that these treatments may induce ANAs is still under investigation and remains an open question, as has already been discussed. The known carcinogenic potential of both treatments could also involve alterations in the immune reactivity of patients, if recent studies in animals are applicable to humans. Finally, exposure of patients over many years to therapies that produce short-term alterations in the function of lymphocytes could have quite unforeseen long-term effects.

SUMMARY

Research in the field of photoimmunology has resulted mainly in isolated observations and in only a few instances has there been a concerted attempt to thoroughly explore one area of interest. Photocarcinogenesis in animals, the immune responses to UV-DNA, and the effects of radiation on lymphocytes are examples where the threads of a developing picture can be discerned.

However, in most other instances only one or two unconnected facts are known and much work must be done to put those facts into some perspective. A fundamental problem in many studies has been the imbalance between the quality and extent of photobiologic and immunologic investigation and nowhere is this more apparent than in diseases such as PMLE and photallergy. The photobiologic aspects of these conditions have received much attention and are at least partially understood, but the immunologic aspects have been so neglected that it is still not fully established that immune mechanisms are involved. However, it is hoped that this situation will change as increased interest is shown in this area of research and more basic observations are made at a cellular and molecular level.

All the disease entities considered to have a photoimmunologic pathogenesis are skin diseases. It is interesting that there have been no suggestions that photoimmunology may be involved in the pathogenesis of any ocular diseases. Nonionizing radiation is absorbed by various components of the eye and immune mechanisms have been invoked in a number of ocular diseases, but it appears that either there is no connection or else the possibility has not been considered.

Finally, almost without exception, observations in photoimmunology have been concerned with the effects of UV radiation. Longer wavelengths of nonionizing radiation, particularly in the visible range, have been shown to be active in other biologic systems and it is quite possible that they also influence immune function. This would appear to be an interesting area for study.

ACKNOWLEDGMENTS. This work was supported by NIH Grant #AM 25924-02 and by funds from the Arthur O. and Gullan M. Wellman Foundation.

REFERENCES

1. Levine, L., Seaman, E., Hammerschlag, E., et al. (1966): Antibodies to photoproducts of deoxyribonucleic acid irradiated with ultraviolet light. *Science* **153**:1666–1667.
2. Tan, E. M. (1968): Antibodies to deoxyribonucleic acid irradiated with ultraviolet light: detection by precipitins and immunofluorescence. *Science* **161**:1353–1354.
3. Natali, P. G., and Tan, E. M. (1971): Immunological detection of thymidine photoproduct formation *in vivo*. *Radiat. Res.* **46**:506–518.
4. Tan, E. M., Stoughton, R. B. (1969): Ultraviolet light alteration of cellular deoxyribonucleic acid *in vivo*. *Proc. Natl. Acad. Sci. U.S.A.* **62**:708–714.
5. Tan, E. M., and Stoughton, R. B. (1969): Ultraviolet light induced damage to desoxyribonucleic acid in human skin. *J. Invest. Dermatol.* **52**:52:537–542.
6. Tan, E. M. (1971): Production of potentially antigenic DNA in cells. In: *Immunopathology, 6th International Symposium*, edited by P. A. Miescher, pp. 346–349. Grune & Stratton, New York.
7. Tan, E. M., Freeman, R. G., and Stoughton, R. B. (1970): Action spectrum of ultraviolet light-induced damage to nuclear DNA *in vivo*. *J. Invest. Dermatol.* **55**:439–443.
8. Jarzabek-Chorzelska, M., Zarebska, Z., Wolska, H., et al. (1976): Immunological phenomena induced by UV rays. *Acta Derm. Venereol. (Stockh.)* **56**:15–18.

9. Ten Veen, J. H., and Lucas, C. J. (1970): Induction of antinuclear antibodies by ultraviolet irradiation. *Ann. Rheum. Dis.* **29**:556–558.

10. Natali, P. G., and Tan, E. M. (1973): Experimental skin lesions in mice resembling systemic lupus erythematosus. *Arthritis Rheum.* **16**:579–589.

11. Davis, P., Russell, A. S., and Percy, J. S. (1976): Antibodies to UV light denatured DNA in systemic lupus erythematosus: detection by filter radioimmunoassay and clinical correlations. *J. Rheumatol.* **3**:375–379.

12. Zarebska, Z., Jarzabek-Chorzelska, M., Rzesa, G., et al. (1978): Antigenicity of DNA induced by photoaddition of 8-methoxypsoralen. *Photochem. Photobiol.* **27**:37–42.

13. Łyanson, S., Greist, M. C., Brandt, K. D., et al. (1979): Systemic lupus erythematosus. *Arch. Dermatol.* **115**:54–56.

14. Millns, J. L., McDuffie, F. C., Muller, S. A., et al. (1978): Development of photosensitivity and an SLE-like syndrome in a patient with psoriasis. *Arch. Dermatol.* **114**:1177–1181.

15. Bjellerup, M., Bruze, M., Forsgren, A., et al. (1978): Antinuclear antibodies during PUVA therapy. *Acta Derm. Venereol.* (*Stockh.*) **59**:73–75.

16. Stern, R. S., Morison, W. L., Thibodeau, L. A., et al. (1979): Antinuclear antibodies and oral methoxsalen photochemotherapy (PUVA) for psoriasis. *Arch. Dermatol.* **115**:1320–1324.

17. Jacobs, S. E. (1965): Pemphigus erythematosus and ultraviolet light. *Arch. Dermatol.* **91**:139–141.

18. Cram, D. L., and Winkelmann, R. K. (1965): Ultraviolet-induced acantholysis in pemphigus. *Arch. Dermatol.* **92**:7–13.

19. Cram, D. L., and Fukuyama, K. (1972): Immunohistochemistry of ultraviolet-induced pemphigus and pemphigoid lesions. *Arch. Dermatol.* **106**:819–824.

20. Michel, B., and Ko, C. S. (1977): An organ culture model for the study of pemphigus acantholysis. *Br. J. Dermatol.* **96**:295–302.

21. Gschnait, F., Pehamberger, H., and Holubar, K. (1978): Pemphigus acantholysis in tissue culture: studies on photoinduction. *Acta Derm. Venereol.* (*Stockh.*) **58**:237–239.

22. Alani, M. D., and Dunne, J. H. (1973): Effects of long wave ultraviolet radiation on photosensitizing and related compounds. II. In vitro binding to soluble epidermal proteins. *Br. J. Dermatol.* **89**:367–372.

23. Herman, P. S., and Sams, W. M., Jr. (1971): Requirement for carrier protein in salicylanilide sensitivity: the migration-inhibition test in contact photoallergy. *J. Lab. Clin. Med.* **77**:572–579.

24. Kochevar, I. E., and Harber, L. C. (1977): Photoreactions of 3,3',4',5-tetrachlorosalicylanilide with proteins. *J. Invest. Dermatol.* **68**:151–156.

25. Morison, W. L., and Parish, J. A. (1981): The *in vivo* effect of PUVA on lymphocyte function. *Br. J. Dermatol.,* **104**:405–413.

26. Parrish, J. A., and Morison, W. L. (1979): Comparative effects of *in vitro* exposure to nonionizing radiation on viability of T and B lymphocytes (abstract). *J. Invest. Dermatol.* **72**:206.

27. Fleischmann, P. (1905): Die bei der Prazipitation beteiligten substanzen in ihrem Verhalten gegenuber photodynamischen stoffen. *Munch. Med. Wochenschr.* **52**:693–694.

28. Battisto, J. R., Pringle, R. B., and Nungester, W. J. (1953): The effect of ultraviolet irradiation on immune serum. *J. Infect. Dis.* **92**:85–88.

29. Kleczkowski, A. (1954): Inactivation of antibodies by ultraviolet radiation. *Br. J. Exp. Pathol.* **35**:402–443.

30. Pappenheimer, A. M. (1917): Experimental studies upon lymphocytes. I. The reactions of lymphocytes under various experimental conditions. *J. Exp. Med.* (*Baltimore*) **25**:633–650.

31. Morison, W. L., Parrish, J. A., Anderson, R. R., et al. (1979): Sensitivity of mononuclear cells to UV radiation. *Photochem. Photobiol.* **29**:1045–1047.

32. Morison, W. L., Parrish, J. A., McAuliffe, D. J., et al. (1980): Sensitivity of mononuclear

cells to UV radiation: effect on subsequent stimulation with phytomehagglutinin. *Photo-chem. Photobiol.* **32**:99–102.
33. Horowitz, S., Cripps, D., and Hong, R. (1974): Selective T cell killing of human lymphocytes by ultraviolet radiation. *Cell. Immunol.* **14**:80–86.
34. Yew, F. H., and Johnson, R. T. (1978): Human B and T lymphocytes differ in UV-induced repair capacity. *Exp. Cell Res.* **113**:227–231.
35. Cripps, D. J., Horowitz, S., and Hong, R. (1978): Spectrum of ultraviolet radiation on human B and T lymphocyte viability. *Clin. Exp. Dermatol.* **3**:43–50.
36. Rocklin, R. E. (1973): Production of migration inhibitory factor by nondividing lympho-cytes. *J. Immunol.* **110**:674–678.
37. Lindahl-Kiessling, K., and Safwenberg, J. (1972): Mechanism of stimulation in the mixed lymphocyte culture. In: *Proceedings of the 6th Leukocyte Culture Conference*, edited by M. R. Schwarz, pp. 623–638. Academic Press, New York.
38. Rollinghoff, M., and Wagner, H. (1975): Secondary cytotoxic allograft response *in vitro*, I. Antigenic requirements. *Eur. J. Immunol.* **5**:875–879.
39. Levis, W. R., Lincoln, P. M., and Dattner, A. M. (1978): Effect of ultraviolet light on dinitrochlorobenzene- specific antigen-presenting function. *J. Immunol.* **121**:1496–1500.
40. Morison, W. L., Parrish, J. A., McAuliffe, D. J., et al. (1980): Sensitivity of mononuclear cells to PUVA: effect on subsequent stimulation with mitogens and on exclusion of trypan blue dye. *Clin. Exp. Dermatol.*, in press.
41. Kruger, J. P., Christophers, E., and Schlaak, M. (1978): Dose-effects of 8-methoxypsoralen and UVA in cultured human lymphocytes. *Br. J. Dermatol.* **98**:141–144.
42. Scherer, R., Kern, B., and Braun-Falco, O. (1977): UVA-induced inhibition of proliferation of PHA-stimulated lymphocytes from humans treated with 8-methoxypsoralen. *Br. J. Dermatol.* **97**:519–527.
43. Scherer, R., Kern, B., and Braun-Falco, O. (1977). The human peripheral lymphocyte—a model system for studying the combined effect of psoralen plus black light. *Klin. Wochenschr.* **55**:137–140.
44. Wulf, H. C., and Wettermark, G. (1977): Toxic effects of 8-methoxypsoralen on lymphocyte division. *Arch. Dermatol. Res.* **260**:87–92.
45. Edelson, R., Jacobs, D., Brin, M., et al. (1977): Lymphocyte sensitivity to 8-methoxy-psoralen (8-MOP) and ultraviolet A (UVA) (abstract). *Clin. Res.* **25**:281A.
46. Berger, C., and Edelson, R. (1979): Effects of 8-methoxypsoralen (8-MOP) and ultraviolet A (UVA) on helper T-cell activity (abstract). *J. Invest. Dermatol.* **72**:198.
47. Evans, R. G., and Norman, A. (1968): Unscheduled incorporation of thymidine in ultraviolet-irradiated human lymphocytes. *Radiat. Res.* **36**:287–298.
48. Berliner, J., Himes, S. W., Aoki, C. T., et al. (1975): The sites of unscheduled DNA synthesis within irradiated human lymphocytes. *Radiat. Res.* **63**:544–552.
49. Nikesch, W., and Norman, A. (1972): Studies of ultraviolet radiation damage in human leukocytes with a fluorescent probe. In: *Book of Abstracts, VI International Congress of Photobiology*, p. 329. Bochum, Germany.
50. Schmoeckel, C., Scherer, R., Dern, B., et al. (1978): The cytolytic effect of PUVA treatment on PHA-stimulated human peripheral lymphocytes. *Acta Derm. Venereol. (Stockh.)* **58**:203–211.
51. Laurens, H. (1928): The physiological effects of radiation. *Physiol. Rev.* **8**:1–87.
52. Spode, E. (1955): Studies on radiation reaction of the blood. V. Radiation experiment with UVC radiation. *Strahlentherapie* **96**:595–598.
53. Spode, E. (1956): Research on blood reactions to radiation. *Strahlentherapie* **99**:482–488.
54. Morison, W. L., Parrish, J. A., Bloch, K. J., et al. (1979): In vivo effect of UV-B on lymphocyte function. *Br. J. Dermatol.* **101**:513–520.
55. Ortonne, J. P., Claudy, A., Alario, A., et al. (1978): Impairment of thymus derived rosette forming cells during photochemotherapy (psoralen-UVA). *Arch. Dermatol. Res.* **262**:143–151.

56. Haftek, M., Glinski, W., Jablonska, S., et al. (1979): T lymphocyte E rosette function during photochemotherapy (PUVA) of psoriasis. *J. Invest. Dermatol.* **72**:214–218.

57. Cormane, R. H., Hamerlinck, F., and Siddiqui, A. H. (1979): Immunologic implications of PUVA therapy in psoriasis vulgaris. *Arch. Dermatol. Res.* **265**:245–267.

58. Fraki, J. E., Eskola, J., and Hopsu-Havu, V. K. (1979): Effect of 8-methoxypsoralen plus UVA (PUVA) on lymphocyte transformation and T cells in psoriatic patients. *Br. J. Dermatol.* **100**:543–550.

59. Morison, W. L., Parrish, J. A., Bloch, K. J., et al. (1979): Transient impairment of peripheral blood lymphocyte function during PUVA therapy. *Br. J. Dermatol.* **101**: 391–398.

60. Harper, R. A., Tam, D. W., Vonderheid, E. C., et al. (1979): Normal T-lymphocyte function in psoriatic patients undergoing methoxsalen photochemotherapy. *J. Invest. Dermatol.* **72**:323–325.

61. Wassilew, S. W. (1978): Stimulation of lymphocytes in patients with psoriasis under photochemotherapy. *Arch. Dermatol Res.* **263**:127–134.

62. Kraemer, K. H., and Weinstein, G. D. (1977): Decreased thymidine incorporation in circulating leukocytes after treatment of psoriasis with psoralen and long-wave ultraviolet light. *J. Invest. Dermatol.* **69**:211–214.

63. Carter, D. M., Wolff, K., and Schnedl, W. (1976): 8-Methoxypsoralen and UVA promote sister-chromatid exchanges. *J. Invest. Dermatol.* **67**:548–551.

64. Lambert, B., Morad, M., Bredberg, A., et al. (1978): Sister chromatid exchanges in lymphocytes from psoriasis patients treated with 8-methoxypsoralen and longwave ultraviolet light. *Acta Derm. Venereol. (Stockh.)* **58**:13–16.

65. Wolff-Schreiner, E. C., Carter, D. M., Schwarzacher, H. G., et al. (1977): Sister chromatid exchanges in photochemotherapy. *J. Invest. Dermatol.* **69**:387–391.

66. McGovern, V. J. (1961): The mechanism of photosensitivity; an experimental study. *Arch. Dermatol.* **83**:40–51.

67. Grof, P., and Kovacs, A. (1967): On the mode of action of UV-light; effects of UVA-rays on mast cells in vivo. *Acta Physiol. Acad. Sci. Hung.* **32**:35–44.

68. Valtonen, E. J. (1968): Studies of the mechanism of ultra-violet erythema formation. V. Changes in the fine structure of mast cells of the skin during the process of ultra-violet erythema caused by waveband UV-C. *Acta Derm. Venereol. (Stockh.)* **48**:203–211.

69. Valtonen, E. J. (1961): The effect of ultra-violet radiation of some spectral wavebands on the mast cell count in the skin; an experimental study in mice. *Acta Pathol. Microbiol. Scand.* **1961** (Suppl. 151):1–95.

70. Konrad, K., Gschnait, F., Honigsmann, H., et al. (1976): UVA-mediated psoralen–tissue interactions: subcellular events (abstract). *J. Invest. Dermatol.* **66**:258.

71. Haniszko, J., and Suskind, R. R. (1963): The effect of ultraviolet radiation on experimental cutaneous sensitization in guinea pigs. *J. Invest. Dermatol.* **40**:183–191.

72. Jessup, J. M., Hanna, N., Palaszynski, E., et al. (1978): Mechanisms of depressed reactivity to dinitrochlorobenzene and ultraviolet-induced tumors during ultraviolet carcinogenesis in BALB/c mice. *Cell. Immunol.* **38**:105–115.

73. Maughan, G. H., and Smiley, D. F. (1978): The effect of general irradiation with ultraviolet light upon the frequency of colds. *J. Prevent. Med. (Baltimore)* **2**:69–77.

74. Barenberg, L. H., Friedman, I., and Green, D. (1926): The effect of ultraviolet irradiation on the health of a group of infants. *J. AMA* **87**:1114–1117.

75. U. S. Department of Commerce (1967): *Effect and Use of Ultraviolet Radiation—U.S.S.R.* U. S. Department of Commerce, Joint Publications Research Service, Washington, D.C.

76. Kripke, M. L. (1974): Antigenicity of murine skin tumors induced by ultraviolet light. *J. Natl. Cancer Inst.* **53**:1333–1336.

77. Fisher, M. S., and Kripke, M. L. (1977): Systemic alteration induced in mice by ultraviolet light irradiation and its relationship to ultraviolet carcinogenesis. *Proc. Natl. Acad. Sci. U.S.A.* **74**:1688–1692.

78. Kripke, M. L., Budmen, M. B., and Fidler, I. J. (1977): Production of specific macrophage activating factor by lymphocytes from tumor-bearing mice. *Cell. Immunol.* **30**:341–352.
79. Lill, P. H., and Fortner, G. W. (1978): Identification and cytotoxic reactivity of inflammatory cells recovered from progressing or regressing syngeneic UV-induced murine tumors. *J. Immunol.* **121**:1854–1860.
80. Kripke, M. L., and Fisher, M. S. (1976): Immunologic parameters of ultraviolet carcinogenesis. *J. Natl. Cancer Inst.* **57**:211–215.
81. Spellman, C. W., Woodward, J. G., and Daynes, R. A. (1977): Modification of immunological potential by ultraviolet radiation. *Transplantation* **24**:112–119.
82. Kripke, M. L., Lofgren, J. S., Beard, J., Jessup, J. M., and Fisher, M. S. (1977): In vivo immune responses of mice during carcinogenesis by ultraviolet irradiation. *J. Natl. Cancer Inst.* **59**:1227–1230.
83. Fisher, M. S., and Kripke, M. L. (1978): Further studies on the tumor-specific suppressor cells induced by ultraviolet radiation. *J. Immunol.* **121**:1139–1144.
84. Daynes, R. A., and Spellman, C. W. (1977): Evidence for the generation of suppressor cells by ultraviolet radiation. *Cell. Immunol.* **31**:182–187.
85. Palaszynski, E. W.. and Kripke, M. L. (1978): Induction of immunologic anergy to UV-induced tumors with grafts of UV-irradiated skin. In: *Program and Abstracts, 6th Annual Meeting of the American Society for Photobiology, Burlington, Vermont, June 11–15, 1978*, p. 75.
86. Roberts, L. K., Schmitt, M., and Daynes, R. A. (1979): Tumor-susceptibility generated in mice treated with subcarginogenic doses of 8-methoxypsoralen and longwave ultraviolet light. *J. Invest. Dermatol.* **72**:306–309.
87. Nairn, R. C., Nind, A. P. P., Guli, E. P. G., et al. (1971): Specific immune response in human skin carcinoma. *Br. Med. J.* **4**:701–705.
88. Blewitt, R. W., Aparicio, S. R., Burrow, H. M., et al. (1978): Failure to detect circulating IgG or IgM antibodies to basal cell carcinoma by immunofluorescence. *Acta Derm. Venereol. (Stockh.)* **58**:82–83.
89. De Moragas, J. M., Winkelmann, R. K., and Jordon, R. E. (1970): Immunofluorescence of epithelial skin tumors, I. Patterns of intercellular substance. *Cancer* **25**:1399–1403.
90. De Moragas, J. M., Winkelmann, R. K., and Jordon, R. E. (1970): Immunofluorescence of epithelial skin tumors, II. Basement membrane. *Cancer* **25**:1404–1407.
91. Muller, H. K., and Sutherland, R. C. (1971): Epidermal antigens in cutaneous dysplasia and neoplasia. *Nature* **230**:384–385.
92. Hersh, L., Fukuyama, K., Inoue, N., et al. (1977): Immunofluorescent studies of epidermal protein during UV induced carcinogenesis. *Virchows Archiv.* [*Cell. Pathol.*] **24**:157–164.
93. Dellon, A. L., Potvin, C., Chretien, P. B., et al. (1975): The immunobiology of skin cancer. *Plast. Reconstr. Surg.* **55**:341–354.
94. Marshall, V. (1974): Premalignant and malignant skin tumours in immunosuppressed patients. *Transplantation* **17**:272–275.
95. Koranda, F. C., Dehmel, E. M., Kahn, G., et al. (1974): Cutaneous complications in immunosuppressed renal homograft recipients. *J. AMA* **229**:419–424.
96. Penn, I. (1975): The incidence of malignancies in transplant recipients. *Transplant. Proc.* **7**:323–326.
97. Walder, B. K., Jeremy, D., Charlesworth, J. A., et al. (1976): The skin and immunosuppression. *Aust. J. Dermatol.* **17**:94–97.
98. Hoxtell, E. O., Mandel, J. S., Murray, S. S., et al. (1977): Incidence of skin carcinoma after renal transplantation. *Arch. Dermatol.* **113**:436–438.
99. Hill, B. H. R. (1976): Immunosuppressive drug therapy as a potentiator of skin tumors in five patients with lymphoma. *Aust. J. Dermatol.* **17**:46–48.
100. Nathanson, R. B., Forbes, P. D., and Urbach, F. (1976): Modification of photocarcinogenesis by two immunosuppressive agents. *Cancer Letters* **1**:243–247.

101. Koranda, F. C., Loeffler, R. T., Koranda, D. M., et al. (1976): Increased cutaneous carcinogenic induction with ultraviolet radiation and immunosuppressive agents (abstract). *J. Invest. Dermatol.* **68**:269.

102. Dupuy, J. M., and Lafforet, D. (1974): A defect of cellular immunity in xeroderma pigmentosum. *Clin. Immunol. Immunopathol.* **3**:52–58.

103. Lafforet, D., and Dupuy, J. M. (1975): Inhibitory factors of lymphocyte proliferation in serum from patients with xeroderma pigmentosum. *Clin. Immunol. Immunopathol.* **4**:165–173.

104. Harber, L. C., Holloway, R. M., Wheatley, V. R., et al. (1963): Immunologic and biophysical studies in solar urticaria. *J. Invest. Dermatol.* **41**:439–443.

105. Sams, W. M., Jr. (1970): Solar urticaria: studies of the active serum factor. *J. Allerg.* **45**:295–301.

106. Horio, T. (1978): Photoallergic urticaria induced by visible light. Additional cases and further studies. *Arch. Dermatol.* **114**:1761–1764.

107. Hawk, J. L. M., Eady, R. A. J., Challoner, A. V. J., et al. (1979): Raised blood histamine levels in solar urticaria associated with mast cell degranulation (abstract). *J. Invest. Dermatol.* **72**:282.

108. Soter, N. A., Wasserman, S. I., Pathak, M. A., et al. (1979): Solar urticaria: release of mast cell mediators into the circulation after experimental challenge (abstract). *J. Invest. Dermatol.* **72**:282.

109. Ramsay, C. A. (1977): Solar urticaria treatment by inducing tolerance to artificial radiation and natural light. *Arch. Dermatol.* **113**:1222–1225.

110. Duke, W. W. (1926): Physical allergy as a cause of dermatoses. *Arch. Dermatol. Syphilol.* **13**:176–186.

111. Epstein, S. (1942): Studies in abnormal human sensitivity to light, III. Passive transfer of light hypersensitivity in prurigo aestivalis. *J. Invest. Dermatol.* **5**:285–287.

112. Epstein, S. (1942): Studies in abnormal human sensitivity to light, IV. Photoallergic concept of prurigo aestivalis. *J. Invest. Dermatol.* **5**:289–298.

113. Shaffer, G., Cahn, M. M., and Levy, E. J. (1959): Polymorphous light eruption. A discussion of its pathogenesis and the therapeutic action of the antimalarials in this disease. *J. Invest. Dermatol.* **32**:363–366.

114. Epstein, J. H. (1972): Photoallergy. *Arch. Dermatol.* **106**:741–748.

115. Mühlmann, I., and Akobjan, A. (1930): Experimenteller Beitrag zur Atiologie der Prurigo aestivalis. *Arch. Dermatol. Syphilol.* (*Berlin*) **159**:318–323.

116. Lester, R. S., Burnham, T. K., Fine, G., et al. (1967): Immunologic concepts of light reactions in lupus erythematosus and polymorphous light eruptions. *Arch. Dermatol.* **96**:1–10.

117. Fisher, D. A., Epstein, J. H., Kay, D. N., et al. (1970): Polymorphous light eruption and lupus erythematosus. *Arch. Dermatol.* **101**:458–461.

118. Jansen, C. T. (1977): Elevated serum immunoglobulin levels in polymorphous light eruptions. *Acta Derm. Venereol.* (*Stockh.*) **57**:331–333.

119. Chorzelski, T., Jablonska, S., and Blaszczyk, M. (1969): Immunopathologic investigations in lupus erythematosus. *J. Invest Dermatol.* **52**:333–338.

120. Horkay, I., and Meszaros, Cs. (1971): A study of lymphocyte transformation in light dermatoses. *Acta Derm. Venereol.* (*Stockh.*) **51**:268–270.

121. Horkay, I., Tamasi, P., and Csongor, J. (1973): UV-light induced DNA damage and repair in lymphocytes in photodermatoses. *Acta Derm. Venereol.* (*Stockh.*) **53**:105–108.

122. Raffle, E. J., MacLeod, T. M., and Hutchinson, F. (1973): In vitro lymphocyte studies in chronic polymorphic light eruption. *Br. J. Dermatol.* **89**:143–147.

123. Jung, E. G., and Bohnert, E. (1974): Chronisch polymorphe Lichtdermatose. *Dermatologica* **148**:209–212.

124. Jansen, C. T., and Helander, I. (1976): Cell-mediated immunity in chronic polymorphous light eruptions. *Acta Derm. Venereol.* (*Stockh.*) **56**:121–125.
125. Cripps, D. J., and Enta, T. (1970): Absorption and action spectra studies on bithionol and halogenated salicylanilide photosensitivity. *Br. J. Dermatol.* **82**:230–242.
126. Horio, T. (1976): The induction of photocontact sensitivity in guinea pigs without UVB radiation. *J. Invest. Dermatol.* **67**:591–593.
127. Harber, L. C., Targovnik, S. E., and Baer, R. L. (1967): Contact photosensitivity patterns to halogenated salicylanilides in man and guinea pigs. *Arch. Dermatol.* **96**:646–656.
128. Willis, I., and Kligman, A. M. (1968): The mechanism of photoallergic contact dermatitis. *J. Invest. Dermatol.* **51**:378–384.
129. Epstein, S. (1968): Chlorpromazine photosensitivity; phototoxic and photoallergic reactions. *Arch. Dermatol.* **98**:354–363.
130. Jung, E. G., Dummler, U., and Immich, H. (1968): Photoallergie durch 4-chlor-2-hydroxybenzesuare-*n*-butylamid. *Arch. Klin. Exp. Dermatol.* **232**:403–412.
131. Amos, H. E. (1973): Photoallergy: a critical survey. *Trans. St. John's Hosp. Dermatol. Soc.* **59**:147–151.
132. Horio, T., and Ofuji, S. (1976): The fate of tetrachlorosalicylanilide in photosensitized guinea pigs. *Acta Derm. Venereol. (Stockh.)* **56**:367–371.
133. Osmundsen, T. E. (1969): Photopatch testing. *Trans. St. John's Hosp. Dermatol. Soc.* **55**:160–173.
134. Harber, L. C., and Baer, R. L. (1972): Pathogenic mechanisms of drug-induced photosensitivity. *J. Invest. Dermatol.* **58**:327–342.
135. Epstein, J. H., Fukuyama, K., and Fye, K. (1970): Effects of ultraviolet radiation on the mitotic cycle and DNA, RNA and protein synthesis in mammalian epidermis in vivo. *Photochem. Photobiol.* **12**:57–65.
136. Epstein, J. H., and Fukuyama, K. (1975): Effects of 8-methoxypsoralen-induced phototoxic effects on mammalian epidermal macromolecule synthesis in vivo. *Photochem. Photobiol.* **24**:325–330.
137. Guilhou, J. J., Meynadier, J., and Clot, J. (1978): New concepts in the pathogenesis of psoriasis. *Br. J. Dermatol.* **98**:585–592.

IV

*Photosensitized and Abnormal
Reactions of Human Skin*

11

Mechanisms of Photosensitization to Drugs in Humans

L. C. Harber, I. E. Kochevar, and A. R. Shalita

Drug-induced photosensitivity refers to adverse cutaneous reactions that result from either combined or successive exposure to certain chemicals and light. Although the word "drug" is properly used in reference to chemicals administered for therapeutic purposes, with regard to "drug-induced photosensitivity," this term has been expanded to include chemicals used for various other purposes, such as sweeteners (1), topical antibacterial agents (2), perfumes (3), and industrial (4), and agricultural (5) products.

Photosensitization to drugs includes three types of reactions in humans: phototoxic, photoallergic, and drug-induced photosensitivity diseases. In phototoxic reactions, photosensitization can occur in all individuals provided that they are exposed to sufficient doses of both the photosensitizing chemical and the appropriate wavelengths of radiation. Phototoxic reactions are independent of immunologic mechanisms. Drug-induced photoallergic reactions also require appropriate doses of drug and radiation and are believed to involve a cell-mediated immunologic response. In addition to the phototoxic and photoallergic reactions, the administration of a drug may result in a disease state in which photosensitivity is a major component of the clinical picture. Examples include porphyria cutanea tarda, systemic lupus erythematosus, and pellagra.

In this chapter historical, clinical, and mechanistic aspects of the three types of drug-induced photosensitivity in humans will be discussed.

L. C. Harber and I. E. Kochevar • Department of Dermatology, Columbia University College of Physicians and Surgeons, New York, New York 10032. *A. R. Shalita* • Division of Dermatology, Department of Medicine, State University of New York, Downstate Medical Center, Brooklyn, New York 11203. Present address for Dr. Kochevar: Department of Dermatology, Harvard Medical School, Massachusetts General Hospital, Boston, Massachusetts 02114.

DRUG-INDUCED PHOTOTOXIC REACTIONS

History

The classic experiments of Raab in 1900 (6) have served as the basis for the photobiologic principles of drug-induced phototoxicity. He observed that when paramecia were exposed to either sunlight alone or to the chemical acridine in the dark there was no adverse reaction. However, when these unicellular organisms were exposed to an acridine solution and then exposed to sunlight, a lethal reaction ensued. Irradiation of acridine prior to adding it to the organisms and incubation in the dark had no effect. Raab further noted that the reaction was dose dependent (i.e., related to the duration of exposure to sunlight as well as to the concentration of acridine).

In 1904, Tappeiner and Jodlbauer (7) demonstrated that oxygen was required for this response to acridine and light and termed the reaction "photodynamic" in contrast to photochemical reactions such as those that occur on x-ray film. Later, Blum (8) expanded these studies to mammalian systems. Subsequently, similar principles have been applied to photobiologic reactions in viruses, bacteria, and fungi. Studies by Oginsky et al. (9) and Mathews (10) demonstrated that 8-methoxypsoralen was a photosensitizer in bacteria in the absence of oxygen. Thus phototoxic reactions are not necessarily photodynamic.

In humans, certain phototoxic agents have been used therapeutically. Psoralens from natural sources were used for centuries to induce pigmentation (11) and are currently used in psoriasis phototherapy (Chapter 22). Phototoxicity induced with chemicals for therapeutic purpose was introduced for patients with diseases such as rickets, skin cancer, psoriasis, and psychosis (12).

Phototoxicity as an adverse reaction to a therapeutic drug was first recognized and studied when sulfanilamide was widely used as an antibiotic (13, 14). In recent years chemicals that induce phototoxicity in humans have been identified through clinical experience (15) and phototoxicity testing (16). Some of the more important ones are listed in Table 11-1.

Clinical Features

The clinical features presented by patients with phototoxic reactions vary considerably, but certain generalizations can be made. The lesions are confined exclusively to the areas of skin exposed to light (29). In most cases these include the face, pinnae of the ears, the V of the neck, and nuchal area. Hairy portions of the body are usually protected, but the scalp of balding persons is particularly susceptible. A dermatitis confined to the dorsa of the hands and anterior aspects of the legs is often suggestive of a phototoxic reaction. The palms and soles of submental portion of the chin, however, are almost never involved.

Table 11-1. Chemicals Inducing Phototoxicity in Humans

Chemical	Reference
Aminobenzoic acid derivatives	17
Anthiaquinone dyes	18, 19
Chlorothiazides	20
Chlorpromazine	21, 22
Coal tar derivatives: Anthracene, acridine, phenanthrene, pyrene	4, 23
Nalidixic acid	24
Phenothiazine	25
Protriptyline	16
Psoralens	3, 12
Sulfanilamide	14, 15
Tetracyclines	26, 27, 28

The morphology of phototoxic reactions also varies. Certain photo-sensitizers, such as the components of coal tars, produce a burning, painful sensation ("tar smarts") during or shortly after UVA exposure (4). For other phototoxic chemicals the acute phase occurs hours after exposure and is characterized by erythema, edema, or vesiculation. After repeated injury, chronic changes appear, including scaling and lichenification (increased thickening and more pronounced skin lines). Reactions to some photosensitizers, such as the psoralens, are characterized by marked hyperpigmentation (increased melanin production) (3, 30).

Factors Affecting Phototoxic Reactions in Humans

Theoretically, phototoxic reactions should occur in 100% of the population if sufficient doses of drug and appropriate wavelengths of light are present. However, these reactions have been found to be quite variable in a population exposed to the same agent. Several factors may influence individual responses to phototoxic agents. These include differences between individuals in absorption and metabolism of the phototoxic agent and differences in the penetration of light into the skin.

A chemical that is applied topically can act as photosensitizing agent only if cutaneous absorption occurs since the necessary photoreactions do not occur on the skin surface. Thus, the cutaneous response will vary according to the skin site because of differences in the thickness of the stratum corneum and the number of adnexal glands. In addition, percutaneous absorption of the same chemical varies when it is applied in different vehicles (31). Increased temperature and humidity also enhance ultraviolet (UV) injury (32) and phototoxic responses (33). The mechanism for this effect may be through augmentation of the percutaneous absorption of the phototoxic drug or increased UV penetration.

The phototoxic potential of a drug could be altered if it were metabolized into a compound which was either more or less phototoxic. However, the role of cutaneous and bacterial enzymes in metabolizing phototoxic drugs has not been extensively studied. Numerous other factors are involved when phototoxic drugs are administered systemically. Thus, the rate of absorption, metabolism, and excretion could influence the phototoxic potential by affecting the persistence and concentration of the drug in the skin.

The amount and localization of melanin and keratin are important determinants in the magnitude of a phototoxic response since they determine the depth of penetration into skin of UV radiation. Phototoxic reactions are considerably less severe in blacks when compared to Caucasians (4).

In addition to the presence of the drug in the skin, an adequate dose of the appropriate wavelengths of light is required. The action spectrum for most phototoxic compounds includes the UVA range (34) or visible light range. However, some drugs elicit phototoxicity with UVB radiation (35).

Mechanisms of Action

Studies of the mechanisms by which phototoxic chemicals cause cellular injury have been performed in many different in vitro systems. The knowledge gained from these studies has been integrated into general classifications of phototoxicity mechanisms.

Classification. As mentioned above, phototoxic chemicals are divided by their requirement for oxygen into photodynamic (oxygen-dependent) and nonphotodynamic (oxygen-independent) sensitizers. There is little information about the oxygen requirement for most of the chemicals that have been reported to be phototoxic in humans, anthracene (36), hematoporphyrin (37), and protoporphyrin (38), an endogeneous photosensitizer, have been found to be photodynamic. Psoralens (39) photochemically combines with DNA in the absence of oxygen, and the formation of toxic photoproducts from chlorpromazine (40) and protriptyline (41) has been reported to be independent of oxygen.

Photodynamic sensitizers interact with oxygen in two ways to produce oxidized molecules (42). In Type I photooxidation, the excited triplet state of the sensitizer reacts with oxygen to form radicals which can react further. In Type II photooxidation, the excited triplet state transfers its energy or an electron to oxygen to produce a reactive oxygen species (singlet oxygen or superoxide anion), which subsequently oxidizes cell components. Photoporphyrin photosensitizes oxidative damage to cell membranes by a Type II process (43). Other photodynamic sensitizers oxidize DNA (44), protein (45), and membrane components (46) by one or both of these mechanisms.

Phototoxicity mechanisms have also been classified by the intracellular site of damage. The major targets are believed to be DNA and cell membranes (both plasma and lysosomal), although other possible sites should not be excluded. DNA damage after exposure of cells to a photosensitizer and appropriate wavelengths of light is monitored by methods including unscheduled DNA synthesis, which indicates repair of DNA, covalent linking of the photosensitizer to isolated DNA, and formation of cross-links between DNA strands.

The membrane-damaging potential of a photosensitizer is often assayed by red blood cell photohemolysis because DNA and intracellular organelles are not present in this system. Both photodynamic (47) and nonphotodynamic (48, 49) sensitized hemolysis have been reported. Protoporphyrin-photosensitized hemolysis has been studied as a model for photodynamic sensitizers. Irradiation of protoporphyrin and red blood cells results in polyunsaturated fatty acid oxidation (50, 51), decreased enzyme activities and active transport (52), membrane protein cross-linking (53) and oxidation (51), and potassium efflux (51). Photosensitized lipid (43) and protein oxidation (51) have been postulated as the primary event in the membrane damage that disrupts the osmotic equilibrium of the intact cell.

Similar events may occur when phototoxic compounds are sequestered in lysosomes. Allison et al. (36) demonstrated that anthracene and other phototoxic compounds were localized primarily in cytoplasmic lysosomes in monkey kidney cells. Exposure of these anthracene-treated cells to 360-nm radiation resulted in significantly increased acid phosphatase activity, indicating that the lysosomes had ruptured. No such hydrolytic activity could be demonstrated in the absence of UV radiation. Lipid peroxidation and enzyme release had previously been reported after UV irradiation of lysosomes (54).

Psoralen Phototoxicity. Phototherapy using psoralens will be discussed elsewhere (Chapter 22); consequently, the mechanism of psoralen phototoxicity will be only briefly reviewed here. Psoralen molecules which are intercalated between base pairs in DNA photochemically form monoadducts and cross-links (12, 39, 55). These products are formed by cycloaddition of the 3,4 double bond of the furan ring and 4′,5′ double bond of the lactone ring with pyrimidine carbon–carbon double bonds. Therefore, the photoadducts and cross-links are based on cyclobutyl ring structures. DNA synthesis is inhibited, and repair by cellular enzymes has been reported (56). The steps between the photochemical events and the cutaneous phototoxicity are not clear. Psoralens can also inactivate enzymes by a photodynamic process (57, 58) and photosensitize membrane damage (59).

Chlorpromazine Phototoxicity. Clinical reports of photosensitivity to chlorpromazine appeared shortly after its introduction in the 1950s (21, 22). Evidence for both phototoxic and photoallergic reactions was reported (22). Conflicting data have appeared regarding the wavelength range that is required to elicit a reaction; some investigators (21, 59) report positive reactions with wavelengths below 320 nm and others (22, 60, 61) with wavelengths above 320 nm. An action spectrum for phototoxicity which extended from 320 to 340 nm with a maximum at 330 nm was determined in mice after intradermal injection of chlorpromazine (62). The lack of correlation between the chlorpromazine absorption spectrum (absorption maximum 305 nm in water) and the action spectra determined in humans and mice may be due to light-filtering effects in the skin and metabolism of chlorpromazine to compounds that absorb at longer wavelengths and are phototoxic. Recent studies by Ljunggren and Moeller (63) showed that two metabolites or chlorpromazine were more potent phototoxic agents than chlorpromazine itself. In addition, these investigators demonstrated that chlorpromazine solutions irradiated prior to injection into the test animals produced toxic responses (40). Consequently, it appears that stable photoproducts of chlorpromazine may be the actual agents eliciting cutaneous phototoxicity. Chlorpromazine is phototoxic to macrophages (48) and photomutagenic to mammalian cells (64) and bacteria (65).

The dominant subcellular location of chlorpromazine has not been identified, although it is known to bind to proteins (66), intercalate with DNA (67), and bind to cell membranes (68) in the dark. Photochemical reactions of chlorpromazine with these three sites have also been reported. Chlorpromazine has been demonstrated to form covalent photoadducts with both single- and double-stranded DNA (69, 70) and with RNA (69). Photoinitiated cleavage of viral DNA (71) and repair of chlorpromazine-photosensitized DNA damage have been reported (71, 72). However, chlorpromazine-sensitized photodynamic killing of *Escherichia coli* was reported to not involve DNA damage (73). Photoaddition of chlorpromazine to protein has been demonstrated (70).

Chlorpromazine causes membrane damage by a nonphotodynamic process as indicated by its ability to photosensitize the lysis of red blood cells both in the presence and absence of oxygen (48, 49). A stable photoproduct may be the actual lytic agent. However, oxygen was required for chlorpromazine-photosensitized disruption of liposomes composed of lecithin (74).

In summary, chlorpromazine has been demonstrated to be phototoxic in many systems involving DNA, proteins, and membranes. How these results are related to phototoxicity in humans has not been determined.

Coal Tar Phototoxicity. Coal tar extracts, and other materials derived from crude coal tar are complex mixtures of aromatic hydrocarbons and heterocyclic aromatic hydrocarbons. Their ability to cause phototoxic reactions is well established (4, 75). Seven chemical components have been identified as photosensitizers; namely, anthracene, β-methylanthracene, pyrene, fluoranthene, benzpyrene, acridine, and phenanthrene (76, 77). Many others did not produce phototoxic reactions under the conditions tested. The action spectra for pitch and 5% crude coal tar were in the range of 340–430 nm (4) and 350–400 nm (78), respectively. Erythemal reactions after application of acridene and anthracene were observed after irradiation in the 340–380-nm range (4). Despite the fact that all these mixtures and compounds absorb radiation between 280 and 320 nm, no abnormal reactions were observed in the normal erythemal range. Restriction of skin blood supply before and during the irradiation eliminated both "smarting" and the erythema response to pitch and anthracene (4), possibly indicating the photodynamic nature of the reaction. The subcellular site of photobiologic damage sensitized by coal tar components has not been well defined. Anthracene photosensitizers both lysosomal and plasma membrane changes (36) and causes photodestruction of tryptophan and glutathione (28). Benzo(a)pyrene photochemically couples with DNA bases (79).

Tetracycline Phototoxicity. Demethylchlortetracycline is a more potent phototoxic chemical than the parent compound, tetracycline (26, 27, 80). Action spectrum experiments of demethylchlortetracycline phototoxicity in hairless mice demonstrated that 350–420-nm radiation was effective, with the greatest response being obtained at 400 nm (81). Only normal erythema responses were obtained at 325 nm and shorter wavelengths even though the chemical absorbed radiation at these wavelengths. Studies in humans also indicated the phototoxic reactions were obtained with radiation above 320 nm (60, 82).

Demethylchlortetracycline photosensitized hemolysis of erythrocytes (83), indicating that it was capable of inducing membrane damage. It also photosensitized the destruction of glutathione but not that of tryptophan (84).

Sulfanilamide Phototoxicity. Sulphanilamide was the first drug recognized to induce both phototoxic and photoallergic reactions (13). Its action spectrum in humans, as determined after intradermal injection, has been reported to be in the UVB range (60, 85), which correlates well with its absorption spectrum. In mice the action spectrum had a sharp maximum at 375–400 nm (81). A photooxidation product, *p*-hydroxylaminobenzene sulfonamide, elicited erythema when intradermally injected into guinea pigs and was proposed as the active toxic compound (86). Sulfonalamide also photosensitized the destruction of glutathione (84).

Mediators of Inflammation in Phototoxic Reactions

The agent (or agents) that may play a role in the erythematous response observed in a phototoxic reaction have been investigated. Mediation by an agent sensitive to protease inhibitors rather than the antihistamines was determined for chlorpromazine phototoxicity in mice (62). However, chlorpromazine-induced histamine release from guinea pig skin irradiated in vitro (87). Histamine was indicated as a mediator of sulfanilamide photo-toxicity (86). Biosynthesis of prostaglandins was enhanced in vitro when skin in microsomal fractions were irradiated at 254 nm in the presence of 8-methoxypsoralen, coal tar (88), and demethylchlortetracycline (89). In vivo, 8-methoxypsoralen and irradiation with UVA did not increase skin levels of the arachidonic acid metabolites measured (90). An inhibitor of prostaglandin synthesis, indomethecin, also failed to inhibit the phototoxic reaction to 8-methoxypsoralen and UVA irradiation (91, 92). There still remains much to be learned about how the initial photochemical events are translated into the inflammatory response that is described as phototoxicity.

DRUG-INDUCED PHOTOALLERGIC REACTIONS

Drug-induced photoallergy is a cutaneous photosensitivity reaction which requires an immunologic response. Other photosensitivity diseases, such as solar urticaria and polymorphous light eruption, may also involve an immune response (93, 94). However, because these diseases are not drug-photosensitized, they are discussed in Chapter 12. The overall mechanism proposed for photoallergy is

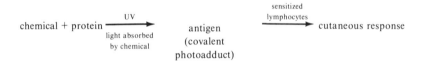

The chemical in the skin absorbs photons and is converted to a stable or unstable photoproduct. The photoproduct binds to soluble or membrane-bound protein to form an antigen. A delayed-type hypersensitivity response ensues which results in the cutaneous reaction.

In this section the historical and clinical aspects of drug-induced photoallergy will be reviewed. The immunologic and biochemical data regarding photoallergy will be discussed.

History

Photoallergy was first differentiated from phototoxicity by Epstein in 1939 (13) for reactions to sulfanilamide. From experimental studies in humans and clinical observations he postulated that one form of sulfanilamide photosensitivity involved an allergic (immunologic) response. Interest in photoallergy increased when Wilkinson in 1961 (95) reported 53 cases of contact photosensitivity following exposure to the antimicrobial agent 3,3′,4′,5-tetrachlorosalicylanilide (TCSA). Because of the widespread use of

Table 11-2. Chemicals Reported to Induce Photoallergy

Chemical	Reference
Aminobenzoic acids	103
Bithionol	104, 105
Chlorpromazine (thorazine)	22
Chlorpropamide (diabinese)	106
Fentichlor	107
Halogenated salicylanilides	95, 108
Jadit	96
6-Methylcoumarin	109
Musk ambrette	110
Promethazine (phenargan)	111
Sulfonilamide	13
Thiazides	112

TCSA and related salicylanilides in soaps and other household agents, thousands of individuals were affected. Jadit, an antimycotic widely used in Europe, which is chemically related to TCSA, was reported to be a photoallergen (96).

Induction of experimental photoallergic contact dermatitis in guinea pigs was first reported by Schwarz and Schwarz-Speck (97) in 1957 using sulfanilamide. Vinson and Borselli (98) induced contact photoallergy with tribromosalicylanilide (TBS) and related compounds (99). More recently, contact photoallergy to chlorpromazine (49, 100) and musk ambrette (101) was experimentally induced. In 1968 Willis and Kligman (102) reported the experimental induction of photoallergic contact sensitization to halogenated salicylanilides and related chemicals in human volunteers.

Table 11-2 lists many of the chemicals that have been reported to cause photoallergic contact dermatitis in humans.

Clinical Features

Cutaneous lesions resulting from photoallergic contact dermatitis can occur on any region of the body when a sufficiently high concentration of photosensitizing chemical and a sufficiently high dose of the appropriate wavelength of radiation are present. The cutaneous sites most frequently involved also include the normally light-exposed areas such as the face, ears, V of the neck, the backs of the hands, extensor surfaces of the arms, and, in women, the anterior aspects of the legs. In contrast, the submental area, eyelids, scalp, antecubital fossae, and palms are usually spared.

The morphology of drug-induced photodermatoses varies depending on several factors, including the route of exposure to the compound and the specific photosensitizer. For example, early phases of photoallergic contact

Table 11-3. Mechanisms of Drug-Induced Photosensitivity:
Comparison of Phototoxic and Photoallergic Reactions[a]

Reaction	Phototoxic	Photoallergic
Incidence	Usually relatively high (theoretically 100%)	Usually very low
Clinical changes	Usually like sunburn	Varied morphology
Reaction possible on first exposure	Yes	No
Incubation period necessary after first exposure	No	Yes
Development of persistent light reaction	No	Yes
"Flares" at distant previously involved sites possible	No	Yes
Cross-reactions to structurally related agents	No	Frequent
Broadening of cross-reactions following repeated photopatch testing	No	Possible
Concentration of drug necessary for reaction	High	Low
Chemical alteration of photosensitizer	Sometimes	Yes
Covalent binding with carrier protein	No	Yes
Passive transfer	No	Possible
Lymphocyte stimulation test	No	Possible
Macrophage migration inhibition test	No	Possible

[a] Modified from Harper and Baer (34).

dermatitis due to halogenated salicylanilides are usually eczematous. Lichenification and thickening can develop later. In contrast, the reaction from an
ingested agent would probably have more edema and less vesiculation.

   The clinical diagnosis of photoallergic contrast dermatitis, suspected by
history and physical examination, can be confirmed by photopatch testing
(113). This is a procedure in which the patient is deliberately exposed to the
suspected chemical under controlled conditions and subsequently irradiated
with UVA. When tested in sufficiently high concentration most, but not all
(101, 109), compounds known to be associated with photoallergic reactions
elicit a phototoxic reaction. However, few phototoxic compounds are
photoallergic. Compounds reported to elicit phototoxic and photoallergic
reactions are summarized in Table 11-3.

   Action spectrum studies in humans have been reported. Cripps and Enta

(114) determined action spectra for three halogenated salicylanilides. Their spectra, in general, showed good correlation above 340 nm with the absorption spectra of the ionized form of the chemicals. Their action spectrum for bithionol (114) extended to wavelengths 30 nm longer than the absorption spectrum. Action spectra for halogenated salicylanilides measured by Freeman and Knox (115) were in the wavelength range of the absorption spectra for the compounds tested. However, the magnitude of response did not closely follow the absorption maxima. Significantly, at wavelengths in the normal erythema range, less energy was usually required to elicit a reaction with the compound applied than without it. This result suggests that wavelengths below the UVA range may also contribute to photoallergic reactions.

In laboratory studies, correlation was found between the index of sensitivity of the halogenated salicylanilides in humans and guinea pigs (108, 113). TCSA had the highest index of photosensitization. Bithionol, dibrominated salicylanilides, and tribromosalicylanilide were next, and hexachlorophene and trichlorocarbanilide had the lowest index of photosensitivity. Cross-reactions to structurally analogous compounds have been reported (96, 108), especially following repeated photopatch testing.

Another condition, called "persistent light reactivity," has been demonstrated to occur in some individuals originally sensitized to photoallergic compounds (34, 116). These individuals remain sensitive to radiation, especially UVB, long after they have apparently ceased contact with the offending compound and consequently must avoid normal levels of light exposure, often for years. Although mechanisms for this disease have been proposed (117, 118), none has yet been established.

Mechanisms of Action

Photoallergic contact dermatitis is believed to involve a delayed-type hypersensitivity immunologic mechanism. With the exception of the obligatory role of light causing the conjugation of the chemical (hapten) with a carrier protein, photoallergy has the characterisitics of allergic contact dermatitis. The evidence to support such a cell-mediated immune response rests on results of experiments in guinea pigs, in humans, and in in vitro cell systems.

Photoallergy to halogenated salicylanilides (98, 99), chlorpromazine (100), and musk ambrette (101) has been induced in guinea pigs and to TCSA in humans (102). In guinea pigs, contact photoallergy to TCSA was passively transferred from sensitized animals to nonsensitized guinea pigs (119). Mononuclear peritoneal exudate cells collected from guinea pigs photosensitized to TCSA were injected intraperitoneally into nonsensitive animals. The injected guinea pigs, when challenged 24 hr later, reacted to the combination of TCSA and UVA radiation, alone or TCSA alone evoked no response. Additional experimental evidence in support of a delayed hypersensitivity mechanism included the in vitro demonstration by Jung et al. (120) of lymphocyte transformation of cells from patients sensitive to Jadit with a photochemically formed Jadit–albumin complex. A positive macrophage migration inhibition assay was demonstrated with the photoadduct of TSCA and albumin (120, 121).

Three photoallergic compounds have been demonstrated to covalently bond to protein upon photoexicitation, namely TCSA (222, 223), chlorpromazine (224), and Jadit (120). The chemical moiety produced by light absorption that actually reacts with skin proteins to form the antigen has not clearly been determined in any of these cases and may vary among compounds. However, indirect evidence in the case of trichlorosalicylanilide indicates that the stable photochemical dechlorination products do not combine with protein without further irradiation (108). Other likely reactive species are the excited states (singlet and triplet) and the free radicals formed by chlorine loss.

TCSA photodechlorinates in alkaline solution with the initial loss of chlorine from the salicylic acid ring (125, 126). In pH 7 buffered solution, chlorine loss from the aniline ring is also observed (126). It has been established that TCSA must noncovalently bond to a protein before photochemically adding to it (123) and that TCSA covalently bonds to multiple sites on albumin (118). In addition, TCSA photosensitizes the oxidation of histidines in albumin (123).

In summary, these results are consistent with a delayed-type hypersensitivity mechanism for photoallergy to topically applied chemicals. However, additional research is required to further characterize the stress in the immunologic process using current techniques and to establish the structure of the complete antigen.

DRUG-INDUCED PHOTOSENSITIVITY DISEASES

Drug-Induced Porphyria

It was demonstrated in laboratory animals that porphyrin synthesis is induced following the feeding of a variety of drugs (127–129). However, it was not appreciated until relatively recently that photosentizing porphyrias could occur in humans from diverse chemical and hormonal exposures. There are now two types of porphyria in humans that are associated with photosensitivity and are known to be induced or exacerbated by drugs. Both are hepatic in origin and both are characterized by a markedly increased production of uroporphyrin. Porphyria cutanea tarda is more frequent in the United States and usually associated with alcoholism or hormonal therapy (130). The second, variegate porphyria, is rare. Clinical characteristics of variegate porphyria include many features of both acute intermittent porphyria and porphyria cutanea tarda (131).

Porphyia cutanea tarda is clinically associated with multiple signs and symptoms in addition to photosensitivity. The earliest clinical feature is usually an increased skin fragility manifested by bruises on the dorsa of the hands (132). This results in numerous shallow, denuded sites with subsequent ulcerations, crusts, and scars. Discrete vesicles (blisters) may be seen also. Increased facial hirsutism and periocular hyperpigmentation are frequently presenting signs (see Chapter 12). Late cutaneous findings include areas of hypo- and hyperpigmentation of the face, ears, neck, and hands as well as scarring and hair loss (alopecia). Invariably, there is liver damage (133), which is usually mild, but often associated with deposition of iron in liver cells. Large amounts of uroporphyrin and coproporphyrin are present in the urine and feces. Both of these porphyrins fluoresce reddish orange when excited with light in the 400-nm range. Each can be quantitated by its specific absorption and emission spectral properties (134).

Major clinical interest in acquired or toxic hepatic porphyria occurred in 1956. It related to a report of 2000 new cases of porphyria cutanea tarda occurring in Turkey. Epidemiologic studies by Cam and Nigogosyan (135) centered about wheat that had been delivered to Turkey and treated with an antifungal agent, hexachlorobenzene. Those individuals who ingested the wheat, which had been intended for planting, developed marked photosensitivity and red urine. Analysis indicated that the urine contained both uroporphyrin and coproporphyrin. All of the clinical signs and symptoms associated with porphyria cutanea tarda were also noted. Subsequent studies in 1961 by Ockner and Schmid (136) showed that rats fed a diet of hexachlorobenzene also had an increased hepatic synthesis of uroporphyrin and coproporphyrin that could be detected in their urine and feces.

Porphyria cutanea tarda was reported by Bleiberg in 26 men employed in an industrial plant manufacturing chlorinated phenols used as herbicides (137). Following the use of industrial hygiene measures to prevent direct contact with these chemicals, the porphyria disappeared. Other chemicals known to induce or exacerbate porphyria cutanea tarda in humans are noted in Table 11-4.

The occurrence of drug-induced porphyria in humans during the 1950s was followed by a reexamination of other chemicals known to induce

Table 11-4. Agents Reported to Provoke or Aggravate
Porphyria Cutanea Tarda in Humans

Di- and trichlorophenols
Estrogens (natural and synthetic) diethystilbesterol
Ethyl alcohol
Hexachlorobenzene
2-Benzyl-4,6-dichlorophenol
2,3,6,7-Tetrachlorodibenzodioxin

Table 11-5. Examples of Porphyrogenic Activity of Drugs Tested in
Chick Embryo Cell Cultures

Pharmacologic action	Compounds tested	Porphyrogenic activity
Hypnotics and sedatives	Meprobamate	+
	Sedormid	+
	Barbiturates	+ to ++
	Sulphonal	++
Anticonvulsants	Hydantoins	± to +
	Succinimides	+ to ++
Analgesics and antirheumatics	Phenylbutazone	0
	Probenecid	+
Antibiotics	Chloramphenicol	+
	Griseofulvin	+++
Hypoglycemic agents	Tolbutamide	±
Other drugs	Chloroquine	0
	Isoniazid	+
Sex steroids	Testosterone	+
	Estradiol	+
	Progesterone	++
Other chemical agents	2-Allyl-2-Isopropyl-acetamide	++
	Hexachlorobenzene	++
	Lindane	++++
	Chlordane	++++

porphyria in animals. Elegant studies by Granick and Urata in 1963 first demonstrated that drugs could induce δ-aminolevulinic acid (ALA) synthetase (138), the rate-limiting enzyme of the heme synthesis. It was based on an in vitro system that employed the use of chick embryo liver cells. When these cells were cultured on cover slips, prophyrin synthesis could be measured in 24–28 hr using fluorescent microscopy. Different chemicals had marked differences in their inducing properties (Table 11-5). Granick deduced that steric factors were important and that they affected the induction of ALA synthetase, the rate-limiting enzyme of porphyrin (heme) synthesis. He suggested that the synthesis of this mitochondrial enzyme was controlled by an operator gene that could be regulated by an aporepressor (139). The aporepressor could be inhibited by selected chemicals, which would then result in increased or uncontrolled ALA synthetase activity.

Sex steroids and their 5B-metabolites have been shown to be potent inducers of hepatic ALAs in the chick embryo (139) and, in addition, various oral contraceptive hormones possess similar induction properties (140). Levere has shown that hepatic ALA activity is increased in selected males receiving stilbesterol therapy for carcinoma of the prostate (141, 142). Several studies have demonstrated the association of porphyria cutanea tarda with estrogen ingestion (143, 144). Statistically, there is a markedly increased incidence of porphyria cutanea tarda in women that can be associated with the ingestion of birth control pills.

Recent studies by Felsher et al. (145) indicate that selected individuals have a genetically determined decreased activity of uroporphyrinogen decarboxylase (Uro-D) inherited in an autosomal dominant pattern. In these patients all the classical signs, symptoms, and biochemical findings of porphyria cutanea tarda are present without an associated drug history. In other individuals, estrogen and/or ethanol appear to unmask or induce a relative deficiency of Uro-D activity. Whether or not this enzyme deficiency results in a compensatory increase in ALA synthetase activity remains to be determined.

Further studies have led to the following biochemical classification of three different structural groups of chemicals that induce ALA synthetase: barbiturates and allylisopropylacetamide; DDC and griseofulvin; and finally the sex-steroid hormones and their metabolites (139, 146–148). Another group of compounds, the chlorinated insecticides such as DOT and Lindane, have been shown to be inducers as well. These diverse compounds all have the property of enhancing the production of porphyrins in the chick embryo liver and some have the same effect in mammalian liver as well.

Drug-Induced Lupus Erythematosus and Pellagra

Lupus erythematosus and pellagra are both diseases in which photo-sensitivity may be a prominent, but not necessarily constant, feature of the clinical picture. They are particularly intriguing to consider because, while they may be induced by drugs, each occurs in patients in whom there is no history of drug exposure. Of further interest is the observation that some drugs, such as isoniazid, may induce either lupus or pellagra, although to our knowledge this has never been reported in the same patient.

Lupus Erythematosus. Lupus erythematosus derives its name from the classically described "butterfly" rash over the malar area of the face, which is now know to occur in less than half the patients with the disease (149). Traditionally lupus has been divided into two distinct forms. Discoid lupus erythematosus is generally limited to the skin, the characteristic lesions being atrophic reddish or hyperpigmented plaques on the face and scalp. More widespread forms of the disease may involve the trunk, extremities, and mucous membranes. The more severe and potentially fatal form of the disease is systemic lupus erythematosus (SLE), where multisystem involvement is a prominent feature, including the skin, lungs, heart, joints, and kidneys. The disease occurs predominantly in females. The specific etiology of SLE remains unknown, and apart from the drug-induced phenomena described here, the pathogenesis of this disease has been attributed to bacteria, viruses, lysosomes, hormones, and genetic factors (150).

Table 11-6. Drugs Associated with the Induction or
Exacerbation of Systemic Lupus Erythematosus in Humans

Diphenylhydantoin	p-Aminosalicylic acid
Griseofulvin	Penicillin
Guanoxan	Phenylbutazone
Hydralazine	Procainamide
Isonicotinic hydrazide	Propylthiouracil
Isoquinaze	Reserpine
Alpha methyldopa	Streptomycin
Methylphenylethylhydantoin	Sulfonamides
Methylthiouracil	Tetracycline
Oral contraceptives	Trimethadone

There is considerable evidence in the the recent literature, however, to suggest that the final common pathway in what may be a multifactorial etiology is the production of autoantibodies, particularly to DNA, which result in the formation of immune complexes (151). These immune complexes are deposited in basement membranes and activate complement. Chemotactic complement products result in an accumulation of neutrophils which phagocytize the complexes and release lysosomal cathepsins, resulting in basement membrane damage.

A wide variety of drugs has been implicated in the production of an SLE-like syndrome. Some of the more frequently implicated drugs are listed in Table 11-6. It should be noted, however, that the drug-induced SLE syndromes are usually reversible upon discontinuation of the drug and rarely cause the immune complex type of renal disease that is a prominent feature of spontaneously occurring SLE. In addition, the serologic abnormalities in the drug-induced syndrome are more limited. Antibodies to denatured (single-stranded) DNA or deoxyribonucleoprotein frequently occur in both drug-induced and spontaneous SLE, but antibodies to native DNA and the Sm nuclear antigen, which occur in spontaneous SLE, have not been convincingly demonstrated in the drug-induced syndrome.

An attractive hypothesis to explain the role of drugs in the induction of SLE is that they combine with DNA to form an immune complex. This complex has an increased index of sensitization, which has been particularly well studied by Tan in the case of hydralazine (152) and by Blomgren et al. in the case of procainamide (153). With regard to the hydralazine-induced lupus syndrome, Tan has demonstrated that the drug probably complexes with deoxyribonucleoprotein and is resistant to in vitro destruction by proteolytic enzymes. He suggests that this might be a mechanism for enhancing the immunogenicity of nucleoprotein (152).

Even more intriguing is the potential role of radiation in the pathogenesis of drug-induced SLE. Heat-denatured DNA and ^{14}C-procainamide were incubated with methylene blue, protoporphyrin, or riboflavin with subsequent exposure to visible light. The data indicated that an almost linear relationship existed between the binding of drug to DNA and the time period of photooxidation (153). This drug-DNA complex possessed structual changes which were immunologically recognizable when assayed by complement fixation. The immunogenicity of the complex, however, was no greater than that observed with denatured DNA alone (153). Although photooxidation was used only as a tool for binding drug to DNA in these experiments, the prospect that this may serve as a model for future investigation is encouraging.

Finally one must consider the possible role of radiation in the pathogenesis of SLE even in the absence of a known drug. Baehr et al. (154) observed that some of their patients with SLE appeared to have contracted their disease immediately following sunexposure, whereas they had no prior history of photosensitivity. In addition, patients with SLE studied by these investigators experienced exacerbation of their disease following sunburn. In general, however, one can detect photosensitivity in no more than 30% of patients with SLE.

Pellagra. Since 1952 (155) a pellagra-like syndrome has been reported in certain patients receiving therapy with isoniazid (INH). Classically, pellagra is characterized by dermatitis, dementia, and diarrhea. The cutaneous lesions are usually symmetric and occur in areas of the body subject to mild forms of trauma, such as friction, heat, and sunlight. In the traditional form of the disease, the skin lesions are usually the first to be noted and are characterized by redness, scaling, and hyperpigmentation. The healing process is slow and characterized by a desquamation or shedding of the superficial, darkened skin with the appearance of healthy, pink skin underneath.

Frequently, inflammation of the oral and rectal mucosae follows the skin manifestations. An accompanying feature is red, painful swollen tongue. Diarrhea is common and probably represents involvement of other areas of the gastrointestinal tract. Neurologic manifestations usually follow, but may occur without skin or digestive tract symptoms. They vary according to the severity of the disease, from weakness and malaise to delirium.

Since the classic observations of Goldberger et al. in 1915 (156), pellagra has been recognized as a dietary deficiency disease. Diets poor in protein, especially if poor in tryptophan and niacin, result in a deficiency of the coenzymes diphosphopyridine nucleotide (NADP) and triphosphopyridine nucleotide (NADPH). These compounds are essential factors in energy transport through their role as hydrogen acceptors in the oxidation–reduction reaction of cellular metabolism. A deficiency of these vital cofactors could lead to alterations in cellular metabolism which would retard mechanisms involved in injury repair. One would expect this to be particularly true in tissues with either high energy requirements, such as the brain, or in rapidly proliferating cells, such as occur in the skin in gastrointestinal mucosa. Thus, this might explain the predilection of the disease for these sites. In addition, several other drugs have been reported to be associated with the induction of pellagra. The role of INH in inducing a pellagra-like syndrome is thought to be competitive inhibition between the drug and nicotinamide (157), the latter being required for the synthesis of NADP and NADPH. Of further interest is the observation that 6-mercaptopurine, which also inhibits NADP synthesis, also causes a pellagra-like eruption (158). A similar syndrome has been reported in patients receiving 5-fluorouracil, a drug that can inhibit the conversion of tryptophan to niacin (150).

SUMMARY

Drug-induced photosensitivity refers to adverse cutaneous responses which follow the combined or successive exposure to certain chemicals and radiation. At present two distinct mechanisms, phototoxic and photoallergic, are known to mediate these reactions. In addition, drug-induced photo-sensitivity diseases have been documented to include porphyria, lupus erythematosus, and pellagra.

ACKNOWLEDGMENTS. This study was supported by Grant No. ES01041 from the National Institutes of Health, Columbia University Cancer Research Center Grant No. CA-13696 from the National Cancer Institute, and the Shiseido Co., Tokyo.

REFERENCES

1. Lamberg, S. I. (1967): A new photosensitizer, the artificial sweetner cyclamate. *J. AMA* **201**:747–750.
2. Wilkinson, D. S. (1961): Photodermatitis due to tetrachlorosalicylanilide. *Br. J. Dermatol.* **73**:213–219.
3. Harber, L. C., Harris, H., Leider, M., et al. (1964): Berloque (berlock) dermatitis. *Arch. Dermatol.* **90**:572–576.
4. Crow, K. D., Alexander, E., Buck, W. H. L., et al. (1961): Photosensitivity due to pitch *Br. J. Dermatol.* **73**:220–232.
5. Birmingham, D. J., Key, M. M., Tubich, G. E., et al. (1961): Phototoxic bullae among celery harvesters. *Arch. Dermatol.* **83**:73–87.
6. Raab, O. (1900): Uber die Wirkung fluorescierender Stoffe auf Infusorien. *Z. Biol.* **39**:524.
7. Tappeiner, H. V., and Jodlbauer, A. (1904): Die sensibilizierende Wirkung fluroescierender Substanzer. *Dtsch. Arch. Klin. Med.* **80**:524.
8. Blum, H. F. (1941): *Photodynamic Action and Diseases Caused by Light.* Reinhold, New York.
9. Oginsky, E. L., Green, G. S., Griffith, D. G., et al. (1959): Lethal photosensitization of bacteria with 8-methoxypsoralen to long wavelength ultraviolet radiation. *J. Bacteriol.* **78**:821–833.

10. Mathews, M. M. (1963): Comparative study of lethal photosensitization of *Sarcina lutea* by 8-methoxypsoralen and by toluidine blue. *J. Bacteriol.* **85**:322–328.

11. Pathak, M. A., Kramer, D. M., and Fitzpatrick, T. B. (1974): Photobiology and photochemistry of furocoumarins (psoralens). In: *Sunlight and Man: Normal and Abnormal Photobiologic Responses,* edited by M. A. Pathak, L. C. Harber, M. Seiji, et al., pp. 131–141. Univ. of Tokyo Press, Tokyo.

12. Blum, H. F. (1964): *Photodynamic Action and Diseases Caused by Light.* Hofner, New York.

13. Epstein, S. (1939): Photoallergy and primary photosensitivity to sulfanilamide. *J. Invest. Dermatol.* **2**:43–51.

14. Peterkin, G. A. (1945): Skin eruptions due to the local application of sulphonamides. *Br. J. Dermatol.* **57**:1–9.

15. Magnus, I. A. (1976): *Dermatological Photobiology,* pp. 213–217. Blackwell, London.

16. Forbes, P. D., Urbach, F., and Davies, R. E. (1978): Phototoxicity testing of fragrance raw materials, *Fd. Cosmet. Toxicol.* **15**:55–60.

17. Emmett, E. A. (1979): Phototoxicity from exogenous agents. *Photochem. Photobiol.* **30**:429–436.

18. Hjorth, N., and Moeller, H. (1976): Phototoxic textile dermatitis. *Arch. Dermatol.* **112**:1445–1447.

19. Gardiner, J. D., Dicksen, A., MacLeod, T. M., et al. (1972): The investigation of photocontact dermatitis in a dye manufacturing process. *Br. J. Dermatol.* **86**:264–271.

20. Sams, W. M., Jr., and Epstein, J. H. (1967): The experimental production of drug phototoxicity in guinea pigs. I. Using sunlight. *J. Invest. Dermatol.* **48**:89–94.

21. Epstein, J. H., Brunsting, L. A., Peterson, M. C., et al. (1957): Study of photosensitivity occurring with chlorpromazine therapy. *J. Invest. Dermatol.* **28**:329–338.

22. Epstein, S. (1968): Chlorpromazine photosensitivity: phototoxic and photoallergic reactions. *Arch. Dermatol.* **98**:354–363.

23. Foerster, H. R., and Schwartz, L. (1939): Industrial dermatitis and melanosis due to photosensitization. *Arch. Dermatol.* **39**:55–68.

24. Ramsay, C. A., and Obreshkova, E. (1974): Photosensitivity from nalidixic acid. *Br. J. Dermatol.* **91**:523–528.

25. De Eds, F., Wilson, R. H., and Thomas, J. O. (1940): Photosensitization by phenothiazene. *J. AMA* **114**:2095–2097.

26. Morris, W. E. (1960): Photosensitivity due to tetracycline derivatives. *J. AMA* **172**:1155–1156.

27. Falk, M. S. (1960): Light sensitivity due to demethylchlortetracycline. *J. AMA* **172**:1156–1157.

28. Harber, L. C., Tromovitsh, T. A., and Baer, R. L. (1961): Studies on photosensitivity due to demethylchlortetracycline. *J. Invest. Dermatol.* **37**:189–193.

29. Domonkos, A. N. (1975): *Andrew's Diseases of the Skin,* Chap. 3, pg. 40. W. B. Saunders, Philadelphia.

30. Lerner, A. B., Denton, C. R., and Fitzpatrick, T. B. (1953): Clinical and experimental studies with 8-methoxypsoralen in vitiligo. *J. Invest. Dermatol.* **20**:299–314.

31. Kaidbey, K. H., and Kligman, A. M. (1974): Topical photosensitizers. Influence of vehicles on penetration. *Arch. Dermatol.* **110**:868–870.

32. Freeman, R. G., and Knox, J. M. (1964): Influence of temperature on ultraviolet injury. *Arch. Dermatol.* **89**:858–864.

33. Levine, G. M., and Harber, L. C. (1969): The effect of humidity on the phototoxic response to 8-methoxypsoralen in guinea pigs. *Acta Derm. Venereol. (Stockh.)* **49**:82–86.

34. Harber, L. C., and Baer, R. L. (1972): Pathogenic mechanisms of drug-induced photosensitivity. *J. Invest. Dermatol.* **58**:327–342.

35. Breza, T. S., Halprin, K. M., and Taylor, J. R. (1975): Photosensitivity to vinblastine. *Arch. Dermatol.* **111**:1168-1170.
36. Allison, A. C., Magnus, I. A., and Young, M. R. (1966): Role of lysosomes and of cell membrane in photosensitization. *Nature* **209**:874-878.
37. Giese, A., and Grossman, E. B. (1946): Sensitization of cells to heat by visible light in the presence of photodynamic dyes. *J. Gen. Physiol.* **29**:193-202.
38. Fleischer, A. S., Harber, L. C., Cook, J. S., et al. (1966): Mechanisms of *in vitro* photohemolysis in erythropoietic protoporphyria. *J. Invest. Dermatol.* **46**:505-509.
39. Masajo, L., Rodighiero, G., Caporale, G., et al. (1974): Photoreactions between skin-photosensitizing furocourmarins and nucleic acids. In: *Sunlight and Man: Normal and Abnormal Photobiologic Responses,* edited by M. A. Pathak, L. C. Harber, M. Seiji, et al., pp. 369-387. Univ. of Tokyo Press, Tokyo.
40. Ljunggren, B. (1977): Phenothiazine phototoxicity: toxic chlorpromazine photoproducts. *J. Invest. Dermatol.* **69**:383-386.
41. Kochevar, I. E. (1980): Possible mechanisms of toxicity due to photochemical products of protriptyline. *Toxicol. Appl. Pharmacol* **54**:258-264.
42. Foote, C. S. (1976): Photosensitized oxidation and singlet oxygen: consequences in biological systems. In: *Free Radicals in Biology,* edited by W. A. Pryor, pp. 85-134. Academic Press, New York.
43. Lamola, A. A., Yamane, T., and Trozzolo, A. M. (1973): Cholesterol hyproperoxide formation in red cell membranes and photohemolysis in erythropoietic protoporphyria. *Science* **1979**:1131-1133.
44. Lochmann, E. R., and Micheler, A. (1973): Binding of organic dyes to nucleic acids and the photodynamic effect. In: *Physicochemical Properties of Nucleic Acids,* edited by J. Duchesne, Vol. I, pp. 223-267. Academic Press, New York.
45. Spikes, J. D., and MacKnight, M. L. (1970): Dye sensitized photooxidation of proteins. *Ann. N.Y. Acad. Sci.* **171**:149-162.
46. Girotti, A. (1975); Photodynamic action of bilirubin in human erythrocyte membranes. *Biochemistry* **14**:3377-3383.
47. Hsu, J., Goldstein, B. D., and Harber, L. C. (1971): Photoreactions associated with *in vitro* hemolysis in erythropoietic protoporphyria. *Photochem. Photobiol.* **13**:67-77.
48. Johnson, B. (1974): Cellular mechanisms of chlorpromazine photosensitivity. *Proc. R. Soc. Med.* **67**:871-873.
49. Kochevar, I. E., and Lamola, A. A. (1979): Chlorpromazine and protriptyline photo-toxicity: photosensitized, oxygen independent red cell lysis. *Photochem. Photobiol.* **29**:791-796.
50. Goldstein, B. D., and Harber, L. C. (1972): Erythropoietic protoporphyria: lipid per-oxidation and red cell membrane damage associated with photohemolysis. *J. Clin. Invest.* **51**:892-902.
51. Schothorst, A. A., van Steveninck, J., Went, L. N., et al. (1972): Photodynamic damage of the erythrocyte membrane caused by protoporphyrin in protoporphyria and in normal red blood cells. *Clin. Chim. Acta* **39**:161-170.
52. Dubbelman, T. M. A. R., de Goeij, A. F. P. M., and van Steveninck, J. (1980): Protoporphyrin-induced photodynamic effects on transport processes across the membrane of human erythrocytes. *Biochim. Biophys. Acta* **595**:133-139.
53. Girotti, A. (1979): Protoporphyrin-sensitized photodamage in isolater membranes of human erythrocytes. *Biochemistry* **18**:4403-4411.
54. Desai, I. D., Savant, P. L., and Tappel, A. L. (1964): Peroxidation and radiation damage to isolated lysosomes. *Biochim. Biophys. Acta* **86**:277-285.
55. Song, P. -S., and Tapley, K. J., Jr. (1979): Photochemistry and photobiology of psoralens. *Photochem. Photobiol.* **29**:1177-1197.
56. Cole, R. S., Levithan, D., and Sinden, R. R. (1976): Removal of psoralen interstrand

cross-links from DNA of *Escherichia coli*: mechanism and genetic control. *J. Mol. Biol.* **103**:39–59.

57. Poppe, W., and Grossweiner, L. I. (1979): Photodynamic sensitization by 8-methoxypsoralen via the singlet oxygen mechanism. *Photochem. Photobiol.* **22**:217–219.

58. Goyal, G. C., and Grossweiner, L. I. (1979): The effect of DNA binding on initial 8-methoxypsoralen photochemistry. *Photochem. Photobiol.* **29**:847–850.

59. Satanove, A., and McIntosh, J. S. (1967): Phototoxic reactions induced by light doses of chlorpromazine and thoridazine. *J. AMA* **200**:121–124.

60. Kaidbey, K. H., and Kligman, A. M. (1978): Identification of systemic phototoxic drugs by human intradermal assay. *J. Invest. Dermatol.* **70**:272–274.

61. Schultz, K. H., Wiskemann, A., and Wulf, K. (1956): Klinische und experimentelle Untersuchungen uber die photodynamische Worksamkeit von Phenotheizinderivaten, insbesundere von Megaphen. *Arch. Klin. Exp. Dermatol.* **202**:285–298.

62. Hunder, J. A. A., Blutani, L. K., and Magnus, I. A. (1970): Chlorpromazine photosensitivity in mice: its action specrum and the effect of anti-inflammatory agents. *Br. J. Dermatol.* **82**:157.

63. Ljunggren, B., and Moeller, H. (1977): Phenathiazine phototoxicity: an experimental study in chlorpromazine and its metabolites. *J. Invest. Dermatol.* **68**:313–317.

64. Kelly-Garvert, F., and Legator, M. S. (1973): Photoactivation of chlorpromazine: cytogenetic and mutagenic effects. *Mutat. Res.* **21**:101–105.

65. Jose, J. G. (1979): Photomutagenesis by chlorinated phenathiazine tranquilizers. *Proc. Natl. Acad. Sci. U.S.A.* **76**:469–472.

66. Starples, D. (1974): The binding of chlorpromazine to human serum albumin. *J. Pharm. Pharmacol.* **26**:640–641.

67. Kantesaria, P., and Marfey, P. (1975): The effect of chlorpromazine in some properties of DNA in solution. *Physiol. Chem. Phys.* **7**:53–67.

68. Kwant, W. O., and Suman, P. (1969): The membrane concentration of a local anasthetic (chlorpromazine). *Biochim. Biophys. Acta* **183**:530–543.

69. Kahn, G., and Davis, B. P. (1970): *In vitro* studies on long wavelength ultraviolet light-dependent reactions of the skin photosensitizer chlorpromazine with nucleic acids, purines and pyrimidines. *J. Invest. Dermatol.* **55**:47–52.

70. Rosenthal, I., Ben-hur, E., Prager, A., et al. (1978): Photochemical reactions to chlorpromazine: chemical and biochemical implication. *Photochem. Photobiol.* **28**:591–594.

71. Day, R. S., and Dimattina, M. (1977): Photodynamic action of chlorpromazine in adenovirus 5: repairable damage and single strand breaks. *Chem. Biol. Interact.* **17**:89–97.

72. Jose, J. G., and Yielding, K. L. (1978): Photosensitive cataractogens, chlorpromazine and methoxypsoralen, cause DNA repair synthesis in lens epithelial cells. *Invest. Ophthalmol. Vis. Sci.* **17**:687–691.

73. Matsuo, I., Ohkido, M., Fujita, H., et al. (1980): Chlorpromazine photosensitization: failure to detect any evidence for involvement of DNA damage in the photodynamic killing of *Escherichia coli* in the presence of chlorpromazine. *Photochem. Photobiol.* **31**:175–178.

74. Copeland, E. S., Alving, C. R., and Grenan, M. M. (1976): Light-induced leakage of spin label marker from liposomes in the presence of phototoxic phenothiazines. *Photochem. Photobiol.* **24**:41–48.

75. Kaidbey, K. H., and Kligman, A. M. (1977): Clinical and histological study of coal tar phototoxicity in humans. *Arch. Dermatol.* **113**:592–595.

76. Burckhardt, W. (1939): Zeer Frage der Photosensibilisierunden wirkung des Teers. *Schweiz. Med. Wochenschr.* **69**:83.

77. Foerster, H. R., and Schwartz, L. (1939): Industrial dermatitis and melanosis due to photosensitization. *Arch. Dermatol. Syphilol* **39**:55–68.

78. Everett, M. A., and Miller, J. V. (1961): Coal tar and ultraviolet light II. Cumulative effects. *Arch. Dermatol.* **84**:937–940.

79. Blackburn, G. M., and Fenwick, R. G., Lockwood, G., et al. (1977): Photoproducts from DNA pyrimidine bases and polycyclic aromatic hydrocarbons. *Nucleic Acids Res.* 4:2487–2494.

80. Epstein, J. H., Tuffanelli, D. L., Seibut, J. S., et al. (1976): Porphyrialike cutaneous changes induced by tetracycline hydrochloride photosensitization. *Arch. Dermatol.* 112:661–666.

81. Stratigos, J. D., and Magnus, I. A. (1968): Photosensitivity by demethylchlortetracycline and sulfanilamide. *Br. J. Dermatol.* 80:391–405.

82. Schorr, W. F., and Monash, S. (1963): Photo-irradiation studies of two tetracyclines. *Arch. Dermatol.* 88:440–443.

83. Freeman, R. G. (1970): Interaction of phototoxic compounds with cells in tissue culture. *Arch. Dermatol.* 102:521–526.

84. Schothorst, A. A., Suurmond, D., and de Luster, A. (1979): A biochemical screening test for the photosensitizing potential of drugs and disinfectants. *Photochem. Photobiol.* 29:531–537.

85. Blum, H. F. (1941): Studies of photosensitivity due to sulfanilamide. *J. Invest. Dermatol.* 4:159–173.

86. Aoki, K, and Saito, T. (1974): Studies in the mechanism of photosensitivity caused by sulfa drugs. In: *Sunlight and Man: Normal and Abnormal Photobiologic Responses,* edited by M. A. Pathak, L. C. Harber, M. Seiji, et al., pp. 431–444. Univ. of Tokyo Press, Tokyo.

87. Sam, S. K., and Tomlinson, D. R. (1976): Chlorpromazine-induced histamine release from guinea pig skin in vitro—a photosensitive reaction. *Arch. Dermatol. Res.* 255:219–223.

88. Lord, J. T., Zeboh, V. A., Poitier, J., et al. (1976): The effects of photosensitizers and ultraviolet irradiation on the biosynthesis and metabolism of prostaglandins. *Br. J. Dermatol.* 95:397–406.

89. Lord, J. T., Zeboh, V. A., Blick, G., et al. (1978): The effects of photosensitizing antibiotics and ultraviolet irradiation on the biosynthesis of prostaglandins. *Br. J. Dermatol.* 98:31–38.

90. Warin, A. P. (1978): The ultraviolet erythemas in man. *Br. J. Dermatol.* 98:473–477.

91. Morison, W. L., Paul, B. S., and Parrish, J. A. (1977): The effects of indomethacin on long-wave ultraviolet-induced delayed erythema. *J. Invest. Dermatol.* 68:130–133.

92. Gschnait, F., and Pehamberger, H. (1977): Indomethacin does not affect PUVA induced erythema. *Arch. Dermatol. Res.* 259:109

93. Epstein, J. H. (1972): Photoallergy. A review. *Arch. Dermatol.* 106:741–748.

94. Morison, W. L., Parrish, J. A., and Epstein, J. H. (1979): Photoimmunology. *Arch. Dermatol.* 115:350–355.

95. Wilkinson, D. S. (1961): Photodermatitis due to tetrachlorosalicylanilide. *Br. J. Dermatol.* 73:213–219.

96. Fregert, S, and Moller, H. (1964): Photocross-sensitization among halogenhydroxybenzoic acid derivatives. *J. Invest. Dermatol.* 43:271–274.

97. Schwarz, J, and Schwarz-Speck, M. (1957): Experimentelle Untersuchungen zur Frage der Photoallergie der Sulfonamide. *Dermatologica* 114:232–243.

98. Vinson, L. J., and Borselli, V. F. (1966): A guinea pig assay of the photosensitizing potential of topical germicides. *J. Soc. Cosmet. Chem.* 17:123–130.

99. Harber, L. C., Targovnik, S. E., and Baer, R. L. (1967): Contact photosensitivity to halogenated salicylanilides: in man and guinea pigs. *Arch. Dermatol.* 96:646–656.

100. Schwartz, K. F. (1969): Experimentelle Unterschungen zur Photoallergic gegen Sulfanilamid und Chlorpromazine. *Dermatologica (Suppl.)* 139:1–88.

101. Kochevar, I. E., Zalar, G. L., Einbinder, J., et al. (1979): Assay of contact photosensitivity to musk ambrette in guinea pigs. *J. Invest. Dermatol.* 73:144–146.

102. Willis, I., and Kligman, A. M. (1968): The mechanism of photoallergic contact dermatitis. *J. Invest. Dermatol.* 51:378–384.

103. Mathias, C. G. B., Maicbac, H. I., and Epstein, J. (1978): Allergic contact photodermatitis to para-aminobenzoic acid. *Arch. Dermatol.* 114:1665–1666.

104. O'Quinn, S., Kennedy, C. B., and Isbell, K. H. (1967): Contact photodermatitis due to bithionol and related compounds. *J. AMA* **199:**125–128.
105. Jillson, O. F., and Baughman, R. D. (1963): Contact photodermatitis from bithionol. *Arch. Dermatol.* **88:**409–418.
106. Hitselberger, J. F., and Fosnaugh, R. P. (1962): Photosensitivity due to chlorpropamide. *J. AMA* **180:**62–63.
107. Burry, J. M. (1967): Photoallergies to fentichlor and multifungin. *Arch. Dermatol.* **95:**287–291.
108. Morikawa, F., Nakayama, Y., Fukuda, M., et al. (1974): Techniques for evaluation of phototoxicity and photoallergy in laboratory animals and man. In: *Sunlight and Man: Normal and Abnormal Photobiologic Responses,* edited by M. A. Pathak, L. C. Harber, M. Seiji, et al., pp. 529–557. Univ. of Tokyo Press, Tokyo.
109. Kaidbey, K. H., and Kligman, A. M. (1978): Photocontact allergy to 6-methylcoumarin. *Contact Derm.* **4:**277–282.
110. Raugi, G. J., Storrs, F. S., and Larsen, W. G. (1979): Photoallergic contact dermatitis to men's perfume. *Contact Derm.* **5:**251–260.
111. Sidi, E., Hincky, M., and Gervais, A. (1955): Allergic sensitization and photosensitization to Phenergan cream. *J. Invest. Dermatol.* **24:**345–352.
112. Harber, L. C., Lashinsky, A. M., and Baer, R. L. (1959): Skin manifestations of photosensitivity due to chlorothiazide and hydrochlorothiazide. *J. Invest. Dermatol.* **33:**83–84.
113. Harber, L. C., Baer, R. L., and Bickers, D. R. (1974): Techniques of evaluation of phototoxicity and photoallergy in biologic systems, including man, with particular emphasis on immunologic aspects. In: *Sunlight and Man: Normal and Abnormal Photobiologic Responses,* edited by M. A. Pathak, L. C. Harber, M. Seiji, et al., pp. 515–528. Univ. of Tokyo Press, Tokyo.
114. Cripps, D. J., and Enta, T. (1970): Absorption and action spectrum studies on bithionol and halogenated salicylanilide photosensitivity. *Br. J. Dermatol.* **82:**230–242.
115. Freeman, R. G., and Knox, J. M. (1968): The action spectrum of photocontact dermatitis caused by halogenated salicylanilides and related compounds. *Arch. Dermatol.* **97:**130–136.
116. Giovinazzo, V. J., Harber, L. C. Armstrong, R. B., et al. (1980): Photoallergic contact dermatitis to must ambrette: clinical report of two patients with persistent light reactor patterns. *J. Am. Acad. Dermatol.* **3:**384.
117. Willis, I., and Kligman, A. M. (1968): The mechanism of the persistent light reactor. *J. Invest. Dermatol.* **51:**385–394.
118. Kochevar, I. E. (1979): Photoallergic responses to chemicals. *Photochem. Photobiol.* **30:**437–442.
119. Harber, L. C., and Baer, R. L. (1969): Mechanisms of drug photosensitivity reactions. *Toxicol. Appl. Pharmacol. Suppl.* **3:**58–67.
120. Jung, E. G., Dummler, V., and Immich, H. (1968): Photoallergie durch 4-chlor-2-hydroxy-benzoesaure-*n*-butylamide II. *Arch. Klin. Exp. Med.* **232:**403–412.
121. Herman, P. S., and Sams, W. M., Jr. (1970): Carrier protein specificity in salicylanilide sensitivity. *J. Invest. Dermatol.* **54:**438–439.
122. Herman, P. S., and Sams, W. M., Jr. (1971): Requirement for carrier protein in salicylanilide sensitivity: the migration inhibition test in contact photoallergy. *J. Lab. Clin. Med.* **77:**572–579.
123. Kochevar, I. E., and Harber, L. C. (1977): Photoreactions of 3,3′,4′,5-tetrachloro-salicylanilide with proteins. *J. Invest. Dermatol.* **68:**151–156.
124. Jung, E. G., Hornke, J., and Hajdu, P. (1968): Photoallergie durch 4-chlor-2-hydroxy-benzpesauer-*N*-butylamid. I. *Arch. Klin. Exp. Dermatol.* **233:**287–295.
125. Coxon, J. A., Jenkins, F. P., and Welti, D. (1965): The effect of light on halogenated salicylanilide ions. *Photochem. Photobiol.* **4:**713–718.

126. Herman, P. S., and Sams, W. M., Jr. (1971): Requirement for carrier protein in salicylanilide sensitivity: the mitgration inhibition test in contact photoallergy. *J. Lab. Clin. Med.* **77**:572–579.

127. DeMatteis, F. (1967): Disturbances of liver porphyrin metabolism caused by drugs. *Pharmacol. Rev.* **19**:523–557.

128. Kappas, A., Song, C. S., Levere, R. D., et al. (1968): Induction of δ-aminolevulinic acid synthetase in vivo in chick embryo liver by natural steroids. *Proc. Natl. Acad. Sci. U.S.A.* **61**:509–513.

129. Stonard, M. D. (1974): Experimental hepatic porphyria induced by hexachlorobenzene as a model for human symptomatic porphyria. *Br. J. Haematol.* **27**:617–625.

130. Harber, L. C., and Bickers, D. R. (1975): The porphyrias: basic science aspects, clinical diagnosis and management. In: *Yearbook of Dermatology, 1975,* edited by F. D. Malkinson and R. W. Pearson, pp. 9–47. Year Book Publishers, Chicago.

131. Eales, L. (1963): Porphyria as seen in Cape Town: a survey of 250 patients and some recent studies. *S. Afr. J. Lab. Clin. Med.* **9**:151–162.

132. Brunsting, L. A., Mason, H. L., and Aldrich, R. A. (1951): Adult form of chronic porphyria with cutaneous manifestations: report of 17 additional cases. *J. AMA* **146**:1207–1212.

133. Watson, C. J. (1960): The problem of porphyria: some facts and questions. *N. Engl. J. Med.* **263**:1205–1215.

134. Watson, C. J., Lowry, P. T., Schmid, R., et al. (1951): Manifestation of different forms of porphyria in relation to chemical findings. *Trans. Assoc. Am. Physicians* **64**:345–352.

135. Cam, C., and Nigogosyan, G. (1963): Acquired toxic porphyria cutanea tarda due to hexachlorobenzene intoxication. *J. AMA* **183**:88–91.

136. Ockner, R. K., and Schmid, R. (1961): Acquired toxic porphyria cutanea tarda due to hexachlorobenzene. *Nature* **189**:499.

137. Bleiberg, J., Wallen, M., Brodkin, R., et al. (1964): Industrially acquired prophyria. *Arch. Dermatol.* **89**:793–797.

138. Granick, S., and Urata, G. (1963): Increase in activity of delta-aminolevulinic acid synthetase in liver mitochondria induced by feeding of 3,5-dicarbethozl-1,4-dihydro-collidine. *J. Biol. Chem.* **238**:821–827.

139. Granick, S. (1966): The induction in vitro of the synthesis of δ-aminolevulinic acid synthetase in chemical porphyria: a response to certain drugs, sex hormones and foreign chemicals. *J. Biol. Chem.* **241**:1359–1375.

140. Rifkind, A. B., Gillette, P. N., Song, C. S., et al. (1970): Induction of hepatic δ-aminolevulinic acid synthetase by oral contraceptive steroids. *J. Clin. Endocrinol. Metab.* **30**:330–335.

141. Levere, R. D. (1967): Porphyrin synthesis in hepatic cirrhosis: increase in δ-aminolevulinic acid synthetase. *Biochem. Med.* **1**:92–99.

142. Levere, R. D. (1966): Stilbesterol-induced porphyria: increase in hepatic δ-aminolevulinic acid synthetase. *Blood* **28**:569–572.

143. Zimmerman, T. S., McMillin, J. M., and Watson, C. J. (1966): Onset of manifestations of hepatic porphyria in relation to the influence of female sex hormones. *Arch. Intern. Med.* **118**:229–240.

144. Warin, R. P. (1963): Porphyria cutanea tarda associated with estrogen therapy for prostatic carcinoma. *Br. J. Dermatol.* **75**:298–299.

145. Felsher, B. F., Norris, M. E., and Shih, J. C. (1978): Red cell uroporphyrinogen decarboxylase in prophyria cutanea tarda. *N. Engl. J. Med.* **299**:1095–1098.

146. Granick, S., and Kappas, A. (1967): Steroid induction of prophyrin synthesis in liver cell culture I. *J. Biol. Chem.* **242**:4587–4593.

147. Kappas, A., and Granick, S. (1968): Steroid induction of porphyrin synthesis in liver cell culture II. *J. Biol. Chem.* **243**:346–351.

148. De Matteis, F. (1971): Drugs and porphyria. *S. Afr. J. Lab. Clin. Med.* **18**:126–133.

149. Talbott, J. H. (1974): *Collagen-Vascular Diseases.* Grune & Stratton, New York.
150. Harber, L. C., and Baer, R. L. (1972): Pathogenic mechanisms of drug-induced photosensitivity. *J. Invest. Dermatol.* **58**:327–342.
151. Rodman, G. P. (ed.) (1973): Primer on the rheumatic diseases. *J. AMA (Suppl)* **224**:701–805.
152. Tan, E. M. (1974): Drug-induced autoimmune disease. *Fed. Proc.* **33**:1894–1897.
153. Bromgren, S. E., Condemi, J. J., and Vaughan, J. H. (1972): Procainamide-induced lupus erythematosus. Clinical and laboratory observations. *Am. J. Med.* **52**:338–348.
154. Baehr, G., Klemperer, P., and Schifien, A. (1935): A diffuse disease of the peripheral circulation. *Trans. Assoc. Am. Physician* **50**:139–155.
155. McConnell, R. B., and Cheetham, H. D. (1952): Acute pellagra during isonazid therapy. *Lancet* **263**:959–960.
156. Goldberger, J., Waring, C. H., and Willets, H. D. (1915): The prevention of pellagra: a test diet among institutional inmates. *Public Health Rep.* **30**:3117–3131.
157. Harber, L. C., Baer, R. L., and Bickers, D. R. (1974): Photosensitization to drugs. Clinical features and mechanisms of action. In: *Proceedings of the International Conference on Photosensitization and Photoprotection,* pp. 211–220. Kanehara Shuppan, Tokyo.
158. Ludwig, G. D., and White, C. (1960): Pellagra induced by 6-mercaptopurine. *Clin. Res.* **8**:212.

12

Photodermatoses

H. Ippen

Under the term photodermatoses or light-dependent (light-influenced) skin diseases we intend to deal here with those changes in the skin that are caused, initiated, or aggravated by light. The structure of the skin is complex and its possible modes of reaction numerous. Therefore, it is not surprising that a large number of such skin diseases has been described. It is thus necessary to have as logical a classification as possible based on physiologic photoreaction. These reactions will be described briefly by way of introduction.

Every biochemical and structural change in the skin resulting from the action of light presupposes the fulfilment of a number of conditions which influence the localization, the type, and the course of all cutanecus photoreactions. Light-dependent skin changes occur only in those areas that are not largely protected from light either for anatomical reasons (hairiness or fold-formation, e.g., in the rima ani) or by clothing. The protection afforded by clothing requires cautious assessment, however, since thin textiles and those made of synthetic fibers may admit large quantities of light, so that with a high degree of light sensitivity it is possible for skin changes to occur in apparently covered zones.

Light must reach the living cells of the skin. The occurrence of all photoreactions is decisively influenced by penetration, especially in areas where a thick horny layer (palms of the hand, soles of the feet, nails) absorbs, reflects, or scatters those quantities of light that are otherwise photochemically and thus photobiologically active in the epidermis. Quality and quantity of the cutaneous photoreactions therefore depend on the penetration of light of individual wavelengths into the different layers of the skin (see Chapter 6).

H. Ippen • Hautklinik and Poliklinik, Kliniken der Universität Gottingen, Gottingen, West Germany.

The light penetrating the skin must be biologically active. The law of Grotthus and Draper must naturally also apply in skin photobiology, namely that the only wavelengths able to cause reactions are those that are absorbed by the reacting system.

The biologically active light must be present in adequate quantity. For sunlight this rule applies primarily to the ultraviolet (UV) components, since the ratio of UVB to UVA can differ greatly in relationship to climate, time of day, and season. Photobiologic effects, such as delayed erythema, caused primarily by UVB, can also be caused by large doses of UVA (see Chapter 8). Because sun may have a considerably greater amount of UVA than UVB, an apparent displacement of the "action spectrum" for sunburn occurs. The actual spectral sensitivity of the skin is unchanged; the apparent shift is because the solar spectrum is rich in the longer wavelengths. In addition, many photoreactions of the skin show such efficient recovery or repair that despite the general validity of the law of reciprocity (constant effect given constant product of intensity and time) very low intensity of light over sufficiently long periods does not necessarily show the same effect as high intensity over correspondingly short periods of time.

MORPHOLOGY OF LIGHT DAMAGE TO NORMAL SKIN AS A BASIS FOR THE CLASSIFICATION OF PHOTODERMATOSES

The exact etiology of most photodermatoses is not known and therefore all classifications are somewhat theoretical and arbitrary, but they are helpful in providing a framework to discuss likely pathophysiologic processes. The morphology of the reactions of normal skin to UV radiation may serve as a basis for classification. Acute light damage to the skin is characterized by (1) erythema, edema, more rarely (intraepidermal) blistering, and very rarely necroses; and (2) focal thickening of the horny layer, desquamation, hyperpigmentation (suntan), more rarely depigmentation, and very rarely scarring. Chronic light damage, i.e., actinic skin degeneration, by contrast, shows the following symptoms: (1) connective tissue degeneration (elastosis) and atrophy of the epidermis, (2) poikiloderma (hyper- and hypopigmentation together with telangiectasia), (3) focal hyperkeratoses (actinic keratoses), precanceroses, (4) squamous cell carcinoma, basal cell carcinoma, melanosis precarcinomatosa, melanoma, and questionably keratoacanthoma.

Because a great number of photodermatoses are similar to the acute or chronic form of light damage, it may be concluded that these diseases involve basically similar fundamental pathophysiologic processes, and that the skin's own intrinsic (autochthonous) light-sensitive structures or substances play the pathogenic leading role in such photodermatoses. I have therefore termed this group of photodermatoses, which corresponds morphologically to sunburn or chronic light damage to the skin, *photo-auto-reactions.*

In the case of the second group of photodermatoses, on the other hand, the morphology differs to a greater or lesser extent from UV-induced reactions of normal skin. Thus we may find here something like the following types of rashes or symptoms: wheals and papules, eczema and lichenification, prurigo type changes, subepidermal bullae, scleroderma-like changes, and many others. For these photodermatoses, it may be assumed that fundamental photochemical reactions take place with substances not normally found in the skin or at least not normally reacting photochemically there. I have termed this type *photo-hetero-reactions*. In individual cases, e.g., in the case of photoallergic eczema, the basic photochemical process has occurred in a substance foreign to the skin.

For the third group it is necessary to consider the topography of the skin changes: the photo-auto-reactions are strictly limited to the skin exposed to light, although it must be borne in mind that in the case of a high degree of light sensitivity, in xeroderma pigmentosum for instance, even small light quantities reaching the skin through relatively thin clothing can have a provocative effect. The photo-hetero-reactions are also limited to skin exposed to the light. However, in an allergic pathogenesis, such as in photoallergic eczema (and solar urticaria), "dissemination phenomena" occur. These are probably due to the fact that photochemically formed antigen–antibody complexes or immunocompetent cells reach the skin protected from light and likewise cause skin changes there, albeit not very marked ones.

There are dermatoses which occur on skin areas completely protected from the light, e.g., psoriasis, but which nevertheless often reveal a distinct light-provocation. This third group was termed *photo-Koebner-phenomena*

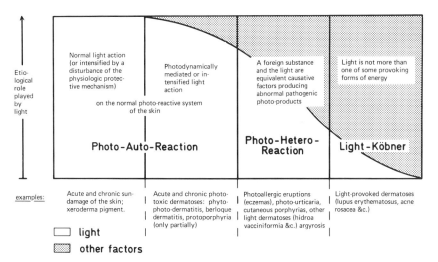

Fig. 12-1. Significance of light in the different types of photodermatoses.

by Gross (1) since an "isomorphic stimulant effect" (Koebner's isomorphic phenomenon) is involved. In general, Koebner's phenomena describe the appearance of disease-specific skin changes in response to nonspecific stimuli, such as can be observed in a large number of skin diseases, and especially in psoriasis vulgaris and lichen planus. The dermatoses listed in this group do not represent photodermatoses in the true sense insofar as light is not a fundamental pathogenic factor as it is in the case of the other two groups. Light energy in this case is only one of many possible provocative factors, among which rubbing and scratching, surface injuries, and burning or even irritation by chemicals can be listed. Accordingly, no wavelength specificity is discernible in this group as a general rule.

This classification of the light-dependent dermatoses can be presented in schematic form (Fig. 12-1).

PHOTO-AUTO-REACTIONS (Table 12-1)

According to present knowledge, the photodermatoses corresponding morphologically to the normal photoreactions of the skin occur in two ways: (1) through disturbance of the normal protective mechanism against the effects of radiation, and (2) through an increase in the quantity of active light energy occurring via photosensitization processes. In both cases the physiologic light-induced changes in the skin occur in more marked form and/or more rapidly. Prototypes of these two pathogenic mechanisms are xeroderma pigmentosum and the internally released phototoxic reaction (e.g., to Declomycin), respectively. In the first case there is severe chronic light damage with malignomas, occurring in childhood instead of at 60, 70, or 80 years of age; in the second case the result is a severe sunburn, with all its sequelae, occurring after perhaps a 5-min exposure to the sun instead of after an hour. Basically, however, each of the pathogenic mechanisms may lead to acute and to chronic photodermatoses, as following examples in Table 12-2 show.

Photo-auto-reactions Resembling Chronic Light Damage

Xeroderma Pigmentosum (2–17). This rare photodermatosis results from inherited enzyme defects in the "dark repair" system of the skin. Whereas in persons with healthy skin a large portion of the thymine dimers produced in the prickle cells by UVB is removed in a multienzyme process, in patients with xeroderma pigmentosum this repair process is disturbed by the absence or deficiency of one of the repair enzymes. Clinically this dermatosis is expressed, in its typical course, by the appearance of acute pellagroid erythema of the infant's or young child's skin where it is exposed to the light. In these areas all the signs of chronically light-affected skin appear more rapidly, with densely packed, brownish black, 2–5-mm melanin spots

Table 12-1. Photodermatoses Related to Exogenous Factors

Class	Group or substance	Type of reaction	Remarks and references[e]
Drugs			
Psychopharmacals	Chlordiazepoxide[a]	Photoallergic	[1]
	Antiepileptics[a] (Tridione, Dilantin)	Photoallergic	Cofactor?
		Prophyria cutanea tarda	[2,3]
	Barbiturates	Phototoxic[b]	By systemic application
	Phenothiazines	Phototoxic, melanosis	[4]
	Amitriptylin	Photoallergic[b]	[5]
	Quietidin	Phototoxic	[6]
	Pyritinol	Photoallergic[b]	
	Hematoporphyrin	Phototoxic	
Antihistamines	Phenothiazines	Photoallergic	By topical application
	Diphenylmethoxyethylamines	Photoallergic	Diphenhydramin [7], carbinoxamin, chlorphenoxamin
Local anesthetics	Cyproheptadin	Photoallergic[b]	[8]
	Procaine and related drugs	Photoallergic	[9]
Antineuralgics	Salicylates[a]	Photoallergic	
	Phenylbutazone[a]	Photoallergic	[10]
	Gold salts	Metal deposition (chrysiasis)	
Antidiabetics	Sulfinamides	Photoallergic	Mainly carbutamide
	Sulfonylureas	Photoallergic	Tolbutamide, chlorpropamide
Anticontraceptives	All combinations of estrogens and gestagens[a]	Porphyria cutanea tarda	Cofactor? [11]
		Hyperpigmentations	Chloasma-like
Estrogens	Only stilbestrol and related substances[a]	Photoallergic[b]	Cofactor? [12]
		Porphyria cutanea tarda	Cofactor; mainly in the therapy of prostate cancer
		Porphyria cutanea tarda	

(*Continued*)

Table 12-1. (cont.)

Class	Group or substance	Type of reaction	Remarks and References[e]
Cardiovascular drugs	Quinidine	Photoallergic[b]	[13]
	Amiodarone	Hyperpigmentation	[14]
	Hypertensives (see Diuretics below)		
Laxatives	Triacetyl-diphenolisatin (TDI)	Photoallergic	Lichen planus-like
Diuretics	(Hydro)chlorothiazid	Photoallergic[b]	[15]
	Quinethazone	Photoallergic	
Dermatologicals	Furocoumarins	Phototoxic	See also plants, foods, and drugs
	Coal tar	Phototoxic	
	Dithranol[a]	Phototoxic	
	Thioxolon	Phototoxic	[16]
Antibiotics	Tetracyclines	Phototoxic	Demeclocycline and others
	Griseofulvin[a]	Photoallergic	
		Porphyria cutanea tarda	
Sulfonamides	Only older drugs(?)	Photoallergic	External and internal
Antimycobacterials	Isonicotinic hydrazide	Pellagra	
		Porphyria cutanea tarda	
	Ethionamide	Photoallergic[b]	Cofactor?
		Pseudo-LE	[17]
	p-Aminosalicylic acid[a]	Photoallergic[b]	
	Thiambutosine	Phototoxic, melanosis	
	Clofazimine	Phototoxic	[18]
	Chloroquine	Photoallergic[b]	[19]
	Quinine	Photoallergic[b]	[20]
Antiprotozoals	Quinoline-methanols	Phototoxic	[21]
	Flavoquine	Phototoxic, melanosis	[22]
	Mepacrine[a]	Phototoxic	
	Stilbamidine[a]	Photoallergic	

Antimicrobials **with heavy metals**	Arsenicals	Phototoxic Photoallergic[b]	[23] Neoarsphenamine
	Silver salts	Pigmentation (argyrosis)	
Topical antiseptics	Chlorophenylphenol	Photoallergic	[24]
	Hexachlorophene	Photoallergic	[25]
	Fenticlor	Photoallergic	
	Bithionol	Photoallergic	
	Halogen-salicylamides	Photoallergic	Antimycotics [26], buclosamid [27, 28]
	Halogen-salicylanilides	Photoallergic	Tribromsalan [29]
Urinary antiseptics	Chlorhexidine	Photoallergic[b]	[30]
	Phenazopyrine[a]	Melanosis	[31]
	Nalidixic acid	Phototoxic	Porphyria cutanea tarda-like bullosis [32]
Cytotoxics	Vinblastine	Photoallergic[b]	[33]
	5-Fluorouracil	Phototoxic[b] Photoprotective[b]	[34] [35]
	Triethylene melamine	Photoallergic[b]	
Cosmetics and ***related products*** **Antibacterial soaps,** **antiseptics,** **deodorants**	See Topical antiseptics	Photoallergic	
Perfumes, toilet **waters**	Furocoumarins		
	Bergamot and other essential oils	Phototoxic	Berloque type hyperpigmentation [36] Also as constituents of other cosmetics; see Face cosmetics
Face cosmetics	Furocoumarins	Phototoxic	Chloasma-like hyperpigmentation [37]

(Continued)

Table 12-1. (cont.)

Class	Group or substance	Type of reaction	Remarks and references[e]
	Petrolatum (tarcontaining)	Phototoxic	Riehl melanosis
Lipsticks, makeup	Eosin and other dyes	Phototoxic	Also photoallergic reactions?
Hair cosmetics	Coal tar	Phototoxic	Hyperpigmentation
	Quinine	Photoallergic[b]	
Aftershaves	Azulene	Phototoxic	Hyperpigmentation
Sunscreens	p-Aminobenzoic acid esters	Photoallergic	
	Digalloyl trioleate	Photoallergic	
	Phenylbenzimidazoles, phenylbenzoxazoles	Phototoxic[b]	Mallorda acne?
Detergents	Optical brighteners	Photoallergic	[38]
Tattoos (yellow)	Cadmium salts	Photoallergic[b]	[39]
Foodstuffs and beverages			
Vegetables	*Atriplex hortensis* (garden orach)	Phototoxic	Betanidine?
	Psoralea esculenta	Phototoxic	Furocoumarins
	Psoralea corylifolia (bavachi)	Phototoxic	Furocoumarins
	Ficus carica	Phototoxic[c]	Fresh fruits only
	Citrus acida (Persian lime, lemon)	Phototoxic	Peels only (?) hyperpigmentation by skin contact
	Pastinaca sativa (parsnip)	Phototoxic[c,d]	Furocoumarins
Liquors and soft drinks	Artificial sweeteners	Photoallergic	See artificial sweeteners

	Plant extracts	Phototoxic	
Artificial sweeteners	Cyclamate	Photoallergic	
Restricted to animals	Fagopyrum (buckwheat)	Phototoxic	Angelica, etc., in liquors [40] [41, 42] Fagopyrismus by fagopyrine
	Hypericum (St. John's wort)	Phototoxic	Hypericismus by hypericin
	Lippia rehmanni and other plants	Phototoxic	Lippia icterus (geeldikkop)

a Photodependent action doubtful.
b Type of reaction uncertain.
c Mostly bullous type (phyto-photo-dermatitis) by direct skin contact.
d Also other plants of this family such as parsley, dill, or celery.
e References

1. Arch. Dermatol. **91**:362 (1965).
2. Arch. Dermatol. **85**:420 (1962).
3. Z. Hautkr. **29**:173 (1960).
4. Dermatologica **129**:183 (1964).
5. Bor. ven. Szle. **43**:121 (1967).
6. Arch. Dermatol. **107**:427 (1973).
7. Arch. Dermatol. **110**:249 (1974).
8. J.A.M.A. **216**:526 (1971).
9. Arch. Dermatol. **92**:591 (1965).
10. Experientia **30**:451 (1974).
11. Hautarzt **26**:53 (1975).
12. Arch. Dermatol. Res. **253**:53 (1975).
13. Cutis **17**:72 (1976).
14. Ann. Dermatol. Syphiligr. (Paris) **102**:277 (1975).
15. Arch. Dermatol. **93**:346 (1966).
16. Med. Welt. 1298 (1959).
17. Bull. Soc. Fr. Dermatol. Syphiligr. **73**:51 (1966).
18. Atti Soc. Ital. Dermatol. **41**:106 (1966).
19. Leprosy Rev. **23**:6 (1962).
20. Z. Hautkr. **29**:203 (1960).
21. J. Med. Chem. **11**:366 (1968).
22. Bull. Soc. Fr. Dermatol. Syphiligr. **82**:319 (1975).
23. J. Gen. Virol. **3**:63 (1968).
24. Arch. Dermatol. **106**:711 (1972).
25. Br. Med. J. **2**:566 (1974).
26. Wz. Actol Dermatol. Monatsschr. **161**:459 (1975).
27. C. C. Thomas, Springfield, Ill. (1972). Herman-Sams: Soap Photo-dermatitis.
28. Contact Dermatitis **1**:263 (1975).
29. J. Invest. Dermatol. **63**:227 (1974).
30. Dermatologica **143**:376 (1971).
31. Ann. Intern. Med. **72**:89 (1970).
32. Am. J. Med. **58**:576 (1975).
33. Arch. Dermatol. **111**:1168 (1975).
34. Arch. Dermatol. **97**:14 (1968).
35. Arch. Klin. Exp. Dermatol. **234**:204 (1969).
36. Hautarzt **22**:535 (1971).
37. Hautarzt **23**:21 (1972).
38. Br. J. Dermatol. **85**:61 (1971).
39. Ann. Intern. Med. **67**:984 (1967).
40. Dtsch. Gesundheitswesen 308 (1954).
41. Br. J. Dermatol. **80**:200 (1968).
42. Lancet **2**:1273 (1969).

Table 12-2. Pathogenic Mechanisms That Lead to Photodermatoses

	Acute form	Chronic form
Disturbance of the normal protective mechanism	Acute erythema reaction in infants with xeroderma pigmentosum	Full clinical picture of xeroderma pigmentosum
Photosensitization	Acute phototoxic tar reaction, e.g., in road workers	Tar and pitch skin

completely dominating the picture at first. Depending on the severity of the disease, precanceroses, carcinomas, melanomas, and basaliomas often occur before age 10 and the patient may die from skin cancers during the second decade of life.

A special form can be differentiated in early childhood in which, in addition to severe skin changes, severe cerebral disturbances are also present. It is called idiotie xérodermique (de Sanctis–Cacchione syndrome). The life expectancy of these patients is even shorter. On the other hand, patients with "pigmented xerodermoid," a further special form of this group, often reach a more advanced age, since the changes occur later and are less marked. According to the observations of Jung and Schnyder (9), a different type of disturbance of the repair system may be involved here, while a special form differentiated by Cleaver (2) revealed absolutely no disturbance of the repair system.

Tar and Pitch Skin (18–24). In classifying the chronic skin changes that occur following many years of contact with tar or pitch, certain reservations are necessary because carcinogenic tar components also play some part in the pathogenesis of hyperpigmentation, precanceroses ("pitch warts"), and carcinomas (Fig. 12-2). As a result, carcinomas can occur in areas definitely not exposed to the light (for instance, the scrotal cancer of chimney sweeps). Nevertheless, in most patients a definite preference is indicated for the zones exposed to light. Depending on the composition of the tar and as a result of the combination with acne-type efflorescences, the clinical picture more closely resembles Hoffmann–Habermann melanodermatitis. However, in

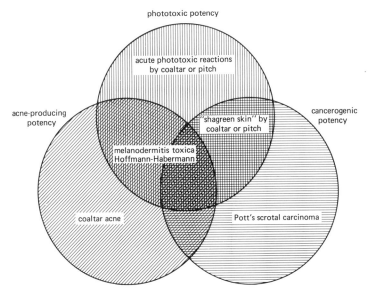

Fig. 12-2. Cutaneous reactions from coal tar and pitch.

most chronic tar damage to the skin a substantial part is played in its pathogenesis by the phototoxic effect of some hydrocarbons, especially anthracene.

Possibly connected with the tar-induced melanodermatitis toxica is the hitherto little-clarified "Mallorca acne," observable in vacationers after using certain sunburn protectants (25). It is characterized by the appearance of acne-like lesions and speckled hyperpigmentation in the exposed skin. All such patients I have seen had used sunburn protectants containing benzimidazole or benzoxazole derivatives as UV filters. One representative of this class of materials, 2-*p*-tertiary butyl-phenyl-1,3-benzoxazole, which is no longer used as a light filter, has long been known to have a marked acne-producing effect.

Pseudomilium Colloidale and Related Conditions (26–37). These are dermatoses that are morphologically and etiologically similar to chronic light damage to the skin.

Elastosis nodularis with cysts and comedones (Favre–Racouchot) is characterized clinically by yellowish sebaceous cysts occurring predominantly periorbicularly, and histologically by coarsely nodular elastosis deep in the dermis. When these lesions occur near the surface of the skin they have the appearance of a comedo. This type of alteration, which is observed relatively frequently in patients with porphyria cutanea tarda, probably constitutes a special form of chronic light damage where the normal picture has been modified by constitutional and exogenic factors (e.g., mineral oil products or cosmetics).

In the case of *pseudomilium colloidale* (Wagner–Pelizzari) there are close topographic and morphologic relationships with chronic light damage to the skin. A constitutional component (disturbance in protein metabolism?), however, is probably involved, as shown by the fact that it runs in families. On the other hand, cases have also been described in which the skin changes occurred not only on the face but also on the hands subsequent to the use of mineral oils and hydroquinone (29, 33) and simultaneous marked exposure to light. Clinically the exposed areas of the skin show densely packed, roundish or angular, yellow to brownish modules or more rarely patches, which stand out histologically as subepidermal, almost cell-free, sharply circumscribed deposits. Recent histochemical and electron microscopic investigations suggest that the deposited material bears no close relationship to connective tissue, parenchyma, serum components, or amyloid, but is probably formed from the "structural glycoprotein" of secretory elements of the fibroblasts.

Finally we should mention *hyalinosis cutis et mucosae* (Urbach–Wiethe lipoproteinosis). This hereditary disturbance of protein metabolism usually begins in childhood. That it also occurs in the oral mucosa argues against a true photodermatosis. Lipoproteinosis was earlier often included in this group, probably because of its morphologic similarity to pseudomilium.

Erythropoietic protoporphyria (see below) may also be accompanied by similar skin changes. In no case of this disorder, however, have I observed involvement of the mucous membrane.

In this connection we must also mention *granuloma actinicum.* As O'Brien (35) was able to prove convincingly, this form of alteration, earlier described under various other names (e.g., granuloma anulare or atypical necrobiosis lipoidica), represents an annularly progressive granuloma within elastotically altered skin in which the pathologic material is largely removed. Thus this foreign-body granuloma is to be viewed as a reparative process accompanying chronic light damage to the skin.

Photo-auto-reactions Resembling Acute Light Damage ("Sunburn-Type Photodermatoses")

The clinical picture for acute chemical phototoxic skin reactions can differ greatly depending on the mode of application of the photosensitizer, so that sometimes the morphologic relationships to sun-exposed sites are barely recognizable. The three major photodermatoses found in this group are (1) acute sunburn-type reaction (dermatitis phototoxica), (2) pigment dermatosis of the berloque dermatitis type (photodermatitis pigmentaria), and (3) striate vesicular to bullous reaction of the meadow-dermatitis type [photodermatitis bullosa (striata), phytophotodermatitis]. However, these differences are certainly only apparent, for, according to the mode of application, one and the same substance or group of substances may cause all three forms. This is particularly well illustrated by the example of furocoumarins: if these phototoxic substances are taken orally, as medicaments or food, dermatitis phototoxica results; if they act upon the skin in an alcohol solution, e.g., as a component of eau de cologne, a photodermatitis pigmentaria develops. If, on the other hand, they get onto or into the skin as aqueous plant juices, then this leads to a photodermatitis (bullosa) striata.

The most plausible explanation for this phenomenon was given as long ago as 1940 by Bergamasco (38), who suggested that according to the mode of application and / or the speed of penetration, the phototoxic substances are found in the outer prickle cells or deep in the epidermis (i.e., in the neighborhood of the melanocytes) or in the dermis (Fig. 12–3). Naturally exceptions are possible, but these can mostly be explained by rapid downward, vertical penetration (e.g., in the case of tar), or transport from the bloodstream to the epidermis (e.g., hyperpigmentation following an internal dose of furocoumarin). The basic photochemical processes occurring in the phototoxic reactions will not be pursued further here, and the reader is referred to Chapter 11. It must be emphasized here, however, that there are two different types of photosensitizers, namely those that are non-oxygen-dependent, such as furocoumarins [but see (39)], and those that are oxygen

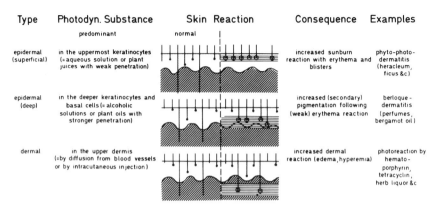

Type	Photodyn. Substance	Skin Reaction	Consequence	Examples
	predominant	normal		
epidermal (superficial)	in the uppermost keratinocytes (=aqueous solution or plant juices with weak penetration)		increased sunburn reaction with erythema and blisters	phyto-photo-dermatitis (heracleum, ficus &c)
epidermal (deep)	in the deeper keratinocytes and basal cells (= alcoholic solutions or plant oils with stronger penetration)		increased (secondary) pigmentation following (weak) erythema reaction	berloque-dermatitis (perfumes, bergamot oil)
dermal	in the upper dermis (=by diffusion from blood vessels or by intracutaneous injection)		increased dermal reaction (edema, hyperemia)	photoreaction by hemato-porphyrin, tetracyclin, herb liquor &c

Fig. 12-3. Types of photodynamic skin reaction (photosensitization).

dependent, such as the porphyrins. It is usually not possible to distinguish these two types of reactions on gross morphologic grounds. The dermatologist cannot always tell whether an erythematous phototoxic reaction was caused by furocoumarins used as medicaments or originating in foodstuffs; by porphyrins, as in the case of erythropoietic protoporphyria; or by hemato-porphyrin, as in the famous Meyer–Betz autoexperiment. Even a bullous reaction resulting from tar photosensitization shows neither macroscopic nor histologic differences by comparison with a bullous phytophotodermatitis resulting from plant juices containing furocoumarin.

Acute Phototoxic Reaction Resembling Sunburn (Dermatitis Photo-toxica). In these cases internal administration (oral or parenteral, probably also by inhalation in the case of tar) of a photosensitizer results in acute erythema with or without edema of the skin exposed to the sun some hours or even 2–3 days later. In contrast to normal sunburn, this photosensitization reaction may occur after very brief sun exposure. Instead of the usual erythema threshold times of 10–60 min, these phototoxic reactions can occur, under the same climatic conditions, after exposure to the sun for as little as 1–3 min. Still more striking is the appearance of a phototoxic reaction in the case of a person remaining exclusively in the shade. These reactions differ from sunburn in that they may also be caused by exposure to the sun through window glass, i.e., largely in the absence of UVB.

Photodermatitis Pigmentaria (Berloque Dermatitis) (40–47). The characteristic signs of this photodermatosis are very sharply demarcated macules of light brown to dark brown hyperpigmentation that frequently occur on the neck in the form of downward-running drops like necklace pendants (berloque, breloque). They are brought about predominantly by cosmetics (eau de cologne, perfume, refresher tissues) with a high content of bergamot oil and other furocoumarin-rich (citrus) oils. According to the mode of application of these cosmetics, in addition to this droplike form (from perfume, etc., running down) it is possible to observe specks (resulting from dabbing, e.g., behind the ears), splashes (from spraying with these preparations), lines (from pencils), or areal pigmentation marks (resulting from rubbing). Apart from the often bizarre morphology, another factor that facilitates diagnosis is an early (erythematous) inflammatory stage. However, this often remains unnoticed, since in the case of this phototoxic reaction the acute sunburn is usually less impressive than the resulting pigmentation. Hyperpigmentation may persist for months and even years as a result of a relatively marked pigment incontinence (melanin phagocytosis in the dermis). Failure to observe the erythematous early stage and the marked persistence of the pigmentation distinguish a special form of photodermatitis pigmentaria, namely cosmetic-induced chloasma. This constitutes a more or less sharply delimited striped or areal brownish hyperpigmeation with varied localization on the face. The forehead and cheekbone region are commonly involved, sometimes as a result of a single application, but frequently also a result of the regular use of a cosmetic containing a photosensitizer (skin cream, face lotion, etc.). These pigmentation marks frequently last for years. Today, furocoumarins are probably the most frequent cause of this disorder, while in earlier days tar-containing petrolatum (Riehl melanosis) and perhaps azulenes were more frequently involved.

Photodermatitis (Bullosa) Striata (Phytodermatitis, "Meadow Dermatitis") (48–58). This type of phototoxic reaction also is occasionally observed following the administration of furocoumarin solutions in alcohol for therapeutic purposes and as a result of the action of preparations containing tar. Nevertheless, aqueous plant juices are the most frequent causative agents. For phytophotodermatitis in the narrow sense, i.e., for phototoxic reactions caused by external action of plant juices, furocoumarins are easily the most common causative photosensitizers. These substances, among which we mention here psoralen, 5-methoxypsoralen (bergapten), 8-methoxypsoralen (xanthotoxin), and 5,8-dimethoxypsoralen (isopimpinellin), are particularly widespread in two plant families, namely the Rutaceae (*Dictamnus, Ruta graveolens,* and species of *Ficus* and *Citrus*) and the Umbelliferae (e.g., *Ammi, Angelica, Apium,* or *Heracleum*). In addition, the species of *Psoralea* should be mentioned from among the Leguminosae. The widely distributed *Heracleum* spp. must be regarded as the most important plants, among which *H. sphondylium* (Wiesenbärenklau, meadow parsnip, cow parsnip, hogweed, pigweed) occurs everywhere in meadows and at roadsides. If, for instance, when picking or lying on such a plant the juice enters the skin, and if a part of the skin so impregnated is subsequently exposed to the sun, then within a few hours a mostly transient and relatively painless erythema develops in these frequently striped and occasionally even leaf-shaped areas, giving rise after a few more hours or even days to round or elongated 1–10-cm translucent blisters. These acute changes disappear after a few days, leaving hyperpigmentation and hypopigmentation.

Whereas this species of *Heracleum* only exceptionally, e.g., in the case of soldiers on exercise (56), leads to a photodermatitis in relatively large groups of people, two other species of *Heracleum, H. giganteum* and especially *H. mantegazzianum* (Riesenbärenklau, Herkules plant, giant hogweed), are occasionally the cause of an outbreak of "caustic injuries." This plant, originating in the Caucasus, is often to be found growing wild over large tracts in Central Europe. Children play among these plants and also fashion blowpipes out of the flower stalks, which are up to 4 m long. The use of these pipes explains the not infrequently observable ring-shaped blisters around the mouth.

If the term phytophotodermatitis is interpreted in a wider sense, however, it is necessary to include those phototoxic reactions that are caused by internal administration. A large number of substances is involved here: furocoumarins apparently only very rarely (e.g., via herbal liquors containing *Angelica*), anthracene derivatives (fagopyrism or hypericism in cattle caused by *Hypericum* or *Fagopyrum*), and as yet unidentified substances (betanidine?) in atriplicism caused by *Atriplex hortensis,* etc. Also included, finally, is "geeldikkop" (Lippia icterus—see below), which is caused by phylloerythrin.

Phenothiazine Melanosis (59–64). The hyperpigmentation of light-exposed skin observed following large doses of some phenothiazines, especially chlorpromazine, may have a pathogenesis differing from time of a true phototoxic reaction. Following doses over 300 mg per day an acute sunburn-type reaction is observed, as in the case of other phototoxic drugs, but following a total dose of about 1 kg of the medication a hyperpigmentation finally develops that contains not only melanin but also conversion products of chlorpromazine. The precise pathogenic mechanism could be viewed as a primary process in which a free radical is formed by chlorpromazine by photochemical dechlorination. Subsequently the radical reacts with melanin (acting as a radical scavenger) so that the hyperpigmentation comes about via melanin–phenothiazine complexes (see also Photoallergic Eczema below).

Pellagra and Related Dermatoses (65–75). In pellagra an acute dermatitis often occurs following relatively marked exposure to light. Dark red erythemas appear with a squamous hyperkeratosis accentuated at the edges. These erythemas are found predominantly on the skin exposed to light (especially periorally, on the dorsa of the hands and forearms, and also on the neck—"Casal's collar"). Stomatitis, enteritis, and neurologic symptoms are common. Causal factors involved in addition to nicotinic acid deficiency resulting from unbalanced nutrition are probably an antivitamin effect (resulting from isonicotinic acid hydrazide or a diet predominantly of maize?) and also alcoholism and therapy with antiepileptics. The ultimate, pathogenically active phototoxic metabolite is not yet known. A number of observations, principally the occurrence of pellagra-type skin reactions in disturbances of indole metabolism, as in the Hartnup syndrome (see below) or the carcinoid syndrome, suggest that this phototoxic substance is a metabolite of tryptophan. Comaish and Cooper (67) observed a rapid disappearance of the skin changes following local application of a 1% niacinamide ointment, suggesting that a phototoxic substance of this kind is formed in the skin itself as a result of (local?) nicotinamid deficiency.

In this connection the "light-band substance" of Kimmig et al. (71) should be mentioned. It consists of a tryptophan derivative [N-(β-indol-3-yl-acryloyl)-glycin] and is considered to play a causal role in photodermatoses, especially chronic polymorphous light eruptions (see below). In the congenital metabolic disturbance termed Hartnup syndrome, in addition to a photodermatosis resembling pellagra but resistant to vitamin B therapy, there are cerebellar symptoms. Recent investigations have indicated disturbances of amino acid metabolism. Probably the substances responsible for the photoreactions in the skin are accumulated metabolites of phenylalanine and, especially, of tryptophan. (See Photopathology and Tryptophan Metabolism, and Seckel Syndrome later in this chapter).

PHOTOREACTIONS IN PORPHYRIAS (76-100) (Table 12-1)

Porphyria Cutanea Tarda and Other Hepatic Porphyrias

Porphyria cutanea tarda (porphyria hepatica chronica) represents a hereditary or acquired disturbance of hepatic porphyrin metabolism with pathologic excretion of various highly carboxylated porphyrins, predominantly in the urine. It occurs most commonly in males, and usually only at a relatively advanced age. The skin changes, developing periodically, usually in late summer or autumn, consist of an increased susceptibility to mechanical injury and the formation of subepidermal blisters in the skin areas exposed to the light (especially the dorsa of the hands, more rarely the face, neck, and lower legs). Independently of the time of year, elastosis (particularly in the region of the eyebrows), hypertrichosis, scleroderma-type changes, and ulcerations may occur in these skin areas. The existence of a relationship between the degree of porphyrin excretion and degree of the skin changes cannot be detected with certainty.

The skin changes in porphyria variegata are similar to those in porphyria cutanea tarda. In this disease, too, the liver is thought to be the site of pathologic porphyrin formation. Periodically, however, in contrast to tarda, large quantities of porphyrin precursors (especially porphobilinogen) are also formed and pathologic quantities of porphyrins are excreted in the stool. In addition, in the course of this hereditary disease, acute attacks of the acute intermittent porphyria type also occur.

In acute intermittent porphyria, which also is hereditary and in which the pathologically increased formation of porphyrin precursors in the liver is very marked, skin changes virtually do not occur.

Porphyria Erythropoietica Congenita Günther

In contrast to the diseases previously mentioned, in this case large quantities of porphyrins are formed in the bone marrow. In this very rare hereditary disease the porphyrins are likewise excreted predominantly in the urine. The skin changes largely correspond to those in porphyria cutanea tarda, but, beginning in childhood, lead to marked scleroderma-type hardening of the skin exposed to the light, with increasing mutilation of the extremities and scarring alopecia.

Erythropoietic Protoporphyria

This hereditary disturbance of porphyrin metabolism, also localized in the bone marrow [for secondary(?) liver participation, see (77, 83, 88, 92)], shows no pathologic porphyrin excretion in the urine, but only in the stool. The skin changes can be definitely distinguished clinically from the other porphyrin diseases. Acute sunburn-like erythemas on the exposed skin following exposure to the sun normally occur in early youth. Also, not infrequently, but independent of these reactions as well, changes may occur that are reminiscent of a solar urticaria or even of a chronic polymorphic light eruption with predominantly papulous alterations. Some of the patients develop, on the bridge of the nose, the upper lip, and knuckle region of the dorsa of the hands, slightly reddened or skin-colored, roughly tesselated infiltrates showing great similarity to Urbach-Wiethe lipoproteinosis but not affecting the mucosa.

Phototoxic Reactions Resulting from Exogenous Introduction of Porphyrin

In the case of some women injected intravenously with 0.5–1.0 g of hematoporphyrin for purposes of carcinoma diagnosis I found a high degree of photosensitivity persisting for weeks or months (90). It was expressed in acute, often itchy, sunburn-type erythematoedematous reactions in those skin areas that were exposed to sunlight. As an expression of a high degree of UVA sensitization the same manifestations also occurred behind window glass, so that these patients had to live for a period of weeks in a darkened room. These findings are thus in full agreement with the famous autoexperiment of Meyer–Betz and show that at least hematoporphyrin, like all other phototoxic compounds—the furocoumarins or tar, for instance—is capable of releasing a phototoxic reaction in UVA and short-wave visible radiation in which the erythematoedematous components of sunburn are in the foreground. Apart from various case reports on local phototoxic reactions following subcutaneous injection of hematoporphyrin, it is important to mention the intensive investigations of McGrae and Perry (94), further proving that hematoporphyrin is capable of releasing typical phototoxic reactions.

Lippia Icterus

Lippia icterus is a photodermatosis occurring in sheep, not in humans. This disease, also called "geeldikkop" (yellow thick head) consists of an icterus and acute phototoxic manifestations, particularly swellings, affecting the less hairy skin, predominantly of the head. The icterus results from a disturbance in bile ducts, This leads to an intestinal resorption of the phylloerythrin produced from chlorophyll in the food, which, as porphyrin, causes the acute phototoxic reaction in the skin (79,85).

Summary

If we consider the photodermatoses occurring with a pathologic increase of porphyrin in the body, we find that they may be divided quite easily into two groups: (1) Disturbances with typical acute phototoxic reactions, particularly the reactions in the case of exogenous uptake of porphyrin, sometimes the erythropoietic protoporphyria, and "geeldikkop." (2) Diseases presenting neither the typical picture of an acute phototoxic reaction nor a picture of chronic light damage as the xeroderma pigmentosum. To this group belong first and foremost porphyria cutanea tarda, porphyria congenita, and porphyria variegata.

A middle position is occupied by erythropoietic protoporphyria. Here we have not only the erythematous form with the typical acute phototoxic reaction or the predominantly chronic lipoproteinosis-type form, but also patients in whom both groups of symptoms may occur simultaneously.

Above all, however, light and electron microscopic studies of various authors show that the tissue changes in the various porphyrias differ only quantitatively, and not qualitatively (80). Histologic findings and clinical symptoms permit us to deduce the following conclusions or hypotheses:

1. The fundamental reaction in all photoreactions induced by porphyrins or occurring in porphyrias is an acute phototoxic reaction proceeding most probably via a singlet oxygen mechanism ("photodynamically").

2. The localization of this initial reaction is determined by the "pharmacokinetics" of the pathologically increased porphyrins. These in their turn depend on their physical (solubility, charge) and chemical (chelating ability, affinity for the body's own substances or structures of the tissues) characteristics, as well as on their distribution in the serum and in the erythrocytes.

3. In the case of exogenous introduction of hematoporphyrin or phylloerythrin, large quantities of such porphyrins with evidently little affinity to the body's own substances or structures lead, via the serum, to a largely uniform saturation of the outer dermis with these sensitizers and thus to a similar reaction as that, for instance, resulting from Declomycin or anthracene (or coal tar).

4. If, on the other hand, the serum contains porphyrins, either formed in the body or released locally from the erythrocytes by photohemolysis, with an affinity to certain skin structures, then the initial phototoxic reaction may be limited to a single type of cell or tissue.

5. Earlier investigations repeatedly pointed to the role of the blood vessels of the dermis in porphyrias. As a result of recent investigations cited, such vascular damage can now, with a high degree of probability, be placed in the endothelial cells. The (endogenous) porphyrins are apparently deposited there from the serum and then invoke the phototoxic reaction with light in the Soret band (about 385–415 nm) reaching these cells.

6. As a result of this damage to the endothelial cells there may be an alteration in permeability with formation of the hyaline material that occurs particularly in protoporphyria but also in other porphyrias.

7. The disturbance in permeability can, however, also lead via reparative processes (thickening of the basal membrane) to reduced function of the vessel and thus to a deterioration in the blood supply to these areas of the skin. This would explain the sclerodermoid changes, including ulceration and mutilation, which occur in tarda and congenita.

8. Above all, a reduced blood supply could explain the fact that, especially in the cases of tarda and congenita, even after a number of years, the skin changes do not resemble those occurring with chronic light damage. Most striking of all is the fact that development toward basaliomas and carcinomas in these two forms of porphyria appears to be an extremely rare occurrence.

9. This phenomenon is evidently a result of the specific localization of the basic phototoxic process in the endothelial cells (and the space separating the dermal connective tissue from the sensitized photoreaction?). Further, the reduced blood supply to the skin exposed to the light caused by the damage to the vessels can also result in an increasing oxygen deficiency and thus to a reduction in the "photodynamic" reaction (i.e., proceeding via singlet oxygen).

It can be established from the observations cited and from the conclusions and considerations derived from them that probably all light-conditioned skin changes in the various porphyrias are phototoxic in nature, but a number of resultant processes following the primary damage to the endothelial cells cause chronic skin changes, which differ substantially from a chronic form of light damage.

PHOTO-HETERO-REACTIONS

All skin changes caused by light in which the fundamental photochemical processes proceed neither directly nor via a phototoxic or photodynamic mechanism in the physiologic "light receptors" (i.e., the photosensitive components or structures of the normal skin) can be termed photo-hetero-reactions. Since in these cases pathogenic photoproducts are produced from abnormal skin components or from substances not normally reacting photochemically, the dermatoses of this group can be clinically distinguished from the photo-auto-reactions by the fact that they are macro- and micromorphologically different from acute and chronic light damage to normal skin.

In the most simple case such a photo-hetero-reaction can lead to a light-dependent color change in the skin, as for instance in argyrosis (see below). In addition, allergenically active photoproducts (photoallergy) may develop. In the case of the remaining photodermatoses of this group, so little is as yet known about the basic photopathologic processes that their classification in the photo-hetero-reactions was determined exclusively on the basis of clinical criteria—no similarity with the physiologic light reactions and no general provocation by light as one of many agents that injure the skin (photo-Koebner).

Photoreactions of Extraneous Substances in the Skin

Argyrosis and Chrysiasis (101–106). To illustrate these very simple photo-hetero-reactions we first mention photochemical deposition, in partic-ular of silver (argyrosis) and gold (chrysiasis), in the skin. In both cases a slate-gray discoloration occurs, predominantly in zones exposed to the light, when silver or gold derivatives have been administered for therapeutic reasons. Pathogenicity is related to the photographic process. The metal derivative is transported by the serum and diffused into the tissue. It is reduced by light, finely distributed and irreversibly precipitated in the connective tissue as a result of "argyrophily" of these fibers.

Phototherapy of Icterus (107–115). Phototherapy of hyperbilirubinemia of infants could be considered another example of this type of photo-hetero-reaction. In this case the extraneous substance is excess bilirubin in the tissues. The dermal connective tissue acts as a matrix for the photochemical process, which is probably the explanation for the fact that different photoproducts occur in this process from those occurring with illumination of bilirubin in solutions (see Chapter 16).

Solar Urticaria (116–122)

Solar urticaria is a form of physical urticaria in which an urticarial skin reaction occurs as a result of the action of light of varying wavelength. In a considerable number of patients there is a noticeable decrease in skin reaction during the late summer. Exhaustion of the causal substance or tachyphylaxis has been argued as the possible cause of this phenomenon (116). The basic pathogenic processes in solar urticaria are evidently very variable and can best be illustrated by reference to the scheme adopted by Harber et al. (117). In

Table 12-3. Pathogenic Processes in Solar Urticaria

Type	Causal wavelengths, nm	Passive transfer	Reverse passive transfer	Remarks
I	285–320	+	+	Allergic pathogenesis
II	320–400	–	–	Pathogenesis unknown, no serum factor demonstrable
III	400–500	–	–	As II [see also (121)]
IV	400–500	+	–	Pathogenesis unknown; probably allergic
V	280–500	–	–	As II
VI	400	–	–	Induced by elevated protoporphyrin 9 in erythrocytes (= urticarial form of erythropoietic protoporphyria)

accordance with this scheme these photodermatoses can be subdivided on the basis of the causal wavelengths and the results of passive transfer experiments as given in Table 12-3.

The inherently reasonable assumption of a light-induced allergic reaction of the immediate type is largely excluded for several of these types of reaction on the basis of numerous observations in which the scheme was based. Among the different types, a photoallergic mechanism of this kind is the most likely one in the case of Type I, the UVB urticaria, and could arguably exist in the case of Type IV. Possibly allergic mechanisms are further discussed in Chapter 11. On the other hand, in many cases the observations appear to support a light-induced (phototoxic?) release of histamine, e.g., from mastocytes (116). In any case, attempts at finding the causal photochemically altered substance by exact determination of the action spectrum have not been successful. Such investigations are further complicated by the fact that a proportion of the patients show widely differing results in repeated determinations of the action spectrum (121) and that acute erythema and whealing reactions can be caused by different wavelengths. All in all, solar urticaria remains a largely unexplained photodermatosis. Intensive investigations have raised more questions than they have answered.

Photoallergic Eczema and Its Sequelae

Photoallergic Eczema (123–159). Clinically, this dermatosis has a morphology and course similar to allergic contact eczema stemming from other causes. Even the restriction to skin areas exposed to the light may not be clearly identifiable in severe cases owing to the phenomenon of dissemination to the remainder of the skin. Like simple allergic contact eczema, photo-allergic contact eczema can proceed via different stages (reddening, papules, blisters, wetness, scabs, and scales) and, above all, become chronic. The decisive difference from an allergic eczema such as a chromate eczema is the fact that in addition to a substance acting as a prohapten, the light is also necessary for the occurrence of skin changes. Electromagnetic radiation may transform a substance, either by photochemical oxidation or by the formation of radicals, into a true hapten, which can then react with protein to form a complete antigen. Such a mechanism was first demonstrated for sulfanilamide, which is converted to the corresponding hydroxylamine by photooxidation:

$$p - H_2N - C_6H_4 - SO_2 - N{<}^H_H \longrightarrow p - {}^{HO}_H{>}N - C_6H_4 - SO_2 - NH_2$$

In persons photoallergic to sulfanilamide, skin changes were also caused by in vitro illumination of sulfanilamide solutions prior to exposure. Because of the short-lived nature of the photochemical intermediates, photoallergies proceeding via free radical mechanisms have been elucidated further only in exceptional cases (e.g., in the case of triacetyldiphenol isatin).

Several conclusions can be made from established facts and clinical observations: Any photosensitive substance intended for human application must be considered as a potential photoallergen, especially if in vitro illumination is accompanied by a shift of absorption to longer wavelengths (126). A photoallergic eczema cannot be elucidated as to its cause by means of the usual epicutaneous test. The photopatch test is much more important for diagnosis: pretreatment of the skin with the substance suspected of causal involvement (mostly under the conditions of the normal epicutaneous test) and subsequent illumination, especially with UVA.

In photocontact allergy, distinction must be made between two different forms, the "florid" form and the "latent" form (126). So long as the causal substance is still in the skin, then the photoallergy is florid: illumination on its own will lead to an eczematous reaction. If, on the other hand, contact occurred some time previously, then latent photoallergy can be detected only under the conditions of the photopatch test, that is, after pretreatment of the skin and subsequent illumination. Therefore, as opposed to normal contact allergy, in the case of florid photoallergy, the exclusion of the substance responsible does not suffice to make the eczema disappear. It is more important in this phase to also exclude light. Severe cases must remain in a darkened room.

Photopathology of Oral Contraceptives (160–163). Among the millions of women taking hormonal contraceptives over a period of years there are isolated cases of patients with light-dependent skin changes in whom these hormonal preparations are suspected of being the cause. Some of the patients have shown symptoms of porphyria cutanea tarda (see above). In these cases the estrogen component of the medication probably contributes to a disturbance in porphyrin metabolism and subsequent photosensitivity. In other women in whom there were no clinical or biochemical indications of porphyria, the clinical picture corresponds most closely to various forms of chronic polymorphous light eruption (see below). Here, too, the estrogen components are allegedly implicated. Nevertheless, it should be remembered that millions of women use these medications and this type of side effect is rare. The contraceptives may, therefore, act to provoke latent dermatoses rather than be primary causative agents.

Persistent Light Reactors and Actinic Reticuloid (133, 134, 144, 164–179). In a small proportion of cases, photocontact allergy does not change into the latent phase but leads to recurrences of light-induced eczema even years after apparent elimination of the photoallergen. The manner in which a proportion of these patients become "persistent light reactors" remains largely unexplained. One assumption is that residual quantities of the causal substance remain in the skin for years, forming allergenic photoproducts there at each renewed exposure to the light. A more likely explanation concerns the existence of specific lymphocytes that have become altered as a result of the first photoallergic outburst in such a way that, with each renewed exposure to light, the cells react to autochthonous cell structures which result from light exposure. Clinically, persistent light reactors can react to each adequate exposure to light (usually to UVA) with eczematous skin changes in the zones exposed to the light. In a proportion of the cases, an exclusively erythematous reaction appears following exposure to very small doses of light. This photosensitivity can be so severe that patients sometimes have to live for years in a weakly illuminated room and can go out only at night.

After a period of years this condition may gradually change into actinic reticuloid, although this condition can also develop after a contact eczema or without the prior existence of any dermatosis or photosensitivity. Conversely, not every persistent light reactor develops into the actinic reticuloid patient. This is particularly true for female patients. Actinic reticuloid, in fact, appears to occur almost exclusively in older males. It has shown a marked increase in occurrence in recent years. This photodermatosis is characterized by massive infiltration and reddening, strictly limited to exposed skin. Often there are marked polygonal grooves in the erythematous patches caused by the relative absence of pathologic changes in the sun-protected wrinkles of the skin. On the sides of the neck this characteristic arrangement of skin changes results in rhombic to almost square papules. The high degree of photosensitivity seen in many of these patients can lead to the development of skin changes on the shoulders and upper parts of the thorax if the clothing is not completely light-impervious, and in very severe cases to a situation where the only skin areas remaining completely free are those that are completely protected from the light, like the insides of the thighs or the armpits. But even in these areas specific skin changes can be caused by brief periods of illumination with UVB, UVA, and short-wave visible light.

Histologically, actinic reticuloid has similarities with (pre)malignant immunocytopathologic conditions. This poses considerable diagnostic and nosologic problems by confusion with the classical malignant granulomatoses (mycosis fungoides, Hodgkin disease) and lymphomas (reticuloses, reticulosarcomas, etc.). As originally described (170), a chronic eczema may appear in the early stage, but then more cells appear, with granulocytes and eosinophils increasingly giving way to histiocytes conspicuous under light and electron microscopes (175). In addition, lymphoid and reticulum cells and numerous mast cells and plasma cells are found. The changes occur mostly in bands, more rarely in nodules, in the upper dermis, but may in isolated places penetrate like Pautrier abscesses into the sometimes atrophic epidermis. The composition of the infiltrates varies. Hyperchromatic cells occur relatively frequently, but more atypical features and mitoses occur only rarely. The clinical picture may fluctuate between a relatively monotonous reticulosis-like state and more granulomatous changes, recalling not only a mycosis fungoides but sometimes even a lymphogranulomatosis.

Chronic Polymorphous Light Eruption (180–201)

This term was proposed in 1900 by Rasch as a collective term for the earlier-described eczema solare, Hutchinson's summer prurigo, and other related, predominantly eczema-type, erythematous and papulopruriginous photodermatoses. The result was that in earlier years and even today a considerable number of the cases that are difficult to classify are included under this term. Conversely, a not inconsiderable proportion of patients formerly published as having that diagnosis would today, after further diagnostic investigation (provocation tests, histology, porphyrin analysis, etc.), be given other diagnoses, such as photoallergic eczema and actinic reticuloid, Jessner–Kanof "lymphocytic infiltration," and erythropoietic protoporphyria.

Chronic polymorphous light eruption is a photodermatosis affecting predominantly female patients in the second or third decade of life and is occasionally observed to run in families. The skin changes appear chiefly in sites regularly exposed to the sun, most often on the middle of the face, the dorsa of the hands, and the neck and shoulders. The skin changes appear a few hours or days after exposure to the sun, beginning usually in the early spring and occurring periodically or else persisting until the autumn. They have occasionally been observed to occur in the winter, especially following marked exposure such as may occur in winter sports. Morphologically, the skin changes may be focal or disseminated and sharply demarcated to relatively diffuse. Generally only one of the many morphologic types mentioned occurs in the individual patient. The morphology shows a markedly varied—"polymorphous"—picture: (a) circumscribed, acute to chronic erythema with or without scaliness; (b) reddish, 2–3-mm papules either densely grouped or irregularly disseminated over the zones exposed to the light; (c) isolated, compact, almost skin-colored papules up to 8 mm in size, and in their residual, excoriated sites (prurigo); (d) clinical picture ranging from subacute eczema to diffuse lichenification with papules and excoriations of the neurodermatitis type; (e) sharply circumscribed, 5–30-mm, bright- to livid-red, superficial or heavily infiltrated plaques, predominantly in the middle of the face.

Such a varied morphology is the reason why, initially, almost every photodermatosis has been referred to as chronic polymorphous light eruption. Further distinction on morphologic grounds is most easily made in the case of prurigo aestivalis and hydroa vacciniformia. By contrast, distinction from lupus erythematosus can frequently be made only on the basis of the disease course, and in the case of erythropoietic protoporphyria on the basis of porphyrin determination in the erythrocytes. Photocontact eczema can be detected by means of the photopatch test. Actinic reticuloid apparently occurs exclusively in older males, and can usually be detected histologically.

The pathogenesis of chronic polymorphous light eruptions is still largely unclarified. Although localization and course have the character of a photodermatitis, provocation tests have given such widely differing results, especially with regard to causal range of wavelengths, that these investigations give little indication of basic pathogenic processes. Therefore the question remains unanswered as to whether the basic pathogenic process in this photodermatosis is immunologic in nature (181, 188), whether it is based on a metabolic disturbance, or whether we are dealing with a hodgepodge of various photodermatoses with varying etiology and pathogenesis. The therapy of chronic polymorphous light eruptions is unsatisfactory. In addition to sun protection, hardening by exposure to sunlight or PUVA therapy, chloroquine and numerous other preparations, thalidomide, and beta-carotene have recently been proposed. No treatment is completely satisfactory.

Hydroa Vaccinoforme (202–206)

In contrast to chronic polymorphous light eruption, hydroa vacciniforme presents a morphologically and probably also pathogenetically uniform clinical picture. Ignoring all of the cases incorrectly published under this name, one is left with a morphologically well-defined dermatosis clearly outlined at the time of its initial description (203) whose occurrence seems largely confined to children. The skin changes most often occur acutely on the face and arms following substantial sun exposure, but can occur anywhere. The skin changes consist of isolated or grouped 1–2-mm blisters with narrow reddish areolae, occasionally in markedly herpetiform arrangement on large red plaques. The covering of the blisters is at first fairly firm and the pruritus slight. Nevertheless, the changes almost always lead via a scab stage to a permanent, markedly vacciniform scar. Similar changes can also occur in the mucous membrane of the mouth. The process often subsides abruptly in adolescence. The cause is not known. A phototropic virus infection is suspected by some clinicians.

Dermatitis Vernalis Aurium Burckhardt (207)

Like hydroa vacciniforme, this photodermatosis occurs predominantly or even exclusively in children and can develop acutely in occasionally epidemic proportions. The lesions usually follow the first relatively marked exposure to the sun in the spring and occur on the upper edge of the external ears. It is morphologically reminiscent of chilblains but may occasionally also exhibit vesiculation to pustule formation. Etiology and pathogenesis are unclear.

Photodermatitis Multiformis Acuta (Ippen) (208)

This photodermatosis, which appears to be rather common, was recently differentiated from chronic polymorphic light eruption. In contrast to the latter, papules, vesicles, and often cockades (target-like lesions) develop within hours after exposure to the first strong sun in areas that are not usually exposed to sunlight. Thus the face and generally the dorsa of the hands remain free from lesions in most of the patients (predominantly young and middle-aged females). The rash clears within a few days even if sun exposure is continued; often the next attack is not to be expected until the following year. The etiology is unknown. Sometimes this dermatosis occurs in relatives. A development of tolerance (desensitization) is therapeutically used by stepwise increased exposure to artificial sunlamps.

OTHER PHOTOSENSITIVE SKIN DISEASES

Bloom Syndrome (209–212)

This probably recessive-autosomal disease with spontaneous chromosomal instability (212) is marked by a proportionate nanosomia, a tendency toward malignant systemic diseases, endocrinic disturbances, and cutaneous manifestations. The latter consist of persistent telangiectatic, lupus erythematosus-like, sun-induced skin changes on the face and forearms, and marked "mottled discoloration." Photosensitivity can additionally be expressed in a bullous cheilitis actinica.

Cockayne Syndrome (213)

Likewise occurring together with nanosomia is Cockayne syndrome, characterized by numerous and variable deformities, mental retardation, auditory and vocal defects, and also retinitis pigmentosa. In these patients there is, as a rule, an acute, often bullous photodermatosis of the exposed skin. Subsequent scab formation and scarring occasionally leads to skin changes recalling the Werner syndrome. In the few cases investigated widely, varying metabolic disturbances were found, including an increased excretion of glycine, alanine, and arginine. Disturbances in metabolism of the aromatic amino acids and tryptophan have not been detected.

Disseminated Superficial Actinic Porokeratosis (214–216)

In this not uncommon photodermatosis, individual foci appear morphologically and microscopically similar to porokeratosis of Mibelli. However, whether this dominantly inherited photodermatosis is, as assumed by its original describer (214), only a variant of Mibelli porokeratosis appears to be uncertain, especially since predominantly women are affected and hitherto, also in contrast to the true porokeratosis of Mibelli, no transition to a squamous cell carcinoma has been described. If we further consider the patients with a "true" Mibelli porokeratosis apparently show no photosensitivity or susceptibility to photoprovocation of further foci, then the porokeratosis of Chernosky probably ought to be numbered among the photo-heteroreactions as an independent photodermatosis rather than among the photo-Koebner phenomena.

Clinically, flat, yellow to reddish foci (though mostly they are only up to 10 mm in size) are sharply circumscribed by a horny side wall. These lesions appear in large numbers (predominantly on the parts of the extremities exposed to the light) following marked exposure to sunlight. In general they do not disappear, especially since the center gradually atrophies. Renewed exposure to sunlight can lead to marked reddening of the old foci and the appearance of new ones.

Rothmund and Thomson Syndromes (217, 218)

These two syndromes show such similar symptoms that many authors assume them to be identical. Clinically a poikiloderma develops in early childhood and shows a certain preference for sun-exposed sites. In addition, cataract formation (developing in childhood) and further deformities of the skin and other organs occur. An increasing mottling develops in the affected zones, recalling striae gravidarum, and later an increasing atrophy with telangiectasia follows.

Seckel Syndrome (219)

This apparently very rare deformity syndrome is worthy of mention here because, on the one hand, it is found alongside proportionate nanosomia as are Bloom or Cockayne syndromes, but, on the other hand, it can, according to an observation of Piñol Aguadé et al., show a disturbance of tryptophan metabolism (among other things), like Hartnup syndrome. Besides a hypotrichosis and numerous organic and skeletal deformities, a photodermatosis with acute erythema and edema of the exposed skin areas occurs periodically with this syndrome, apparently disappearing without consequences.

Dermatosis Atrophicans Maculosa (220)

Recently, Stevanovic reported on four male patients who had altered skin in all sun-exposed sites since childhood. The changes were reminiscent of a combination of ichthyosiform erythroderma, mild xeroderma pigmentosum, and chronic radiodermatitis, and on the elbows and knees reminiscent of an epidermolysis bullosa dystrophicans. No metabolic disturbances of any kind were detected. This photodermatosis in probably sex-linked.

Werner Syndrome (Progeria Adultorum) (221–223)

In contrast to the Rothmund–Thomson syndrome but otherwise very similar as regards cutaneous symptoms, and atrophy (and often also sclerosis) of the skin in the Werner syndrome usually begins only in adult life. In addition to the skin of the face and upper extremities, the lower legs in particular are also affected. Cataracts develop and other deformities may also occur.

PHOTO-KOEBNER PHENOMENA

In numerous dermatoses, occasional, frequent, or more or less regular descriptions have been given of an unfavorable influence of sun exposure. If all those dermatoses in which isolated cases of such light provocation had been reported were listed, this chapter would be virtually like a dermatologic textbook. Therefore only those skin diseases will be mentioned that do not comprise photodermatoses but in which photoprovocation has been observed so often that they occasionally or more frequently give the impression of being a photodermatosis sensu strictu because they affect predominantly the skin areas exposed to the light. Since such photoprovocation can occur in psoriasis or lichen planus (among other conditions), that is, dermatoses with frequent isomorphic stimulatory effects (Koebner phenomena), this group of light-provocable skin diseases will be brought together under the general term "photo-Koebner phenomena."

Collagen Diseases

Lupus Erythematosus (LE) (194, 224–226). Very frequently photoprovocation is observed in the case of chronic cutaneous LE. In many patients, with the first substantial exposure to sun in the summer, numerous 5–50-mm, round, well-demarcated, slightly atrophic, often depigmented lesions with hyperkeratotic edges may occur. Such a case of LE with acute exacerbation is occasionally accompanied by distinct disturbances in the general condition, although light-induced transition to true systemic lupus erythematosus (SLE) is considered doubtful. However, there is no doubt that sun exposure can cause severe skin disease and precipitate systemic symptoms in persons with SLE. With regard to therapy, clear differentiation between excerbated discoid lupus erythematosus (DLE) and the acute SLE provoked by light is absolutely essential. The usual general clinical and serologic criteria are effective here in confirming or excluding a diagnosis of SLE.

Dermatomyositis. Patients with this disease may have photosensitivity which is expressed by the occurrence of persistent erythemas on sun-exposed aspects of the neck and shoulders. Occasionally a worsening of the general symptoms is observed following substantial exposure to sun.

Viral Infections (227, 228)

The fact that various viral infections of the skin (e.g., smallpox) have the capacity for photoprovocation has already been referred to in the case of hydroa vacciniforme. Another excellent example is recurrent cutaneous herpes simplex infection. It may occur as "herpes solaris" following relatively marked exposure to sun. Sun-induced recurrent herpes simplex is especially frequent near the lips. Occasionally, however, an attack also occurs on large areas of exposed skin, particularly on the face. Normally, large doses of sun exposure are required for such provocation. An ability for photoprovocation in viral tumors has not yet been established with certainty. If, however, the virus dependence of keratoacanthoma is conclusively proved (this lesion occurs predominantly in sun-exposed skin), then other skin tumors appearing predominantly in sun-exposed skin, especially basalioma and melanosis circumscripta praecarcinomatosa of Dubreuilh, ought also to be intensively investigated from these aspects.

Psoriasis and Seborrheic Skin Conditions (229–232)

Following marked exposure to UV radiation, e.g., in the case of excessive doses during phototherapy, psoriasis can be made worse and may progress to erythroderma. Occasionally erythrodermic psoriasis is confined to exposed sites. In the rare instances where the face is involved, from time to time either relief or exacerbation is reported by the patients as a result of sun exposure. It is striking that in many psoriasis patients susceptible to photoprovocation a more exudative-seborrhoid psoriasis is present. Some patients with perioral dermatitis and older patients with seborrheic dermatitis and acne rosacea frequently suffer a deterioration in the skin condition when exposed to UV radiation. This is not true for cases of acne vulgaris, which is often favorably affected by sun. Finally, photoprovocation is occasionally reported in persons with pityriasis rubra pilaris. In view of the mode of spread of this dermatosis from uncovered to covered skin areas, however, these reports appear rather dubious.

Other Dermatoses Provoked by Light (233–242)

Among the numerous dermatoses for which photoprovocation has been reported, in the case of lichen planus this may be taken as certain but rare. It is possible though, that lichen tropicus actinicus is in fact a variant of this dermatosis. It is also noteworthy that apparently high exposure doses are required for such provocation and that dark-skinned persons are more prone to be affected. A clear susceptibility to provocation is further shown by many patients with dyskeratosis follicularis Darier or with certain forms of pemphigus. In the last-mentioned group photosensitivity relates almost exclusively to the so-called benign familial pemphigus of Hailey–Hailey, which today is usually treated as a special form of the dyskeratosis of Darier, and pemphigus seborrheicus erythematosus Senear–Usher, in which a spectrum exists and some patients appear to have LE.

Finally to be mentioned here are some dermatoses in which photoprovocation has been reported for the most part only in isolated cases or whose classification is uncertain: purpura "solaris," livedo reticularis, or tinea faciei. To be mentioned also is the photosensitivity that occasionally occurs in mycosis fungoides; this can certainly pose therapeutic and diagnostic problems. A marked sensitivity of the pityriasis rosea of Gilbert to relatively high doses of sun has also been observed.

SUMMARY

Photopathology and Tryptophan Metabolism
(65, 71, 72, 176, 187, 243–254)

Basic photopathologic research will be improved by advances in photochemistry and photobiology and further investigations on the normal and abnormal metabolism of tryptophan and its metabolites. A large number of particularly interesting substances appears in the metabolism of this amino acid. These include not only photosensitive indole derivatives like indolyl acetic acid and the pigmentation inhibitor melatonin, but also kynurenic acid (176, 248, 249) and N'-formylkynurenine (250–252), which have recently been shown to exert a photohemolytic effect. Kynureninase deficiency may be pathogenically important in various photodermatoses (65).

For some photodermatoses there is a possibility of a disturbance in this particular branch of metabolism, although unanswered questions remain and the pathophysiology of most photodermatoses is still a mystery. These include photo-auto-reactions such as pellagra (72) or Hartnup disease, photo-hetero-reactions such as hydroa vacciniforme and actinic reticuloid (176), as well as chronic polymorphous light eruption with unknown action spectra (71). In considering a possible role of tryptophan and its metabolites it must be remembered that the isolation of the primary photochemical reactions in the various photodermatoses has not been possible. Walrant's group (250–252) was able to show that the N'-formylkynurenine produced by UVB photo-oxidation of tryptophan can sensitize further photooxidation of tryptophan by UVA, i.e., an "internal photosensitization." Of further importance is the observation of Nilsson et al. (246), who detected a singlet oxygen pathway for kynurenic acid photohemolysis. Other phototoxic compounds (chlorpromazine or Declomycin) operate as excited triplet sensitizers. Hematoporphyrin may react via both pathways. More information is needed.

These few points, and the cited literature, are intended merely to indicate that this area of basic photobiologic and biochemical research can be expected to provide important new knowledge in the future relating to the effect of radiation on the skin and the pathogenesis of the photodermatoses.

Photochemistry of the Cell Membrane, Intercalation, and Other Phenomena (255-281)

A variety of different molecular mechanisms may be involved in photosensitization. Basic work in many disciplines, including cancer research, will add to our understanding of photodermatoses. In this framework it is only possible to make a few points and direct the interested person to the appended literature.

Ultraviolet damage of cell membranes resulting in hemolysis is probably an example of the fact that entirely different mechanisms can ultimately invoke the same biologic phenomenon: on the one hand photooxidation of lipids, especially cholesterol, but on the other hand also protein reactions like the loss of spectrin and the cross-linking of other proteins (265). It seems possible that further clarification of these membrane changes is obtainable from clinical observations. We might mention here, for instance, the differences—recently largely clarified—that exist between the photostable protoporphyrin-rich erythrocytes in lead poisoning and the photolabile "fluorocytes" in erythropoietic protoporphyria (271, 296). Further, clarification of the protection of carotenoids in this particular porphyria should provide suggestions about the nature of the effect of light on cells or membranes.

We mention also our observations on the effect of chloroquine, which is used therapeutically in various photodermatoses, on the erythrocytes in erythropoietic porphyria congenita (268). When this medication was administered in small doses to two patients there was not only a transient sharp rise in porphyrin excretion in the urine, but also a substantial rheologic alteration in the red blood cells. While these cells were highly inflexible prior to chloroquine, some weeks after initiation of therapy they exhibited a completely normal elasticity. A similar phenomenon seems to occur in the case of erythropoietic protoporphyria.

Finally, we mention that some skin components may have physiologic and pathologic roles as quenchers or as photosensitizers. In addition to carotenoids, which occur in the skin of every person at least in small quantities, the flavins and bilirubin deserve special attention. A considerable intensification of research on both these groups of substances has occurred over recent years, research that will probably be important not only for the photodermatoses, but also, most importantly, in connection with the question of chronic sun damage to the skin and the question of photocarcinogenesis.

REFERENCES

1. Gross, P. (1956): The Koebner phenomenon in its relationship to photosensitivity. *Arch. Dermatol.* **74**:43–45.
2. Cleaver, J. E. (1972): Xeroderma pigmentosum—variants with normal DNA repair and normal sensitivity to ultraviolet light. *J. Invest. Dermatol.* **58**:124–128.
3. Cleaver, J. E. (1973): DNA repair with purines and pyrimidines in radiation and carcinogen-damaged normal and xeroderma pigmentosum human cells. *Cancer Res.* **33**:362–369.
4. Day, R. S. (1975): Xeroderma pigmentosum variants have decreased repair of ultraviolet-damaged DNA. *Nature* **253**:748–749.
5. Der Kaloustian, V. M., De Weerd-Kastelein, E. A., Kleijer, W. J., et al. (1974): The genetic defect in the de Sanctis–Cacchione syndrome. *J. Invest. Dermatol.* **63**:392–396.
6. Dingman, C. W., and Kanunaga, T. (1976): DNA strand breaking and rejoining in response to ultraviolet light in normal human and xeroderma pigmentosum cells. *Int. J. Radiat. Biol.* **30**:55–66.
7. Dupuy, J. M., Lafforet, D., and Lerrégue, M. (1976): Xeroderma pigmentosum, maladie générale; étude de l'immunité retardée. *Bull. Soc. Fr. Dermatol. Syphligr.* **83**:311–314.
8. Goth-Goldstein, R. (1977): Repair of DNA damage by alkylating carcinogens is defective in xeroderma pigmentosum-derived fibroblasts. *Nature* **267**:81–82.
9. Jung, E. G., and Schnyder, U. W. (1970): Xeroderma pigmentosum and pigmentiertes Xerodermoid. *Schweiz. Med. Wochenschr.* **100**:1718–1726.
10. Lynch, H. T., Frichot, B. C., and Lynch, J. F. (1977): Cancer control in xeroderma pigmentosum. *Arch. Dermatol.* **113**:193–195.
11. Maher, V. M., Ouellette, L. M., Curren, R. D., et al. (1976): Frequency of ultraviolet light-induced mutations is higher in xeroderma pigmentosum variant cells than in normal human cells. *Nature* **261**:593–595.
12. Meffert, H., Barthelmes, H., Diezel, W., et al. (1976): Xeroderma pigmentosum und Antigenität UV-bestrahlter DNS. *Dermatol. Monatsschr.* **162**:300–305.
13. Ramsay, C. A., Coltart, T. M., Blunt, S., et al. (1974): Prenatal diagnosis of xeroderma pigmentosum. *Lancet* **2**:1109–1112.
14. Ramsay, C. A., and Gianelli, F. (1975): The erythemal action spectrum and deoxyribonucleic acid repair system in xeroderma pigmentosum. *Br. J. Dermatol.* **92**:49–56.
15. Sutherland, B. M., and Oliver, R. (1975): Low levels of photoreactivating enzyme in xeroderma pigmentosum variants. *Nature* **257**:132–134.
16. Setlow, R. B., Faulcon, F. M., and Regan, J. D. (1976): Defective repair of gamma-induced DNA damage in xeroderma pigmentosum cells. *Int. J. Radiat. Biol.* **29**:125–136.
17. Tennstedt, D., and Lachapelle, J. M. (1977): Kératoacanthomes et xéroderma pigmentosum. *Ann. Dermatol. Venerol.* **104**:98–102.
18. Crow, K. D., Alexander, E., Buck, W. H. L., et al. (1961): Photosensitivity due to pitch. *Br. J. Dermatol.* **73**:220–232.
19. Everett, M. A., Daffer, E., and Coffey, C. M. (1961): Coal tar and ultraviolet light. I. *Arch. Dermatol.* **84**:473–476.
20. Everett, M. A., and Miller, J. V. (1961): Coal tar and ultraviolet light. II. Cumulative effects. *Arch. Dermatol.* **84**:937–940.
21. Forbes, P. D., Davies, R. E., and Urbach, F. (1976): Phototoxicity and photocarcinogenesis: comparative effects of anthracene and 8-methoxypsoralen in the skin of mice. *Food Cosmet. Toxicol.* **14**:303–306.
22. Kaidbey, K. H., and Kligman, A. M. (1977): Clinical and histologic study of coal tar phototoxicity in humans. *Arch. Dermatol.* **113**:592–595.
23. Wiskemann, A., and Hoyer, H. (1971): Zur Phototoxicitität von Teerpräparaten. *Hautarzt* **22**:257–258.

24. Wulf, K., Unna, P. J., and Willers, M. (1963): Experimentelle Untersuchungen über die photodynamische Wirksamkeit von Steinkohlenteerbestandteilen. *Hautarzt* **14**:292–297.
25. Hjorth, N., Sjolin, K.-E., Sylvest, B., et al. (1972): Acne aestivalis-Mallorca acne. *Acta Derm. Venereol. (Stockh.)* **52**:6163.
26. Brust, B. (1977): Uber das Pseudomilium colloidale. *Dermatol. Monatsschr.* **163**:484–489.
27. Carli-Basset, C., Fauchier, C., Despert, F., et al. (1976): Maladie de Urbach–Wiethe. A propos d'un cas avec étude ultrastructurale. *Bull. Soc. Fr. Dermatol. Syphiligr.* **83**:358–360.
28. Fanta, D., and Niebauer, G. (1976): Aktinische (senile) Komedonen. *Z. Hautkr.* **51**:791–797.
29. Findlay, G. H., Morrison, J. G. L., and Simson, I. W. (1975): Exogenous ochronosis and pigmented colloid milium from hydroquinone bleaching creams. *Br. J. Dermatol.* **93**:613–622.
30. Francis, R. S. (1975): Lipoid proteinosis: a case report. *Radiology* **117**:301–302.
31. Garrel, J., Millet, J. P., Jeanney, J.-C., et al. (1975): Colloid milium. *Ann. Dermatol. Syphiligr. (Paris)* **102**:399–400.
32. Hashimoto, K., Katzman, R. L., Kang, A. H., et al. (1975): Electron microscopical and biochemical analysis of colloid milium. *Arch. Dermatol.* **111**:49–59.
33. Holzberger, P. C. (1960): Concerning adult colloid milium. *Arch. Dermatol.* **82**:711–716.
34. Kastl, J., and Horacek, J. (1973): Favre–Racouchot's disease with the formation of secondary osteomas. *Csl. Dermatol.* **48**:191–194.
35. O'Brien, J. P. (1975): Actinic granuloma. An annular connective tissue disorder affecting sun- and heat-damaged (elastotic) skin. *Arch. Dermatol.* **111**:460–477.
36. Pisani, M., and Ruocco, V. (1977): La ialinosi della cute e delle mucose (su di un caso con carattere di fotosensibilitá). *Biorn. Minerva Dermatol.* **112**:293–298.
37. Rook, A. (1976): Lipoid proteinosis: Urbach–Wiethe's disease. *Br. J. Dermatol.* **94**:341–342.
38. Bergamasco A. (1940): Le fotodermatosi. *Arch. Ital. Dermatol.* **16**:131–154.
39. Poppe, W., and Grossweiner, L. I. (1975): Photodynamic sensitization by 8-methoxypsoralen via the singlet oxygen mechanism. *Photochem. Photobiol.* **22**:217–219.
40. Forbes, P. D., Urbach, F., and Davies, R. E. (1977): Phototoxicity testing of fragrance raw material. *Food Cosmet. Toxicol.* **15**:55–60, 265.
41. Frain-Bell, W., and Zaynoun, S. (1975): The oil of bergamot photopatch test. *Contact Dermatol.* **1**:245.
42. Ippen, H., and Tesche, S. (1971): Zur Photodermatitis pigmentaria Freund (Berloque Dermatitis, "Eau de Cologne Pigmentation"). *Hautarzt* **22**:535–536.
43. Ippen, H., and Tesche, S. (1972): Das "Chloasma" ausserhalb der Gravidität. *Hautarzt* **23**:21–25.
44. Jung, E. G. (1976): Furocumarine in Kosmetika. *Dtsch. Med. Wochenschr.* **101**:29.
45. Marzulli, F. N., and Maibach, H. I. (1970): Perfume phototoxicity. *J. Soc. Cosmet. Chem.* **21**:695–715.
46. Nolting, S., and Koch-Schulte, U. (1975): Ein Beitrag zum Bild der Berloque-Dermatitis. *Z. Hautkr.* **50**:721–723.
47. Zaynoun, S., Hall, J., Johnson, B. E., et al. (1974): A study of Bergamot photosensitivity. *Br. J. Dermatol.* **91**(Suppl. 10):14–15.
48. Altobella, L. (1971): Contributo allo studio delle fotodermatosi da Bergaptene. Considerazioni a proposito di una epidemia fra operai addetti alla raccolta del sedano (celery). *Arch. Ital. Dermatol.* **37**:39–47.
49. Camm, E., Buck, H. W. L., and Mitchell, J. C. (1976): Phytophotodermatitis from *Heracleum mantegazzianum*. *Contact Dermatol.* **2**:68–72.
50. Dijk, E., and Berrens, L. (1964): Plants as an etiological factor in phytophotodermatitis. *Dermatologica* **129**:321–328.
51. Giese, A. C. (1971): Photosensitization by natural pigments. *Photophysiology* **6**:77–129.

52. Hegnauer, R. (1964/1973): *Chemotaxonomie der Pflanzen.* Birkhauser Verlag, Basel/ Stuttgart.

53. Ippen H. (1973): Verätzungen beim Baden. Ein differentialdiagnostischer Beitrag. *Dtsch. Med. Wochenschr.* **98:**2048-2049.

54. Pathak, M. A., Daniels, F., and Fitzpatrick, T. B. (1962): The presently known distribution of furocoumarins (psoralens) in plants. *J. Invest. Dermatol.* **39:**225-239.

55. Prinz, L., and Köstler, H. (1976): Ein Bericht über drei Fälle von toxischer Phytophoto-dermatitis durch *Heracleum mantegazzianum* (Riesenherkulesstaude). *Dermatol. Monats-schr.* **162:**881-886.

56. Qadripur, S. A., and Gründer, K. (1975): Kasuistischer Beitrag über eine Gruppener-krankung mit Photodermatitis bullosa striata pratensis (Oppenheim). *Hautarzt* **26:**495-497.

57. Reichel, K. (1976): Welche Gräser bzw. Pflanzen verursachen bei uns am häufigsten Dermatitis pratensis? *Schrifttum Praxis* **7:**176.

58. Sommer, R. G., and Jileson, O. F. (1967): Phyto-photodermatitis (solar dermatitis from plants). Gas plant and wild parsnip. *N. Engl. J. Med.* **276:**1484-1486.

59. Copeland, E. S., Alving, C. R., and Grenan, M. M. (1976): Light-induced leakage of spin lable marker from liposomes in the presence of phototoxic phenothiazines. *Photochem. Photobiol.* **24:**41-48.

60. Ippen, H. (1958): Über eine lichtabhängige Reaktion im Blutserum. Ein Beitrag zur Photoallergie. *Klin. Wochenschr.* **36:**587.

61. Leterrier, F. (1976): Interaction of Chlorpromazine with biological membranes. A photochemical study using spin labels. *Biochem. Pharmacol.* **25:**2469-2474.

62. Ljunggren, B., and Möller, H. (1977): Phenothiazine phototoxicity: an experimental study on Chlorpromazine and its metabolites. *J. Invest. Dermatol.* **68:**313-317.

63. Ljunggren, B., and Möller, H. (1977): Phenothiazine phototoxicity: an experimental study on Chlorpromazine and related tricyclic drugs. *Acta Derm. Venereol. (Stockh.)* **57:**325-329.

64. Raffle, E. J., MacLeod, T. M., Hutchinson, F., et al. (1975): Chlorpromazine photo-sensitivity. *Arch. Dermatol.* **111:**1364-1365.

65. Binazzi, M., and Calandra, P. (1971): Identification of an error in the tryptophan-niacin pathway in carriers of some dermatoses conditioned or aggravated by sunlight. *Arch. Klin. Exp. Dermatol.* **239:**368-376.

66. Castiello, R. J., and Lynch, P. J. (1972): Pellagra and the carcinoid syndrome. *Arch. Dermatol.* **105:**574-577.

67. Comaish, J. S., and Cooper, M. (1977): Isoniazid-incuded pellagra. *Arch. Dermatol.* **113:**986-987.

68. Des Groseilliers, J. P., and Shiffman, N. J. (1976): Pellagra. *Can. Med. Assoc. J.* **115:**768-790.

69. Dogliotti, M., Liebowitz, M., Downing, D. T., et al. (1977): Nutritional influences on pellagra on sebum composition. *Br. J. Dermatol.* **97:**25-28.

70. Gupta, O. P. (1977): Study of anemia in cases of pellagra with hemosiderosis of liver. *J. Assoc. Physicians India* **25:**261-265.

71. Kimmig, J., Shicherling, W., Tschesche, R., et al. (1958): *N*(-β-(Indolyl-3)-acryloyl)-glycin. Isolierung aus Harn und Synthese. *Z. Physiol. Chem.* **311:**234-238.

72. Larregue, M., Degos, R., Schnibler, L., et al. (1970): Erythème pellagroide avec trouble du métabolisme du tryptophane. *Bull. Soc. Fr. Dermatol.* **77:**885-887.

73. Stratigos, J. D., and Katsambas, A. (1977): Pellagra: a still existing disease. *Br. J. Dermatol.* **96:**99-106.

74. Tahmoush, A. J. (1976): Hartnup disease. *Arch. Neurol.* **33:**797-807.

75. Tarlow, M. J., Seakins, J. W. T., Lloyd, J. K., et al. (1972): Absorption of amino acids and peptides in a child with a variant of Hartnup disease and coexistent coeliac disease. *Arch. Dis. Child.* **47:**798-803.

76. Bickers, D. R., Keogh, L., Harber, L. C., et al. (1976): The effect of environmental light exposure on drug-induced porphyria in the rat. *Photochem. Photobiol.* **24**:551–553.

77. Bloomer, J. R., Philips, M. J., Davidson, D. L., et al. (1975): Hepatic disease in erythropoietic protoporphyria. *Am. J. Med.* **58**:869–882.

78. Cauzzo, G., Gennari, G., Jori, G., et al. (1977): The effect of chemical structure on the photosensitizing efficiencies of porphyrins. *Photochem. Photobiol.* **25**:389–395.

79. Eakins, M. N., and Slater, T. F., (1975): Biochemical studies on bile secretion. In: *Proceedings of the 2nd NATO Advanced Study Institute on the Biliary System, Denmark, August, 1975.* pp. 38–41.

80. Epstein, J. H., Tuffanelli, D. L., and Epstein, W. L. (1973): Cutaneous changes in the porphyrias—a microscopic study. *Arch. Dermatol.* **107**:689–698.

81. Goeij, A. F. P. M., de Ververgaert, P. H. J. T., and van Steveninck, J. (1975): Photodynamic effects of protoporphyrin on the architecture of erythrocyte membranes in protoporphyria and in normal red blood cells. *Clin. Chim. Acta* **62**:287–292.

82. Goeij, A. F. P. M., and van Steveninck, J. (1976): Photodynamic effects of protoporphyrin on cholesterol and unsaturated fatty acids in erythrocyte membranes in protoporphyria and in normal red blood cells. *Clin. Chim. Acta* **68**:115–122.

83. Gschnait, F., Konrad, K., Hönigsmann, H., et al. (1975): Mouse model for protoporphyria. I. The liver and hepatic protoporphyrin crystals. *J. Invest. Dermatol.* **65**:290–299.

84. Gschnait, F., Wolff, K., and Konrad, K. (1975): Erythropoietic protoporphyria—submicroscopic effects during the acute photosensitivity flare. *Br. J. Dermatol.* **92**:545–557.

85. Heikel, T. A. J. (1968): Inhibition of biliary secretion by icterogenin and related triterpenes. *Biochem. Pharmacol.* **17**:1079–1097.

86. Honigsmann, H. (1977): Die erythropoetische Protoporphyrie. I. Klinik und Problematik der Pathogenese. *Z. Hautkr.* **52**:495–509.

87. Honigsmann, H. (1977): Die erythropoetische Protoporphyrie. II. Experimentelle Untersuchungen an Modellsystemen: Photosensibilität und Hautveränderungen. *Z. Hautkr.* **52**:541–564.

88. Honigsmann, H. (1977): Die erythropoetische Protoporphyrie. III. Experimentelle Untersuchungen an Modellsystemen: Pathogenese der Leberschadigung. *Z. Hautkr.* **52**:599–621.

89. Hsu, J., Goldstein, B. D., and Harber, L. C. (1971): Photoreactions associated with in vitro hemolysis in erythropoietic protoporphyria. *Photochem. Photobiol.* **13**:67–77.

90. Ippen, H. (1960): Lichtdermatosen und Porphyrin-Photosensibilisierung. *Arch. Klin. Exp. Dermatol.* **210**:496–522.

91. Lightner, D. A. (1974): Photochemistry of pyrroles, bile pigments and porphyrins. *Photochem. Photobiol.* **19**:457–459.

92. MacDonald, D. M., and Nicholson, D. C. (1976): Erythropoietic protoporphyria. Hepatic implications. *Br. J. Dermatol.* **95**:157–162.

93. Magnus, I. A., Janousek, V., and Jones, K. (1974): The effect of environmental lighting on porphyrin metabolism in the rat. *Nature* **250**:504–505.

94. McGrae, J. D., Jr., and Perry, H. O., (1963): Relationship of photodynamic action to phototoxicity determinants of morphologic response. *Arch. Dermatol.* **87**:253–257.

95. Miura, T., Magnus, I. A., Jones, K., et al. (1975): Skin porphyrin and photosensitivity in the porphyric rat. *Dermatologica* **151**:80–88.

96. Nordmann, Y., and Grandchamp, B. (1976): Conjugated effect of light and uroporphyria on porphbilinogen. *Biochem. Med.* **15**:119–125.

97. Runge, W. J. (1972): Photosensitivity in porphyria. *Photophysiology* **7**:149–160.

98. Ryan, T. J. (1975): Erythropoietic protoporphyria: submicroscopic events during the acute photosensitivity flare. *Br. J. Dermatol.* **93**:605.

99. Schothorst, A. A., and de Haas, C. A. C. (1977): Photodynamic effects of protoporphyrin and violet light on fibroblast cultures: damage and repair (abstract). *J. Invest. Dermatol.* **68**:244.

100. Spikes, J. D. (1975): Porphyrins and related compounds as photodynamic sensitizers. *Ann. N. Y. Acad. Sci.* **244**:496–508.

101. Altmeyer, P., and Hufnagl, D. (1975): Chrysiasis: Nebenwirkung einer intramuskulären Goldtherapie. *Hautarzt* **26**:330–333.

102. Cox, A. J. (1973): Gold in dermis following gold therapy for rheumatic arthritis. *Arch. Dermatol.* **108**:655–657.

103. Gracianski, P. de, and Perals, P. (1974): Argyrie cutanée. *Bull. Soc. Fr. Dermatol. Syphiligr.* **81**:303.

104. Kaufmann, J., Gilliet, F., Ott, F., et al. (1975): Lokalisierte Chrysiasis. *Dermatologica* **150**:233.

105. Lofferer, O. (1975): Argyrose. *Dermatol. Monatsschr.* **161**:511.

106. Nasemann, T., Rogge, T., and Schaeg, G. (1974): Licht- und elektronenmikroskopische Untersuchungen bei der Hydrargyrose und der Argyrose der Haut. *Hautarzt* **25**:534–540.

107. Bonnet, R. (1976): Mechanisms of the photodegradation of bilirubin. *Biochem. Soc. Trans.* **4**:222–228.

108. Kapoor, C. L., Murti, C. R. K., and Bajpai, P. C. (1974): Role of human skin in the photodecomposition of bilirubin. *Biochem. J.* **142**:567–573.

109. Land, E. J. (1976): The triplet excited states of bilirubin. *Photochem. Photobiol.* **24**:475–477.

110. McDonagh, A. F. (1975): Thermal and photochemical reactions of bilirubin IXα. *Ann. N. Y. Acad. Sci.* **244**:553–569.

111. McDonagh, A. F. (1976): Phototherapy of neonatal jaundice. *Biochem. Soc. Trans.* **4**:219–222.

112. Pedersen, A. O., Schønheyder, F., and Brodersen, R. (1977): Photooxidation of human serum albumin and its complex with bilirubin. *Eur. J. Biochem.* **72**:213–221.

113. Schaffer, R., Odell, G. B., and Simopoulos, A. P. (1975): *Phototherapy in the Newborn: An Overview*. National Academy of Sciences Printing Office, Washington, D.C.

114. Sisson, T. R. C. (1976): Visible light therapy of neonatal hyperbilirubinemia. *Photochemistry and Photobiology Reviews* **1**:241–268.

115. Tan, K. L. (1977): The nature of the dose–response relationship of phototherapy for neonatal hyperbilirubinemia. *J. Pediatr.* **90**:448–452.

116. Baart de la Faille, H., Brottier, P. B., and Baart de la Faille-Kuyper, E. H. (1975): Solar urticaria: a case with possible increase of skin mast cells. *Br. J. Dermatol.* **92**:102–107.

117. Harber, L. C., Holloway, R. M., Wheatley, V. R., et al. (1963): Immunological and biophysical studies in solar urticaria. *J. Invest. Dermatol.* **41**:439–443.

118. Horio, T. (1977): Solar urticaria: photoallergen in a patient's serum. *Arch. Dermatol.* **113**:157–160.

119. Illig, L., and Kunick, J. (1969, 1970): Klinik und Diagnostik der physikalischen Urticaria. *Hautarzt* **20**:167–178, 499–512; **21**:16–21.

120. Shelley, W. B., and Heaton, C. L. (1976): Pathogenesis of solar urticaria. *Arch. Dermatol.* **112**:850–852.

121. Tödt, D., and Jung, E. G. (1974): Lichturticaria. *Z. Hautkr.* **49**:31–35.

122. Willis, I., and Epstein, J. H. (1974): Solar vs. heat-induced urticaria. *Arch. Dermatol.* **110**:389–392.

123. Amos, H. E. (1973): Photoallergy: a critical survey. *Trans. St. John's Hosp. Dermatol. Soc.* **59**:147–151.

124. Epstein, J. H. (1972): Photoallergy: a review. *Arch. Dermatol.* **106**:741–748.

125. Horio, T. (1976): The induction of photocontact sensitivity in guinea pigs without UVB radiation. *J. Invest. Dermatol.* **67**:591–593.

126. Ippen, H. (1972): Basic mechanisms of photoallergic reactions. In: *Proceedings of the 6th International Congress on Photobiology, Bochum, 1972,* Paper 049.

127. Jung, E. G. (1972): Photoallergie. *Z. Hautkr.* **47**:329–334.

128. Kleiniewska, D., Wolska, H., and Kowalski, J. (1976): Photocontact dermatitis. *Przegl. Dermatol.* **63**:339-343.
129. Nagreh, D. S. (1975): Photodermatitis. Study of the condition in Kuantan, Malaysia. *Contact Dermatol.* **1**:27-32.
130. Ramsay, C. A., and Black, A. K. (1973): Light-sensitive eczemas. *Trans. St. John's Hosp. Dermatol. Soc.* **59**:152-158.
131. Emmett, E. A. (1974): Diphenhydramine photoallergy. *Arch. Dermatol.* **110**:249-252.
132. Horio, T. (1976): Allergic and photoallergic dermatitis from Diphenhydramine. *Arch. Dermatol.* **112**:1124-1126.
133. Burry, J. N. (1974): Fenticlor: actinic reticuloid and antihistamines. *Br. Med. J.* **2**:556-557.
134. Clayton, R., and Feiwel, M. (1976): From fenticlor sensitivity to actinic reticuloid? *Proc. R. Soc. Med.* **69**:379-380.
135. Breit, R. (1975): Photodermatitis from halogenated salicylanilides in Germany. *Contact Dermatol.* **1**:263.
136. Emmett, E. A. (1974): Nature of tribromosalicylanilide photoallergy. *J. Invest. Dermatol.* **63**:227-230.
137. Herman, P. S., and Sams, W. M., Jr. (1972): *Soap Photodermatitis: Photosensitivity to Halogenated Salicylanilides.* C. C. Thomas, Springfield, Ill.
138. Horio, T., and Ofuji, S. (1976): The fate of tetrachlorosalicylanilide in photosensitized guinea pigs. *Acta Derm. Venereol. (Stockh.)* **56**:367-371.
139. Kochevar, I. E., and Harber, L. C. (1977): Photoreactions of 3,3′,4,4′-tetrachlorosalicylanilide with proteins. *J. Invest. Dermatol.* **68**:151-156.
140. Schubert, H., Wurbach, G., and Döring, H.-G. (1977): Untersuchungen über die Afungin-Allergie. *Dermatol. Monatsschr.* **163**:384-386.
141. Tarnick, M. (1975): Sensibilisierung der Haut gegen Monobromsalizylsäure-isopropylamid. *Dermatol. Monatsschr.* **161**:459-461.
142. Frain-Bell, W., and Gardiner, J. (1975): Photocontact dermatitis due to quindoxin. *Contact Dermatol.* **4**:256.
143. Frain-Bell, W. (1976): Photocontact dermatitis due to quindoxin. *Cutis* **18**:654.
144. Johnson, B. E., Zaynoun, S., Gardiner, J. M., et al. (1975): A study of persistent light reaction in quindoxin and quinine photosensitivity. *Br. J. Dermatol.* **93**:21.
145. Scott, K. W., and Dawson, T. A. J. (1974): Photocontact dermatitis arising from the presence of quindoxin in animal feeding stuffs. *Br. J. Dermatol.* **90**:543-546.
146. Zaynoun, S., Johnson, B. E., and Frain-Bell, W. (1976): The investigation of quindoxin photosensitivity. *Contact Dermatol.* **2**:343-352.
147. Gammer, S., and Gross, P. R. (1976): Photoallergy induced by quinidine. *Cutis* **17**:72-74.
148. Groot, W. P. de, and White, J. (1974): Livedo racemosa-like photosensitivity reaction during quinidine durettes medication. *Dermatologica* **148**:371-376.
149. Pariser, D. M., and Taylor, J. R. (1975): Quinidine photosensitivity. *Arch. Dermatol.* **111**:1440-1443.
150. Pariser, R. J., and Pariser, D. M. (1976): Quinidine photosensitivity. *Arch. Dermatol.* **112**:1610-1611.
151. Horio, T., Tagami, H., and Ikai, K. (1975): Photoallergic dermatitis from phenothiazines. *Acta Dermatol. (Kyoto)* **70**:115-121.
152. Lam, S. K., and Tomlinson, D. R. (1976): Chlorpromazine-induced histamine release from guinea-pig skin in vitro: a photosensitive reaction. *Arch. Dermatol. Res.* **255**:219-223.
153. Menighini, C. L., and Angelini, G. (1975): Elastotic and citrine skin following an allergic photocontact dermatitis in a child. *Contact Dermatol.* **1**:301-305.
154. Romaguera, C., Lecha, M., Piñol Aguade, J., et al. (1973): Estudio comparativo de las reacciones cruzadas alergicas y fotoalergicas producidas por el fenergan y la elilenodiamina. *Med. Cutanea* **7**:121-124.
155. Suhonen, R. (1976): Thioridazine photosensitivity. *Contact Dermatol.* **2**:179.

156. Breza, T. S., Halprin, K. M., and Taylor, R. (1975): Photosensitivity reaction to vinblastine. *Arch. Dermatol.* **111**:1168–1170.

157. Kapur, T. R. (1976): Systemic photosensitivity towards cyclophosphamide (Endoxan). A case report. *Indian J. Dermatol. Venereol. Leprol.* **42**:5.

158. Leoni, A., Cogo, R., Schettin, D., et al. (1976): Photodermatitis with mucositis due to Moquizone. A new iatrogenic dermatosis. *Minerva Dermatol.* **111**:182–188.

159. Ljunggren, B. (1977): Psoralen photoallergy caused by plant contact. *Contact Dermatol.* **3**:85–90.

160. Elgart, M. L., and Higdon, R. S. (1971): Photosensitivity caused by oral contraceptives. *Med. Ann. D. C.* **40**:501–503.

161. Horkay, I., Tamasi, P., Prékopa, A., et al. (1975): Photodermatoses induced by oral contraceptives. *Arch. Dermatol. Res.* **253**:53–61.

162. Roberts, D. T., Brodie, M. J., Moore, M. R., et al. (1977): Hereditary coproporphyria presenting with photosensitivity induced by the contraceptive pill. *Br. J. Dermatol.* **96**:549–554.

163. Tamasi, P., Prékopa, A., Dalmy, L., et al. (1974): Photodermatoses induced by estrogens. *Borgyogy Venereol. Szle.* **50**:63–67.

164. Akhoundzadeh, H. (1973): Photo-hématodermie benigne ou "actinoréticulose." *Bull. Soc. Fr. Dermatol.* **80**:625–627.

165. Burry, J. N. (1974): Persistent phototoxicity due to nalidixic acid. *Arch. Dermatol.* **109**:263.

166. Davies, A. K., Hilal, N. S., McKellar, J. F., et al. (1975): Photochemistry of tetra-chlorosalicylanilide and its relevance to the persistent light reactor. *Br. J. Dermatol.* **92**:143–148.

167. Frain-Bell, W. (1975): Die klinischen, histologischen und photobiologischen Eigenarten des aktinischen Reticuloids. *Dermatol. Monatsschr.* **161**:32–37.

168. Gasparini, G., Prandi, G., and Caputo, R. (1976): Aspetti ultrastrutturali di due casi di actinoreticulosi. *Minerva Dermatol.* **111**:667–668.

169. Grupper, C., Bourgeois-Spinasse, J., and Eisenmann, D. (1973): Actino-reticulose chez un psoriasique. *Bull. Soc. Fr. Dermatol.* **80**:266.

170. Ive, F. A., Magnus, I. A., Warin, R. P., et al. (1969): Actinic reticuloid: a chronic dermatosis associated with severe photosensitivity and the histologic resemblance to lymphoma. *Br. J. Dermatol.* **81**:469–485.

171. Mischer, P. (1973): Aktinisches Reticuloid. *Z. Hautkr.* **48**:748.

172. Sapuppo, A., and Baratta, P. F. (1974): Fotodermatosi a decorso protratto recidivante culminata in emoblastosi. *Minerva Dermatol.* **109**:136–143.

173. Schaumburg-Lever, G., and Lever, W. (1976): Actinic reticuloid. *Arch. Dermatol.* **112**:889.

174. Schnitzler, L., Schubert, B., Belperron, P., et al. (1973): Actinoréticulose survenant au décours d'une porphrie cutanée tardive. *Bull. Soc. Fr. Dermatol.* **80**:488–489.

175. Schnitzler, L., Verret, J. L., Schubert, B., et al. (1975): Langerhans cells in actinic reticuloid. *J. Cutan. Pathol.* **2**:170–178.

176. Swanbeck, G., and Wennersten, G. (1973): Evidence for kynurenic acid as a possible photosensitizer in actinic reticuloid. *Acta Derm. Venereol. (Stockh.)* **53**:109–113.

177. Texier, L., Gauthier, O., and Gauthier, Y. (1973): Succession d'une vitiligo, d'un psoriasis et d'une dermatose actinique. *Bull. Soc. Fr. Dermatol.* **80**:369–370.

178. Thomsen, K. (1977): The development of Hodgkin's disease in a patient with actinic reticuloid. *Clin. Exp. Dermatol.* **2**:109–113.

179. Wiskemann, A. (1965): Lichtprovozierbare granulomatöse Reticulose. *Dermatol. Wochenschr.* **151**:1420.

180. Ayala, F., Palombini, L., and Santoianni, P. (1975): Sulla infiltrazione linfocitaria della pelle di Jessner e Kanof. *Minerva Dermatol.* **110**:428–433.

181. Barthelmes, H., and Sönnichsen, N. (1968): Differential diagnosis des chronischen discoiden L. erythematodes und der "lymphocytic infiltration" von Jessner und Kanof durch Immunfluoreszenz-Histologie. *Arch. Klin. Exp. Dermatol.* **232**:384–397.

182. Castrow, F. F., and Cornelison R. L., Jr. (1975): Summer prurigo. *Cutis* **16**:640–641.
183. Frain-Bell, W., Dickson, A., Herd, J., et al. (1973): The action spectrum in polymorphic light eruption. *Br. J. Dermatol.* **89**:243–249.
184. Guilhou, J. J., Barneon, G., Meynadier, J., et al. (1975): Infiltrat lymphocytaire de la peau de Jessner et Kanof. *Bull. Soc. Fr. Dermatol.* **82**:317–319.
185. Herzberg, J. (1973): Wenig bekannte Formen der Neurodermitis. *Hautarzt* **24**:47–51.
186. Heyse, H. (1964): Zum Krankheitsbegriff des chronischen polymorphen Lichtexanthems. Dissertation, Dusseldorf.
187. Horkay, I., and Alfoldy, G. (1972): Angaben über den Serotonin-Stoffwechsel bein chronisch polymorphen Lichtausschlägen. *Z. Hautkr.* **47**:855–858.
188. Jansen, C. T. (1977): Elevated serum immunoglobulin levels in polymorphous light eruptions. *Acta Derm. Venereol. (Stockh.)***57**:331–333.
189. Jessner, M. Kanof, N. B., and Orfuss, A. J. (1953): Lymphocytic infiltration of the skin. *Arch. Dermatol.* **68**:447–449.
190. Jonquières, E. D. L., and e Garrido, R. C. B. (1973): Prurigo actinico familiar. *Med. Cutan. Iber. Lat. Am.* **5**:319–326.
191. Londono, F. (1973): Thalidomide in the treatment of actinic prurigo. *Int. J. Dermatol.* **12**:326–328.
192. Londono, F., and Lopez, M. (1973): La talidomida en el tratemiento del prurigo actinico. *Arch. Argent. Dermatol.* **23**:183–190.
193. Nordlund, J. J., Klaus, S. N., Mathews-Roth, M. M., et al. (1973): New therapy for polymorphous light eruption. *Arch. Dermatol.* **108**:710–712.
194. Panet-Raymond, C., and Johnson, W. C. (1973): Lupus erythematosus and polymorphous light eruption. *Arch. Dermatol.* **108**:785–787.
195. Panfilis, G. de (1976): Infiltrazione linfocitaria cutanea de Jessner e Kanof. *Minerva Dermatol.* **111**:368–370.
196. Raffle, E. J., Macleod, T. M., and Hutchinson, F. (1973): In vitro lymphocyte studies in chronic polymorphic light eruption. *Br. J. Dermatol.* **89**:143–148.
197. Rasch, C. (1900): Om et polymorft (erythematst, vesikulst og ekzematoidt) Lysudslet. *Hospital stidende* **43**:478.
198. Saul, A. (1976): Polymorphous light eruption: treatment with thalidomide. *Australas. J. Dermatol.* **17**:17–21.
199. Szabo, E., Toth-Kasa, I., and Heszler, E. (1976): Reticulin-Antikörper bei Lupus erythematodes und polymorphem Lichtexanthem. *Z. Hautkr.* **51**:353–360.
200. Thune, P. (1976): Chronic polymorphic light eruption. *Acta Derm. Venereol. (Stockh.)* **56**:127–133.
201. Verhagen, A. R. H. B. (1965): *Onderzoekingen bij chronische polymorfe Lichtdermatosen.* Proff Copy, Amsterdam.
202. Altobella, L. (1974): Hidroa vacciniforme de Bazin: a proposito di un' osservazione clinica. *Arch. Ital. Dermatol.* **39**:353–357.
203. Bazin, P. A. E. (1862): *Leçons Théoriques et Cliniques sur les Affections Génériques de la Peau. Troisieme leçon: de l'herpes,* p. 128. E. Baudot, Paris.
204. Dulanto, F. de, and Armijo Moreno, M. (1975): Hidroa vacciniforme. *Actas Dermosifilogr.* **66**:651–658.
205. Jaschke, E., Reinken, L., and Frisch, H. (1975): Hydroa vacciniforme Bazin. *Hautarzt* **26**:11–17.
206. Musger, A. (1971): Zur nosologischen Stellung der als Hydroa vacciniforme bezeichneten Hautveranderungen. *Z. Hautkr.* **46**:1–8.
207. Cabré, J., and Fuertes Fidalgo, M. (1971): Dermatitis primaveral infantil. *Actas Dermosifilogr.* **62**:91–94.
208. ippen, H. (1980): Photodermatitis multiformis acuta. *Dermatol. Monatsschr.* **166**:145–150.
209. Bloom, A. D. (1975): Genetics and cytogenetics of ataxia telangiectasia and Bloom's

syndrome. In: Pediatric dermatology, edited by R. Ruiz-Maldonado. *Mod. Probl. Paediatr.* **17**:6–10.

210. Bourgeois, C. A., Claverley, M. H., Forman, L., et al. (1975): Bloom's syndrome, a probable new case with cytogenetic findings. *J. Med. Genet.* **12**:423–425.

211. Dugois, P., Amblard, P., Jalbert, P., et al. (1974): Le syndrome de Bloom. *Ann. Dermatol. Syphiligr. (Paris)* **101**:5–13.

212. Schroeder, T. M. (1973): Die spontane Chromosomeninstabilität bei den seltenen Erbkrankheiten: Fanconi-Anämie und Bloom-Syndrom. *Dtsch. Med. Wochenschr.* **98**:2213–2215.

213. Brezine, Z. (1976): Cockayne-Syndrom. *Kinderaerztl. Prax.* **44**:259–265.

214. Chernosky, M. E. (1966): Porokeratosis: report of twelve patients with multiple superficial lesions. *South. Med. J.* **59**:289–294.

215. Gutschmidt, E. (1977): Disseminierte superficiale actinische Porokeratose. *Z. Hautkr.* **52**:622–624.

216. Pirozzi, D. J., and Rosenthal, A. (1976): Disseminated superficial actinic porokeratosis. Analysis of an affected family. *Br. J. Dermatol.* **95**:429–432.

217. Hanecke, E., and Gutschmidt, E. (1976): Warty hyperkeratoses, cellular immune defect, and tapetoretinal degeneration in poikiloderma congenitale. *Dermatologica* **152**:331–336.

218. Rodermund, O. E., and Hausmann, D. (1977): Das Thomson-Syndrom (Ein Beitrag zu den congenitalen Poikilodermien). *Dermatol. Monatsschr.* **163**:601–612.

219. Piñol Aguadé, J., Capdevila, J. M., Lecha, M., et al. (1973): Sindrome de Seckel con manifestationes de fotosensibilidad. *Med. Cutan. Iber. Lat. Am.* **5**:327–332.

220. Stevanovic, D. V. (1977): The diffuse and macular atrophic dermatosis. A premature light degenerative heritable condition. *Br. J. Dermatol.* **97**(Suppl. 15):10–11.

221. Bjornberg, A. (1976): Werner's syndrome and malignancy. *Acta Derm. Venereol. (Stockh.)* **56**:149–150.

222. Goldstein, S., and Niewiarowski, S. (1976): Increased procoagulant activity in cultured fibroblasts from progeria and Werner's syndromes of premature ageing. *Nature* **260**:711–713.

223. Kocks, J., Goerz, G., and Gruneklee, D. (1977): Werner-Syndrom (Progeria adultorum). *Z. Hautkr.* **52**:69–71.

224. Cripps, D. J., and Rankin, J. (1973): Action spectra of lupus erythematosus and experimental immunofluorescence. *Arch. Dermatol.* **107**:563–567.

225. Diezel, W., Meffert, H., Günther, W., et al. (1977): Exazerbation des Lupus erythematodes visceralis infolge UV-Bestrahlung. *Dermatol. Monatsschr.* **163**:290–295.

226. Horkay, I., Nagy, E., Tamasi, P., et al. (1975): DNA repair and UV-light sensitivity of the lymphocytes in discoid lupus erythematosus. *Studia Biophys.* **50**:1–6.

227. Castrow, F. F., II, and Wolf, J. E., Jr. (1973): Photolocalized varicella. *Arch. Dermatol.* **107**:628.

228. Gilchrest, B., and Baden, H. P. (1974): Photodistribution of viral exanthema. *Pediatrics* **54**:136–140.

229. Bielicky, T., and Kvicalova, E. (1964): Photosensitive psoriasis. *Dermatologica* **129**:339–348.

230. Frumess, G. M., and Lewis, H. M. (1957): Light-sensitive seborrhoid. *Arch. Dermatol.* **75**:245–248.

231. Helinski, M.: Sonnenstrahlen-Empfindlichkeit in einigen Fällen von Psoriasis. *Z. Hautkr.* **51**:208–210.

232. Mihan, R., and Ayres, S., Jr. (1964): Perioral dermatitis. *Arch. Dermatol.* **89**:803–805.

233. Baden, H. P., and Provan, J. (1977): Sunlight and pityriasis rosea. *Arch. Dermatol.* **113**:377–378.

234. Basset, A., Maleville, J., Grosshans, E., et al: (1973): Lichen actinique tropical ou lupus erythémateux discoide disséminé chez un enfant. *Ann. Dermatol. Syphiligr. (Paris)* **100**:555–556.

235. Brody, H. J., and Castrow, F. F. (1976): Photolocalized tinea facialis. *Cutis* **17**:913–915.
236. Cram, D. L., and Fukuyama, K. (1972): Immunohistochemistry of ultraviolet-induced pemphigus and pemphigoid lesions. *Arch. Dermatol.* **106**:819–824.
237. Lindemayr, W. (1961): Purpura als Symptom erhönter Lichtempfindlichkeit. *Hautarzt* **12**:174–179.
238. Marion, D. F., and Terrien, C. M., Jr. (1973): Photosensitive livedo reticularis. *Arch. Dermatol.* **108**:100–101.
239. Orfanos, C. E., Gartmann, H., and Mahrle, G. (1971): Zur Pathogenese des Pemphigus erythematosus. *Arch. Klin. Exp. Dermatol.* **240**:317–333.
240. Santoianni, P. (1965): Lichen planus actinicus (vel tropicus). *Minerva Dermatol.* **40**:421–427.
241. Volden, G. (1977): Light sensitivity in mycosis fungoides (abstract). *J. Invest. Dermatol.* **68**:255.
242. Went, M., and Rasko, I. (1976): Die Wirkung der UV-Bestrahlung auf die Chromosomen bei der Dyskeratosis follicularis Darier. *Z. Hantkr.* **51**:393–396.
243. Charlier, M., and Hélène, C. (1975): Photosensitized splitting of pyrimidine dimers in DNA by indole derivatives and tryptophan-containing peptides. *Photochem. Photobiol.* **21**:31–37.
244. Handley, S. L., and Miskin, R. C. (1977): The interaction of some kynurenine pathway metabolites with 5-hydroxytryptophan and 5-hydroxytryptamine. *Psychopharmacology* **51**:305–309.
245. McCormick, J. P., Fischer, J. R., Pachlatko, J. P., et al. (1976): Characterization of a cell-lethal product from the photooxidation of trytophan: hydrogen peroxide. *Science* **191**:468–469.
246. Nilsson, R., Swanbeck, G., and Wennersten, G. (1975): Primary mechanisms of erythrocyte photolysis induced by biological sensitizers and phototoxic drugs. *Photochem. Photobiol.* **22**:183–186.
247. Rubaltelli, F. F., Allegri, G., Costa, C., et al. (1974): Urinary excretion of tyrptophan metabolites during phototherapy. *J. Pediatr.* **85**:865–871.
248. Swanbeck, G., and Wennersten, G. (1974): Photohemolytic activity of tryptophan and phenylalanine metabolites. *Acta Derm. Venereol. (Stockh.)* **54**:99–104.
249. Swanbeck, G., Wennersten, G., and Nilsson, R. (1974): Participation of singlet state excited oxygen in photochemolysis induced by kynurenic acid. *Acta Derm. Venereol. (Stockh.)* **54**:433–436.
250. Walrant, P., Santus, R., and Grossweiner, L. I. (1975): Photosensitizing properties of *N*-formylkynurenine. *Photochem. Photobiol.* **22**:63–65.
251. Walrant, P., Santus, R., and Charlier, M. (1976): Role of complex formation in the photosensitized degradation of DNA induced by *N'*-formylkynurenine. *Photochem. Photobiol.* **24**:13–19.
252. Walrant, P., Santus, R., Redpath, J. L., et al. (1976): *N'*-formylkynurenine-photosensitized inactivation of bacteriophage. *Int. J. Radiat. Biol.* **30**:189–192.
253. Wennersten, G., and Brunk, U. (1977): Cellular aspects of phototoxic reactions induced by kynurenic acid. I. Establishment of an experimental model utilizing in vitro cultivated cells. *Acta Derm. Venereol. (Stockh.)* **57**:201–209.
254. Wong, P. W. K. (1976): A defect in tryptophan metabolism. *Pediatr. Res.* **10**:725–730.
255. Alpert, B., and Lopez-Delgado, R. (1976): Fluorescence lifetimes of haem proteins excited into the tryptophan absorption band with synchrotron radiation. *Nature* **263**:445–446.
256. Baird, M. B., Massie, H. R., and Piekielniak, M. J. (1977): Formation of lipid peroxides in isolated rat liver microsomes by singlet molecular oxygen. *Chem. Biol. Interact.* **16**:145–153.
257. Berns, D. S. (1976): Photosensitive bilayer membranes as model systems for photobiological processes. *Photochem. Photobiol.* **24**:117–139.
258. Birks, J. B. (1976): Singlet and triplet mechanisms in photochemistry. *Photochem. Photobiol.* **24**:287–289.

H. Ippen

259. Chan, J. T., and Black, H. S. (1977): Antioxidant-mediated reversal of ultraviolet light cytotoxicity. *J. Invest. Dermatol.* **68**:366–368.
260. Diamond, I. (1977): Photochemotherapy and photodynamic toxicity: simple methods for identifying potentially active agents. *Biochem. Med.* **17**:121–127.
261. Diezel, W., Meffert, H., Höhne, W. E., et al. (1975): Endprodukte der Lipidperoxidation in menschlicher Epidermis: Nachweis, Zunahme nach UV-Bestrahlung, pathogene Bedeutung. *Dermatol. Monatsschr.* **161**:823–830.
262. Dougherty, T. J., Gomer, C. J., and Weishaupt, K. R. (1976): Energetics and efficiency of photoinactivation of murine tumor cells containing hematoporphyrin. *Cancer Res.* **36**:2330–2333.
263. Fesenko, E. E., and Lyubarskiy, A. L. (1977): Effect of light on artificial lipid membranes modified by photoreceptor membrane fragments. *Nature* **268**:562–563.
264. Girotti, A. W. (1976): Bilirubin-sensitized photoinactivation of enzymes in the isolated membrane of the human erythrocyte. *Photochem. Photobiol.* **24**:525–532.
265. Girotti, A. W. (1976): Photodynamic action of protoporphyrin 9 on human erythrocytes: cross-linking of membrane-proteins. *Biochem. Biophys. Res. Commun.* **72**:1367–1374.
266. Gromisch, D. S., Lopez, R., Cole, H. S., et al. (1977): Light (phototherapy)-induced riboflavin deficiency in the neonate. *J. Pediatr.* **90**:118–122.
267. Hawco, F. J., O'Brien, C. R., and O'Brien, P. J. (1977): Singlet oxygen formation during hemoprotein catalyzed lipid peroxide decomposition. *Biochem. Biophys. Res. Commun.* **76**:354–361.
268. Ippen, H., Tillmann, W., Seubert, S., et al. (1978): Porphyria erythropoietica congenita Gunther and chloroquine. *Klin. Wochenschr.* **56**:623–624.
269. Kocerginskij, N. M., Kagan, B. E., Novikov, K. H., et al. (1976): Regulation of membrane reactions by light. *Studia Biophys.* **58**:43–50.
270. Koter, M., Kowalska, M. A., Leyko, W., et al. (1977): ESR radiation studies of erythrocyte membrane–haemoglobin interaction. *Int. J. Radiat. Biol.* **32**:369–374.
271. Lamola, A. A., and Yamane, T. (1973): Cholesterol hydroperoxide formation in red cell membranes and photohemolysis in erythropoietic protoporphyria. *Science* **179**:1131–1133.
272. Lamola, A., Piomelli, S., Poh-Fitzpatrick, M., et al. (1975): Erythropoietic protoporphyria and lead intoxication: the molecular basis for difference in cutaneous photosensitivity. II. Different binding of erythrocyte protoporphyrin to hemoglobin. *J. Clin. Invest.* **56**:1528–1535.
273. Moore, W. M., McDaniels, J. C., and Hen, J. A. (1977): The photochemistry of riboflavin. VI. The photophysical properties of isoalloxazines. *Photochem. Photobiol.* **25**:505–512.
274. Paine, A. J. (1976): Induction of benzo(a)pyrene mono-oxygenase in liver cell culture by the photochemical generation of active oxygen species. Evidence for the involvement of singlet oxygen and the formation of a stable inducing intermediate. *Biochem. J.* **158**:109–117.
275. Pereira, O. M., Smith, J. R., and Packer, L. (1976): Photosensitization of human diploid cell cultures by intracellular flavins and protection by antioxidants. *Photochem. Photobiol.* **24**:237–242.
276. Piomelli, S., Lamola, A. A., Poh-Fitzpatrick, M. B., et al. (1975): Erythropoietic protoporphyria and lead intoxication: the molecular basis for difference in cutaneous photosensitivity. I. Diffusion rates of disappearance of protoporphyrin from the erythrocytes, both in vivo and in vitro. *J. Clin. Invest.* **56**:1519–1527.
277. Puchkov, E. O., Roshchupkin, D. I., and Vladimirov, Yu. A. (1976): Study of the effects of UV-light on biomembranes. VII. Photolysis of SH and S–S groups and lipid photoperoxidation if polyunsaturated fatty acids in isolated erythrocyte membranes. *Studia Biophys.* **60**:1–14.
278. Putvinsky, A. V., Potapenko, A. Ya., Puchkov, E. O., et al. (1977): Study of the effects of ultraviolet light on biomembranes. Increase in the ion permeability of mitochondral and artificial lipid membranes. *Studia Biophys.* **64**:17–32.

279. Roshchupkin, D. I., Pelenitsyn, A. B., Potapenko, A. Ya., et al. (1975): Study of the effects of ultraviolet light on biomembranes. IV. The effect of oxygen on UV-induced hemolysis and lipid photoperoxidation in rat erythrocytes and liposomes. *Photochem. Photobiol.* **21**:63–69.
280. Voet, D. (1977): Intercalation complexes of DNA. *Nature* **269**:285–286.
281. Wennersten, G. (1974): Experimental and Clinical Studies of Photodermatological Problems with Special Reference to the Inhibitory Effect of Beta-carotene on Light-Induced Reactions, and Studies on the Photodynamic Activity of Tryptophan Metabolites, Thesis, Dept. Dermatol., Karolinska Sjukhuset.

BIBLIOGRAPHY

Photobiology and Photopathology

Giese, A. C. (Ed.) (1964–1973): *Photophysiology*, 8 Vols. Academic Press, New York.

Giese, A. C. (1976): *Living with Our Sun's Ultraviolet Rays*. Plenum Press, New York.

Harber, L. C. (1976): Reflections and perspectives concerning cutaneous photobiology. *Arch. Dermatol.* **112**:1668–1670.

Johnson, B. E., Daniels, F., Jr., and Magnus, I. A. (1968): Response of human skin to ultraviolet light. *Photophysiology* **4**:139–202.

Jung, E. G. (1975): Sun and skin. *Dermatologica* **151**:257–267.

Kiefer, J. (Ed.) (1977): *Ultraviolette Strahlen.* W. de Gruyter, Berlin.

Magnus, I. A. (1976): *Dermatological Photobiology. Clinical and Experimental Aspects.* Blackwell, Oxford.

Mier, P. D., and Cotton, D. W. (1976): *The Molecular Biology of Skin.* Blackwell, Oxford.

Olson, R. L., Gaylor, J., and Everett, M. A. (1973): Skin color, melanin and erythema. *Arch. Dermatol.* **108**:541–544.

Pathak, M. A., and Epstein, J. H. (1971): Normal and abnormal reactions of man to light. In: *Dermatology in General Medicine*, edited by T. B. Fitzpatrick, K. A. Arndt, W. H. Clark, Jr., et al. pp. 977–1036. McGraw-Hill, New York.

Piñol Aguade, J., Mascaro Ballester, J. M., Melcior, J. R. G., et al. (1972): *Fotobiologia y Dermatologia.* Masnou, Barcelona.

Smith, K. C. (Ed.) (1976): *Photochemical and Photobiological Reviews*, Vol. 1. Plenum Press, New York.

Urbach, F. (Ed.) (1969): *The Biologic Effects of Ultraviolet Radiation with Emphasis on the Skin.* Pergamon Press, Oxford.

Urbach, F., Forbes, P. D., Davies, R. E., et al. (1976): Cutaneous photobiology: past, present and future. *J. Invest. Dermatol.* **67**:209–224.

Willis, I. (1971): Sunlight and skin. *J. AMA* **217**:1088–1093. *Photochemistry and Photobiology.* Pergamon Press, Oxford. (Two volumes per year.)

Photodermatoses

Barth, J. (1976): Historische und aktuelle Aspekte der Fotosensibilisierung. *Dermatol. Monatsschr.* **162**:961–973.

Daniels, F., Jr. (1965): Diseases caused or aggravated by sunlight. *Med. Clin. North Am.* **49**:565–580.

Epstein, J. H. (1971): Adverse cutaneous reactions to the sun. In: *Yearbook of Dermatology 1971*, edited by F. O. Malkinson and R. A. Pearson, pp. 5–43. Year Book Medical Publishers, Chicago.

Frain-Bell, W. (1973): The photodermatoses. *Recent Adv. Dermatol.* 3:100–133.

Hursthouse, M. W. (1973): Photodermatoses: causes and management. *Drugs* 6:255–260.

Ippen, H., and Goerz, G. (1974): *Photodermatosen und Porphyrien.* Greiter AG, Kressbronn, Germany.

Sutton, R. L., Jr., and Waisman, M. (1977): Dermatoses due to physical agents. *Cutis* 19:513–529.

Wassermann, G. A., and Haberman, H. F. (1975): Photosensitivity: results of investigation in 250 patients. *Can. Med. Assoc. J.* 113:1055–1060.

Photoreactions Caused by Exogenous Factors

Breit, R. (1975): Phototoxische und photoallergische Reaktionen der Haut. *Munch. Med. Wochenschr.* 117:23–28.

Harber, L. C., and Baer, R. L. (1972): Pathogenic mechanisms of drug-induced photosensitivity. *J. Invest. Dermatol.* 58:327–342.

Ippen, H. (1962): Lichtbeeinflusste Arzneimittel-Nebenwirkungen an der Haut. *Dtsch. Med. Wochenschr.* 87:480–488, 544–547.

Jakac, D., and Wolf, A. (1974): Alterazioni fotodinamiche e fotoallergiche della cute devute a medicamenti e cosmetici. *Minerva Dermatol.* 109:29–31.

Jarrat, M. (1976): Drug photosensitization. *Int. J. Dermatol.* 15:317–325.

Kalivas, J. (1970): A guide to the problem of photosensitivity. *J. AMA* 209:1706–1709; 211:1173.

Padilla, H. C. (1973): Fotosensibilidad y yatrogenia en dermatologia. *Med. Cutanea* 7:103–114.

Pathak, M. A., and Fitzpatrick, T. B. (1972, 1973): Photosensitivity caused by drugs. *Ration. Drug Ther.* 6:1–6; *Internist* 14:339–344.

Scheel, L. D. (1973): Photosensitizing agents. In: *Toxicants Occurring Naturally in Foods*, 2nd ed., pp. 558–572. National Academy of Sciences, Washington, D.C.

Stempel, E., and Stempel, R. (1973): Drug-induced photosensitivity. *J. Am. Pharm. Assoc. (N. S.)* 13:200–204.

Storck, H. (1965): Photoallergy and photosensitivity due to systemically administered drugs. *Arch. Dermatol.* 91:469–482.

Tronnier, H. (1974): Lichtdermatosen als Arzeimittelnebenwirkung. *Diagnostik* 7:174–178.

Velasco Pernia, M. (1974): Fotosensibilisacion debida a drogas. *Dermatol. Venez.* 11:281–295.

Widmer, O., Zürcher, K., and Krebs, A. (1976): Cutaneous side effects of systemic drugs. C. Drug induced photosensitivity. D. Drug induced changes in skin colour. *Dermatologica* 152:193–256.

Young, J. W. (1964): A list of photosensitizing agents of interest to the dermatologist. *Bull. Assoc. Milit. Dermatol.* 13:33–35.

V

Photoprotection

13

Photobiology of Carotenoid Protection

N. I. Krinsky

When Sistrom, Griffiths, and Stanier (1) reported that carotenoid pigments protect cells against light under aerobic conditions in the purple-sulfur bacterium *Rhodopseudomonas spheroides*, they proposed that these pigments acted as "chemical buffers" and were oxidized during the process. They suggested that carotenoid epoxides might be the product of this chemical buffering effect. Carotenoid epoxides, however, although widely distributed in nature, have never been observed in bacteria (2). The function of carotenoid epoxides is still unknown but is under active investigation (3).

Since carotenoid epoxides are not present in bacteria, they cannot serve as a basis for a protective role in these organisms. Mathews-Roth and Krinsky (4) have looked for changes in carotenoids in nonphotosynthetic bacteria under conditions in which the carotenoid pigments were acting as protective agents, but could find no evidence for oxidation of the carotenoids. This would seem to indicate that a chemical oxidation, the basis for the chemical buffering hypothesis of Sistrom et al. (1), was not a satisfactory explanation for the mechanism of carotenoid protection. In 1968, Krinsky (5) reviewed the role of carotenoid pigments as protective agents in bacteria (both photosynthetic and nonphotosynthetic), algae, plants, and animals. In almost all cases where a carotenoid deficiency was observed due either to a mutation or an environmental alteration, the resultant organism was light-sensitive under aerobic conditions. An example of an environmental alteration is the effect caused by a large number of herbicides which appear to function by inhibiting carotenoid biosynthesis. Among these herbicides are pyrichlor (6) and various Sandoz chemicals (7, 8). In all of these cases, the inhibition of carotenoid

N. I. Krinsky • Department of Biochemistry and Pharmacology, Tufts University School of Medicine, Boston, Massachusetts 02111.

biosynthesis results in the formation of plants or cultures that cannot survive under illuminated aerobic conditions.

There were four mechanisms proposed by Krinsky (5) to explain how carotenoid pigments protected cells against the harmful effects of visible light. In subsequent years, a better understanding of these mechanisms has been made possible by a clarification of the processes of photochemical oxidations. These are described in detail in Chapter 5; only those reactions related to the mechanism of carotenoid protection will be discussed here.

PHOTOCHEMISTRY

There are two classes of photochemical oxidations, which have been referred to as Type I and Type II by Gollnick and Schenck (9), and these are shown in Fig. 13-1. In both cases, the sensitizer (S) is excited by light to its first excited state (^{1}S), which can then undergo intersystem crossing to form the metastable triplet state (^{3}S). It is the triplet state, with its relatively long lifetime (10^{-8}–10^{-1} sec), that allows a variety of photochemical reactions to occur. Both Type I and Type II reactions can result in photochemical oxidations, although Type I can proceed under anaerobic conditions. It is now apparent that carotenoid pigments act at several points in this series of photochemical reactions. This chapter will deal with the evidence supporting the role of carotenoid pigments as protective compounds in photosensitized systems.

^{1}S-Carotenoid Interaction

As seen in Fig. 13-1, the photochemical reaction consists of the absorption of a photon by the sensitizer (S), forming the singlet excited species of the sensitizer (^{1}S). All of the subsequent reactions are dark reactions. One possibility for carotenoid (CAR) involvement would conceivably be through a ^{1}S-CAR interaction. At first glance, this seems unlikely, for the important function of carotenoids as accessory pigments in photosynthetic systems is

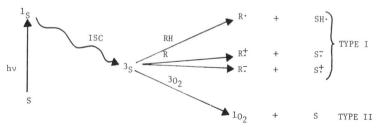

Fig. 13-1. Schematic representation of the reactions involved in Type I and Type II photosensitized oxidations.

carried out by a singlet–singlet energy transfer process from CAR to the photosynthetic sensitizer, chlorophyll (10–12). Nevertheless, Beddard et al. (13) proposed that CAR could interact with ^{1}S, in the form of singlet chlorophyll (^{1}CHL), in the following electron transfer process:

$$CAR + {}^1CHL \longrightarrow CAR^+ + CHL^-$$

A subsequent reaction between the carotene radical cation and a chlorophyll molecule would result in the regeneration of ground-state CAR and a charge-separated pair CHL^- / CHL^+, which might function in the reaction center of photosystem II:

$$CAR^+ + CHL \longrightarrow CAR + CHL^+$$

$$\text{Sum:} \quad {}^1CHL + CHL \longrightarrow CHL^- / CHL^+$$

Their argument (13) is based on the quenching of CHL fluorescence by CAR. However, there is a great deal of evidence (14, 15) that the species responsible for quenching chlorophyll fluorescence is actually a triplet carotenoid, ^{3}CAR. Recently, Mathis et al. (16) have presented very convincing evidence that ^{3}CAR is the quencher of chlorophyll fluorescence in spinach chloroplasts and subchloroplast particles. However, the mechanism of this quenching still remains to be elucidated.

Although rejecting the proposal of Beddard et al. (13) that all CAR is directly involved in the primary charge separation at reaction centers in photosynthetic systems, Searle and Wessels (17) do support the notion that CAR might interact directly with ^{1}CHL to form a long-lived exciplex:

$$CAR + {}^1CHL \rightleftharpoons (CAR^+ \cdot CHL^-)$$

The formation of this exciplex ($CAR^+ \cdot CHL^-$) would reduce the rate of transfer of excitation energy from the reaction center and result in an increased efficiency in the trapping of excitation energy in photosynthetic reaction centers.

^{3}S–Carotenoid Interaction

This is an important area for an understanding of carotenoid function in photosensitized systems, and may, in fact, be the most important from the quantitative point of view (18). Depending on the nature of the photochemical system, the effectiveness of converting ^{1}S to ^{3}S will vary as a function of the intersystem crossing rate for different sensitizers. In photosynthetic systems, the rate is known for chlorophyll and amounts to 0.04% of all the ^{1}S molecules being converted to the [3]S species of chlorophyll (19). In 1957, Fujimori and Livingston (20) first demonstrated that carotenoid pigments had the capacity to quench the triplet state of chlorophyll ([3]CHL) in vitro and there are now many examples of triplet–triplet energy transfer from chlorophyll to carotenoids. The reaction is apparently a direct energy transfer between [3]CHL and the carotenoid:

$$^3\text{CHL} + \text{CAR} \longrightarrow \text{CHL} + {}^3\text{CAR}$$

This form of triplet–triplet energy transfer in photosynthetic systems has been reviewed recently by Cogdell (11) and DeVault and Kung (21). Foote (18) has calculated, based on the high efficiency of the reaction between [3]CHL and beta-carotene, that only 10% of the [3]CHL would survive carotenoid quenching within intact chloroplasts with a local concentration of beta-carotene at 2×10^{-2} M. Unfortunately, comparable data are not available for the many other [3]S compounds that can be quenched by carotenoids. So, for example, Chantrell et al. (22) have studied the quenching of the triplet species of protoporphyrin IX, the pigment that accumulates in erythropoietic porphyria. They used the dimethyl ester of this compound, but the energy exchange between this compound and the carotenoids studied should not be affected. Chantrell et al. (22) studied a series of carotenoid pigments of different polyene lengths, and concluded that beta-carotene gives the maximum quenching of [3]protoporphyrin IX. The relationship between polyene length and carotenoid function will be discussed later.

Free Radical–Carotenoid Interaction

Any [3]S that escapes quenching by carotenoid pigments can then proceed to react in either a Type I or Type II reaction. Type I reactions are redox reactions which frequently result in the formation of radical species that can lead to radical-catalyzed damage. These Type I reactions frequently involve hydrogen or electron abstraction, depending on the nature of both the sensitizer and the prospective hydrogen or electron donor R. In the presence of unsaturated fatty acids, Type I reactions can lead to lipid peroxidation with subsequent cellular damage. There have been a number of suggestions that carotenoid pigments might interact directly with some of the intermediates in lipid peroxidation and act to protect cells against these potentially damaging compounds. Yamane and Lamola (23) reported that red blood cell hemolysis induced by cholesterol hydroperoxide could be inhibited by beta-carotene. In addition, Kellogg and Fridovich (24) observed that beta-carotene inhibited the peroxidation of lipids in a system containing unsaturated lipids and the enzyme xanthine oxidase. Anderson and Krinsky (25) observed that beta-carotene prevented lipid peroxidation under conditions in which radical reactions initiated the formation of lipid peroxides. Some of these results have

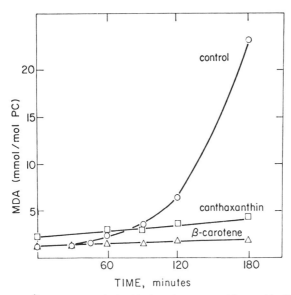

Fig. 13-2. The Fe^{2+}-generated radical oxidation of unsaturated fatty acids. Egg phosphatidylcholine liposomes containing either beta-carotene, canthaxanthin, or no pigment were incubated with 0.1 M $FeCl_2$, and the malondialdehyde (MDA) formed was determined.

been described recently (26) and an example of carotenoid protection against radical oxidations is shown in Fig. 13-2. In this experiment, the extent of lipid peroxidation was quantitated by the appearance of the lipid peroxide product, malondialdehyde. The system contained unsaturated fatty acids present in egg phosphatidylcholine and was supplemented with either beta-carotene or canthaxanthin (4,4′-diketo-β-carotene). Ferrous iron was added to generate free radicals and, as can be seen, the presence of the carotenoid pigments inhibited the onset of radical-induced lipid peroxidation.

Singlet Oxygen–Carotenoid Interaction

The other photochemical reaction involving ^3S is the Type II reaction in which ^3S reacts directly with ground-state oxygen. The reaction proceeds very efficiently since O_2 in its ground state is a paramagnetic molecule which exists as a triplet species, represented as $^3O_2$. The reaction between ^3S and $^3O_2$ proceeds with conservation of spin and the product formed is the $^1\Delta_g$ species of O_2, hereafter referred to as singlet oxygen or $^1O_2$. The reaction is

$$^3S + {}^3O_2 \longrightarrow S + O_2({}^1\Delta_g)$$

This reaction was originally postulated by Kautsky et al. (27), but was not generally accepted until the reports of Foote and Wexler (28) and Corey and

Taylor (29) appeared in which these investigators demonstrated that the products of photosensitized oxidations were identical to those that had been reported when $^1O_2$ was generated either chemically or by use of a radio-frequency discharge apparatus.

The pioneering work of Foote and his collaborators was instrumental in helping to explain the protective action of carotenoid pigments mediated through the quenching of $^1O_2$. This reaction was first demonstrated in 1968 by Foote and Denny (30) in an in vitro system. The effectiveness of this reaction can be evaluated from the quenching constant, which approaches a diffusion-controlled limit and has been determined to be 1.3×10^{10} M^{-1} sec^{-1} in benzene solutions (31). This quenching capacity, found in all carotenoids that have nine or more conjugated double bonds (32), has overshadowed the other mechanisms whereby carotenoid pigments serve as protective agents. In fact, the inhibition of reactions by the addition of carotenoids has occasionally been taken as evidence for $^1O_2$ mechanisms.

In summary, then, it appears that carotenoid pigments can act as protective agents against photosensitized reactions by any of the following mechanisms: (a) Carotenoid quenching of triplet sensitizers, (b) carotenoid inhibition of free radical reactions, (c) carotenoid quenching of $O_2(^1\Delta_g)$. It seems unlikely that a common mechanism will explain these three separate functions, even though they all serve a similar purpose, in terms of protecting cells. The potential mechanisms whereby carotenoid pigments carry out these three reactions are described below.

MECHANISMS OF CAROTENOID PROTECTION

Shortly after the original observations of Sistrom et al. (1) that carotenoid pigments protected cells against photosensitized oxidations, Claes and her collaborators (33, 34) had an opportunity to study this phenomenon in the photosynthetic algae *Chlorella vulgaris*. Her observations, using both the wild-type and mutant stains of this organism, have served as the basis for understanding the mechanism of carotenoid protection.

Chromophore Length and Carotenoid Protection

Among the mutant stains of *C. vulgaris* studied by Claes (33) were several that had defects in their carotenoid synthesizing enzymes. As such, these cells synthesized carotenoids that had either 5, 7, 9, or 11 conjugated double bonds. The ability to protect the cells against photosensitized damage, or the ability to prevent photobleaching of chlorophyll *a* in vitro, was related to the length of the chromophore of the carotenoid pigment (33, 34). A similar relationship to $^1O_2$ quenching was reported by Foote et al. (32) and the data of

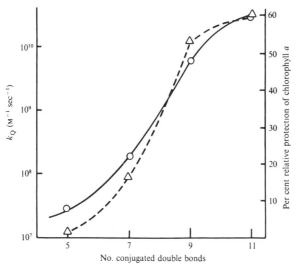

Fig. 13-3. The relationship between carotenoid chromophore length and either $^1O_2$ quenching rates (32) or protection against chlorophyll a photobleaching (33, 34).

both groups are shown in Fig. 13-3. There are now many examples of systems in which the protective action of carotenoid pigments depends on the chromophore length and this subject has been reviewed by Krinsky (12). The conclusions based on both the in vitro and the in vivo work is that carotenoid pigments containing nine or more conjugated double bonds are effective quenchers of $^1O_2$ and protect as well against photosensitized damage in vivo. In contrast, carotenoid pigments containing seven or fewer conjugated double bonds are not as effective in either the in vivo systems or as quenchers of $^1O_2$.

Mathews-Roth and Krinsky (4) extended these observations through the use of a mutant strain of *Micrococcus luteus* (*Sarcina lutea*) whose major carotenoid pigment contained only eight conjugated double bonds. This mutant strain, which also contained a smaller amount of carotenoid pigment per cell, was not protected against the harmful effects of oxygen and an exogenous photosensitizer. The studies were extended by Mathews-Roth et al. (35), who studied the ability of several naturally occurring carotenoid pigments to quench $^1O_2$ and inhibit free radical reactions. The wild-type *M. luteus* contained a pigment with nine conjugated double bonds that was as effective a quencher of $^1O_2$ as either beta-carotene, lutein, or isozeaxanthin. The latter two pigments are carotenoid diols containing 10 and 11 conjugated double bonds, respectively. The carotenoid pigment from the mutant strain, which contains only eight conjugated double bonds, was two to three times less efficient than the wild-type pigment, whereas phytofluene (five conjugated double bonds) and phytoene (three conjugated double bonds) were 100 and 1000 times less efficient than beta-carotene at quenching $^1O_2$.

Carotenoid Triplet Levels

An understanding of the relationship between chromophore length and carotenoid protection has come from the studies of Mathis and Kleo (36) and Bensasson et al. (37). These two groups have been looking at the triplet energy levels of carotenoid pigments as well as other polyenes. Although it has been difficult to obtain direct measurements of the triplet energies of carotenoids, these two groups have presented excellent estimates. As would be expected, based on the calculations of Salem (38), an inverse relationship was found between the number of conjugated double bonds in the polyenes and the triplet energy levels. The data from these publications (36, 37) have been plotted in Fig. 13-4 and clearly display the linear relationship between the length of the conjugated polyene chain and the inverse of the triplet energy level $1/E_t$. The dashed line in this figure represents the inverse energy level of $O_2(^1\Delta_g)$. From this figure, it can be readily concluded that only those carotenoid pigments that contain nine or more conjugated double bonds could be involved in an efficient energy transfer relationship with $^1O_2$, since in those cases the triplet energy level of the carotenoids would lie below that of $^1O_2$. Conversely, the carotenoids of shorter chromophore length would be much less efficient in this process.

As mentioned earlier, carotenoid pigments can also serve as quenchers for various triplet sensitizers, including ^{3}CHL. In Fig. 13-4, the $1/E_t$ of chlorophyll is also plotted; and it can be seen that carotenoid pigments containing seven or more conjugated double bonds should be effective quenchers of ^{3}CHL. This is precisely the relationship that had been observed by Claes (39) for carotenoid protection against the anaerobic photobleaching of chlorophyll, which presumably proceeds through the active participation of ^{3}CHL. Claes (39) demonstrated that the major difference in the ability of carotenoid pigments to protect against chlorophyll photobleaching occurred in pigments containing five double bonds and the results indicated that the carotenoid pigments with seven double bonds were effective protective agents.

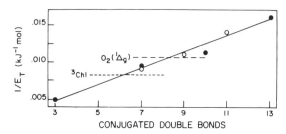

Fig. 13-4.   The relationship between the reciprocal of carotenoid triplet energy level $1/E_T$ and the number of conjugated double bonds in the pigment. Data are taken from Bensasson et al. (37) (●) and from Mathis and Kleo (36) (○). The energy difference between $^1O_2$ and $^3O_2$ (– –) and the triplet energy level of chlorophyll (- - -) are also depicted.

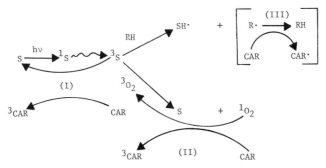

Fig. 13-5. Mechanisms of carotenoid protection against photosensitized oxidations. Carotenoids can either quench triplet sensitizers (I), quench $^1O_2$ (II), or quench free radical intermediates (III).

Radical Quenching

Very little evidence has been presented with respect to the mechanism of radical quenching by carotenoids. There are several reports in the literature dealing with the formation of radical species of carotenoids, but very little evidence that stable radical products can be formed using carotenoids. Much of the recent work has been summarized (26).

SUMMARY

As reviewed in this chapter, carotenoid pigments are very effective compounds for protecting cells against the harmful effects of photosensitized oxidations. The sites of protection are described schematically in Fig. 13-5. Both ^3S and $^1O_2$ can be quenched by carotenoids in energy transfer reactions, generating the ground states of the sensitizer and oxygen, respectively, as well as ^3CAR. In addition, radical species produced in Type I photoreactions can also be quenched by carotenoids. All three mechanisms would therefore serve as protective reactions. The applications of these phenomena are described in Chapter 14.

REFERENCES

1. Sistrom, W. R., Griffiths, M., and Stanier, R. Y. (1956): The biology of a photosynthetic bacterium which lacks colored carotenoids. *J. Cell. Comp. Physiol.* **48**:473–515.
2. Liaaen-Jensen, S. (1979): Carotenoids—a chemosystematic approach, *Pure Appl. Chem.* **51**:661–675.
3. Yamamoto, H. Y. (1979): Biochemistry of the violaxanthin cycle in higher plants. *Pure Appl. Chem.* **51**:639–648.

4. Mathews-Roth, M. M., and Krinsky, N. I. (1970): Studies on the protective function of the carotenoid pigments of *Sarcina lutea*. *Photochem. Photobiol.* **11**:419–428.

5. Krinsky, N. I. (1968): The protective functions of carotenoid pigments. In: *Photophysiology*, vol. 3, edited by A. C. Giese, pp. 123–195, Academic Press, New York.

6. Burns, E. R., Buchanan, G. A., and Carter, M. C. (1971): Inhibition of carotenoid synthesis as a mechanism of action of amitrole, dichlormate and pyriclor. *Plant Physiol.* **47**:144–148.

7. Hilton, J. L., St. John, J. B., Christiansen, M. N., et al. (1971): Interactions of lipoidal materials and a pyridazinone inhibitor of chloroplast development. *Plant Physiol.* **48**: 171–177.

8. Vaisberg, A. J., and Schiff, J. A. (1976): Events surrounding the early development of *Euglena* chloroplasts. 7. Inhibition of carotenoid biosynthesis by the herbicide SAN 9789 (4-chloro-5-(methylamino)-2-(α,α,α-trifluoro-*m*-tolyl)-3(2H) pyridazinone) and its developmental consequences. *Plant Physiol.* **57**:260–269.

9. Gollnick, K., and Schenck, G. O. (1967): Oxygen as a dienophile. In: *1,4-Cycloaddition Reactions*, edited by J. Hamer, pp. 255–344, Academic Press, New York.

10. Blinks, L. R. (1964): Accessory pigments and photosynthesis. In: *Photophysiology*, vol. 1, edited by A. C. Giese, pp. 199–221. Academic Press, New York.

11. Cogdell, R. S. (1978): Carotenoids in photosynthesis. *Phil. Trans. R. Soc. Lond.* [*Biol.*] **284**:569–579.

12. Krinsky, N. I. (1971): Function. In: *Carotenoids*, edited by O. Isler, pp. 669–716. Birkhaüser Verlag, Basel.

13. Beddard, G. S., Davidson, R. S., and Trethewey, K. R. (1977): Quenching of chlorophyll fluorescence by β-carotene. *Nature* **267**:373–374.

14. Mathis, P., and Galmiche, J. M. (1967): Action des gaz paramagnétiques sur un état transitoire induit par un éclair laser dans une suspension de chloroplastes. *C. R. Acad. Sci.* [*D*] (*Paris*) **264**:1903–1906.

15. Mathis, P. (1971): Étude de formes transitoires des carotenoides. Thesis, University of Orsay, France.

16. Mathis, P., Butler, W. L., and Satoh, K. (1979): Carotenoid triplet state and chlorophyll fluorescence quenching in chloroplasts and subchloroplast particles. *Photochem. Photobiol.* **30**:603–614.

17. Searle, G. F. W., and Wessels, J. S. C. (1978): Role of β-carotene in the reaction centres of photosystems I and II of spinach chloroplasts prepared in non-polar solvents. *Biochim. Biophys. Acta* **504**:84–99.

18. Foote, C. S. (1976): Photosensitized oxidation and singlet oxygen: consequences in biological systems. In: *Free Radicals and Biological Systems*, vol. 2, edited by W. A. Pryor, pp. 85–133. Academic Press, New York.

19. Breton, J., and Mathis, P. (1970): Mise en évidence de l'état triplet de la chlorophylle dans des lamelles chloroplastiques. *C. R. Acad. Sci.* [*D*] (*Paris*) **271**:1094–1096.

20. Fujimori, E., and Livingston, R. (1957): Interaction of chlorophyll in its triplet state with oxygen, carotene, etc. *Nature* **180**:1036–1038.

21. DeVault, D., and Kung, M. C. (1978): Interactions among photosynthetic antenna excited states. *Photochem. Photobiol.* **28**:1029–1038.

22. Chantrell, S. J., McAuliffe, C. A., Munn, R. W., et al. (1977): Excited states of protoporphyrin IX dimethyl ester: reaction of the triplet with carotenoids. *J. Chem. Soc.* [*Faraday I*] **73**:858–865.

23. Yamane, T., and Lamola, A. A. (1973): Red blood cell lysis induced by a product of singlet oxygen and cholesterol. In: *Abstracts of the American Society for Photobiology, Sarasota, Florida*, p. 66.

24. Kellogg, E. W., III, and Fridovich, I. (1975): Superoxide, hydrogen peroxide, and singlet oxygen in lipid peroxidation by a xanthine oxidase system. *J. Biol. Chem.* **250**:8812–8817.

25. Anderson, S. M., and Krinsky, N. I. (1973): The inhibition of photosensitized oxidations in liposomes by carotenoid pigments and free radical quenchers. *Fed. Proc.* **32**:562.

26. Krinsky, N. I. (1979): Carotenoid protection against oxidation. *Pure Appl. Chem.* **51**:649–660.

27. Kautsky, H., De Bruijn, H., Neuwirth, R., et al. (1933): Energie-unwandlung an Grenz-flachen. VII. Photosensibilisierte Oxydation als Wirkung eines Aktiven, metastabilen Zustandes des Sauerstoff-moleküls. *Chem. Ber.* **66**:1588–1600.

28. Foote, C. S., and Wexler, S. (1964): Olefin oxidations with excited singlet molecular oxygen. *J. Am. Chem. Soc.* **86**:3879–3880.

29. Corey, E. J., and Taylor, W. C. (1964): A study of the peroxidation of organic compounds by externally generated singlet oxygen molecules. *J. Am. Chem. Soc.* **86**:3881–3882.

30. Foote, C. S., and Denny, R. W. (1968): Chemistry of singlet oxygen, VII. Quenching by β-carotene. *J. Am. Chem. Soc.* **90**:6233–6235.

31. Foote, C. S. (1979): Quenching of singlet oxygen. In: *Singlet Oxygen*, edited by H. H. Wasserman and R. W. Murray, pp. 139–171. Academic Press, New York.

32. Foote, C. S., Chang, Y. C., and Denny, R. W. (1970): Chemistry of singlet oxygen. X. Carotenoid quenching parallels biological protection. *J. Am. Chem. Soc.* **92**:5216–5218.

33. Claes, H. (1960): Interaction between chlorophyll and carotenes with different chromophoric groups. *Biochem. Biophys. Res. Commun.* **3**:585–590.

34. Claes, H., and Nakayama, T. O. M. (1959): Das photoxydative ausbleichen von Chlorophyll *in vitro* in gegenwart von Carotinen mit verschieden chromophoren Gruppen. *Z. Naturforsch.* **14B**:746–747.

35. Mathews-Roth, M. M., Wilson, T., Fujimori, E., et al. (1974): Carotenoid chromophore length and protection against photosensitization. *Photochem. Photobiol.* **19**:217–222.

36. Mathis, P., and Kleo, J. (1973): The triplet state of β-carotene and of analog polyenes of different length. *Photochem. Photobiol.* **18**:343–346.

37. Bensasson, R., Land, E. J., and Maudinas, B. (1976): Triplet states of carotenoids from photosynthetic bacteria studied by nanosecond ultraviolet and electron pulse irradiation. *Photochem. Photobiol.* **23**:189–193.

38. Salem, L. (1966): *The Molecular Orbital Theory of Conjugated Systems*, pp. 379–383. Benjamin, New York.

39. Claes, H. (1961): Energieübertrangung von angeregtem Chlorophyll auf C_{40}-Polyene mit verschiedenen chromophoren Gruppen. *Z. Naturforsch.* **16B**:445–454.

14

Beta-Carotene Therapy for Erythropoietic Protoporphyria and Other Photosensitivity Diseases

M. M. Mathews-Roth

Exposure to ultraviolet (UV) radiation or visible light can have profound effects on the skin of a susceptible individual. The harmful effects of the sunburn spectrum (290–320 nm) are well known. In addition, there are several diseases associated with sensitivity to visible light. An example of one of these diseases is erythropoietic protoporphyria, in which sensitivity to visible light (380–560 nm) is a cardinal sympton. Until recently, no satisfactory way existed for preventing the sensitivity to visible light characteristic of prophyria other than to avoid light exposure. Sunscreens effective in preventing abnormal reactions to light of the sunburn spectrum are ineffective for the prevention of sensitivity to visible light. Observations that the carotenoid pigments of green plants and photosynthetic bacteria played an important role as protective agents against photosensitization by the organisms' own chlorophyll led to the suggestion that these pigments might be of benefit in the treatment of photosensitive diseases characterized by sensitivity to visible light. In this chapter we will discuss the studies in bacteria, plants, and animals that led to the use of carotenoid pigments in the treatment of human photosensitivity, and briefly discuss the clinical pharmacology of the carotenoid pigments. The reader is referred to the books by Karrer and Jucker (1), Goodwin (2), and Isler (3) for a detailed discussion of the chemistry of the carotenoid pigments.

M. M. Mathews-Roth • Channing Laboratory and Department of Medicine, Harvard Medical School , Boston, Massachusetts 02114; and Brigham and Women's Hospital, Boston, Massachusetts 02115.

DEVELOPMENT OF THE IDEA TO USE CAROTENOID
PIGMENTS IN THE TREATMENT OF PHOTOSENSITIVITY

Cartenoid pigments are present along with chlorophyll in every green plant. The chlorophyll plays the central role in photosynthesis, but it has long been noted that other pigments also participate to some degree in the process. Engelmann (4, 5) was the first to observe that carotenoids could act as accessory light-absorbing pigments in photosynthesis. The presence of carotenoids serves a useful role for the plant because, by their absorption at lower wavelengths than chlorophyll, they serve to extend the wavelengths of light that can be used to trap energy for use in photosynthesis. For many years this was thought to be the sole function for the carotenoids present in photosynthetic organisms. Studies by Stanier and his group then suggested a new function for these pigments—that of protection against photosensitization. Additional functions have also been ascribed to the carotenoids present in various organisms, but none of these functions has been convincingly documented (6, 7).

Studies in Bacteria

Sistrom, Griffiths, and Stanier (8) first suggested that carotenoids might be acting as protective agents against photodynamic action in bacteria, as a result of observations they made on the wild type and a certain mutant of *Rhodopseudomonas spheroides*. This mutant, which they called "blue-green," did not produce colored carotenoids, but accumulated the colorless carotenoid precursor phytoene. They found that when the blue-green mutant was grown in the presence of light and air, growth stopped, chlorophyll was destroyed, and the cells were killed. On the other hand, the wild type, with the normal component of carotenoid pigments, is not injured by growth in light and air; in the presence of air, chlorophyll synthesis stops, and the organism grows by aerobic metabolism. It should be noted that the deletion of the carotenoid pigments did not markedly affect the ability of the blue-green mutant to grow photosynthetically in the presence of light in an atmosphere of nitrogen (bacterial photosynthesis is anaerobic); only when light and air were present did the lack of carotenoids give rise to problems.

These workers were able to show that it was the bacteriochlorophyll that was responsible for the lethal photosensitization of the blue-green mutant, and that both oxygen and light were necessary for the destructive reaction to occur (a photodynamic action). They concluded that the carotenoid pigments were functioning as protective agents against this photodynamic killing, and that the bacteriochlorophyll was the endogenous photosensitizer. These findings, that carotenoids can protect against chlorophyll photosensitization, have been confirmed in other photosynthetic bacteria and algae [see (6) for detailed review].

In their report (8), Stanier and his group suggested that the carotenoid pigments of all green plants function as protective agents to prevent photosensitization by chlorophyll. Observations on carotenoidless mutants of higher plants suggest that this indeed may be the case. Koski and Smith (9) and Smith et al. (10) reported studies on a white mutant of corn, which lacked colored carotenoids, and which, when exposed to light, would die when the food supply in the cotyledons was exhausted. Examination of the plants showed that the chloroplasts were destroyed. Anderson and Robertson (11) showed that destruction of chlorophyll was occurring in light in these colorless mutants, and that the presence of carotenoids prevented this destruction. Wallace and Schwarting (12) studied a mutant of sunflowers (HA) that did not contain colored carotenoids. This plant also died when grown in air and light once the food supply in the cotyledons was used up.

Thus, in view of all the data now available, it can be concluded that the carotenoid pigments in all photosynthetic organisms (bacteria, algae, and higher plants) play an important role in protecting these organisms against the seriously damaging effects of photooxidation by their own endogenous photosensitizer, chlorophyll.

With these data as background, it was not surprising that Stanier and his associates also suggested that the carotenoids of nonphotosynthetic bacteria might also play some sort of a protective role in these cells (8) even though these organisms did not seem to contain large amounts of an obvious endogenous photosensitizer, as did the photosynthetic organism. Kunisawa and Stanier (13) induced a colorless mutant of *Corynebacterium poinsettiae*, a nonphotosynthetic bacterium that contains carotenoids. They found that the mutant was killed in the presence of an exogenous photosensitizer (toluidine blue), light, and air, whereas the wild type, which contained colored carotenoids, was not affected by this exposure. Again, they found that this was a photodynamic phenomenon, as oxygen was necessary for the phenomenon to occur; the cells were not killed in the presence of dye and light in a nitrogen atmosphere. They attempted to see whether they could demonstrate the presence of an endogenous photosensitizer in this organism by exposing the wild type and colorless mutant to visible light in the presence of air but with no added photosensitizer. However, this treatment did not kill the cells. They concluded that carotenes indeed could protect the cells against photosensitization with an exogenous photosensitizer, but they could not determine whether this ability were of any use to the cells. Mathews and Sistrom (14, 15) were able to show that nonphotosynthetic bacteria might indeed contain endogenous photosensitizers by exposing wild-type *Sarcina lutea*, another nonphotosynthetic carotene-containing organism, and its colorless mutant to natural sunlight in air for 4 hr. It was found that, at these high intensities (1200 foot-candles at the start of the experiment and 5000 foot-candles at its end), the mutant was killed and the wild type was not. They showed that this was also a photodynamic effect, as the mutant was not killed after exposure to sun in an atmosphere of nitrogen. Since these studies were done (13–15), many other workers have confirmed the protective function of carotenoid pigments in nonphotosynthetic bacteria [see (6) for detailed review].

Ecologic Importance of the Protective Function of Carotenoid Pigments in Photosynthetic Bacteria

Stanier and Cohen-Bazire have pointed out the important role played by carotenoid pigments in the evolution of photosynthetic organisms, both bacteria and higher plants, during the process of the development of porphyrin-containing photosynthetic pigments in these organisms (16, 17). Since porphyrins are powerful photosensitizers (18), it was crucial for photosynthetic organisms to evolve protective mechanisms against photosensitization by their chlorophyll. Hence, carotenoids have proved to be important not only as trappers of additional energy for photosynthesis, but also as the mechanism whereby the plant protects itself against photosensitization by its own chlorophyll in our aerobic atmospheres. Stanier and Cohen-Bazire also suggested that a similar protective function for crotenoid pigments could be postulated for nonphotosynthetic carotenoid-containing bacteria. For example, carotenogenesis in fungi and *Mycobacterium* is stimulated by light, and there is a negative correlation between anaerobiasis and the presence of carotenoids (17). In fact, one finds that organisms that are normally exposed to both light and air contain carotenoid pigments. For example, many aquatic bacteria such, as the *Flavobacterium*, which are normally exposed to light and air contain carotenoid pigments (1, 2, 19, 20). Aquatic organisms of the genera *Vibrio*, *Pseudomonas*, and *Corynebacierium* also contain these pigments (21, 22). On the other hand, most aerobic terrestrial bacteria probably will not be exposed to high light intensities while in the soil; for example, carotenoids are rarely found in coliform organisms. Bacteria commonly found in air would be subject to intense light. Spores are probably resistant to photodynamic killing, and carotenoids are seldom if ever found in the bacilli. Non-spore-forming bacteria commonly found in air will, on the Stanier hypothesis, contain carotenoids. Examples of these organisms are *Mycobacterium*, *Corynebacterium*, *Staphylococcus*, and *Sarcina*, all of which genera contain carotenoids (1, 2, 22). Thus, both in photosynthetic organisms and nonphotosynthetic bacteria, carotenoid pigments play an important role in providing these organisms with protective mechanisms against photosensitization by endogenous photosensitizers that would cause damage to the organisms in the presence of the light and air normally present in their environment.

Studies in Animals

The data presented above indicated that carotenoid pigments have a well-documented ability to protect plants and bacteria against photosensitivity. From these data it seemed sensible to determine whether the administration of carotenoid pigments could prevent photosensitization in patients with those photosensitivity diseases in which the photosensitizer had some resemblance to the endogenous photosensitizer in plants. Such a disease was light-sensitive porphyria, where the porphyrins produced are similar to the porphyrin group of chlorophyll. Preliminary experiments done in the summer of 1961 with L. C. Harber at New York University Medical School seemed to suggest that the onset of erythema to artificial light could be delayed by the oral administration of beta-carotene. A search of the literature revealed that Kesten had been able to delay the onset of erythema in a patient with urticaria solare by the use of beta-carotene (23).

Because of this promising clinical information, it was though worthwhile to develop an animal model in order to test more thoroughly the hypothesis that carotenoids could protect against photosensitization in an animal system. Lipson and Baldes had developed a model of lethal and sublethal porphyrin sensitivity in mice, in which they injected mice intraperitoneally with a derivative of hematoporphyrin and exposed the animals to light (24). At about the same time, Forssberg et al. (25) had devised a Tween-80 suspension of beta-carotene which they administered intraperitoneally to mice 18–24 hr before irradiation, to determine whether lycopene could protect the animals against the lethal effects of x-irradiation.

The photosensitization method of Lipson and Baldes (24) and the carotene suspension of Forssberg et al. (25) were used in an experiment to determine whether carotene could prevent the lethal photosensitivity of injected hematoporphyrin and light exposure (26). Suspensions of beta-carotene in Tween-80 were prepared according to the method of Forssberg et al. (25) and 3 mg of beta-carotene or the equivalent volume of Tween-80 alone was administered intraperitoneally to groups of mice 18–24 hr before injecting them with the hematoporphyrin derivative prepared by the method of Lipson and Baldes (24). Because mice cannot accumulate high levels of carotenoids after oral administration, the beta-carotene was administered parenterally. Prior to exposure to light, these two groups of mice received 1 mg of the hematoporphyrin derivative intraperitoneally. Another group of mice received 1 mg of hematopoyphyrin alone. In addition, dark controls, animals receiving either hematoporphyrin alone or beta-carotene in Tween-80 alone, were included. It can be seen from Table 14-1 that significantly more animals that received the beta-carotene survived the treatment with hematoporphyrin and light than did those that had not received the beta-carotene (26). Thus, beta-carotene was effective in mice in preventing the lethal photosensitivity induced by injection of hematoporphyrin and exposure to visible light.

Table 14-1. Protective Effect of Beta-Carotene on Photosensitization
of Mice by Hematoporphyrin and Visible Light[a]

Group	Light exposure	Number of animals	Number dead	Number alive
Hematoporphyrin[b]	Yes	27	21	6
Hematoporphyrin[b] and carotene[c]	Yes	27	9	18
Hematoporphyrin[b] and Tween 80-saline	Yes	8	7	1
Hematoporphyrin[b]	No	8	0	8
Carotene[c]	No	8	0	8

[a] Data taken from (26).
[b] Animals received 1 mg intraperitoneally before exposure to light.
[c] Carotene was suspended in Tween 80-saline. Animals received 3 mg of beta-carotene intraperitoneally 18–24 hr before exposure to light.

RESULTS OF TREATING PATIENTS SUFFERING FROM ERYTHROPOIETIC PROTOPORPHYRIA WITH BETA-CAROTENE

The observations in bacteria and in animals suggested that it would probably be feasible to administer beta-carotene orally to patients with photosensitivity. For this study, the author entered into collaboration with Drs. T. B. Fitzpatrick, L. C. Harber, E. H. Kass, and M. A. Pathak (27, 28) and later with a number of physicians in different parts of the country [see (29, 30) for list]. The disease we chose to study was erythropoietic protoporphyria (EPP).

Erythropoietic Protoporphyria—Characteristics of the Disease

Erythropoietic protoporphyria (EPP) is a disorder of prophyria metabolism characterized by abnormally elevated levels of protoporphyrin IX in erythrocytes, feces, and plasma, and by sensitivity to visible light (380–560 nm) (31–33). This sensitivity, in which the protoporphyrin was shown to be the photosensitizer, manifests itself by a burning sensation in the skin, followed by varying degrees of erythema and edema. The disease is diagnosed by detecting the presence of abnormally high levels of protoporphyrin in blood and stool by chemical analysis. Contrary to what is found in the other porphyrias, urinary porphyrins remain within normal limits in EPP. When a smear of blood from a patient with EPP is examined under the fluorescence microscope, large numbers of red-fluorescent erythrocytes are seen; these are not seen in normal individuals. In addition, if the skin of the light-exposed areas of the body is examined under the light microscope, an amorphous, homogeneous substance in and around the walls of small blood vessels of the upper papillary dermis is seen (31–33).

For the majority of patients with EPP, other members of their families also have the disease. There have been several genetic studies of EPP patients and their families. It was found that some relatives of the patients had somewhat elevated erythrocyte protoporphyrin levels, but yet were asymptomatic; this suggests the existence of a carrier state for EPP. It was concluded that EPP is genetically transmitted as an autosomal dominant trait with variable penetrance and expressivity (31, 32, 34).

The majority of patients with EPP report that the onset of photosensitivity began in early childhood—usually before age six, some as early as 18 months. The predominant manifestations of sensitivity reported by the patients were, in decreasing order of frequency: burning, swelling, itching, and redness of the skin. Some patients develop shallow, depressed scars over the nose and cheeks and on the backs of the hands, which developed after severe episodes of photosensitivity. Some patients report only subjective symptoms of itching and burning, and have none of the objective changes of redness, swelling, and scarring; these patients are usually dismissed by their physicians as hypochondriacs, when in reality they have EPP. Thus, it is important for the physician to investigate for the presence of EPP in all patients who report itching and burning of the skin on light exposure, even in the absence of objective findings.

The amount of sun exposure a patient with EPP can tolerate before symptoms develop varies. Some report they can tolerate only a few minutes, others say they can tolerate several hours. Characteristically, they report being sensitive to light through window glass. About half of the patients report decreases in photosensitivity during winter, but those who engage in skiing report that the light reflected by the snow can cause severe photosensitivity reactions.

In the majority of cases, EPP appears to be a benign disease. Many patients have a mild degree of anemia characterized by somewhat decreased levels of hemoglobin and hematocrit. This usually requires no treatment (35). There also seems to be an increased incidence of cholelithiasis, with several patients requiring cholecystectomies (31, 32). Chemical analyses of the gallstones detected high levels of protoporphyrin. An occasional patient, however, has been found to develop fatal liver disease, probably due to massive deposition of protoporphyrin in the liver. There are 15 such cases recorded to date (33, 36–41). These patients all had extremely high levels of protoporphyrin, and had abnormal liver function tests, jaundice, and microscopic evidence of cirrhosis. There is some evidence that serious liver disease in EPP might be ameliorated, or at least slowed down, by the administration of cholestyramine (42).

On light microscope examination of liver biopsies from EPP patients, both with and without cholelithiasis, some workers have noted prophyrin deposits in the liver cells and, in some cases, slight fibrotic changes; these were not associated with abnormal liver chemistries (33). Electron microscope examination of liver biopsies from EPP patients revealed that the liver cells of some EPP patients contain either cytoplasmic or mitochondrial inclusions, again in the absence of abnormal liver function tests (43). The significance of these various structural changes and their relationship if any, to the development of serious liver disease are unknown at this time.

The source of the abnormal amounts of protoporphyrin that accumulate in EPP has been under study for several years. Some workers have postulated that a significant amount, it not all, of the protoporphyrin is synthesized in the liver; others have suggested that all the abnormal porphyrin is synthesized by the bone marrow. Recently Piomelli and his collaborators have calculated that all protoporphyrin excreted in the stool can be accounted for by synthesis by the reticulocytes in the bone marrow (44). They showed that there is rapid leakage into the plasma of this protoporphyrin from the reticulocytes during the process of their maturation into erythrocytes, and that the leaked protoporphyrin is rapidly cleared from the plasma by the liver, thus accounting for the protoporphyrin in the stool. They found that circulating erythrocytes of up to about 20 days of age contained protoporphyrin—older ones usually did not. They also suggested that those pathologic liver changes seen in occasional EPP patients which we have just mentioned were secondary to the accumulation in the liver of this protoporphyrin leaked from the erythrocytes and cleared by the liver. They calculated that their theory would hold true even in the presence of a stool porphyrin level equivalent to the erythroid mass. Thus they suggested that there is no need to postulate synthesis of porphyrins by the liver as an integral finding in EPP. Their work also showed that there is only one line of erythrocytes present in EPP, as all reticulocytes were found to fluoresce.

The genetic lesion in EPP has also been studied. Several groups of workers have now found that there are markedly decreased levels of the enzyme ferrochelatase (heme synthetase) in the cells of patients with EPP (45, 46). Enzyme levels have been studied in bone marrow, liver, and skin fibroblasts; decreased levels of enzymes have been found in all these tissues. Decreased levels in the bone marrow would lead to overproduction of protoporphyrin, but apparently not to the point of getting any significant degree of feedback inhibition of ALA synthetase, which would lead to severe anemia. Although many patients with EPP have some degree of anemia, it is very slight, and usually does not need treatment. There has been one reported case of a serious hemolytic anemia in a patient with EPP (47). Some workers have suggested that there might be some episodic overproduction of protoporphyrin by the liver if there were instances of sporadic increases of ALA-synthetase production (perhaps triggered by various chemicals, drugs, alcohol, etc.). Calculations suggest that even though there are decreased levels of ferrochelatase in liver in EPP, there would be enough heme made to keep ALA-synthetase inhibited to avoid constant overproduction of this enzyme, with concomitant increase in protoporphyrin production.

Other workers have suggested that perhaps the high levels of proto-porphyrin occur because of the presence in EPP patients of a defective ferrochelatase, or mRNA for the enzyme, which is destroyed rapidly, and thus protoporphyrin builds up (48).

Thus it would seem that in EPP there is either a decreased amount of, or the presence of a defective, easily destroyed, ferrochelatase or mRNA, which leads to the accumulation of protoporphyrin in reticulocytes. This excess protoporphyrin leaks rapidly into the plasma from the maturing reticulocytes and young erythrocytes. The protoporphyrin is then cleared from the plasma by the liver and excreted into the bile (with or without some recirculation via the enterohepatic circulation). Accumulation of this protoporphyrin in the liver may, in some patients, lead to serious liver disease. The levels of ferrochelatase in the marrow are usually sufficient to allow enough hemo-globin synthesis to take place so as not to lead to serious anemia, and the levels in the liver are sufficient to keep ALA-synthetase inhibited. Further work still needs to be done to determine whether in actuality there may be episodic overproduction of protoporphyrin by the liver in EPP under certain circumstances.

Effect of Beta-Carotene Treatment

The first patient treated, a 10-year-old girl, was first seen in the winter of 1967. At that time she could tolerate only brief exposures to sunlight (30 min or less). Exposure to a carbon-arc light (340–640 nm) produced erythema in 2 min. In June 1968, she was given a preparation of concentrated carrot oil in doses approximately equivalent to 30 mg beta-carotene per day. After a month of carrot oil ingestion, she could tolerate at least 30 min of carbon-arc light and more than 1 hr of sunlight. By the middle of the summer she could play outdoors in the afternoon without experiencing any symptoms of photosensitivity. As is characteristic of the disease, her porphyrins remained elevated throughout the period of treatment. Because the carrot oil was unpleasant to take and caused diarrhea, its use was discontinued. In the summer of 1969, she (and all subsequent patients) was given beta-carotene in the form of 10% beta-carotene "beadlets" (Hoffman-La Roche).

The first patient and two others were successfully treated with this preparation during the summer of 1969 (27, 28). In 1970, since the beadlet preparation had proven effective in our three patients, we enlarged the study to include all the patients of Dr. L. C. Harber and those of other physicians who had contacted us concerning the use of beta-carotene following publication of our first three cases. By the summer of 1975, we had treated 133 patients suffering from EPP with beta-carotene, using a standard protocol adhered to by all participating physicians (29, 30). In July 1975, the U.S. Food and Drug Administration approved the use of beta-carotene for the treatment of EPP and we terminated the collaborative study at this time.

We have used the following starting dosage schedule of beta-carotene: 1–4 years of age, 60–90 mg/day; 5–8 years, 90–120 mg/day; 9–12 years, 120–150 mg/day; 13–15 years, 150–180 mg/day; and 16 years and older, 180 mg/day. The average dose for the patient's age should be administered for 4–6 weeks, and the patient should be instructed not to increase sun exposure either for 4 weeks or until some yellow discoloration of the skin, especially of the palms of the hands, is noted. Then, exposure can be increased cautiously and gradually until the patient determines the limits of exposure to light that can be tolerated without the development of symptoms. If the degree of protection is not sufficient, the daily dose of carotene should be increased by 30–60 mg for children under 16, and up to a total of 300 mg/day for those over 16 years of age. If after 3 months of therapy at these higher doses (blood carotene levels should reach at least 800 μg/dl) no significant increase in tolerance to sunlight exposure has occurred, it can be assumed that beta-carotene therapy will not be effective for that patient, and the medication should be discontinued.

To determine the efficacy of the treatment with beta-carotene, patients were given detailed questionnaires each time they visited the physician for physical examinations and blood tests as described in the protocol. These visits occurred several times before and at 4–6-week intervals during therapy. The questionnaires recorded the length of time the patient could tolerate exposure to sunlight without the development of symptoms, and from the data obtained before and during therapy, a protection index was calculated (29, 30).

Table 14-2 shows the effect of treatment with beta-carotene on the tolerance to sun exposure of the 133 patients we studied. Eighty-four percent of the patients increased their ability to tolerate sunlight exposure by a factor of 3 or more without the development of symptoms.

Table 14-2. Effect of Beta-Carotene on Tolerance to Sunlight of Patients with Erythropoietic Protoporphyria[a]

Number of patients	Percent	Protection index[b]
10	16	1[c]
12		2[c]
27		3–5
39		6–10
15	84	11–15
6		16–20
24		>21
Total 133	100	

[a] Data taken from (29, 30).
[b] Protection index is defined as the number of minutes of summer sunlight tolerated without the development of symptoms after therapy, divided by the number of minutes of summer sunlight tolerated without the development of symptoms before therapy. An index of less than 3 represents no improvement.
[c] Patients showed little or no improvement despite blood carotene levels of at least 400 μg% following intake of highest dose appropriate for their ages.

On the average, it took between 1 and 2 months for the patients who received benefit from carotene therapy to notice increased tolerance to sun exposure. The majority are now engaging in outdoor activities which they were unable to do before therapy started, many stating that they spend more time in the sun since taking beta-carotene. This seemed to be especially gratifying to the children, who, previous to carotene therapy, were unable to play out-of-doors to any great extent; now the majority can spend hours outside with their friends.

Many patients stated that they were able to develop a suntan for the first time in their lives. Indeed, the results of tests with artificial light sources indicate that patients with EPP react normally to sunburn radiation (290–320 nm) when tested with that radiation alone. However, because of the presence of light of 380 nm and above in natural sunlight, which light causes symptoms, the patient with EPP has never been able to tolerate sun exposure long enough to develop a tan. It was the impression of several of the patients that the acquisition of the tan, plus the beta-carotene, added to their protection from the sun's effects.

The majority of the patients have noted that when they are taking beta-carotene, those reactions from the sun that do occur are less severe in intensity and duration than before therapy. Not only have the patients increased the time that they can remain in the sun symptom-free, but they also do not develop significant numbers of cutaneous lesions during their increased exposure time.

We found that the patients' blood and stool porphyrin levels were not affected by the ingestion of large amounts of beta-carotene. Thus, treatment with beta-carotene ameliorates photosensitivity in EPP, but has no effect on the biochemical lesion in this disease.

Because of the difficulties in the subjective evaluation of therapeutic effect and of setting up a controlled double-blind study in the particular case of beta-carotene and EPP, we decided to use phototesting with polychromatic light from 380 to 560 nm (as opposed to monochromatic light) as an objective measure of clinical improvement. Using a xenon-arc lamp under the conditions we have developed (29), we have not yet found a patient with EPP who did not develop immediate erythema when exposed to this light. A few patients develop, in addition to erythema, wheals, itching, and burning, but the erythema is the reproducible phenomenon. Table 14-3 records the average for each patient of three phototests done before treatment with beta-carotene was begun, and the average of those phototests done during treatment, after blood carotenoid levels had reached at least 400 μg/dl. The number of tests was large, and clearly established the reliability and reproducibility of the tests. We found that tolerance to xenon-arc light exposure increased in those patients who reported benefit from beta-carotene therapy, but no increased tolerance to this radiation has been found in patients reporting no improvement (Table 14-3; note patient 8). Other workers have also noted increased

Table 14-3. Tolerance to Xenon-Arc Light (Phototest) Measured
before Therapy and during Therapy[a]

	Minutes to develop minimal erythema	
Patient	Before therapy	After therapy
1	20	40
2	20	40
3	0.5	7
4	20	30
5	10	20
7	5	10
8	5	5
9	15	30
10	5	30
11	3	45
12	5	15
13	5	30
14	5	20
15	5	20
16	10	20
34	5	10
35	5	25
37	5	15
38	10	25
39	2	10
42	5	15

[a]Data given in this table are taken from (29), where also a description of the phototesting technique is given. The data are the average for each patient of three tests done before treatment was started and the average after treatment of those tests done after blood carotenoid levels have reached at least 400 μg%. Individuals who do not have protoporphyria or other forms of photosensitivity will not develop erythema to at least 45 min of exposure to the filtered xenon-arc light, according to the described technique.

tolerance to polychromatic xenon-arc light after treatment with beta-carotene (49, 50). Thus, phototesting with polychromatic xenon-arc light can serve as an objective method of determinig improvement in tolerance to light (51).

It should be noted that we did not find a definite relationship between the ability to tolerate a given amount of xenon-arc light and the ability to tolerate a given amount of sunlight. Response to artificial light shows a qualitative but not a quantitative relationship to response to sunlight.

We have found 16 other studies reporting increases in tolerance to sunlight in over three-quarters of patients with EPP treated with high doses of beta-carotene (49, 50, 52–65). One study reporting little or no improvement has also appeared (66); however, these workers used a much lower dosage of beta-carotene than recommended. Later, some of the patients from the unsuccessfully treated group were given higher doses of beta-carotene by another investigator and the patients noted some increased tolerance to sun while taking the higher doses (67). These results emphasize the importance, as mentioned above, of individualizing dosage to each patient, and increasing the dose until the patient reports some improvement. The problem of individualizing treatment is important to the conduct of a controlled trial and makes double-blinded designs almost impossible. At a minimum, such trials should use a dose of beta-carotene large enough to produce amelioration of symptoms in the majority of patients (a minimum period of 3 months' treatment at doses giving blood levels of at least 800 μg/dl; for adults at least 180 mg/day should be given).

From our results, and those of the other workers cited above, it can be concluded that beta-carotene, when administered in sufficiently high doses, can be an effective therapy for ameliorating photosensitivity in most patients with EPP.

BETA-CAROTENE THERAPY IN OTHER PHOTOSENSITIVITY DISEASES

Since beta-carotene seemed to be effective in preventing photosensitivity in EPP, it seemed logical to see whether it could prevent photosensitivity in other photosensitivity diseases. Several workers have investigated this possibility.

Seip et al. (68) and Sneddon (69) reported some success in treating patients suffering from congential porphyria (Gunther disease) with beta-carotene. We also have treated with beta-carotene two children having this disease, and have noted some improvement. New lesions were significantly decreased in number and severity, and the patients have been able somewhat to increase their sun exposure (70).

Wennerstein and Swanbeck treated eight patients with polymorphous light eruption (PMLE) with beta-carotene and found an increase in the minimal erythema dose (tested with an appropriately filtered xenon-arc lamp) of all the patients after treatment (50, 71). Jansen (72) treated 66 patients, 55 of whom improved as judged by patients' questionnaires and physicians' examinations. Nordlund et al. found that a topical sunscreen had to be used in conjunction with oral beta-carotene to get an effective therapeutic result in a severe case of PMLE (73). During the course of the collaborative study, we have treated 27 patients with PMLE with high doses of beta-carotene (30). Nine of these patients increased their ability to tolerate exposure to sunlight by more than a factor of 3 (Table 14-4). Only two of these nine patients reported marked improvement in their photosensitivity with the use of beta-carotene alone; the other seven had to use a sunscreen in addition to the beta-carotene. (None of the 27 patients with PMLE had received any benefit from the use of nonopaque sunscreens alone.) The remaining 18 patients reported no improvement with the use of both oral beta-carotene and the topical sunscreen.

Thune (74) administered beta-carotene to 17 patients with PMLE and

Table 14-4. Effect of Beta-Carotene on Tolerance to Sunlight of 39
Patients with Various Forms of Photosensitivity Other than EPP[a]

	Number of patients with given protection index (PI)[b]						
Diagnosis	PI = 1	2	3–5	6–10	11–15	16–20	>21
Polymorphous light eruption	12	6	5[c,d]	2[e,f]	1[e]	0	1[c,f]
Solar urticaria	5	0	1[f,h]	0	0	0	0
Hydroa aestivale	1	1	0	0	0	0	1[e,g]
Porphyria cutanea tarda	1	0	0	0	0	0	0
Actinic reticuloid	2	0	0	0	0	0	0

[a] Data taken from (30).
[b] Protection index is defined in Table 14-2. Patients with protection indices of 1 and 2 showed little or no improvement despite blood carotene levels of at least 400 μg% following intake of highest dose of beta-carotene for their ages.
[c] One patient reporting a protection index of 4 and one patient reporting a protection index of 24 stated they did not need to use a topical sunscreen in conjunction with beta-carotene ingestion. All other PMLE patients needed both beta-carotene and topical sunscreen to achieve the stated protection.
[d] Three patients were in the study for one summer, two patients for two summers.
[e] One summer in study.   [g] Boy, 7 years old.
[f] Two summers in study.   [h] Woman, 40 years old.

found "a significant increase in minimal erythema dose for unfiltered (xenon) light at the 5% level of probability." However, only five of the 17 patients had a protection index of more than 3 with respect to sunlight exposure, a much lower rate than found by the above two authors, and more in line with our findings. He also could not show a direct correlation between the protection index obtained for artificial light and that obtained for sunlight exposure, as we also had been unable to do for EPP. Thune also found, as we have, that some patients benefitted from the combined therapy of oral beta-carotene and topical sunscreen.

Parrish et al. (75) found a similar low rate of improvement (six out of 19) in patients with PMLE treated with beta-carotene, and Haeger-Aronsen et al. (64) reported improvement in 15 out of 18 patients treated.

Porphyria cutanea tarda is successfully treated by phlebotomy, but this treatment is occasionally contraindicated. We treated one patient with this disorder with beta-carotene in the hope of decreasing the appearance of new cutaneous lesions, which in this condition are porphyrin-induced photo-injury. However, examination of the patient's skin and the patient's own report after 2 months of beta-carotene therapy showed no appreciable decrease in the number of new lesions formed.

Kobza et al. reported that beta-carotene alone had no effect in the treatment of two cases of actinic reticuloid and three cases of solar urticaria (76). We treated six cases of solar urticaria, three cases of hydroa aestivale, and two cases of actinic reticuloid with high doses of beta-carotene. Only one patient with solar urticaria and one patient with hydroa aestivale reported noticeable relief (Table 14-4). Both stated that they obtained improvement without the use of a topical sunscreen.

Bickers et al. noted that two patients with hydroa vacciniforme developed no new lesions when taking beta-carotene (77).

In summary, beta-carotene treatment may be of some use in congenital porphyria, if given in high doses starting when the patients are very young. However, carotene treatment seems of limited use in PMLE, solar urticaria, hydroa aestivale, and hydroa vaccineforme; we would recommend it only after other treatment modalities have failed. The treatment seems to be of no use in either porphyria cutanea tarda or actinic reticuloid.

Two independent observations suggested that perhaps carotenemia might have an effect on a normal individual's response to sunlight. Bendes (78) observed that the presence of carotenemia in children undergoing helio-therapy for tuberculosis prevented sunburn, and Sandler (79) found that carotenemia facilitated tanning of the skin. These observations, plus our success with beta-carotene in the treatment of EPP, led us to conduct a controlled trial to determine whether the administration of high doses of beta-carotene would alter the normal fair-skinned individual's response to sunlight. It was found that high doses of beta-carotene had a small but statistically significant effect in increasing the minimal erythema dose for eliciting erythema produced by natural sunlight. However, the observed effects were too small to recommend the use of beta-carotene as a protective agent for sunburn (80). It was also found that the men in the group taking carotene in this study developed more pigmentation (tanning) than did the men in the placebo group, thus confirming the findings of Bendes (78) and Sandler (79).

Anyan (81) reported that a young girl who had been carotenemic while hypothyroid had not been able to tan while in this condition. Once she became euthyroid after appropriate treatment, her carotenemia disappeared and the ability to tan returned. These findings are not necessarily at variance with ours; perhaps, as Anyan suggests, marked, long-standing carotenodermia may protect the skin to such a degree that tanning may become hard to induce. In addition, one does not know the effects of hypothyroidism itself on tanning. Unfortunately, serum carotenoid levels were not given. Also, it is difficult to compare the degree of sun exposure of this youngster to the degree of sun exposure of the patients in our study. As we mentioned above, many of our EPP patients report tanning for the first time because of their new-found ability to stay out in the sun. Some actually sunbathe on the beach. None have reported not being able to tan. These observations would all support our findings and those of Bendes (78) and Sandler (79) that tanning increases and burning decreases in carotenemic individuals. However, more work needs to be done to elucidate the extent of the ability of carotenoids to alter the skin's reaction to sunburn.

SOME ASPECTS OF THE CLINICAL PHARMACOLOGY
OF BETA-CAROTENE

Role of Beta-Carotene in Human Nutrition

In spite of the current availability and use of synthetic vitamin A either in foods or in vitamin supplements, carotenoid vitamin A precursor-containing foods are still a very significant source of this vitamin in the diets of humans, particularly in developing countries. Diets in various parts of the world vary greatly in their content of vitamin A, either available directly in meat, fish, eggs, or dairy foods, or as the various provitamins A in vegetable sources. Beta-carotene is the most important vitamin A precursor, mainly because of its prevalence in plants widely consumed by humans and livestock, and because it is the provitamin A with the greatest activity (82).

In addition to availability in the diet, several other factors, such as severe dietary deficiency in protein, the amount, nature, and dispersion of dietary fat, and the nitrate content of the food, may influence the absorption and utilization of beta-carotene and other provitamins (82–87).

The transformation of beta-carotene to vitamin A (retinol) in the animal (plants are not thought to contain vitamin A as such) is thought to occur by cleavage of the carotene molecule at the central double bond (88, 89) or by cleavage of the conjugated chain adjacent to one beta-ionone ring followed by sequential oxidative removal of fragments consisting of 2–5 carbon atoms (90, 91). The activity of the enzyme carotene deoxygenase isolated from rat and human intestinal mucosa and also from liver seems to suggest that the cleavage of the molecule at the central double bond is the more important mechanism for metabolism of carotene in the mammal (91, 92).

Many studies have shown that the main point of conversion of ingested carotenoids is the intestinal mucosa. Conversion also occurs to a fairly significant degree in the liver. It was suggested that lung might also be a site of conversion, but data from heart–lung preparations have not confirmed this (93). Greenberg et al. suggest that sebacceous glands may convert beta-carotene to vitamin A (94–96).

Traditionally, it has been thought that only plants and bacteria can synthesize carotenoids from simple precursors (2); recently some evidence has been presented that bovine corpus luteum tissue could synthesize beta-carotene from acetate in vitro (97). Further confirmation of this finding must be obtained before the present view of no carotenoid synthesis in animals can be abandoned.

The manner in which carotenoids are excreted is not clear. Hashimoto (98) claims that none is excreted in the urine. Hess and Meyers (99) found that urine got yellower within ¾ hr after giving concentrated carrot extract. Unfortunately, they did not chemically extract the urine to determine the presence of carotenoids. Almond and Logan (100) made the same observation and attempted to chemically extract the urine. They extracted a yellow pigment, but this was found not to be carotene. We also looked for carotenoids in the urine of EPP patients taking carotene, and also found that the yellow pigment contained in the urine did not seem to be a carotenoid on spectrophotometric or chromatographic analysis. More work certainly needs to be done on the question of the excretion of carotenoids.

Toxicity Studies

The results of studies we have conducted on patients with EPP treated with beta-carotene and on normal volunteers given similar doses of beta-carotene for a 10-week period in our study on carotene and sunburn radiation (29, 30, 80) have confirmed reports in the literature that the ingestion of large amounts of pure beta-carotene has not led to toxic side effects (101, 102). Some of our patients have been taking carotene for 9 years, with no appearance to date of toxicity. We detected no abnormalities in blood sugar or blood urea nitrogen in either EPP patients or normal volunteers, nor have the above-mentioned workers who are using beta-carotene in the treatment of EPP reported any toxicity. All but one patient with EPP in our study had normal total bilirubin and serum glutamate-oxaloacetate transaminase levels. This one patient had fairly consistently elevated levels of these parameters before as well as during therapy, but never complained or gave a history of liver disease. He has not responded to carotene therapy, and has sustained high levels of blood and stool porphyrins. As we mentioned above, although serious liver disease is seen in some cases of EPP, this patient is the only one in our group to demonstrate significant liver function test abnormalities. Another patient has had his gall bladder removed, but his liver function tests were normal.

The complete blood count was not affected by carotene intake. Many of the patients with EPP had a mild anemia (35). This was not worsened or improved by carotene intake. Leukopenia has been reported in patients who ingested large amounts of carrots (103, 104). This phenomenon was found to reverse itself when the patient stopped eating an abnormal amount of carrots. We found no evidence of leukopenia in any of our patients or volunteers. The absence of this finding in our study strengthens the suggestion of earlier workers that the leukopenia was probably due to substances other than beta-carotene present in the carrots (101, 102). Indeed they reported that the administration of pure beta-carotene did not induce leukopenia in a patient who had experienced leukopenia after eating large amounts of carrots (101, 102).

Methemoglobinemia has recently been shown to result from the consumption of large amounts of carrot juice (105). This is another example of the toxicity of large amounts of vegetables and their products, and a reason why we do not encourage photosensitive patients to become carotenemic by ingesting large amounts of these foods.

None of our patients were found to develop abnormally high levels of serum vitamin A. This confirms what has been repeatedly reported in the literature, that individuals ingesting large amounts of beta-carotene do not develop hypervitaminosis A (101, 102, 106).

Magnus and his collaborators report that one patient treated with beta-carotene reported an increase in hay fever attacks and another reported swelling of the tongue and face (76). We found no such reactions in our patients. However, it should be kept in mind that an occasional patient could be allergic to some of the other components of the beadlet preparation (gelatin, antioxidants, etc.). Perhaps such patients should be given crystalline beta-carotene in vegetable oil, to determine whether indeed the reaction was caused by beadlet components. If the adverse reaction disappears, then the patient can continue to take the carotene in oil, if ingestion of carotene has benefitted his photosensitivity. Thus, it would seem that the only "side effect" from the ingestion of large amounts of beta-carotene is carotenodermia, the yellowish coloration of the ski observed in many people who ingest large amounts of the pigment.

Carotenoids have been found in human milk (107, 108), and there are at least two reported instances of breast-fed infants becoming carotenemic on their carotenemic mothers' milk (100, 109). It also seems that carotenoids can cross the placental barrier. DeBuys reports that two children of a carotenemic mother were born carotenemic with no apparent side effects (110). Claussen and McCoord suggest that 1 mg of carotenoid/kg fetus/day crosses the placenta (111). Claussen reports the presence of some carotenoid in the cord blood at birth (112). After birth, the amount of carotenoid present is dependent on the child's diet.

We recently studied the livers of two patients who had been taking beta-carotene for photosensitivity. There was no evidence of any accumulation of large amounts of either beta-carotene or vitamin A in the liver by chemical analysis, or evidence of morphologic alterations attributable to carotenoids or vitamin A accumulation on light microscopic examination (113).

Carotenemia and Carotenodermia

Hess and Myers (99) noted that people who consumed large amounts of carrots and other vegetables often developed a yellow color of their skin; they used the term "carotenemia" for this condition. The phenomenon of yellow skin color was probably first noted by Baeltz (114), who called it aurantiasis cutis; he did not, however, make the connection between a diet abnormally high in carotene-containing foods and the yellow skin color. Apparently Hess and Myers were the first to do so. In actuality, carotenodermia is the more accurate term for the phenomenon of yellow skin coloration by the ingestion of large amounts of carotenoid pigments; carotenemia literally means carotene in the blood. Carotenemia has been thoroughly reviewed in the past (104, 115, 116); we will note only highlights about this condition here.

Mammals can be divided into three groups according to their ability to accumulate carotenoids after oral administration in blood and tissues as carotenoids (not vitamin A): (a) those that can accumulate a mixture of carotenoids; (b) those that accumulate predominately carotenes, as opposed to xanthophylls; and (c) those that cannot accumulate any carotenoids (2). Humans, the fox, the fitchert, and possibly the badger and roedeer are examples of the first group; cattle, horses, dogs, sheep, buffalo, deer, antelope, caribou, and hedgehog are examples of the second; and goats, swine, hares and the common laboratory animals, mice, rats, rabbits, and guinea pigs, are examples of the third group. Castle (117) studied a strain of rabbit which carried a recessive gene for "yellow fat," or the ability to accumulate carotenoids.

In humans, the most common cause of carotenemia and carotenodermia is over-indulgence in carotenoid-containing vegetables and fruits. The predominant pigment found in the serum is the predominant pigment of the vegetable eaten. Usually this is beta-carotene. There has been a report of high levels of lycopene, the principal pigment of the tomato, in a patient whose dietary indiscretion was tomato juice (118). There have been a few cases reported in which carotenemia and carotenodermia have developed in individuals whose vegetable intake is not abnormal. It seems that these patients have a genetic inability to split carotenoids into vitamin A to the same degree as the normal individual (116, 119–121). These patients have low to normal serum vitamin A levels, and may or may not show symptoms of vitamin A deficiency (116, 119–121).

The development of carotenodermia seems to be quite variable; different individuals on essentially the same diet can vary in the degree of carotenodermia they develop (104). Factors that seem to influence the development of carotenodermia, besides the amount of carotenoid-containing foods ingested, are the amount, nature, and dispersion of lipid in the diet, the digestability of the carotenoid-containing food, and the general adequacy of nutrition and level of protein in the diet (82). It has been found that the ingestion of mineral oil definitely decreases the absorption of carotenoids (and for that matter also that of vitamin A). The time of development of carotenemia and carotenodermia from the onset of increased carotenoid intake varies widely, depending on the amount of and kind of carotenoid-containing foods ingested. In our studies of EPP patients and normal volunteers taking pure beta-carotene and on otherwise normal diets, we found that development of carotenodermia occurred between 1½ to 3 months, but the development of serum carotene levels above normal values occurred within 1 month. Those taking the higher doses from the beginning (180 mg/day) developed carotenemia and carotenodermia somewhat earlier. Some development of carotene tolerance, manifested by decrease in blood levels of carotene after several months of therapy, has been noted by some workers (95, 122). We have not found any conclusive evidence of this kind of phenomenon in our patients or subjects, but we have noted that some individuals, even on fairly high doses, never achieve as high a level as do others on the same dose. This may indicate the variation in different individuals' ability to absorb carotene.

Clinical observation of patients with carotenodermia has long demonstrated that this coloration is most obvious in those areas of the body with a prominent amount of horny layer, such as the palms of the hands, soles of the feet, knees, and other areas of skin that are subject to mechanical irritation. Gandy (123, 124) also suggested that in addition to areas subject to mechanical irritation, carotenoids are deposited in greater amounts in areas subject to irritation by physical factors, including light. The observation that light may play a part in regulating the intensity of carotenodermia was suggested by Klose (125). He observed that carotenodermia was confined to areas exposed to light in infants fed carrots, and suggested that this might be due to the influence of light. He found that in a group of infants given the same food, carotenodermia developed only in those infants whose cribs were kept near the window. Interestingly, the findings of Edwards and Duntley on the distribution of carotene in the skin of the whole body fairly well parallels those areas of the body exposed to light (126). These findings are interesting in view of the protective function of carotenoids. They might suggest a function of the carotenoid pigments normally present in skin; that is, a certain level of protective pigments is always present to "balance" the potential photosensitizing pigments such as cytochromes and other heme pigments which are also always present. Thus, in conditions of increased light exposure, the body might increase the deposition of carotenoids in light-exposed areas; if there was sufficient carotene present in the diet, this would be seen as some carotenodermia in the light-exposed areas, explaining the findings of Klose. It is known that visible light can penetrate through the epidermis into the dermal layer (127). As skin contains potential photosensitizers as we pointed out above, it would indeed seem important that exposed skin have some kind of protective mechanism to guard against photosensitization. I suggest that this protective mechanism is provided by the normally occurring carotenoid pigments.

It is intriguing to think that there might be some increase of carotenoid pigments in light-exposed areas, in view of the protective function of the carotenoids. However, other than the observations of Klose (125), there are no data to suggest that light really does play a role in increasing the deposition of carotenes in the skin of humans. Interestingly, in certain bacteria and fungi, light indeed does play a role in the deposition of carotenoids (128). The possibility remains that carotenoids are more prevalent in light-exposed areas simply because there is more horny layer in these areas. In addition, those areas of the body exposed to light are also usually exposed to mechanical irritation, resulting in increased formation of horny layer, so it is hard to say which factor could be more important. It would seem that certain physical and probably also anatomical factors influence the development of the horny layer. Because of the affinity of carotenoids for the horny layer, the pigments are predominant in those areas of marked horny layer deposit. If the diet is high in carotenoids, carotenodermia becomes most marked in these areas. Grof et al. suggest a histamine-mediated mechanism to explain the deposit of carotene in these areas (129). I suggest that perhaps such a mechanism is not necessary, since the carotenoids naturally accumulate in skin cells. When physical irritation occurs there is a more rapid division of cells and resultant thickening of the horny layer, and thus accumulation of carotenoids in the area, the degree again being related to the amount of carotenoid intake. However, the Grof suggestion is appealing if there were some mechanism in the skin for the regulation of the level of photoprotector; then some mechanism would be necessary to get more carotenoids into the area susceptible to photosensitization. Clearly, more work is needed to study the factors involved in the development of carotenodermia.

Although the presence of carotenoids in skin has been established by visual and reflectance spectrophotometric observation, until recently no one had chemically isolated carotenoids from skin. Dohi and Ono had observed yellow material in the horny layer of an unstained section of skin (130), and Grof et al. (129) extracted carotenoids from horny layer scraped from the soles and knees of a carotenemic patient. For the chemical isolation of carotenoids from human skin, specimens of abdominal skin were obtained from noncarotenemic individuals at autopsy, and whole skin, epidermis, and dermis were analyzed for the presence of carotenoids (131). We found that the epidermis contained more carotenoids than did the dermis. Some authors have proposed that carotene, which they thought to be present in sebum, is excreted onto the surface of the skin and rubbed into the horny layer (104). However, Greenberg et al. could not demonstrate carotene in sebum, but did find vitamin A (95), and also carotenoids oxidize rapidly when applied to the surface of the skin. In addition, our findings that carotene is present in both layers of the skin, and also the fact that abdominal skin does not have a prominent horny layer, but does contain carotenoids, would tend to militate against this mechanism's, if indeed it exists, playing a prominent part in the accumulation of carotenoids in skin. It is more likely that carotenoids are carried to all the skin cells via the circulation and extracellular fluid, and the pigments enter the cells and bind to membranes. A precedent for this entry into cells and binding to membranes is the finding that carotenoids are present in the membranes of liver cell mitochondria (132). Further studies of the subcellular anatomy of skin are necessary to pinpoint exactly the localization of the carotenoid pigments in the cellular organelles of the various layers.

Another area of the body in which a localized deposit of carotenoids has been found is in a preexisting arcus senilis of the cornea. Giorgio et al. (133) reported the case of a man in whose corneas were found golden-yellow rings, at first thought to be Kayser–Fleischer rings. On more careful examination, however, these rings did not have the characteristics of Kayser–Fleischer rings; nor did the patient have elevated serum copper and ceruloplasmin, or disease of the liver or basal ganglia, factors pathognomonic of Wilson disease, in which Kayser–Fleischer rings occur exclusively. A detailed history elicited from the patient revealed that he ate a diet prominent in vegetables, and in addition consumed daily 1–2 quarts of carrot juice. The serum carotene level at the time of examination was 900 μg%. Neither we nor any of our collaborating physicians have seen any patient or normal subject with a carotenoid-stained arcus senilis, but it is conceivable that, as the number of patients receiving high doses of carotenoids for the treatment of photosensitivity increases, some patients may develop this phenomenon, or smaller amounts of carotenoid deposits in the cornea. Hence the physician should be aware of the existence of this phenomenon. Another ophthalmologic finding was noted in patients receiving high doses of beta-carotene for EPP by deVries-de Mol et al. (134). In a study of 39 patients they noted that treatment with beta-carotene had no effect on the patients' visual acuity, dark adaptation, and color discrimination, all of these parameters being within the normal range. They found no yellow color in the lens. No mention was made of any pigmentation in the cornea. They found that most patients seemed to have "grains" in the macular region, which the authors considered not to be pathologic.

CAROTENOID METABOLISM IN VARIOUS DISEASE STATES

Levels of carotenoids in blood and skin are influenced by several disease conditions. The blood carotene level may be markedly decreased in malabsorption diseases such as steatorrhea and sprue. Workers have found that, although the actual level of carotenoids in blood is not an absolute diagnostic parameter for diseases of malabsorption, the rate at which carotene is absorbed can be used as an indication of the presence of these diseases (135–137). Hence, a carotene loading test has been developed for use as a diagnostic test for malabsorption diseases.

Studies have been conducted on carotenoid levels in various infectious diseases. Carotenodermia has been reported in polio (138) and malaria (104), and lowered carotene absorption (or intake?) in several fevers, pneumonia, sepsis, and grippe (2). Claussen (112) suggested that high levels of carotene might prevent infections, after having observed that infants with high carotene levels develop less severe upper respiratory infections.

High carotene levels have also been reported in castrated males (139) and in retarded children (140). In the latter it seems that the particulate size of the food was an important matter, the smaller the particles the more likely to develop carotenodermia. These children probably do not chew their food well, so large-particle food may pass rather unchanged through the digestive tract.

Jehgers (115) suggested that carotenemia may be present in liver disease. However, Ditlefsen and Stoa (141) found decreased carotene levels in alcoholics (perhaps this may be somewhat related to diet), but patients with cirrhosis and chronic hepatitis had either normal or only moderately decreased carotene levels, with much individual variation. Blood carotene levels were found to be below normal in patients with obstructive jaundice, acute hepatitis and cholecystitis, and secondary carcinoma of the liver. Adlersberg et al. (142) found that carotene absorption was markedly decreased in severe hepatic damage. Interestingly, Newberne et al. found that the administration of carotenoids to rats protected against liver damage induced by aflatoxin (143).

Patients with conditions associated with hyperlipemia have in many cases been found to have concomitant carotenemia and, in some cases, though not all, carotenodermia. Examples are nephrosis, diabetes, and hypothyroidism (104, 111, 115). It is not clear, however, whether the hyperlipemia is the important factor in the increased carotene levels. In nephrosis there is some question about decreased excretion of carotenoids, but since, as noted above, there is disagreement as to whether carotenoids are excreted in the urine, this point is still not settled. Interestingly and for reasons unknown, patients with nephrosis do not often develop carotenodermia.

Carotenemia and carotenodermia have been observed for many years in diabetics, and the question has long been asked as to whether this is due to some role of insulin on carotenoid metabolism. Animal experiments suggested such a role, as it was found that in alloxan diabetic rats there was markedly less conversion of beta-carotene to vitamin A in the isolated intestinal loop (144). Ralli et al. (145, 146) suggested that diabetics had an impaired ability to convert beta-carotene to vitamin A in the liver. However, since that time, studies of carotene tolerance curves in diabetics and normals reveal no difference between them in absorption and conversion of carotene to vitamin A (147, 148). This latter finding would suggest that there is no direct role of insulin on carotenoid metabolism. The carotenemia and carotenodermia which result are probably due to the diet containing ample amounts of vegetables and fruits which most diabetics follow (2). It is interesting to note that, on the other hand, vegetarians do not often develop carotenodermia. This is because their diet in actuality does not contain an overabundance of carotenoid-containing vegetables, as these are low in protein. The vegetarians increase the concentration of high-protein vegetables, such as various seeds and beans, in their diet. These are not very high in carotenoid content.

Carotenemia and carotenodermia are often noted in cases of hypothyroidism. For many years it was suggested that thyroid hormone had some effect on the absorption of carotenoids and their conversion to vitamin A. Studies by Walton et al. (149) suggest that absorption of carotenoids is unimpaired in hypothyroidism, but that the mechanism for the disposal of the carotenoids once they are taken into the body as such ("intrinsic" carotenoids—those carotenoids not split into vitamin A by the intestine, but absorbed into the circulation) was interfered with. They found that the amounts of low-density lipoproteins (S_f 3–9) responsible for carriage of carotenoids in serum are significantly higher in patients with hypothyroidism than in euthyroid patients, and also that this fraction is overloaded with respect to carotene as compared to the concentration of carotene in the S_f 3–9 fraction in euthyroid blood. Absorption and utilization of preformed vitamin A seem to be within normal limits. They suggest that serum lipoprotein levels may be influenced by the level of protein metabolism, which is under the influence of thyroid hormone. Conversion of high S_f to low S_f classes, however, does not seem to be affected by this hormone. These authors suggest that the conversion of absorbed and circulating carotenoids to vitamin A might be dependent on complete catabolism of the S_f 3–9 lipoprotein fraction. Thus it would seem that once carotenoids are absorbed and bound to lipoprotein, there is a defect in the disposal of the carotenoids and their carrier lipoprotein and, as a result, a decrease in the conversion of some of this intrinsic carotene into vitamin A, probably in organs other than the intestinal wall. Clearly, careful carotene absorption and conversion studies, with concurrent lipoprotein metabolic studies on a significantly large number of patients, are needed to establish whether indeed the effect of thyroid hormone is limited to the fate of the "intrinsic" carotenoids, and has no effect on the absorption of carotene and the conversion of some of this absorbed carotene to vitamin A in the intestinal wall.

Page (150) reported menstrual disorders and hypervitaminosis A in women ingesting large amounts of carotenoid-containing food. Two of the women had anorexia nervosa. Several authors have reported carotenemia in anorexia nervosa, which condition also results in menstrual disorders (151–155). Pops and Schwabe suggest that there might be decreased catabolism of beta-lipoproteins in anorexia nervosa, as there is in hypothyroidism, as found by Walton (153). This may indeed be true, as lipoprotein metabolism is so closely linked to protein metabolism, which may be altered in anorexia nervosa. More investigation of lipoprotein metabolism in anorexia nervosa is certainly in order. In all of these cases, Page's included, one cannot rule out the effects of other components of the ingested vegetables in causing some of the "symptoms," such as tiredness, nervousness, and depression, occasionally attributed to carotenemia due to excessive vegetable ingestion, and also found in anorexia nervosa. In our patients taking pure beta-carotene, no such symptoms have developed, and the women patients between 17 and 45 developed no menstrual abnormalities (29, 30). The unusual finding in Page's (150) and Robboy et al.'s (154) patients is that of abnormally high serum vitamin A; all previously published reports of which we are aware indicate that this does not happen if ingested vegetables are the only source of carotenoids. It is not clear whether or not these patients were taking any supplemental vitamins. In studies of this kind, it is important to ascertain (and report) whether or not the patients are taking any supplementary vitamins containing even small amounts of vitamin A. In addition, one must be sure that appropriate corrections are made in the vitamin A assays for the cross-reacting carotene, the latter being especially important when there is carotenemia.

We also examined the carriage of carotenoids in the lipoprotein fractions of normal individuals taking carotene and of normal individuals on a regular diet (156). We found that the amount of carotene in each lipoprotein fraction had increased in the serum from carotenemic individuals, but that the relative increase is significant only in the LDL and HDL fractions. There was no significant difference between the cholesterol levels of each fraction of the sera of carotenemic and noncarotenemic individuals, indicating that there is no increase in serum beta-lipoprotein in carotenemia. We also found, as Krinsky et al. had reported (157), that the majority of the pigments were in the beta-lipoprotein fraction of both the carotenemic and noncarotenemic volunteers.

From the results of our studies and from the data found in the literature, it would seem that there is no marked direct toxicity from the ingestion of large amounts of pure beta-carotene. On the other hand, those individuals developing carotenemia and carotenodermia by means of increased intake of carotenoid-containing foods are at some risk for the development of some hematologic abnormality. They also may encounter other difficulties because of the misdiagnosis of their "jaundice" by a physician unaware of their dietary indiscretions, and unfamiliar with carotenemia.

Because of the potential dangers associated with excessive ingestion of carotenoid-containing foods, we do not recommend that photosensitive patients obtain relief from their photosensitivity by increasing the intake of such foods. Pure beta-carotene, either as the beadlet preparation or as crystalline beta-carotene for those allergic to beadlet components, is indeed the preparation to be recommended.

SUMMARY

In this chapter we have presented evidence to show that carotenoid pigments can exert a protective action against photosensitivity in humans as well as in animal and plant systems. From the evidence available to date, it would seem that administration of high levels of carotenoids is effective for the amerlioration of photosensitivity in the majority of patients with EPP, and does not lead to toxic side effects. Larger numbers of patients with other forms of photosensitivity (PMLE, congenital porphyria, etc.) must be studied before it can definitely be determined whether carotenoids are effective in ameliorating photosensitivity in these conditions.

REFERENCES

1. Karrer, P. and Jucker, E. (1950): *Carotenoids*, translated by E. A. Braude. Elsevier, Amsterdam.
2. Goodwin, T. W. (1952): *The Comparative Biochemistry of the Carotenoids*. Chapman and Hall, London.
3. Isler, O. (1971): *Carotenoids*. Brikhauser Verlag, Basel.
4. Engelmann, T. W. (1883): Farbe und Assimilation. *Bot. Z.* **41**:1–16.
5. Engelmann, T. W. (1884): Untersuchung über die Quantität Beziehunger zwischen Absorption des Lichtes und Assimilation in Pflanzenzellen. *Bot. Z.* **42**:81–93.
6. Krinsky, N. I. (1968): The protective function of carotenoid pigments. In: *Photophysiology*, edited by A. C. Giese, Vol. 3, pp. 123–195. Academic Press, New York.
7. Krinsky, N. I. (1971): Function. In: *Carotenoids*, edited by O. Isler, pp. 669–716. Birkhauser Verlag, Basel.
8. Sistrom, W. R., Griffiths, M., and Stanier, R. Y. (1956): Biology of a photosynthetic bacterium which lacks colored carotenoids. *J. Cell Comp. Physiol.* **48**:473–515.
9. Koski, V. M., and Smith, J. H. C. (1951): Chlorophyll formation in a mutant, white seedling-3. *Arch. Biochem. Biophys.* **34**:189–195.
10. Smith, J. H. C., Durham, L., and Warster, C. F. (1959): Formation and bleaching of chlorophyll in albino corn seedlings. *Plant Physiol.* **34**:340–345.
11. Anderson, I. C., and Robertson, D. S. (1960): Role of carotenoids in protecting chlorophyll from photodestruction. *Plant Physiol.* **35**:531–534.
12. Wallace, R. H., and Schwarting, A. E. (1954): A study of chlorophyll in a white mutant strain of *Helianthus annus*. *Plant Physiol.* **29**:431–436.
13. Kunisawa, R., and Stanier, R. Y. (1958): Studies on the role of carotenoid pigments in a chemoheterotropic bacterium, *Corynebacterium poinsettiae*. *Arch. Mikrosk.* **31**:146–156.
14. Mathews, M. M., and Sistrom, W. R. (1959): Function of carotenoid pigments in non-photosynthetic bacteria. *Nature* **184**:1892.
15. Mathews, M. M., and Sistrom, W. R. (1960): The function of the carotenoid pigments of *Sarcona lutea*. *Arch. Mikrosk.* **35**:139–146.
16. Stanier, R. (1960): Carotenoid pigments—problems of synthesis and function. In: *The Harvey Lectures*, vol. 54, pp. 219–255. Academic Press, New York.
17. Stanier, R., and Cohen-Bazire, G. (1957): Role of light in the microbial world—some facts and speculations. In: *Microbial Ecology, 7th Symposium of the Society of General Microbiology*, edited by R. E. O. Williams and C. C. Spicer, pp. 56–89. Cambridge University Press, Cambridge.
18. Blum, H. F. (1941): *Photodynamic Action and Diseases Caused by Light*. Reinhold, New York.
19. Weeks, O. B., and Garner, R. J. (1967): Biosynthesis of carotenoids in *Flavobacterium dehydrogenans* Arnaudi. *Arch. Biochem. Biophys.* **121**:35.
20. Zobell, C. E., and Feltham, C. B. (1934): Preliminary studies on the distribution and characteristics of marine bacteria. *Bull. Scripps Inst. Ocean. Tech. Ser.* **3**:279–296.
21. Courington, D. P., and Goodwin, T. W. (1955): Carotenoids of marine bacteria. *J. Bacteriol.* **70**:568–571.
22. Hodgkiss, W., Liston, J., Goodwin, T. W., et al. (1954): Isolation and description of two marine microorganisms with special reference to their pigment production. *J. Gen. Microbiol.* **11**:438–450.

23. Kesten, B. M. (1951): *Urticaria solare* (4,200–4,900 Å). *Arch. Dermatol. Syphilol.* **64**:221–228.

24. Lipson, R. L., and Baldes, E. J. (1960): Photodynamic properties of a particular hematoporphyrin derivative. *Arch. Dermatol.* **82**:508–516.

25. Forssberg, A., Lingen, C., Ernster, L., et al. (1959): Modification of X-irradiation syndrome by lycopene. *Exp. Cell Res.* **16**:7–14.

26. Mathews, M. M. (1964): Protective effect of beta-carotene against lethal photosensitization by hematoporphyrin. *Nature* **203**:1092.

27. Mathews-Roth, M. M., Pathak, M. A., Fitzpatrick, T. B., et al. (1970): Beta-carotene as a photoprotective agent in erythropoietic protoporphyria. *N. Engl. J. Med.* **282**:1231–1234.

28. Mathews-Roth, M. M., Pathak, M. A., Fitzpatrick, T. B., et al. (1970): Beta-carotene as a photoprotective agent in erythropoietic protoporphyria. *Trans. Assoc. Am. Physicians* **83**:176–184.

29. Mathews-Roth, M. M., Pathak, M. A., Fitzpatrick, T. B., et al. (1974): Beta-carotene as an oral photoprotective agent in erythropoietic protoporphyria. *JAMA* **228**:1004–1008.

30. Mathews-Roth, M. M., Pathak, M. A., Fitzpatrick, T. B., et al. (1977): Beta-carotene therapy for erythropoietic protoporphyria and other photosensitivity diseases. *Arch. Dermatol.* **113**:1229–1232.

31. Tschudy, D. P., Magnus, I. A., and Kalivas, J. (1971): The porphyrias. In: *Dermatology in General Medicine*, edited by T. B. Fitzpatrick, K. A. Arndt, W. H. Clark, Jr., pp. 1143–1166. McGraw-Hill, New York.

32. Marver, H. S., and Schmid, R. (1972): The porphyrias. In: *The Metabolic Basis of Inherited Disease*, 3rd ed., edited by J. B. Stanbury, J. B. Wyngaarden, and D. S. Fredrickson, pp. 1087–1140. McGraw-Hill, New York.

33. DeLeo, V. A., Poh-Fitzpatrick, M. B., Mathews-Roth, M. M., et al. (1976): Erythropoietic protoporphyria—10 years' experience. *Am. J. Med.* **60**:8–22.

34. Bloomer, J. L., Bonkowsky, H. L., and Ebert, P. S. (1976): Inheritance in protoporphyria: comparison of heme synthetase activity in skin fibroblasts with clinical features. *Lancet* **2**:226–238.

35. Mathews-Roth, M. M. (1974): Anemia in erythropoietic protoporphyria. *J. AMA* **230**:824.

36. Pimstone, N. R., Weber, B. L., Blekkenhorst, G. H., et al. (1976): The hepatic lesion in protoporphyria (PP): preliminary studies of haem metabolism, liver structure and ultrastructure. *Ann. Clin. Res.* **17**:122–132.

37. Meffert, H., Barthelmes, H., Schmidt, B., et al. (1974): Leberheteiligung bei erythropoietischer Protoporphyrie. *Dermatol. Monatsschr.* **160**:748–757.

38. MacDonald, D. M., and Nicholson, D. C. (1976): Erythropoietic protoporphyria: hepatic implications. *Br. J. Dermatol.* **95**:157–162.

39. Cripps, D. J., and Goldfarb, S. S. (1978): Erythropoietic protoporphyria: hepatic cirrhosis. *Br. J. Dermatol.* **98**:349–354.

40. Bloomer, J. R., Phillips, M. J., Davidson, D. L., et al. (1975): Hepatic disease in erythropoietic protoporphyria. *Am. J. Med.* **58**:869–882.

41. Singer, J. A., Plaut, A. G., and Kaplan, M. M. (1978): Hepatic failure and death from erythropoietic protoporphyria. *Gastroenterology* **74**:588–591.

42. Bloomer, J. R. (1979): Pathogenesis and therapy of liver disease in protoporphyria. *Yale J. Biol. Med.* **52**:39–48.

43. Wolff, K., Wolff-Schreiner, E., and Gschnait, F. (1975): Liver inclusions in erythropoietic protoporphyria. *Eur. J. Clin. Invest.* **5**:21–26.

44. Piomelli, S., Lamola, A. A., Poh-Fitzpatrick, M. B., et al. (1975): Erythropoietic protoprophyria and lead intoxication: the molecular basis for difference in cutaneous photosensitivity. I. Different rates of disappearance of protoporphyrin from the erythrocytes, both in vivo and in vitro. *J. Clin. Invest.* **56**:1519–1527.

45. Bottomly, S. S., Tanaka, M., and Everett, M. A. (1975): Diminished erythroid ferrochelatase activity in protoporphyria. *J. Lab. Clin. Med.* **86**:126–131.

46. Bonkowsky, H. L., Bloomer, J. R., Ebert, P. S., et al. (1975): Heme synthetase deficiency in human porphyria—demonstration of the defect in liver and cultured skin fibroblasts. *J. Clin. Invest.* **56**:1139–1148.

47. Porter, F. S., and Lowe, B. A. (1963): Congenital erythropoietic protoporphyria: 1. Case reports, clinical studies and porphyria in two brothers. *Blood* **22**:521–531.

48. Clark, K. G. A., and Nicholson, D. C. (1971): Erythrocyte protoporphyrin and iron uptake in erythropoietic protoporphyria. *Clin. Sci.* **41**:363–379.

49. Krook, G., and Haeger-Aronson, B. (1974): Erythropoietic protoporphyria and its treatment with beta-carotene. *Acta Derm. Venereol. (Stockh.)* **54**:39–44.

50. Wennersten, G., and Swanbeck, G. (1974): Treatment of light sensitivty with carotenoids. *Acta Derm. Venereol. (Stockh.)* **54**:491.

51. Mathews-Roth, M. M., Kass, E. H., Fitzpatrick, T. B. (1979): Phototesting as an objective measure of improvement in erythropoietic protoporphyria. *Arch. Dermatol.* **115**: 1381–1382.

52. Anderson, C. R. (1972): Erythropoietic protoporphyria. *Arch. Dermatol.* **106**:412–413.

53. Baart de la Faille, H., Suurmond, D., Went, L. N., et al. (1972): Beta-carotene as a treatment for photohypersensitivity due to erythropoietic protoporphyria. *Dermatologica* **145**: 389–394.

54. Beckert, E., and Metz, J. (1974): Zur Beta-karotin-behandlung der erythropoetische Protoporphyrie. *Hautarzt* **25**:195–196.

55. Chapel, T. A., Stewart, R. H., and Webster, S. B. (1972): Erythropoietic protoporphyria— report of a case successfully treated with beta-carotene. *Arch. Dermatol.* **105**:572–573.

56. Gschnait, F., and Wolff, K. (1974): Die erythropoetische Protoporphyrie. *Hautarzt* **25**:72–80.

57. Hopsu-Havu, V. K., Terho, P. E., and Hollmen, T. (1973): Erythropoietic protoporphyria— the first case in Finald. *Ann. Clin. Res.* **5**:181–185.

58. Lewis, M. B. (1972): Effect of beta-carotene on serum vitamin A levels in erythropoietic protoporphyria. *Australas. J. Dermatol.* **13**:75–78.

59. Moynahan, E. J., and Leppard, B. (1973): Erythropoietic protoporphyria. *Proc. R. Soc. Med.* **66**:1085–1086.

60. Wurker, I. (1972): Photoporphyrinamische Lichtdermatose bei Vitium Cordis. *Z. Haut. Geschch.* **47**:1006–1007.

61. Ippen, H., Goerz, G., and Botsch, C. (1974): Photoprotection in porphyris and the role of phlebotomy. In: *Sunlight and Man: Normal and Abnormal Photobiologic Responses,* edited by M. A. Pathak, L. C. Harber, M. Seiji, pp. 655–658. Univ. of Tokyo Press, Tokyo.

62. Wiskemann, A. (1974): Topical and systemic protoprotection against prophyrins. In: *Sunlight and Man: Normal and Abnormal Photobiologic Responses,* edited by M. A. Pathak, L. C. Harber, M. Seiji, pp. 669–676. Univ. of Tokyo Press, Tokyo.

63. Zaynoun, S. T., Hunter, J. A. A., Darby, F. J., et al. (1977): The treatment of erythropoietic protoporphyria: experience with beta-carotene. *Br. J. Dermatol.* **97**:663–668.

64. Haeger-Aronsen, B., Krook, G., and Abdulla, M. (1979): Oral carotenoids for photohypersensitivity in patients with erythropoietic protoporphyria, polymorphous light eruptions and lupus erythematodes discoides. *Int. J. Dermatol.* **18**:73–82.

65. Eales, L. (1978): The effects of canthaxanthin on the photocutaneous manifestations of porphyria. *S. Afr. Med. J.* **54**:1050–1052.

66. Corbett, M. F., Herxheimer, A., Magnus, I. A., et al. (1977): The long term treatment with beta-carotene in erythropoietic protoporphyria: a controlled trial. *Br. J. Dermatol.* **97**:655–662.

67. Shafrir, A. (1977): Comments on a case of erythropoietic protoporphyria with onycholysis. *Proc. R. Soc. Med.* **70**:574.

68. Seip, M., Thune, P. O., and Eriksen, L. (1974): Treatment of photosensitivity in congenital erythropoietic porphyria with beta-carotene. *Acta Derm. Venereol. (Stockh.)* **54**:239–240.

69. Sneddon, I. B. (1974): Congenital porphyria. *Proc. R. Soc. Med.* **67**:593–594.
70. Mathews-Roth, M. M. Haining, R. G., and Kinney, T. R. (1977): Beta-carotene treatment of congenital prophyria. *Am. J. Dis. Child.* **131**:366.
71. Swanbeck, G., and Wennersten, G. (1972): Treatment of polymorphous light eruption with beta-carotene. *Acta Derm. Venereol. (Stockh.)* **52**:462–466.
72. Jansen, C. T. (1974): Beta-carotene treatment of polymorphous light eruption. *Dermatologica* **149**:363–373.
73. Nordlund, J. J., Klaus, S. N., Mathews-Roth, M. M., et al. (1973): New therapy for polymorphous light eruption. *Arch. Dermatol.* **108**:710–712.
74. Thune, P. (1976): Chronic polymorphic light eruption; particular wave bands and the effect of carotene therapy. *Acta Derm. Venereol. (Stockh.)* **56**:127–133.
75. Parrish, J. A., Levine, M. J., Morison, W. L., et al. (1979): Comparison of PUVA and beta carotene in the treatment of polymorphous light eruption. *Br. J. Dermatol.* **100**:187–193.
76. Kobza, A., Ramsay, C. A., and Magnus, I. A. (1973): Oral beta-carotene therapy in actinic reticuloid and solar urticaria. *Br. J. Dermatol.* **88**:157–166.
77. Bickers, D. R., Demar, L. K., DeLeo, V., et al. (1978): Hydroa vaccineforme. *Arch. Dermatol.* **114**:1193–1196.
78. Bendes, J. H. (1926): Heliotherapy in tuberculosis. *Minn. Med.* **9**:112–114.
79. Sandler, A. S. (1935): Carotene in prophylactic pediatrics. *Arch. Pediatr.* **52**:391–406.
80. Mathews-Roth, M. M., Pathak, M. A., Parrish, J. A., et al. (1972): A clinical trial of the effects of oral beta-carotene on the responses of human skin to solar radiation. *J. Invest. Dermatol.* **59**:349–353.
81. Anyan, W. P. (1972): Carotenemia. *Arch. Dermatol.* **105**:130.
82. Thompson, S. Y. (1965): Occurrence, distribution and absorption of provitamins A. *Proc. Nutr. Soc.* **24**:136–146.
83. Arroyave, G., Wilson, D., Mendez, J., et al. (1961): Serum and liver vitamin A and lipids in children with severe protein malnutrition. *Am. J. Clin. Nutr.* **9**:180–185.
84. Berger, S., Recheigl, M., Loosli, J. K., et al. (1962): Protein quality and carotenoid utilization. *J. Nutr.* **77**:174–178.
85. Deshmukh, D. S., and Ganguly, J. (1964): Effect of dietary protein content on the internal conversion of beta-carotene to vitamin A in rats. *Indian J. Biochem.* **1**:204–207.
86. Jagannathan, S. N., and Patwardhan, V. N. (1960): Dietary protein in vitamin A metabolism. I. Influence of level of dietary protein on the utilization of orally fed preformed vitamin A and beta-carotene in the rat. *Indian J. Med. Res.* **48**:775–784.
87. Wood, R. D. (1967): Effect of adding nitrate and nitrite to drinking water on the utilization of carotene by growing swine. *J. Anim. Sci.* **26**:510–513.
88. Goodman, D. S., and Huang, H. S. (1966): Biosynthesis of vitamin A with rat intestinal enzymes. *Science* **149**:879–880.
89. Olson, J. A. (1961): The absorption of beta-carotene and its conversion into vitamin A. *Am. J. Clin. Nutr.* **9**:1–12.
90. Glover, J., and Redfern, E. R. (1954): The mechanism of the transformation of beta-carotene into vitamin A *in vivo*. *Biochem. J.* **58**:xv.
91. Glover, J. (1960): The conversion of beta-carotene into vitamin A. *Vitam. Horm.* **18**:371–386.
92. Goodman, D. S. (1967): Metabolism of beta-carotene and vitamin A. *Prog. Biochem. Pharmacol.* **3**:487–497.
93. Olson, J. A. (1964): Biosynthesis and metabolism of carotenoids and related molecules. *J. Lipid Res.* **5**:281–299.
94. Cornbleet, T., and Greenberg, R. (1957): Conversion of carotene to vitamin A by sebacceous glands. *Arch. Dermatol.* **76**:431–433.
95. Greenberg, R., Cornbleet, T., and Jeffay, A. L. (1959): Accumulation and excretion of vitamin A-like fluorescent material by sebacceous glands after the oral feeding of various carotenoids. *J. Invest. Dermatol.* **32**:599–604.

96. Greenberg, R., Cornbleet, T., and Demovsky, R. (1957): Conversion of carotene to vitamin A by sebacceous glands. *Arch. Dermatol.* **76**:17-23.

97. Austern, B. M., and Gawienowski, A. M. (1969): *In vitro* biosynthesis of beta-carotene by bovine corpus luteum tissue. *Lipids* **4**:227-229.

98. Hashimoto, H. (1922): Carotenoid pigmentation of the skin resulting from a vegetarian diet. *J. AMA* **78**:1111-1112.

99. Hess, A. F., and Myers, V. C. (1919): Carotenemia: a new clinical picture. *J. AMA* **73**:1743-1745.

100. Almond, S., and Logan, R. F. L. (1942): Carotinaemia. *Br. Med. J.* **2**:235-241.

101. Niemann, C., and Klein Obbink, H. J. (1954): Biochemistry and pathology of hyper-vitaminosis A. *Vitam. Horm.* **12**:69-99.

102. Ostwald, R., and Briggs, G. M. (1967): Toxicity of the vitamins. In: *Toxicants Occurring Naturally in Foods*, edited by the Food Protection Commission, pp. 183-220. National Science Foundation, Washington, D.C.

103. Gjerlow, J. (1966): Granulocytopeni som folge au karotinemi. *Tidjschr. Norske Legeforen.* **86**:33-34.

104. Josephs, H. W. (1944): Hypervitaminosis A and carotenemia. *Am. J. Dis. Child.* **67**:33-43.

105. Keating, J. P., Lell, M. E., Strauss, A. W., et al. (1973): Infantile methemoglobinemia caused by carrot juice. *N. Engl. J. Med.* **288**:824-826.

106. Hoch, H. (1943): Effect of prolonged administration of carotene in the form of vegetables on the serum carotene and vitamin A levels in man. *Biochem. J.* **37**:430-433.

107. Kon, S., and Mawson, M. E. (1950): *Carotenoids in Breast Milk* Spec. Report. Ser., Med. Res. Council, London, No. 269.

108. Lesher, M., Brody, J. K., Williams, H. H., et al. (1945): Human milk studies. *Am. J. Dis. Child.* **70**:182-192.

109. Thomson, M. L. (1973): Carotenemia in a suckling. *Arch. Dis. Child.* **18**:112.

110. DeBuys, L. R. (1923): Some clinical experiences with carotenemia. *Trans. Mississippi State Med. Assoc.* pp. 133-138.

111. Clausen, S. W., and McCoord, A. B. (1938): The carotenoids and vitamin A of the blood. *J. Pediatr.* **13**:635-650.

112. Clausen, S. W. (1931): Carotenemia and resistance to infection. *Trans. Am. Pediatr. Soc.* **43**:27-30.

113. Mathews-Roth, M. M., Abraham, A. A., and Gabuzda, G. (1976): Beta-carotene content of certain organs from two patients receiving high doses of beta-carotene. *Clin. Chem.* **22**:922-924.

114. Baeltz, I., cited in Miyake, I. (1924): Über Aurantiasis cutic Baeltz. *Arch. Dermatol. Syphilol. (Berlin)* **147**:184-195.

115. Jehgers, H. (1943): Skin changes of nutritional origin. *N. Engl. J. Med.* **228**:678-686.

116. Cohen, L. (1958): Observations on carotenemia. *Ann. Intern. Med.* **48**:219-227.

117. Castle, W. E. (1933): Linkage relations of yellow fat in rabbits. *Proc. Natl. Acad. Sci. U.S.A.* **19**:947-950.

118. Reich, P., Shwachman, H., and Craig, J. M. (1960): Lycopenemia—a variant of carotenemia. *N. Engl. J. Med.* **262**:263-269.

119. McLaren, D. S., and Zekian, B. (1971): Failure of enzymic cleavage of beta-carotene. *Am. J. Dis. Child.* **121**:278-280.

120. Molholm-Hansen, J. (1965): Xanthosis cutis og hyperkarotenoidaemi. *Nord. Med.* **22**:385-388.

121. Sharvill, D. E. (1970): Familial hypercarotenemia and hypovitaminosis A. *Proc. R. Soc. Med.* **63**:605-606.

122. Urbach, C. (1952): Effect of individual vitamins A, C, E and carotene administered at high levels on their concentration in the blood. *Exp. Med. Surg.* **10**:7-20.

123. Gandy, D. T. (1935): Carotenemia and carotenodermia. *South. Med. J.* **8**:444-446.

124. Gandy, D. T. (1964): Carotenemia and carotenodermia. *Medical Records and Annals (Houston)* **47**:274–275.
125. Klose, E. (1919): Hautverfarbung bei Sauglingen und Kleinkindern infolge der nahrung. *Munch. Med. Wochenschr.* **66**:419–420.
126. Edwards, E. A., and Duntley, S. Q. (1939): Pigments and color of living human skin. *Am. J. Anat.* **63**:1–33.
127. Everett, M. A., Yeargers, E., Sayre, R. M., et al. (1966): Penetration of epidermis by ultraviolet light. *Photochem. Photobiol.* **5**:533–542.
128. Batra. P. (1971): Mechanism of light-induced carotenoid synthesis in non-photosynthetic plants. In: *Photophysiology*, edited by A. C. Giese, pp. 47–76. Academic Press, New York.
129. Grof, P., Bodzay, J., and Kovaks, A. (1967): Carotenodermia. *Acta Med. Acad. Sci. Hung.* **24**:129–139.
130. Dohi, D., and Ono, T., cited by Hashimoto, H. (1922): Carotenoid pigmentation of the skin resulting from a vegetarian diet. *J. AMA* **78**:1111–1113.
131. Lee, R., Mathews-Roth, M. M., Pathak, M. A., and Parrish, J. A. (1974): The detection of carotenoid pigments in human skin. *J. Invest. Dermatol.* **64**:175–177.
132. Green, D. E., and Harefi, Y. (1961): The mitochondrion and biochemical machines. *Science* **133**:13–19.
133. Giorgio, A. L., Cartwright, G. E., and Wintrobe, M. M. (1964): Pseudo Kayser–Fleischer rings. *Arch. Intern. Med.* **113**:817–818.
134. DeVries-de Mol, E. C., Went, L. M., and Volker-Dieben, H. J. (1974): Farnsworth–Munsell 100-hue results in a series of patients with long-standing therapeutic carotenemia. In: Color Vision Deficiencies II, International Symposium, Edinburg, 1973. *Med. Prob. Ophthalmol.* **13**:349–352.
135. Feldman, E., and Adlersberg, D. (1959): Response to carotenoid loading in malabsorption states. *Am. J. Med. Sci.* **238**:733–739.
136. Kasper, H., and Hospach, R. (1974): Der diagnostische Wert der Vitamin-A und Carotin-Bestimmung im Serum bei Maldigestion und Malabsorption. *Dtsch. Med. Wochenschr.* **99**:198–200.
137. Onstad, G. R. (1972): Carotene absorption—a screening test for steatorrhea. *J. AMA* **221**:677–679.
138. Linn, H. W. (1954): Xanthosis cutis in poliomyelitis. *Med. J. Aust.* **1**:581–588.
139. Edwards, E. A., Hamilton, J. B., Duntly, S. Q., et al. (1941): Cutaneous vascular and pigmentary changes in castrate and eunuchoid men. *Endocrinology* **28**:119–128.
140. Patel, H., Dunn, H. G., Tischler, B., et al. (1973): Carotenemia in mentally retarded children—incidence and etiology. *Can. Med. Assoc. J.* **108**:848–852.
141. Ditlefson, E.-M. L., and Stoa, K. F. (1954): Vitamin A and carotenoid levels in blood serum with special reference to values observed in disease of the skin. *Scand. J. Clin. Lab. Invest.* **6**:210–216.
142. Adlersberg, D., Kann, S., Maurer, A. P., et al. (1949): Studies on serum carotene in man. *Am. J. Dig. Dis.* **16**:333–337.
143. Newberne, P., Chan, W.-C., and Rogers, A. (1974): Influence of light, riboflavine and carotene on the response of rats to the acute toxicity of aflatoxin and monocrotaline. *Toxicol. Appl. Pharmacol.* **28**:200.
144. Rosenberg, A., and Sobel, A. E. (1953): *In vitro* conversion of carotene to vitamin A in alloxan diabetes. *Arch. Biochem. Biophys.* **44**:326–329.
145. Pariente, A., Present, C., and Ralli, E. P. (1936): A case of carotenemia and diabetes mellitus, with necropsy report and analysis of liver for carotene, vitamin A, total fat and cholesterol. *Am. J. Med. Sci.* **192**:365–371.
146. Ralli, E. P., Brandaleone, H., and Mandelbaum, T. (1934–1935): Studies on the effect of the administration of carotene and vitamin A in patients with diabetes mellitus. I. Effect of the

oral administration of carotene on the blood carotene and cholesterol of diabetic and normal individuals. *J. Lab. Clin. Med.* **20**:1266–1275.

147. Murrill, W. A., Horton, P. B., Leiberman, E., et al. (1941): Vitamin A and carotene. II. Vitamin A and carotene metabolism in diabetics and normals. *J. Clin. Invest.* **20**:395–400.

148. Ramachandran, K. (1973): Beta-carotene metabolism in diabetes. *Indian J. Med. Res.* **61**:1831–1834.

149. Walton, K. W., Campbell, D. A., and Tonks, D. (1965): Significance of alterations in serum lipids in thyroid dysfunction. I. The relation between serum lipoproteins, carotenoids and vitamin A in hypothyroidism and thyrotoxicosis. *Clin. Sci.* **29**:199–215.

150. Page, S. W. (1971): Golden ovaries. *Aust. N.Z. J. Obstet. Gynecol.* **11**:32–36.

151. Crisp, A. H., and Stonehil, E. (1967): Hypercarotenemia as a symptom of weight phobia. *Postgrad. Med. J.* **43**:721–725.

152. Dally, P. J. (1959): Carotenemia occurring in a case of anorexia nervosa. *Br. Med. J.* **2**:1333.

153. Pops, M. A., and Schwabe, A. D. (1968): Hypercarotenemia in anorexia nervosa. *J. AMA* **205**:121–122.

154. Robboy, M. S., Sato, A. S., and Schwabe, A. D. (1974): The hypercarotenemia in anorexia nervosa: A comparison of vitamin A and carotene levels in various forms of menstrual dysfuction and cachexia. *Am. J. Clin. Nutr.* **27**:362–367.

155. Silverman, J. A. (1974): Anorexia nervosa: Clinical observations in a successful treatment plan. *J. Pediatr.* **84**:68–73.

156. Mathews-Roth, M. M., and Gulbrandsen, C. L. (1974): Transport of beta-carotene in serum of individuals with carotenemia. *Clin. Chem.* **20**:1578–1579.

157. Krinsky, N. I., Cornwell, D. G., and Oncley, J. L. (1958): Transport of vitamin A and carotene in human plasma. *Arch. Biochem. Biophys.* **73**:233–246.

15

Topical and Systemic Approaches to Protection of Human Skin against Harmful Effects of Solar Radiation

M. A. Pathak, T. B. Fitzpatrick, and J. A. Parrish

Why is photoprotection of importance to humans? We must be in the light; we cannot be forced to work or live in the dark. The sun is necessary to sustain all life on earth. We are warmed by its rays, and we are able to see with eyes that respond to that portion of the solar spectrum known as visible light. Our skin and blood vessels respond to the electromagnetic spectrum of the sun in the form of sunburn and tanning reactions. Many of our daily rhythms are dependent upon the sunlight. Natural sunlight has always been recognized for, and endowed with, health-giving powers. Yet excessive amounts of this life-supporting radiation can be very damaging to our skin. There are two concerns about the deleterious effects of sun exposure: (1) the acute effects (e.g., sunburn, phototoxicity), and (2) the potential long-term risk of repeated sun exposure, namely, the development of actinic changes (wrinkling, premature aging, irregular thickening and thinning of epidermis, hyper- and hypopigmentation), keratosis, and both nonmelanoma and melanoma skin cancer (1–3).

One of the most important of the many diversified functions of the skin is the protection against solar radiation. To survive the insults of actinic damage resulting from sun exposure, human skin has evolved various defensive mechanisms and these included: the process of keratinization, melanin pigmentation, the preferential accumulation of carotenoids in subcutaneous fat, and the formation of urocanic acid, the deaminated product of histidine.

M. A. Pathak, T. B. Fitzpatrick, and J. A. Parrish • Department of Dermatology, Harvard Medical School, Massachusetts General Hospital, Boston, Massachusetts 02114.

In spite of these natural photoprotective agents, human skin often requires protection by artificial means because not all people of the world are created equal in their capacity to react to sunlight. In the over two billion pigmented people of the world, there exists a natural chromophore, melanin, contained in the epidermis. Melanin limits the penetration and transmission of solar energy into the dermis, and thus minimizes the harmful effects of ultraviolet (UV) and visible radiation. The nearly one billion fair-skinned, "white" population have virtually all the problems associated with sunlight (e.g., acute and chronic effects of sunburn reaction, skin cancer, premature aging of the skin etc.). The onset of the cancerous or abnormal changes in the skin is directly related to the UV intensity and the duration of solar exposure and inversely related to the amount of melanin in the skin.

On the other hand, disorders of skin can also occur in the presence of a normal melanin filter when there is an abnormal light-absorbing mechanism either in the epidermis or in the dermis. The skin of a fair-skinned individual or a pigmented individual may become highly reactive to light when a photosensitizer is present either in the form of: (a) an exogenous agent (e.g., certain drugs, applied topically or given orally); or (b) an endogenously produced metabolite (e.g., increased levels of prophyrins in various porphyrias). Diseases of humans caused or exacerbated by light can also occur in certain situations: (a) when there is an abnormal DNA repair mechanism (e.g., as in the hereditary disease xeroderma pigmentosum, in which individuals develop different kinds of cancers of the skin aggravated by sunlight),or(b) in certain diseases of unknown etiology (e.g., polymorphic photodermatoses and lupus erythematosus) in which there is an abnormal reaction of the skin, and the biochemical and metabolic abnormality is unknown.

Until recently, effective protection against solar radiation has been attempted by various methods. These include: (a) avoidance of sunlight between 10 a.m. and 3 p.m.; (b) promotion of tanning reaction (melanin pigmentation) and increased thickening of the stratum corneum by carefully controlled exposure to sunlight; (c) topical application to the skin of a chemical formulation that will act as a chemical or a physical screen and absorb, scatter, or reflect the damaging radiation impinging on the skin; (d) chemical modification of the stratum corneum so that exogenously applied material (e.g., dihydroxyacetone, 2-hydroxy-1,4-naphthoquinone or lawsone, and 5-hydroxy-1,4-naphthoquinone or juglone) when conjugated with the proteins of stratum corneum will substantially absorb and minimize the penetration of damaging rays; (e) promotion of the natural defenses of the human skin by oral administration of 4,5′,8-trimethylpsoralen or 8-methoxypsoralen and subsequent exposure to UVA radiation (320–400 nm); (f) oral administration of certain agents (e.g., beta-carotene) that selectively block the harmful effects of certain potential photosensitizing agents (e.g., porphyrins) in certain disease conditions.

In this presentation, various artificial methods effective in minimizing or preventing the harmful effects of solar radiation, both in normal individuals and in patients with photosensitivity problems, will be reviewed. The topical and systemic approaches will be discussed to emphasize the extent of protection in certain disease conditions.

THE SOLAR SPECTRUM IMPLICATED IN HUMAN SKIN REACTIONS (1, 2, 4)

For clinical and practical considerations, the solar spectrum at the earth's surface (sea level) consists of wavelengths of electromagnetic energy between 290 and 3000 nm (nanometers). The range of solar radiation implicated in the causation or augmentation of certain skin diseases extends from 290 to 1800 nm. Solar UV radiation of wavelengths shorter than 290 nm are not encountered at sea level, as they are selectively absorbed and filtered out by the ozone layer and molecular oxygen of the stratosphere. The solar radiation spectrum at the earth's surface is subdivided into: ultraviolet radiation (290–400 nm); visible radiation (400–760 nm); and near-infrared radiation of wavelengths longer than 760 nm (see Table 15-1).

The UV radiation from both sunlight and artificial sources is subdivided, both arbitrarily and for convenience, into three bands from the longer to the shorter wavelengths. These are referred to as UVA, UVB and UVC regions (see Chapter 1). The UVA region extends from 320–400 nm. It causes tanning reaction (both immediate tanning or immediate pigment darkening reaction, and delayed tanning reaction or new melanogenesis). UVA can also evoke sunburn reaction; however, the erythemogenic or sunburn-producing capacity of UVA is very weak. About 20–100 J/cm^2 of UVA energy is required to produce a minimally perceptible redness reaction. The intensity of erythema is optimal at approximately 6–10 hr after exposure to UVA, and the exposed sites may remain maximally red for up to 24 hr.

The UVB band extends from 290 to 320 nm. It is often referred to as the sunburn radiation, mid-UV radiation, or erythemal band. UVB radiation is

Table 15-1. Solar Irradiance[a] (at Sea Level on Cloudless Days) in Spectral Bands and for Two Zenith Angles

Spectral band, nm	Zenith angle 0°	Zenith angle 20°
290–320 (UVB)	0.5	0.3
320–400 (UVA)	6.3	5.0
400–760 (visible)	48.9	41.0
720–3000 (infrared)	56.3	49.0

[a]units mW/cm^2.

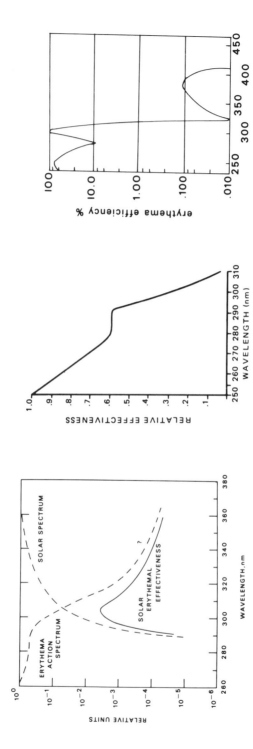

Fig. 15-1. Erythema effectiveness action spectrum curves: Left: Solar erythemal effectiveness. The sunburn curve reaction peaks at 307 nm. Center: Recent studies with monochromatic radiation indicate maximum effectiveness at 250 nm with gradual decreasing effectiveness at longer wavelengths (36, 37). Right: Erythema action spectrum for human skin plotted on a logarithmic vertical axis. Note that UVB (290–320 nm), UVC (λ < 290 nm), and UVA (320–400 nm) are erythemogenic, but with varying effectiveness.

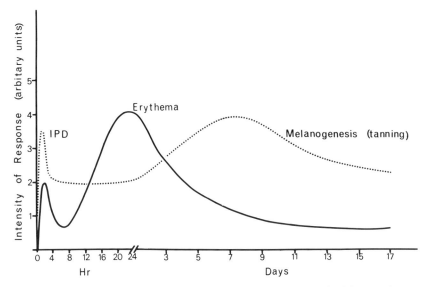

Fig. 15-2. Time course of erythema and tanning response of an average individual (Skin Type III) after a single exposure to solar radiation (90 min or approximately 4 × MED). IPD = immediate tanning reaction and represents photooxidation of preexisting melanin. It is maximum at the end of exposure (60–90 min), then gradually fades; IPD may or may not totally disappear and is dose dependent. The action spectrum for IPD is between 300 and 700 nm, with maximum reaction between 360 and 400 nm. Melanogenesis or delayed tanning reaction involves increased formation, melanization, and transfer of melanosomes. The functional melanocytes are increased in number.

the principal cause of the sunburn reaction (see Chapter 8) (Figs. 15-1 and 15-2). It also is most effective in stimulating pigmentation (melanogenesis or tanning) in the skin. Approximately 20–50 mJ/cm² of UVB energy is required to produce a minimally perceptible erythema reaction. This is also referred to as minimal erythema dose or MED. Exposure of human skin to multiple MEDs (10–15 × MED) can cause marked sunburn reaction that can lead to severe edema and blistering reaction. The erythema reaction is maximal in intensity between 16 and 24 hr after exposure to UVB radiation. Thus, both UVA and UVB are erythemogenic and melanogenic, but the amount of UVA energy required to produce these effects is about 800 to 1000 times than for the UVB region. It should be realized, however, that the amount of solar UVA reaching the surface of the earth is about 20 times greater than that of UVB (5.0–6.0 mW/cm² of UVA as compared to 0.3–0.5 mW/cm² of UVB. The long-term cumulative effects of UVA flux may therefore be as important as the effects of UVB radiation. UVC radiation (germicidal, short-UV or far-UV radiation) comprises wavelengths shorter than 290 nm (200–290 nm). Although UVC radiation from sunlight does not reach the surface of the earth, individuals can encounter this spectrum from artificial UV sources (e.g., germicidal lamps, high-pressure and low-pressure mercury-arc lamps). Radiation in the UVC band from artificial sources is very efficient in causing erythema of normal skin (MED about 5–25 mJ / cm^2) and photokeratitis of the eye. It can also stimulate melanogenesis, but is not as effective as UVB or UVA radiation. The erythema reaction caused by UVC is maximum in intensity within 6–8 hr after exposure.

FACTORS THAT INFLUENCE SUNBURN OR ERYTHEMA REACTION

Incident Solar Flux and Wavelengths

For practical considerations of photoprotection in both normal and disease conditions one has to realize that:

1. Solar radiation of 290–320 nm (UVB) is most damaging to human skin; it is erythemogenic and carcinogenic.

2. UVA radiation is also erythemogenic. Although UVA is 1,000 times less effective than solar UVB in causing sunburn, the amount of solar UVA reaching the surface of the earth is enormously greater than that of UVB.

3. Exposure of skin to longer wavelengths (UVA) may accentuate the effects of shorter wavelengths. The combined effects of UVA and UVB can be additive or augmentative to the erythemogenic and injurious action of UVB.

4. The solar UV flux that reaches the surface of the earth is a function of the solar spectral irradiance at the top of the atmosphere and the subsequent absorption and scattering by the atmosphere. The attenuation of the incident solar flux is a strong function of wavelength. The UV flux is influenced by: (a) changes in ozone concentration; (b) scattering by atmospheric molecules, particles, and aerosols; (c) attenuation by clouds, haze, and smog near the ground (the pollution of the atmosphere significantly decreases the UVB radiation); (d) seasonal variation; (e) air mass (maximum intensity of UV radiation between 10 a.m. and 2 p.m.); (f) altitude (about 4% increase in the flux of UV radiation can occur for every 300 m rise in altitude); (g) latitude (promixity to equator); (h) reflectivity of the ground (reflection by snow and sand increases UV flux).

5. Most of the drug-induced or chemically induced photosensitization reactions (phototoxic and photoallergic) are mediated or activated by UVA radiation. In rare instances, however, UVB may also be implicated.

6. Visible radiation (400–760 nm) is generally innocuous to a normal individual; however, in the presence of certain chemicals (porphyrins, dyes, etc.), this radiation can be quite damaging to the skin.

In photoprotection, therefore, the primary aim should be to filter out the UVB and UVA radiation that impinges on the exposed skin.

The Sun-Reactive Skin Types (2, 5, 6)

When viewed from the perspective of photobiology, the most obvious differences in the skin of various people of the world are: (a) the variation of skin color, and (b) the variation of acute and chronic responses to sun. There is a wide variation in the constitutive (genetic) or intrinsic skin color, and in the facultative or inducible skin color (tanning response). Based on personal history of response to sun and skin color, individuals can be grouped into six sun-reactive Skin Types, and the population at high risk for the development of actinic changes, including skin cancer, can be identified (Table 15-2). Personal history of sunburning and suntanning for the preceding 5–7 years, when carefully recorded, is very helpful in the classification of normal people into the six grades of reactivity (see Table 15-2).

In counseling people on the use of sunscreens for the prevention of sunburn, actinic changes (wrinkling), skin cancer, and various forms of sun sensitivity, the choice and recommendations of sunscreens depend on several factors. The most important consideration should be the reactivity of an individual to sunlight. All people are not endowed with the same degree of sun tolerance. The sun-reactive skin typing system developed by our laboratories (1, 2, 6, 7) is based on ascertaining the personal history of sunburning, peeling, and tanning of an individual following the first 45–60 min of exposure to midday summer sun in early June (Table 15-2).

ACTION SPECTRA OF VARIOUS LIGHT-INDUCED PHOTODERMATOSES

An action spectrum is a plot of the relative efficacy for producing a given abnormal response (e.g., sunburn reaction or an urticarial wheal) as a function of wavelength. In cutaneous photobiology, the action spectrum is a plot of the reciprocal of the UV-radiation against the wavelength to achieve a given degree of response. The action spectrum for a particular biologic response may be helpful in identifying the light absorber or photosensitizer and in prescribing the correct sunscreen for the prevention or amelioration of cutaneous symptoms precipitated by exposure to sunlight. To a clinician, the action spectrum refers to the limits of the wavelength region that are implicated in a given abnormal reaction.

Table 15-3 lists the various diseases and the wavelengths implicated in the causation of this particular response.

TOPICAL SUNSCREENING AGENTS

Until recently, sunscreens were regarded as cosmetics; however, the U.S. Food and Drug Administration has classified them as "drugs" intended to

Table 15-2. Sun-Reactive Skin Types Used in Clinical Practice

Skin type	Skin reactions to solar radiation[a]	Examples
I	Always burns easily and severely (painful burn); tans little or none and peels	People[b] most often with fair skin, blue eyes, freckles; unexposed skin is white
II	Usually burns easily and severely (painful burn); tans minimally or lightly, also peels	People[b] most often with fair skin, red or blond hair, blue, hazel or even brown eyes; unexposed skin is white
III	Burns moderately and tans about average	Normal average Caucasoid; unexposed skin is white
IV	Burns minimally, tans easily, and above average with each exposure; exhibits IPD (immediate pigment darkening) reaction	People with white or light brown skin, dark brown hair, dark eyes (e.g., Mediterraneans, Mongoloids, Orientals, Hispanics, etc); unexposed skin is white or light brown
V	Rarely burns, tans easily and substantially; always exhibits IPD reaction	Brown-skinned persons (e.g., Amerindians, East Indians, Hispanics, etc); unexposed skin is brown
VI	Never burns and tans profusely; exhibits IPD reaction	Blacks (e.g., African and American blacks, Australian and South Indian Aborigines); unexposed skin is black

[a] Based on the first 45–60 min ($\cong$ 2–3 minimum erythema dose) exposure of the summer sun (early June) at sea level.
[b] They may be of Celtic background (Irish or Scottish); others may even have dark hair or brown eyes.

Table 15-3. Action Spectra of Various Normal and Abnormal Responses of Human Skin to Solar Radiation[a]

Condition	Range of effective wavelengths	Maximum reaction, nm
Normal individuals		
Sunburn reaction (solar)	290–320	305–307
Sunburn reaction (artificial light source)	250–320	250
Immediate pigment darkening (IPD) or tanning reaction	320–700	340–380
Delayed tanning (melanogenesis)	290–480	290–320
Photosensitivity		
Phototoxic reaction:		
Oral or internal (drugs)[b]	300–400	320–380
Topical or external (drugs)[c]	300–400	320–380
Phytophotodermatitis (plants)[d]	320–400	320–360
Phototoxicity in chemically induced porphyria or hematoporphyrins	380–600	380–420
Photoallergic reaction:		
Drug-photoallergy (delayed hypersensitivity, topical, or systemic)[e,f]	290–450	320–380
Certain solar urticaria (immediate hypersensitivity)	290–380	290–320 320–400
Persistent photosensitivity (persistant light reactions or actinic reticuloid)	290–400	290–320
Degenerative and neoplastic		
Chronic actinic elastosis	290–400	290–320
Actinic keratosis	290–320	290–315
Basal cell epithelioma	290–320	290–315
Squamous cell carcinoma	290–320	290–315
Malignant melanoma (?)	290–320	290–315
Genetic and metabolic		
Xeroderma pigmentosum	290–320	290–320
Albinism	290–400	290–320
Ephelides (freckles)	290–400	290–320
Erythropoietic porphyria	390–600	390–420
Erythropoietic protoporphyria	390–600	390–420
Porphyria cutanea tarda	390–600	390–420
Variegate porphyria	390–600	390–420
Vitiligo (macules)	290–320	290–315
Hartnup syndrome	290–320	
Cockayne syndrome	290–320	
Darier–White disease	290–320	
Bloom syndrome	290–320	

(continued)

Table 15-3. (cont.)

Condition	Range of effective wavelengths,	Maximum reaction, nm
Rothmund–Thomson syndrome	290–320	
Hailey–Hailey disease	290–320	
Nutritional		
Kwashiorkor	290–400	
Pellagra	290–400	
Viral		
Lymphogranuloma venereum	290–320	
Herpes simplex	290–320	
Miscellaneous (light and abnormal skin or diseases)		
Hydroa aestivale	290–400 infrared	290–320
Hydroa vacciniforme	290–400 infrared	290–320
Polymorphous photodermatoses, including variants such as papules, plaques, and papulo-vesicular, eczematous eruptions	290–400	290–320
Disseminated superficial actinic porokeratosis	290–320	290–320
Discoid lupus erythematosus	290–320	290–320
Systemic lupus erythematosus	290–320	
Dermatomyositis	290–320	
Photosensitive eczema	290–320	

[a] Adapted from (4, and 11).
[b] Oral drugs: Psoralens (8-methoxypsoralen, trimethylpsoralen, psoralen), demethylchlortetracycline (Declomycin), phenothiazines, chlorothiazides, sulfonylureas, sulfonamides, hematoporphyrin, griseofulvin, quinine.
[c] Topical drugs: Coal tar, anthracene.
[d] Certain plants (e.g., fig, wild parsnip, celery, lime, Ammi majus, psoralen, etc.) of Umbelliferae and Rutaceae families.
[e] Topical photoallergic agents: Halogenated salicylanilides (tetrachloro- and tetrabromosalicylanilide, tribromo- and dibromosalicylanilide), Bithionol, Jadit, and other antifungal agents, hexachlorophene, antihistamines, blankophores, sunscreens, PABA derivatives, digalloylloyl trioleate, 6-methylcoumarin, musk ambrette.
[f] Systemic photoallergic agents: sulfonamide, quinethiazone, phenothiazides, promethazine, sulfonylurea, chlorothiazides, oral contraceptives, calcium cyclamate, griseofulvin, chlordiasepoxide hydrochloride (Librium), diphenlhydramine (Benadryl).

protect the structure and function of the human integument against actinic damage (8).

Sun-protective topical preparations are chemical agents in the form of solutions (clear or milky lotions), gels, creams, or ointments that attenuate the deleterious effects on human skin of excessive exposure to UVB (290–320 nm) and UVA (320–400 nm) radiation. The active chemical ingredients(s) of a sunscreen afforα protection by the absorption, reflection, and scattering of the solar radiation impinging on the skin. Sunscreens, therefore, can prevent sunburn, protect the viable cells of the epidermis and dermis against the acute and chronic harmful effects of solar radiation, and help prevent certain photosensitivity reactions and various photodermatoses. Sunscreens can be grouped into two broad categories: topical and oral. (Table 15-4).

The concept of sun protection factor (SPF) was originally proposed by Franz Greiter of Vienna, Austria, and subsequently adopted by the U.S. Food and Drug Administration (8) and certain pharmaceutical companies in Europe and America. It is based on the UV-absorbing properties of the active ingredients(s) of a sunscreen product and is a measure of the effectiveness of a given product. The SPF is defined as the ratio of the least amount of UVB energy (MED) required to produce a minimal erythema reaction through a sunscreen-product film to the amount of energy required to produce the same erythema without any sunscreen treatment:

$$SPF = \frac{MED \text{ of the sunscreen-protected skin}}{MED \text{ of the non-protected skin}}$$

A preparation containing 8% homomenthyl salicylate (SPF 3.5–4.5) has been recommended as a standard to compare against the SPF value of the test product.

Example: (a) MED of the sunscreen-treated skin (e.g., 5% PABA in 70% alcohol) = 180 min (sun) or 360 mJ/cm^2 UVB. (b) MED of the nontreated skin = 15 min (sun) or 30 mJ/cm^2 UVB. Thus the SPF of 5% PABA in alcohol = 180/15 = 12 or 360/30 = 12.

To aid the physician and the consumer in selecting the appropriate

Table 15-4. Sunscreens

Sunscreens	Remarks
Topical	
Chemical: Creams, lotions, or gels containing UV-absorbing chemical filters, such as para-aminobenzoic acid (PABA), PABA esters, benzophenones, cinnamates, etc.; they act as UV-absorbing agents	Cosmetically acceptable
Physical: Containing titanium dioxide, zinc oxide, kaolin, talc, or iron oxide, which act as reflectors and scattering agents, and form and opaque barrier to sunlight	Usually opaque; cosmetically less acceptable
Oral	
Chemical agents (e.g., beta-carotene, chloroquine, etc.) which, upon oral ingestion, act as quenchers of singlet oxygen and/or free radicals, or as stabilizers of the cell membrane	Useful in certain diseases; not yet proven for use against sunburn

sunscreen formulation that is best suited to an individual's reactivity to the sun (see Table 15/2 on skin typing), the FDA has recommended the following product category designations for the sunscreen formulations of various SPF values (8):

Categories of sunscreen products	SPF
Minimal sun protection	>2 and <4
Moderate sun protection	4 to <6
Extra sun protection	6 to <8
Maximal sun protection	8 to <15
Ultra sun protection	15 or greater

Factors That Influence SPF Values

Summarized below is a list of factors that are known to influence the SPF values of sunscreens under both indoor and outdoor (field) conditions:

1. Test subjects: Skin type, melanin content (constitutive and facultative skin color), regional differences in skin thickness.

2. UV intensity: UVB and UVA irradiance, season, latitude, altitude, clouds, smog, time of day, the combined effects of UVB and UVA radiation.

3. Radiation source: Emission spectrum (spectral power distribution) of the UV-radiation source used will greatly influence the SPF values; sun provides a polychromatic continuum source of radiation; low-pressure sunlamps and high-pressure mercury-arc lamps provide a discontinuous line spectrum; solar simulators mimic solar radiation in a narrow spectral range; and monochromators provide a single wavelength only.

4. Concentration (sunscreens): Concentration (g%) of UV-absorbing active ingredient(s); molar absorptivity at 297–307 and 320–400 nm.

5. Vehicle (base): Its composition, properties (lipophilic and hydrophilic nature), emollients, pH, stability to heat, etc.

6. Thickness of the applied film: Uniform application ($2.5 \mu l/cm^2$, 2–2.5 mg/cm^2) assures even protection.

7. Substantivity of the sunscreen: Percutaneous absorption, adsorption, diffusion, conjugation with proteins, ionized and nonionized state of active ingredient(s).

8. Environment: Temperature, high or low humidity, direct and scattered radiation, snow, sand, wind velocity.

9. Sweating: Skin temperature (temperature receptors, heat zones of skin influencing radiation by convection and conduction of heat), rate of production and evaporation of sweat.

10. Swimming: Duration, water (chlorinated vs. salted), and hydrated state of skin.

11. Testing procedure: Application and waiting interval before exposure, test site (back vs. arm), application errors, errors in MED visualization.

12. Impurities and other ingredients: Some act as photosensitizers (*ortho*-amyldimethyl aminobenzoate and 6-methylcoumarin).

Chemical Agents as Topical Sunscreens

Chemical sunscreening agents that are used topically contain various UV-absorbing agents, such as para-aminobenzoic acid (PABA) and its esters, the benzophenones, salicylates, cinnamates, digalloyl-trioleate, etc. (see Table 15-5). The excellent photoprotective properties of PABA in the prevention of sunburn reaction induced by UVB radiation have been carefully documented by several investigators (3, 9–16). The effectiveness of two PABA esters (e.g., isoamyl-*p*-*N*,*N*-dimethyl aminobenzoate or Escalol 506 and 2-ethylhexyl ester of dimethyl aminobenzoate, commonly referred to as Escalol 507 or octyldimethyl PABA) also have been established by several of these investigators. Benzophenone derivatives such as oxybenzone or 2-hydroxy-4-methoxy-benzophenone and sulisobenzone (2-hydroxy-4-methoxy-benzophenone-5-sulfonic acid) have been reported also to be effective sunscreens against UVB and UVA radiation (3, 9, 16, 17). Recently, combination sunscreens containing two or more UV-absorbing agents have been evaluated more extensively to achieve higher protection than that provided by a single ingredient (3). Some of these combination sunscreens are non-PABA derivatives and contain the benzophenone derivative oxybenzone and cinnamates, while others contain the oxybenzone and PABA ester Escalol 507 (3, 14, 18, 19). A combination of dihydroxyacetone (DHA) and lawsone (2-hydroxy-1,4-naphthoquinone) has been reported by Fusaro et al. (20) to protect patients with various types of photosensitivity reactions. The chemical formulations in which sequential application of 3% DHA cream followed by 0.25% lawsone cream changes the color of the stratum corneum such that the transmission of UV and visible radiation is markedly decreased. The DHA and lawsone chemically react and bind to the amino acids of keratin such that the color cannot easily be removed by soap and water, sweating, or swimming. The DHA plus lawsone formulation is, however, not a very effective sunscreen in the UV spectrum (290–320 nm). The color imparted to the stratum corneum does not totally block the transmission of UVB radiation and is cosmetically unacceptable to many patients; it is also cumbersome to use (personal observations).

The chemical sunscreens have certain elegant properties and these include the following: (a) they are able to selectively absorb and screen sunburn-producing UV radiation (290–320 nm); (b) they do not completely prevent the transmission of UVA radiation (320–400 nm) that can stimulate tanning reaction; (c) they are colorless and cosmetically acceptable; (d) most

Table 15-5. Evaluation of Sunscreens under Indoor and Outdoor Conditions

Formulation ingredients	Commercial name	SPF values[a]		Resistance to[b]	
		Indoor solar simulator	Outdoor sun	Sweating	Water immersion
PABA sunscreens					
5% Para-aminobenzoic acid in 50–70% ethyl alcohol	PreSun	10–15	6	Good	Poor
	Pabanol	10–15	6–8	Good	Poor
	Coppertone Supershade (1978)	10–12	4–6	Poor	Poor
	Sunbrella	10	6	Good	Poor
Esters and derivatives of PABA					
2.5% Glyceryl PABA + 2.5% octyldimethyl PABA + 2.5% oxybenzone	Total Eclipse	15–18	9–12	Excellent	Good
7% Octyldimethyl PABA + 3% oxybenzone	Supershade 15 (1979)	15–18	6–9	Excellent	Good
3.3% Iso-amyl-p-N,N-dimethyl amino-benzoate (Escalol 506, padimate A)	Block Out	>6–8	6	Good	Fair
	PABA Film	>6–8	4–6	Good	Fair
2.5% Glyceryl PABA + 2.5% octyldimethyl PABA (Escalol 507)	Spectraban	>6–8	4–6	Good	Fair
	Eclipse	>8–10	4–6	Fair	Fair
2.5% Octyldimethyl PABA (Escalol 507) + 3% dioxybenzone	Sungard	6	4–6	Poor	Poor
3.3% Octyldimethyl PABA (Escalol 507) in ammonium acrylate-acrylate polymer	Sundown	8–10	4–6	Good	Fair
3.3% Octyldimethyl PABA	Sea & Ski	7–8	3–4	Poor	Poor
5% Homomenthyl salicylate + amyl-p-dimethyl aminobenzoate	Aztec	6	2–4	Poor	Poor
Non-PABA chemical sunscreens					
10% 2-Hydroxy-t-methoxybenzophenone 5-sulfonic acid	UVAL	10	4	Poor	Poor
5% Ethyl-hexyl-p-methoxycinnamate + 3% 2-hydroxy-3,4-methoxybenzophenone +	TI-Screen cream. Piz Buin—Exclusive,	20–22.5	10–13	Excellent	Good

Active ingredients	Product (Company)				
5% Ethyl-hexyl-*p*-methoxycinnamate + 3% 2-hydroxy-4-methoxybenzophenone	Piz Buin 4	6–8	4–6	Fair	Fair
	Piz Buin 6,	18–20	8–10	Excellent	Good
8% Homomenthyl salicylate	TI-Screen lotion / Coppertone 2	3–4	<2	Poor	Poor
Combination sunscreens					
5% PABA + 5% padimate-O +3% oxybenzone	PreSun-15 (Westwood)	15–20	10	Good	Fair
7% Padimate-O +3% oxybenzone	Supershade-15 (Plough, Inc.)	20	9	Excellent	Good
3% Padimate-O + 2.5% benzophenone 3	MMM-What A Tan (3M Company)	15	12	Excellent	Fair
3% 2-hydroxy-4-methoxy-benzophenone + 5% ethyl-hexyl-*p*-methoxycinnamate	TI-Screen Cream (TI Pharmaceuticals)	20	13	Excellent	Good
Phenyl-benzimidazole-5-sulfonic acid + padimate-O	Clinique-19 (Clinique Labs.)	15–19	7	Good	Fair
2.5% glyceryl PABA + 2.5% octyldimethyl PABA + oxybenzone	Total Eclipse (Herbert Labs.)	15	9	Good	Good
2-phenyl-benzimidazole-5-sulfonic acid + 6-methyl-2-phenyl benzoxazole	Deléal-10 (Cutter Labs.)	25	8	Good	Good
Ethyl-hexyl-*p*-methoxycinnamate + 2-hydroxy-4-methoxybenzophenone + methyl benzylid camphor	Piz Buin 8 (Grieter A.G.)	18	9	Excellent	Good
3.3% Octyldimethyl PABA	Sundown (Johnson & Johnson Co.)	8–10	4–6	Good	Fair
10% 2-Hydroxy-4-methoxybenzophenone	UVAL (Dorsey Labs.)	8–12	6	Poor	Poor
Physical sunscreens					
Titanium dioxide, zinc oxide, kaolin, talc, iron oxide, etc.	A-Fil	6–8	4–6	Fair	Fair
	RVPaque	6–8	2–4	Poor	Poor
	Shadow	4–6	2–4	Poor	Poor
	Reflecta	6–8	4–6	Fair	Fair
	Covermark	6–8	4–6	Fair	Fair

[a] Determined under static or passive exposure conditions without the stress of sweating, swimming, etc.
[b] Based on the SPF values: excellent, >6; good, 4–6; fair, 2–4 poor, <2.

of them are innocuous to skin (nonsensitizing) and do not cause appreciable discoloration of clothing.

Physical Agents as Sunscreens

The physical sunscreens (also referred to as sunshades or parasols) contain opaque powders, such as titanium oxide, zinc oxide, kaolin, or talcum, that scatter both the UV and visible radiation (290–760 nm); in contrast to chemical sunscreens, most of the protection derives from this scattering rather than absorption of photons. Examples of certain physical sunscreens are listed in Table 15-6. The opaqueness of titanium dioxide, zinc oxide, etc. makes these physical sunscreens invariably effective and nonsensitizing sunscreens for filtering a broad spectrum of solar radiation. They are generally used for providing extra protection to certain areas of the body that burn easily (nasal mucosa, nose bridge, inframammary region, lips). They are ideal for minimizing the sunlight-induced pigment darkening of skin in patients with melasma. Cosmetically, however, they are not as acceptable as chemical sunscreens that are invisible. They cause discoloration of clothes and may occasionally be so occlusive that the patient may develop miliaria or folliculitis.

Adverse Effects of Sunscreens

Certain sunscreening formulations containing UV-absorbing chemicals (e.g., certain esters of PABA) may cause selective burning (smarting) and may occasionally cause contact dermatitis or allergic contact photodermatitis (16, 21, 22). The contact irritation reaction may be enhanced during the period of sun exposure. They also have certain limitations in rendering total protection to individuals who are abnormally sensitive to solar radiation. Generally, most of the chemical sunscreens absorb and filter out a narrow band of solar radiation (mostly 290–320 nm) and rarely act as a broad-spectrum sunscreen to minimize or prevent the harmful effects of UVA (320–400 nm) and visible radiation (400–760 nm).

Reported adverse effects from topical sunscreens include:

Table 15-6. Physical Sunscreens

Ingredients
    Titanium dioxide, zinc oxide, kaolin, talc, iron oxide, etc.
Examples
    A-Fil (Texas Pharmacol Company)
    RVP, RVPaque (Paul B. Elder Company)
    Shadow (Beauty Counselors)
    Reflecta, different shades (Texas Pharmacol Company)
    Covermark, different shades (Lydia O'Leary)

1. Contact dermatitis: PABA, certain PABA esters (*ortho*-amyldimethyl aminobenzoate), certain benzophenones, and cinnamates are implicated.

2. Photocontact dermatitis (phototoxic and delayed-hypersensitivity reactions): PABA, certain PABA esters (glyceryl PABA), iso-amyl-dimethyl-PABA, and *ortho*-amyldimethyl aminobenzoate are implicated (21, 22). Cutaneous reactions to sunscreens containing PABA and PABA esters may at times be cross-reactions resulting from a primary sensitization to benzocaine rather than to the ester. Occasionally, the impurities of the *ortho* derivatives of aminobenzoic acid present in PABA-containing sunscreens may be sensitizing agents. Some of the sunscreens may contain a synthetic fragrance ingredient 6-methylcoumarin (6-methyl-1,2-benzpyrone), which has been reported by Kaidbey and Kligman (23) to induce photoallergic reactions. In certain European countries, especially in France, manufacturers of sunscreen products are exploiting the consumers' craze for the promotion of tanning reaction by incorporating low concentrations of 5-methoxypsoralen (bergapten), a known photosensitizing and photocarcinogenic agent. Occasionally, the antioxidants used as preservatives, the quality of lanolin, and other ingredients such as almond oil, cocoa butter, etc. can be sensitizing agents in sunscreen preparations.

3. Cross-photosensitivity reactions: patients allergic to benzocaine, procaine, para-phenylenediamine and sulfonamides may undergo allergic reactions to PABA. Patients receiving antihypertensive or diuretic drugs (e.g., Diuril or chlorothiazides) or sulfonamides that may cross-react with PABA may develop eczematous dermatitis (21, 22).

4. Discoloration and staining of clothes (e.g., PABA sunscreens).

TOPICAL SUNSCREENS IN HEALTH AND DISEASES (CLINICAL CONSIDERATIONS)

No perfect topical sunscreen preparation is available; however, habitual use of effective sunscreens decreases the risk of acute sunburn and helps to minimize (or prevent) the risk of premature aging of skin and UV-induced skin cancers. In addition, the regular use of broad-spectrum sunscreens (combination sunscreens containing two or more agents that absorb both UVB and UVA radiation) would ameliorate or help prevent certain photo-dermatosis reactions in those disease entities outlined in Table 15-3.

Sunscreens for Normal Individuals

The choice and recommendation of a sunscreen depend upon several factors. The most important consideration should be the individual's reactivity to sunlight (see Tables 15-2, 15-5, and 15-7).

Table 15-7. Photoprotectants in Health and Diseases (25)

Radiation	Situations for which photoprotectants should be used	Photoprotectant indicated	
		Topical	Oral
Nonvisible: germicidal (λ <280 nm) UVC	Prevention against radiation from artificial light in operating rooms and industrial facilities	Benzophenones	None
Nonvisible: Sunburn (290–320) UVB	Prevention of sunburn, polymorphous photodermatitis, ? prevention of skin cancer	5% para-aminobenzoic acid in 50–70% ethanol; 4% ethyl-hexyl-para-methoxy-cinnamate + 3% 2-hydroxy-4-methoxy-cinnamate + 5.5% 2-phenylbenzimidazole sulfonic acid (triethanol amine salt) in cream base	Psoralens: 8-methoxypsoralen 4,5',8-trimethyl-psoralen
Nonvisible: long-wave (320–400 nm) UVA	Melasma, photosensitivity to drugs, polymorphous photodermatitis	Titanium dioxide in colored, opaque sunscreens	None
Visible (400–760 nm)	Melasma, erythropoietic protoporphyria	Titanium dioxide in colored, opaque sunscreens	Beta-carotene (60–180 mg daily)

It should be realized that the deleterious effects of sunlight exposure are cumulative, and can lead to a degeneration of skin (actinic elastosis) or more serious health, effects such as malignant melanoma and nonmelanoma skin cancers (basal cell and squamous cell carcinoma). These latter effects have been increasing at an alarming rate since World War II, and there is a considerable need to educate the adult and the school-age populations regarding effective methods for protection and precautions against these deleterious effects. People with fair skin, blue eyes, with or without freckles, who burn easily and tan poorly (Skin Types I and II), should be given those sunscreens that have a high protection facter (8 or more) listed on the label. Table 15-5 summarizes a list of such agents. Individuals with Skin Types III and IV who prefer to be tanned may be recommended sunscreening agents that carry a protection factor of 4.

Sunscreens for Patients with Photosensitivity Disorders

The clinical diagnosis should help to delineate the range of solar radiation involved in the causation of abnormal response. The spectral reactivity of patients with various types of photosensitivity disorders is given in Table 15-3 and should serve as a guide for recommending the proper sunscreen. In many instances, the patient may require combination therapy with two sunscreens. A combination of an effective alcoholic solution of PABA (e.g., PreSun) and a cream containing benzophenone (e.g., Piz Buin Exclusive Extrem Cream) can often yield protection that is greater than that achieved by any single sunscreen absorber currently available.

Guidelines and Principles of Photoprotection

Certain guidelines and general principles of photoprotection listed below are helpful in recommending the desired formulations for both normal individuals and patients with photosensitivity disorders (see Table 15-6).

1. *Type of sunscreen*: The commercially available chemical sunscreens can be grouped into two broad categories (see Tables 15-5 and 15-7): PABA (para-aminobenzoic acid) and its derivatives, and the non-PABA derivatives (e.g., those containing benzophenones, cinnamates, etc.).

Individuals who are sensitive to certain drugs and manifest cell-mediated delayed-hypersensitivity reactions should not be prescribed sunscreens containing PABA or its derivatives (including the sodium or potassium salts of PABA and the esters of PABA). Patients receiving antihypertensive or diuretic drugs (e.g., Diuril or chlorothiazide) may cross-react with PABA sunscreens and develop contact and even photocontact-type eczematous dermatitis from PABA derivatives. It is very rare to find patients sensitive to benzophenone, sunscreens, although occasionally a patient using benzophenone may complain of a "burning or smarting" sensation during sun exposure.

2. *Sun protection factor (SPF)*: SPF helps the physician and the consumer in selecting the type of sunscreen best suited for his/her complexion, response to UV radiation, and the type of outdoor activity that can be enjoyed when the product is applied to the skin. The SPF (e.g., 2, 4, 6, 8, etc.) indicates the number of minimal erythema doses (MEDs) a given product can screen during sun exposure and render total protection against the development of erythema reaction.

Generally, an average MED of UVB radiation for an individual with Skin Type I or II is in the range of 25 mJ/cm^2 (±5). An SPF value of 6, for example, signifies that the product will at the least afford total protection up to an exposure dose of 150 mJ/cm^2 (±30). In the northern latitudes of the United States, extending approximately from 23.5° to 50° N, an equivalent dose of 1 MED (25–30 mJ/cm^2) can be achieved in approximately 10–20 min during the months of June and July, depending upon the proximity of the place to the equator. A product with an SPF of 6 can provide protection for a sunbathing period of 60–120 min. Fair-skinned individuals (Skin Types I and II) should always be prescribed sunscreens with an SPF value exceeding 6 or 8. It should be pointed out that a stress of sweating, swimming, or prolonged sunbathing in hot and humid weather markedly affects the SPF value; invariably, the applied product is easily washed off, and the subject is vulnerable to sunburn.

3. *SPF—indoor vs. outdoor field tests*: It should also be emphasized that the determination of SPF in most instances is carried out under laboratory conditions with artificially produced UV radiation, which simulates natural radiation only in a narrow spectral range. The SPF of a product determined under laboratory conditions does not represent the true sun protection factor value. In reality, it represents the UVB protection factor for artificial sources. The SPF values determined under laboratory conditions may not take into account the stress of sweating, swimming, humidity, temperature, and the effects of direct and indirect scattered radiation and infrared radiation, etc., that contribute significantly to the dimunition of the SPF value. Described in Table 15-5 are examples of SPF values of various commercially available sunscreens. The SPF values were determined under field conditions and under indoor conditions without the stress of sweating or swimming. It is obvious that the SPF values determined under field conditions are always significantly lower than those determined under indoor conditions.

4. *SPF—stress of sweating and swimming*: Many of the commercially available sunscreen formulations cannot withstand the stress of sweating and water immersion. Their "substantivity" appears to be poor; they are either easily eluted after sweating or washed off after swimming. *Substantivity of a sunscreen is related to the physicochemical properties of diffusion and*

adhesion, defined, e.g., as the capacity of the UV-absorbing agent to remain
absorbed or chemically conjugated with the proteins of the stratum corneum.
It is practically defined as resistance to loss of sunscreen during swimming or
sweating. Substantivity is markedly influenced by the vehicle.

The stress of sweating stimulated by vigorous exercise for 30 min under
dry or humid conditions significantly lowers the SPF value. The ability of
various products to resist sweating stress is listed in Table 15-5 under column 5
(gradations are based on SPF values: excellent, >6; good, 4–6; fair, 2–4; and
poor, <2).

The stress of swimming in a chlorinated pool or in ocean water for 15–20
min significantly lowers the SPF value. Many sunscreens are easily washed
off. Highly protective formulations that totally resist sweating and water
immersion are ideal, but are not yet available. The ability of formulations to
partially resist water immersion is given in Table 15-5 under column 6
(gradations are based on SPF values: excellent, >6; good, 4–6 fair, 2–4; and
poor, <2).

Only a few brand-name formulations presently available on the market
have this quality, which can be labeled as "substantive to the skin," and resist
elution after perspiration or swimming. It is important to realize that the
substantivity of most of these formulations (Table 15-5) has not been
evaluated under rigid outdoor test conditions. In the absence of such
information, it is best to advise the consumer and the patient to reapply the
formulation after profuse sweating or swimming.

5. *Combined effects of UVA and UVB radiation*: Although solar UVB
radiation is primarily known to cause the sunburn, it should be emphasized
that UVA radiation is also erythemogenic. The minimal erythema dose
(MED) of UVA radiation for an average individual (Skin Type III) may range
from 20 to 100 J/cm^2. Although UVA is 1000 times less effective than solar
UVB in causing sunburn, it should be recognized that solar UVA irradiance is
approximately 100 times more than that of UVB around midday during the
summer months. Sun exposure of long duration (>90 min) may result in
erythema from both UVB and UVA radiation. Furthermore, the effects of
UVA may be additive or augmentative to the erythemogenesis of UVB (2).

6. *The vehicle or the base*: A vehicle, or base, of a sunscreen is as
important as the high molar extinction coefficient and substantivity of its
light-absorbing active ingredient(s). The base composition of different creams
and lotions (oil-in-water or water-in-oil base) determines the lipophilic or
hydrophilic nature and in many ways affects the ability of the sunscreen to be
substantive to the stratum corneum. The addition of emollients can, in certain
instances, decrease the ability of the active sunscreen agent to diffuse or to
remain adsorbed on the stratum corneum. For example, 5% solution of
PABA in 70% ethanol is quite substantive to the skin; it protects individuals
for nearly 3 hr of sunbathing (protection facter 12 MEDs). The same PABA

solution when mixed with emollients becomes a less effective sunscreen (protection factor 5–6 MEDs).

Alcoholic solutions and alcoholic gels of PABA and its esters are now increasingly used as sunscreens. They can be used as "colognes" or after-shave lotions, but they often impart a burning and stinging sensation. Children in particular do not like or appreciate the topical application of an alcoholic lotion, and patients with inflamed or eczematous skin should not be prescribed such formulations. The eyes should be protected against the stinging sensation of alcohol.

Certain manufacturers (e.g., Sundown, Johnson & Johnson) have used ammonium acrylate and acrylate copolymer as the water-resistant base for incorporating the active ingredient of a sunscreen (octyl-dimethyl-para-aminobenzoic acid). The manufacturers claim that such lotions provide an invisible water-resistant protective film on the skin; however, when used under outdoor test conditions, these, too, have certain limitations in consumer acceptance. These lotions form a nonuniform dry film that easily cracks, and people do burn (see Table 15-5).

PIGMENTATION OR TANNING REACTION (1, 4, 6)

Melanin pigmentation stimulated by exposure to solar radiation involves immediate tanning reaction (photooxidation of melanin) and delayed tanning response (formation of new pigment, or melanogenesis) (Fig. 15-2). Sun-induced tanning (suntanning), or melanogenesis, is maximally stimulated by UVB. While UVA is also melanogenic, it is less so than UVB; however, repeated exposures of UVA (approximately 20–30 J/cm^2 daily for 7 days) can stimulate melanogenesis quite effectively without the discomforts of sunburn (e.g., erythema, edema, desquamation). The mode of this increased tanning reaction is discussed elsewhere (6).

Many manufacturers and consumers believe that sunscreening lotions promote or accelerate tanning reaction. The entire advertising program is at times geared toward this erroneous claim. No sunscreen product can give "a deeper suntan" or "a longer-lasting suntan." Melanogenesis or tanning reaction is not induced or augmented by topical sunscreens. The ability to produce melanin pigment is genetically predetetmined by the functional capacity of a person's melanocytes. Individuals with Skin Types I and II are genetically less capable of stimulating tanning reaction than individuals with Skin Types III–VI. For fair-skinned individuals, who burn easily and subsequently peel, and tan little or minimally (Skin Types I and II), repeated efforts to coax a tan may induce irreversible skin damage (wrinkling, aging, keratoses, and eventually skin cancer).

Although the tanning reaction is most effectively stimulated by UVB (290–320 nm) radiation, it should be recognized that UVA radiation (320–400 nm) is also melanogenic (6). Increased tanning following sun exposure may be the result of direct or indirect stimulation and the increased population of the melanocytes. The melanocytes are activated by the UVB as well as by the UVA radiation and not by any ingredient in the sunscreen preparations. The melanocytes increase in number, and, in turn, lead to the increased formation, melanization, and transfer of newly synthesized melanosomes. The potent or most effective sunscreens (SPF>12) do not permit enhanced tanning reaction. Sunscreens (suntanning lotions) that are less effective (SPF 4) may facilitate tanning reaction with minimal discomforts of severe sunburn only in those individuals who can tan well (Skin Types III–VI).

Immediate tanning reaction and delayed tanning reaction observed in the presence of topically applied sunscreens are the result of photooxidation of the preexisting melanin, and subsequently there is stimulation of new pigment formation (melanogenesis) by UVA radiation. Pigmentation or tanning reaction can be best achieved by daily and well-controlled exposures. Skin sites treated with topical application of an effective sunscreen (e.g., PABA) generally show a minimal tanning response in comparison to the control, untreated but exposed skin; however, a few well-controlled sun exposures (four to six, each for 60–90 min) following the topical application of the sunscreen can eventually generate an effective tanning response in the same individual. Individuals anxious to develop a "healthy suntan" can achieve the desired effect by minimizing the discomforts of the sunburn reaction (erythema, edema, and desquamation) by the topical application of UVB-absorbing sunscreens and optimizing the melanogenic potential of UVA radiation.

TOPICAL SUNSCREENS: THEIR PROPERTIES AND LIMITATIONS (2, 3, 9–12, 14, 16, 18, 19)

At present, the most effective sunscreening agents are as follows: (a) the alcoholic solution of para-aminobenzoic acid (5% PABA in 50–70% ethyl alcohol), (b) the nonalcoholic combination sunscreen lotions containing PABA esters and benzophenones, and (c) the non-PABA sunscreening creams or lotions containing benzophenones and cinnamates (see Tables 15-5 and 15-7). After a single application, these preparations provide satisfactory protection against sunburn under varying conditions (sunbathing for prolonged periods under dry and humid conditions, and after sweating and while skiing).

Alcoholic solutions of PABA provide a practical method for prophylaxis against repeated exposures to sunlight inasmuch as a single application can be used each morning in reducing UV-radiation exposure dose and diminishing chronic sun-damaged skin and possibly basal cell and squamous cell carcinoma in the high-risk population (Skin Types I–III). The disadvantages of these alcoholic solutions of PABA are: (a) "drying" of the skin; (b) stinging sensation in children and people with thin skin and flushed face; (c) occasional development in a few patients of contact eczematous dermatitis; (d) yellow staining of the clothes, especially after sun exposure.

The esters of PABA (Escalol 506 and 507), however, do not cause discoloration of clothing. When two PABA esters are used in concentrations ranging from 2.5% to 3.3%, they are quite effective sunscreens, but they do cause irritation of the exposed skin. The formulations containing only one ester of PABA (2.5% Escalol 506 or 507), although less effective than 5% PABA in 70% ethanol, are recommended for normal individuals who wish to minimize the discomforts of sunburn reaction and yet desire to acquire a gradual tan (Skin Types III and IV).

Alcoholic preparations containing 5% PABA or PABA esters are partially substantive to skin. PABA penetrates the cells of the stratum corneum and, because it is a zwitterion (a dipolar ion), it can remain adsorbed on the proteins of the stratum corneum through hydrogen bonding. PABA esters (Escalol 507) appear to resist water elution better than PABA. Although the bulk of the active ingredient of the applied formulation is washed off after the skin is immersed in water (as in swimming), a certain residual fraction of PABA as well as PABA ester is left on the surface of the stratum corneum and within the horny cells to the extent that the residual sunscreen provides partial, if not total, protection to an individual (equivalent to 2 or at the most 3 MEDs); however to reassure total protection, it is best to recommend reapplication of the sunscreen after a stress of swimming or profuse sweating.

Topical formulations in an oily cream base containing two or more UV-absorbing ingredients, such as 4% ethylhexyl-p-methoxy cinnamate, 3% 2-hydroxy-4-methoxybenzophenone, and 5.5% 2-phenylbenzimidazole sulfonic acid, appear to be also very effective formulations in the protection of human skin against the harmful effects of UVB and, to a certain extent, UVA radiation up to 380 nm (see Tables 15-5 and 15-7). These formulations are also effective for use in ski areas of snow-covered, UV-reflecting mountains at high altitudes (4, 14). These non-PABA formulations containing benzophenones and cinnamates are more popular in the European market and are reported to protect normal individuals against the sunburn spectrum under varying stress conditions of prolonged sunbathing, profuse sweating induced by exercise in hot and humid weather, and swimming in fresh or sea water (14).

The topical sunscreens effective in the prevention of sunburn reaction induced by 290–320-nm radiation have not proven highly effective in the prevention of phototoxic and photoallergic reactions induced by long-wave UV and visible radiation, (e.g., demethylchlorotetracycline-induced phototoxic reaction). The phototoxic reaction induced by topical application or oral ingestion of psoralens (methoxsalen and trioxsalen) can be reduced with topical sunscreens containing benzophenones (see Tables 15-5 and 15-6) (2, 3, 7, 24).

TOPICAL PROTECTION AGAINST GERMICIDAL RADIATION (UVC)

Most sunscreens are designed to block erythemogenic rays of the sun (290–320 nm). The effectiveness of commercially available screening formulations against the short-wave UV rays ($\lambda < 280$ nm) which normally are not encountered at the earth's surface has not been thoroughly evaluated, and systemic studies to develop such screens have not been conducted. Short-wave UV radiation (254 nm emitted by low-pressure mercury-arc lamps) reduces visible airborne bacteria and is widely used for its microbicidal effect in tissue-culture laboratories, food preparation plants, hospital ventilation systems, and operating rooms.

As little as 5–7 times the MED of UVB radiation from artificial sources or from sunlight may cause marked redness accompanied by pain, swelling, and even blistering reaction; on the other hand, hundreds of MEDs of UVC cause no more than moderate redness and rarely a blistering reaction.

Twenty topically applied sunscreen formulations containing PABA, benzophenones, thymine, urocanic acid, PABA esters, etc., were evaluated for their ability to block short-wavelength (254 nm) UV radiation by measuring their ability to prevent erythema from developing on the germicidal lamp-exposed backs of volunteers in the laboratory and operating rooms. Only the 2-hydroxy-4-methoxybenzophenone-5-sulfonic acid (10%) in a cream base was found to be an excellent screen (25, 26). PABA, PABA esters, and other agents were not effective in protecting skin against germicidal radition. The effectiveness of benzophenone derivatives in the protection against the short-wavelength (254 nm), UVB (290–320 nm), and the long-wavelength (320–380 nm) UV radiation suggests that they may be distinctive "broad-spectrum" sunscreens (see Table 15-5 for sunscreens containing benzophenones).

SYSTEMIC PHOTOPROTECTION

The development of systemic photoprotectants that could reduce the reaction of skin to sunburn radiation has long been hoped for, but has not proven successful. Agents such as PABA, antihistamine compounds such as triprolidine exhibiting UV absorption in the 283–290 nm range, acetyl salicylic acid, vitamins A, C (ascorbic acid), and E (α-tocopherol), certain unsaturated fatty acids that are easily photooxidized, and certain steroids have been suggested as systemic photoprotectants (see Table 15-8). Their effectiveness in preventing UVB-induced sunburn reaction is mostly anecdotal and has not been carefully evaluated in a controlled double-blind study. The three oral photoprotective agents of limited effectiveness are beta-carotene, chloroquine, and certain psoralens (8-methoxypsoralen and 4,5′,8-trimethyl-psoralen) (see Table 15-8).

Beta-Carotene (27–29)

Beta-carotene is recommended for the amelioration of photosensitivity reactions in patients with erythropoietic protoporphyria (EPP) and other porphyrias, such as erythropoietic prophyria. This disease, which is a dominant genetic trait, appears in early childhood, and unless the afflicted patients, and especially the children, avoid even the briefest exposure to the sun, a severe photosensitivity reaction with erythema, swelling, itching, and even vesicles often leading to scarring will develop. Beta-carotene is a natural constituent of many plants, including common foods such as carrots, tomatoes, and oranges. Only beta-carotene, which absorbs primarily in the

Table 15-8. Natural and Systemic Photoprotective Agents

Agent	Range[a]	Effectiveness
Melanin	UVB, UVA	Good
Keratin	UVB, UVC	Fair
Urocanic acid	UVB, UVC	Fair
Carotenoids (β-carotene)	UVA, visible	Good
Psoralens (8-methoxypsoralen and trimethylpsoralen)	UVB, UVA	Fair to good
Antioxidants ascorbic acid, alpha tocopherol (vitamin E)	UVB	Poor and questionable
Chloroquine	UVB, UVA	Fair to good
Antihistamines (triprolidine, etc.)	UVB	Poor and questionable
Unsaturated fatty acids	UVB	Poor and questionable
Steriods	UVB	Poor and questionable
Para-aminobenzoic acid	UVB	Questionable and not proven
Para-aminosalicylic acids	UVB	Questionable and not proven
Acetyl salicylic acids	UVB	Poor and questionable

[a]UVB = 290–320 nm; UVA = 320–400 nm.

visible spectrum of light (360–500 nm) with a maximum absorption at 450 to 475 nm, has been shown to be very effective as a systemic photoprotective agent; it is particularly so in patients with EPP, who are extremely sensitive to visible radiation (27–29). Our earlier study of three patients with EPP first reported in 1970 (27) has now been extended to over 100 patients, all of whom have shown subjective as well as objective improvement in their tolerance to sunlight and exposure to 400-nm radiation (28, 29) (see Chapter 14). Beta-carotene may also be recommeded for the amelioration of cutaneous photosensitivity reactions in other types of porphyrias (e.g., erythropoietic porphyria and porphyria cutanea tarda).

Recommendations for treatment at the present time are that oral ingestion of synthetic beta-carotene be regulated to maintain blood carotene levels between 600 and 800 μg/100 ml (usually a dose of 120–180 mg/day for adults). Children under the age of 12 receive 30–90 mg/day.

Beta-carotene (Solatene by Hoffmann-La Roche) should be prescribed as follows:

Children: 30–90 mg/day for 1–8 years of age
90–120 mg/day for 9–16 years of age
Adults: 120–180 mg/day, can be increased to 250 mg/day

The protective effect of beta-carotene is evidenced after 6 weeks of therapy. Even on such adequate doses, patients with EPP may develop some reaction (e.g., itching and burning) to sun exposure, and each patient must carefully establish his/her tolerance limits to sun exposure. A subsequent increment in the oral dose of beta-carotene does seem to provide increased protection. In addition, the topical application of UVB and UVA-absorbing sunscreens is also helpful. The safety of beta-carotene usage during pregnancy has not been determined. No adverse effects have been reported at these recommended doses. Nonetheless, we recommend that before therapy and at frequent intervals (6–9 months) the following tests be made: (a) complete blood count and reticulocyte count, (b) BUN, (c) SGOT, (d) alkaline phosphatase, (d) carotene, (e) vitamin A, and (g) total bilirubin.

Most patients take beta-carotene only during the spring and summer seasons. Maximal effect of the drug as measured by increased tolerance to sunlight seems to occur after 1–3 months of therapy, and may last 1 or 2 months after cessation of therapy. Protection appears to coincide with the slow development and slow resolution of carotenemia.

The mechanisms by which beta-carotene is effective in protecting EPP patients from photosensitivity are unknown. It does not appear to act as a sunscreen that filters out 400–700-nm radiation, but acts as a quenching agent for free radicals and excited-singlet oxygen that are believed to be generated in protoporphyrin photosensitizing reactions (27–29). Other factors involved may include the relationship between plasma proteins and protoporphyrin levels, between plasma protein and beta-carotene and the interrelationship between these two systems, and, finally, the effects of these factors on the time levels of these substances.

Beta-carotene, when applied topically or given orally, is not an effective agent for preventing sunburn reaction induced by UVB radiation. Patients with polymorphic light eruptions, including solar urticaria and hydroa aestivale, appear to derive only limited benefits with systemic beta-carotene (28, 29).

Antimalarials (Chloroquine) (1, 2, 30–34)

Antimalarials have been used for a number of years to treat diverse entities other than malaria, and these include lupus erythematosus (LE), polymorphous light eruptions (PMLE), and solar urticaria. Chloroquine (Aralen) and hydroxychloroquine (Plaquenil) are substituted 4-amino quinolines; quinacrine (Atabrine) is an acridine compound. Antimalarials are valuable therapeutic agents but are not first-line drugs of choice and should be used only after conservative measures (topical sunscreens) have been tried. The recommended maintenance dosage is 200 mg/day for hydroxychloroquine, 250 mg/day for chloroquine, and 100–300 mg/day for quinacrine. Patients should not remain on antimalarials indefinitely, and as their disease improves, the drug should be discontinued. A complete ophthalmologic examination with paracentral red field testing should be performed prior to therapy and at 4-month intervals. Treatment with antimalarials for a prolonged period has been shown to result, not frequently, in retinopathy. These drugs bind avidly to melanin and are deposited along the uveal tract and retinal pigment epithelium.

The mechanisms of action of antimalarials in treating LE and PMLE photosensitizing reactions are unknown. The MED in normal individuals as well as patients with discoid LE is not altered by chloroquine therapy, and it is doubtful that these drugs work merely via physical sunscreen effect. However, these drugs have been shown to inhibit a variety of enzyme systems, to be potent inhibitors of histamine, and to have anti-inflammatory properties. Their effects in the immune system have been well studied; they do not affect either the primary or secondary antibody response or tests of delayed hypersensitivity, and have been shown to weakly inhibit complement activity and dissociate antigen–antibody reactions in in vitro test procedures.

Chloroquine is selectively taken up and concentrated with lysosomes and has been shown to inhibit the lysosomal degradation of mucopolysaccharides; whether or not it also inhibits the degradation of other macromolecules is not known. Initially, both chloroquine and quinacrine were shown to stabilize the lysosomal membrane and to retard the release of hydrolytic enzymes. Recently, however, evidence has appeared that indicates the chloroquine may also labilize the lysosomal membrane (2).

Both chloroquine and quinacrine have been shown to bind to and stabilize double-stranded DNA, preventing its heat denaturation and retarding enzymic depolymerization (2, 30). They are thought to intercalate between DNA pairs and have been shown to sensitize tumor cells to alkylating agents investigated by researchers in the field of cancer chemotherapy (2, 30, 31, 33, 34).

Indications for Chloroquine Use. These drugs are not used as the first line of therapy. When used for rheumatoid arthritis of SLE, they are usually given in combination with either salicylates or small doses or corticosteriods. When used for cutaneous LE, PMLE, or solar urticaria, they are usually administered only when other measures have failed; a patient with the extensive facial scarring disease LE, however, might be started on antimalarials. The recommended dosage is 250–500 mg/day for chloroquine, 200–400 mg/day for hydroxychloroquine, and 100–200 mg/day for quinacrine.

Guidelines for Chloroquine Use

1. Prior to therapy: (a) Twenty-four-hour urines should be collected for uro- and coproporphyrins to rule out preexisting porphyria cutanea tarda. (b) Baseline laboratory tests should include complete blood counts, G-6-PD levels, BUN, creatinine, and routine tests of hepatic function. (c) Ophthalmologic examinations as specified by the technique of Percival and Behrman are essential (32).

2. At 6-month intervals, both laboratory and ophthalmologic tests should be repeated.

3. Total dosage of these drugs should not exceed 200 g. Careful records of cumulative dosages must be maintained.

4. For PMLE and solar urticaria, antimalarials should be given for active periods only. As the disease is brought under control, attempts should be made to discontinue the medication. Often a remission will follow which may then be prolonged with more conservative therapy.

5. For discoid LE, the usual indication is in case of progressive, chronic, extensive, and scarring lesions which are cosmetically unacceptable to the patient.

6. Often when a given antimalarial fails, another may be utilized with success.

7. Exacerbations are not refractory to a second or third course of antimalarial therapy.

Oral Psoralens

The use of oral psoralens, e.g., 8-methoxypsoralen (8-MOP) and 4,5′,8-trimethylpsoralen (TMP), may increase tolerance to sunlight only when the administration of the drug is followed by exposure of the skin to sunlight or to UVA radiation emitted by artificial sources (35) (see Table 15-7). In blond or freckled persons with Skin Types II and III (and even albino patients) who suffer painful reactions to sunlight, 8-MOP can aid in increasing resistance to solar damage. Certain patients with polymorphic photodermatosis and vitiligo (idiopathic leukoderma) may also be benefitted by the indirect protective action of 8-MOP. This protective action appears to be related to the thickening of the horny layer and increased formation and melanization of melanosomes by the pigment-producing cells, the melanocytes. To increase tolerance to sunlight and/or to enhance melanin pigmentation, the patient is advised to take two or three capsules (10 mg each) of methoxsalen (8-methoxypsoralen) or trioxsalen tablets (4,5′,8-trimethylpsoralen, 20 mg) 2 hr before measured periods of exposure to sunlight or UV radiation from high-intensity UVA sources. The therapy is continued for a maximum period of 2 weeks. The exposure schedule to sunlight or to UVA sources can be shown as in Table 15-9.

Well-controlled studies have carefully documented that orally administered furocoumarins such as 8-MOP might afford increased tolerance to sun exposure, probably by providing secondary protection through increased synthesis of melanin and increased formation of keratinized stratum corneum (24). The melanin-laden thickened epidermis decreases the transmission of damaging UV radiation. Despite these objective data, 8-MOP or TMP has not received wide support as a systemic agent to increase tolerance to sunlight. Perhaps the most overriding factor in its limitation as a systemic photo-protectant is the fact that it requires a "breaking-in" period to build up two natural defenses of the body (the increased production of melanin and keratin). Patients do not want to go through the bother of 10 or 15 days of carefully controlled exposures to obtain the gradual increment in tan that will lead to secondary and more durable protection.

MANAGEMENT OF ACUTE AND CHRONIC SUN-INDUCED REACTIONS

Acute Sunburn

Individuals with acute sunburn reaction manifesting severe erythema, edema, and painful blistering reaction may obtain relief with ice-cold compresses of Burow's solution diluted 1:10 with plain tap water. One may recommend tepid tub baths with or without nonirritating additives (e.g., bath oils). The topical application of sterile petrolatum also helps to minimize excessive drying and burning sensations. Topical fluorinated steroids (0.025%), such as triamcinolone ointment or cream, applied three or four times daily under compresses may be recommended. Steroid-induced vasoconstriction may reduce the erythema, itching and burning sensation, and discomfort. Severe sunburn or dangerous accidental overexposure should be treated with systemic corticosteroids. Oral prednisone beginning with 40–60 mg and tapering over 4–8 days will minimize the severe sunburn reaction.

Table 15-9. Schedule to Increase Sun Tolerance with Oral Psoralens[a]

Exposure[b]	Light skin color (Skin Types I and II)	Medium skin color (Skin Types III and IV)
Initial	15 min, 1.5–2.0 J/cm^2 [c]	20 min, 2.0–2.5 J/cm^2 [c]
Second	20 min, 2.0–2.5 J/cm^2	25 min, 2.5–3.0 J/cm^2
Third	25 min, 2.5–3.0 J/cm^2	30 min, 3.0–4.0 J/cm^2
Fourth	30 min, 3.0–4.0 J/cm^2	35 min, 4.0–4.5 J/cm^2
Subsequent	Gradual increment	Gradual increment

[a] Sunglasses that filter out UVA radiation should be worn soon after ingestion of the drug and for an additional 8-hr period after exposure. Lips should be protected with a lipstick containing and effective sunscreen.
[b] Increment in exposure in based on the absence of erythema and tenderness at 24 and 48 hr after each exposure.
[c] UVA exposure only (320–400 nm).

Preventive Measures

It is always helpful to instruct the patient to avoid sunlight exposure between 10 a.m. and 3 p.m. Confinement of the patient in a darkened room for several days may often be beneficial for an early recovery. Patients with photosensitivity disorders may obtain protection against sunlight with adequate clothing. Closely woven brown, orange, green, yellow, or red fabrics are generally good screens for protection. White, thinly knit cotton, or synthetic fabrics should not be recommended, as they can be permeable to erythema-producing radiation, especially when they are wet from water or perspiration.

Many normal individuals (adults as well as children) may encounter localized, acute, and chronic effects of sunburn reaction (e.g., the nose and lips of lifeguards, sailors on duty, etc.). In such instances, it is best to recommend topical application of opaque sunscreens containing zinc oxide to the nose and lips. Although such formulations are cosmetically not elegant, they do adhere to the skin and resist the elution effects of perspiration and swimming (see Table 15-6). Macleod and Frain-Bell (15) have recommended a combination of a benzophenone (Mexenone) and a physical sunscreen (zinc oxide, kaolin, titanium dioxide, and ferric oxide) for the most effective protection when normal individuals or patients must have prolonged protection. Certain lipsticks (colored or light-reflecting) are also beneficial in minimizing the sun-induced changes of the lips, (dryness, exfoliation, chapping, etc.).

Patients with allergic hypersensitivity to chemicals or drugs must be advised to obtain sunscreens that do not contain the implicated sensitizer or the cross-reacting sensitizer. Patients with hypersensitivity to hair dyes, sulfonamides, procaine, or benzocaine should strictly avoid the use of sunscreens containing para-aminobenzoic acid or esters of PABA (21). Most proprietary sunburn remedies contain local anesthetics, such as benzocaine, together with antiseptics, emollients, and perfumes. These should not be recommended to patients who are sensitive to PABA or who are receiving antihypertensive or diuretic drugs. Their use must be weighted against the hazard of sensitization to benzocaine (21).

ACKNOWLEDGMENTS. This study was supported by Grant 2-R01-CA-05003-22 awarded by the U.S. National Cancer Institute, DHEW.

REFERENCES

1. Pathak, M. A., and Epstein, J. H. (1971): Normal and abnormal reactions to light. In: *Dermatology in General Medicine*, edited by T. B. Fitzpatrick, K. A. Arndt, W. H. Clark, Jr. et al., pp. 977–1036. McGraw-Hill, New York.

2. Parrish, J. A., White, H. A. D., and Pathak, M. A. (1979): Photomedicine. In: *Dermatology in General Medicine*, 2nd ed., edited by T. B. Fitzpatrick, A. Z. Eisen, K. Wolff, et al., pp. 942–994. McGraw-Hill, New York.

3. Pathak, M. A., Fitzpatrick, T. B., and Parrish, J. A. (1979): Photosensitivity and other reactions to light. In: *Harrison's Principles of Internal Medicine*, 9th ed., edited by K. J. Isselbacher, et al., pp. 255–262. McGraw-Hill, New York.

4. Pathak, M. A. (1974): Physical units of radiation and some common terms used in photobiology. In: *Sunlight and Man: Normal and Abnormal Photobiologic Responses*, edited by M. A. Pathak, L. C. Harber, M. Seiji, et al. (T. B. Fitzpatrick, consulting editor), pp. 815–818. University of Tokyo Press, Tokyo.

5. Fitzpatrick, T. B. (1976): In: *Halocarbons: Environmental Effects of Chlorofluoromethane Release*, p. 123. Committee on Impacts of Stratospheric Change. Assembly of Mathematical and Physical Sciences, National Research Council, National Academy of Sciences, Washington, D. C.

6. Pathak, M. A., Jimbow, K., and Szabo, G., et al. (1976): Sunlight and melanin pigmentation. In: *Photochemical and Photobiological Reviews*, Vol. 1, edited by K. C. Smith, pp. 211–239. Plenum Press, New York.

7. Parrish, J. A., Pathak, M. A., and Fitzpatrick, T. B. (1971): Prevention of unintentional overexposure in topical psoralen treatment of vitiligo. *Arch. Dermatol.* **104**:281–283.

8. Federal Register (1978): Sunscreen Drug Products for Over-the-Counter Human Drugs: Proposed Safety, Effective and Labeling Conditions. Department of Health, Education and Welfare, U. S. Food and Drug Administration. Vol. 43, No. 166, 08/25/78.

9. Pathak, M. A., Fitzpatrick, T. B., and Frenk, E. (1969): Evaluation of topical agents that prevent sunburn: superiority of para-aminobenzoic acid and its ester in ethyl alcohol. *N. Engl. J. Med.* **280**:1459–1463.

10. Willis, I., and Kligman, A. M. (1969): Evaluation of sunscreens by human assay. *J. Soc. Cosmet. Chem.* **20**:639.

11. Willis, I., and Kligman, A. M. (1970): Aminobenzoic acid and its esters. *Arch. Dermatol.* **102**:405–417.

12. Langer, A., and Kligman, A. M. (1972): Further sunscreen studies of aminobenzoic acid. *Arch. Dermatol.* **105**:851–855.

13. Cripps, D. J., and Hegedus, S. (1974): Protection factor of sunscreens to monochromatic radiation. *Arch. Dermatol.* **109**:202–204.

14. Fitzpatrick, T. B., Pathak, M. A., and Parrish, J. A. (1974): Protection of the human skin against the effects of the sunburn ultraviolet (290–320 nm). In: *Sunlight and Man: Normal and Abnormal Photobiologic Responses*, edited by M. A. Pathak, L. C. Harber, M. Seiji, et al. (T. B. Fitzpatrick, consulting editor), pp. 751–765. University of Tokyo Press, Tokyo.

15. Macleod, T. M., and Frain-Bell, W. (1971): The study of the efficacy of some agents used for the protection of the skin from exposure to light. *Br. J. Dermatol.* **84**:266–281.

16. Kaidbey, K. H., and Kligman, A. M. (1978): Laboratory methods for appraising the efficacy of sunscreens. *J. Soc. Cosmet. Chem.* **29**:525–536.

17. Knox, J. M., Guin, J., and Cockerell, E. G. (1957): Benzophenones. Ultraviolet light absorbing agents. *J. Invest. Dermatol.* **29**:435–444.

18. Sayre, R. M., Desrochers, D. L., and Marlowe, E. (1978): The correlation of indoor solar simulator and natural sunlight testing of sunscreen products. *Arch. Dermatol.* **114**:1649–1651.

19. Sayre, R. M., Marlowe, E., Poh Agin, P., et al. (1979): Performance of six sunscreen formulations of human skin. *Arch. Dermatol.* **115**:46–49.

20. Fusaro, R. M., Runge, W. J., and Johnson, J. A. (1972): Protection against light sensitivity with dihydorxyacetone-naphthoquinone. *Int. J. Dermatol.* **11**:67–70.

21. Fisher, A. A. (1977): The presence of benzocaine in sunscreens containing glyceryl PABA (Escalol 106). *Arch. Dermatol.* **113**:1299–1300.

22. Toby-Mathias, C. G., Maibach, H. I., and Epstein, J. H. (1978): Allergic contact photodermatitis to para-aminobenzoic acid. *Arch. Dermatol.* **114**:1665–1666.

23. Kaidbey, K. H., and Kligman, A. M. (1978): Contact photoallergy to 6-methylcoumarin in proprietary sunscreens. *Arch. Dermatol.* **114**:1709–1710.

24. Fitzpatrick, T. B., Pathak, M. A., Harber, L. C., et al (1974): An introduction to the problem of normal and abnormal responses of man's skin to solar radiation. In: *Sunlight and Man: Normal and Abnormal Photobiologic Responses,* edited by M. A. Pathak, L. C. Harber, M. Seiji, et al. (T. B. Fitzpatrick, consulting editor), pp. 3–14. University of Tokyo Press, Tokyo.

25. Parrish, J. A., Pathak, M. A., and Fitzpatrick, T. B. (1971): Protection of skin from germicidal ultraviolet radiation in the operating room by topical chemicals. *N. Engl. J. Med.* **284**:1257–1258.

26. Parrish, J. A., Pathak, M. A., and Fitzpatrick, T. B. (1972): Topical protection against germicidal radiation. *Arch. Surg.* **104**:276–283.

27. Mathews-Roth, M. M., Pathak, M. A., Fitzpatrick, T. B. et al. (1970): Beta-carotene as a photoprotective agent in erythropoietic protoporphyria. *N. Engl. J. Med.* **282**:1231–1234.

28. Mathews-Roth, M. M., Pathak, M. A., Fitzpatrick, T. B., et al. (1974): Beta-carotene as an oral photoprotective agent in erythropoietic protoporyria. *J. AMA* **228**:1004–1008.

29. Mathews-Roth, M. M., Pathak, M. A., Fitzpatrick, T. B., et al. (1977): Beta-carotene therapy for etythropoietic protoporphyria and other photosensitivity diseases. *Arch. Dermatol.* **113**:1229–1232.

30. Allison, J. L., O'Brien, R. L., and Hahn, F. E. (1965): DNA reactions with chloroquin. *Science* **149**:1111–1113.

31. Allison, J. L., O'Brien, R. L., and Hahn, F. E. (1965): Nature of the deoxyribonucleic acid–chloroquine complex. In: *Antimicrobial Agents and Chemotherapy,* edited by G. L. Hobby, pp. 310–314. American Society for Microbiology, Ann Arbor, Michigan.

32. Percival, S. P., and Behrman, J. (1967): Ophthalmological safety of chloroquine. *Br. J. Ophthalmol.* **53**:101–109.

33. Rubin, M., Berstein, H. N., and Zvaifler, N. J. (1963): Studies on the pharmacology of chlorquine. Recommendations for the treatment of retinopathy. *Arch. Ophthalmol.* **70**:470–481.

34. Sams, W. M., Jr. (1976): Chloroquine: its use in photosensitive eruptions. *Int. J. Dermatol.* **15**:99–111.

35. Imbrie, J. D., Daniels, F., Bergeron, L., et al. (1959): Increased erythema threshold six weeks after a single exposure to sunlight plus oral methoxsalen. *J. Invest. Dermatol.* **32**:331–337.

36. Everett, M. A., *et al.* (1965); *Arch. Dermatol.* **92**:713–719 (1965).

37. Freeman, R. G. *et al.* (1966): *J. Invest. Dermatol.* **67**:586–592 (1966).

VI

Therapeutic Photomedicine

16

Phototherapy of Hyperbilirubinemia

T. R. C. Sisson and T. P. Vogl

Jaundice occurs in about half of all newly born infants, and is the visible expression of high concentrations of bilirubin in the circulating plasma. Bilirubin, a tetrapyrrole pigment derived from the heme moiety of hemoglobin, is carried in plasma bound primarily to albumin; small amounts may also be bound to red cell membranes. If the production of bilirubin exceeds the infant's ability to conjugate and excrete it, this pigment accumulates in the circulation, a condition called "hyperbilirubinemia," and thence is deposited in the skin and other tissues. If the amount of bilirubin in the plasma exceeds the available binding sites, it is believed to circulate in a free (unbound or loosely bound) form that can enter and damage the neural tissue of the brain, especially the basal ganglia.

Bilirubin is particularly toxic to cells of the central nervous system, and on reaching those cells, may produce irreversible brain damage known as *bilirubin encephalopathy*. The term *kernicterus* is reserved for the most severe forms of damage: deafness, cerebral palsy, or death. Strictly speaking, the presence of kernicterus can be established only at autopsy by observing the yellow staining of the basal ganglia. However, the definition given previously is often used, and will be used herein.

Severe jaundice of the newborn must be reduced promptly in order to prevent brain damage. At present, only two types of treatment are available that possess a high degree of effectiveness: exchange transfusion, in which the

T. R. C. Sisson • Department of Pediatrics, Rutgers University School of Medicine, Perth Amboy, New Jersey 08861. *T. P. Vogl* • Departments of Radiology and Pediatrics, Columbia University College of Physicians and Surgeons, New York, New York 10027. Present address: Nutrition Coordinating Committee, Office of the Director, National Institute of Health, Bethesda, Maryland 20205.

infant's entire blood volume is replaced with bilirubin-free blood; and phototherapy, irradiation of the infant with visible light. Exchange transfusion has been in use since the mid-1940s, and phototherapy since late in the 1950s.

HISTORICAL PERSPECTIVE

One hundred years ago, when Americans were less well educated but no less gullible than now, a craze swept the country that rivaled today's diet fads (1). A mania for the use of blue light (sunlight filtered through blue glass) followed publication of studies by Augustus J. Pleasonton (2), a Civil War General and amateur scientist, who claimed that exposure to blue light would cure arthritis and a number of other afflictions, as well as increase the germination and yield of plants and the fecundity of domestic animals.

As things do, this bit of lunacy passed, except in tiny groups of color-therapy adherents who periodically have surfaced over the decades. Occasionally, a physician of some prominence might speak in its favor (3). The use of colored light had lost scientific credence by the turn of the century, when Finsen, on impeccable scientific principles, promoted natural sunlight (4) and later artificial ultraviolet (UV) radiation from carbon-arc lamps (5) for the treatment of tuberculosis of the skin. Thus, the use of colored light—phototherapy—gave way to heliotherapy, a far more respectable modality at the time.

The greater credibility granted heliotherapy was based on two factors: demonstrated effectiveness in the treatment of tuberculosis, and a somewhat mystical regard for God's natural light in the promotion of good health (an uncritical esteem which exists to some degree today).

In 1938 the German chemist, Hans Fischer, observed that bilirubin in solution, when exposed to light, decomposes and becomes colorless (6). This observation supported the later finding of Cremer and his associates (7).

The nursing sister in charge of Cremer's hospital nursery reported to him that the jaundice of infants in the sunlit part of the room faded after a short period of exposure. Cremer tested her observation in a controlled manner with intermittent exposures to sunlight and found that not only did the yellow color of exposed skin fade, but that the serum bilirubin concentrations of the infants were reduced. This was the first indication that the sera of jaundiced infants were photosensitive and that the concentration of bilirubin in these sera was reduced by photooxidation. Cremer then designed an apparatus utilizing the radiation of eight fluorescent lamps emitting blue light. These lamps were chosen because part of their emission was in the range of absorption of bilirubin (420–480 nm). Jaundiced infants were exposed to the lamps and successful reduction of visible jaundice and hyperbilirubinemia was demonstrated. The report of these studies is the first scientific record of the use of phototherapy in neonatal hyperbilirubinemia (8).

The fact that high blood levels of bilirubin cause severe brain damage from the toxic effects of bilirubin on neurons was well known at the time. The simplicity, demonstrable effectiveness, and seeming lack of morbidity from phototherapy stood in marked contrast to the significant mortality then associated with exchange transfusion via the umbilical vein, the only method of treatment available. Consequently, phototherapy rapidly gained favor in Europe and South America, but not in the United States, probably because of the thorough disrepute of colored light as a therapeutic principle. In the United States a decade was to pass before the widespread acceptance of phototherapy. Despite a number of papers (9–16) published during this period documenting the clinical advantages of phototherapy, it met with massive disinterest from American physicians.

In 1967, Lucey, Ferriero, and Hewitt reported, and the following year published (17), their study of the *prevention* of hyperbilirubinemia in premature infants by the use of light irradiation—prophylactic phototherapy. This report had a stunning impact on pediatric practice. The attitude toward phototherapy quickly swung from disdainful indifference to enthusiastic, if uncritical, acceptance.

No devices for the application of phototherapy to neonates were commercially available, and at first most units were homemade. Several manufacturers soon produced hoods of more or less appropriate design, containing 8–10 fluorescent lamps arranged as a canopy over infant incubators and bassinets, relying principally upon descriptions of Cremer's and Lucey's units. Unfortunately, the proliferation of phototherapy hoods was not accompanied by very much understanding of the characteristics of fluorescent lamp phosphors, the spectral radiance of the several lamp types in use, their thermal output, or the small but significant UV radiation emitted. Indeed, some physicians were under the mistaken impression that UV radiation *was* the appropriate light for neonatal phototherapy. Perhaps the most alarming aspect of the extravagant interest in this new mode of treatment was the general state of ignorance among clinicians concerning the photobiologic effects of intense and prolonged irradiation on the newly born, who were exposed to these high levels of visible light radiation.

Fortunately, it is now appreciated that, although ubiquitous, visible light is not necessarily harmless. The last few years have been marked in medical circles by concern for, and study of, the biologic effects of visible light beyond the photooxidation of bilirubin, and by an interest in photobiology as a broad discipline with many potential applications, only exemplified by phototherapy of the neonate. Studies of clinical treatment of jaundice in the newborn have also stimulated research in the metabolism, binding, transport, and biologic fate of bilirubin and related pigments, and facilitated other therapeutic applications of light.

Phototherapy cannot completely replace exchange transfusion for the reduction of hyperbilirubinemia. When the production of the pigment outstrips the infant's capacity to conjugate and/or excrete bilirubin, notably in Rh hemolytic disease of the newborn, exchange transfusions are necessary. The use of phototherapy as an adjunctive treatment has served to reduce the number of repeat exchange transfusions formerly found necessary.

BILIRUBIN

Bilirubin, a straight-chain tetrapyrrole, is derived principally from the catabolism of the heme moiety by oxidation of the α-methene bond in the reticuloendothelial cells of the liver. Smaller amounts result from catabolism of erythrocytes in the spleen and from the bone marrow secondary to the incomplete formation of erythrocyte precursors [18]. Bilirubin is a lipid-soluble, nonpolar substance that, upon entering the blood stream, is normally bound by albumin and transported to the liver. There it is conjugated with glucuronic acid and excreted into the bile. Bilirubin in the neonate generally circulates almost entirely in the unconjugated, nonpolar, lipid-soluble form, bound to two sites on albumin molecules [19]: a primary site of strong affinity with a binding constant of 3×10^7 (carrying the bulk of the bilirubin) and a secondary and weaker site with a binding constant of 10^6. The second site is therefore occupied only if the bilirubin:albumin molar ratio exceeds unity or if other endogenous or exogenous compounds compete successfully for the stronger binding site. To a minor degree, bilirubin is also bound to red cell membranes. When all possible binding sites are occupied, the pigment is believed to circulate as free molecules. Thus, once hyperbilirubinemia has become excessive (at an uncertain and variable plasma concentration), the brain may be damaged. This is known to be due to the entry of divalent bilirubin (acid) into neuron membranes. There bilirubin binds to phospholipids, causing distortion of the cell and, as the bound pigment precipitates, leads to the cell's eventual destruction [20].

Broderson [21] formulated the process that establishes equilibrium of bilirubin concentration between plasma and tissue:

$$\text{bilirubin–albumin} + 2H \rightleftharpoons \text{bilirubin–membrane} + \text{albumin}$$
$$\text{(anion)} \qquad\qquad\qquad \text{(acid)}$$

He considers the bilirubin–membrane complex to be a solid with fixed chemical potential, as represented by the following equation:

$$\frac{[\text{bilirubin–albumin}][H^-]^2}{[\text{reserve albumin}]} = K$$

The left side of this equation is an expression of the molar ratio of bound bilirubin (unconjugated plasma bilirubin concentration) to that of reserve albumin (albumin–bilirubin binding capacity) times the squared hydrogen ion concentration (plasma pH). Equilibrium of bilirubin in plasma with that in tissue occurs when $K \approx 3 \times 10^{-15}$ M^2. If the value of the left side of the equation exceeds K, bilirubin will be transported from plasma to tissues. Thus the numerical value of the left side of the equation indicates the toxicity of the plasma bilirubin.

Nearly all tissues having collagen and fat cells will accept bilirubin, especially the skin and subcutaneous fatty tissues. It is this deposit that accounts for the visible expression of hyperbilirubinemia.

Albumin-bound bilirubin cannot cross the blood-brain barrier and thus cytotoxicity and bilirubin encephalopathy are prevented. However, many components of extracellular fluid affect the bilirubin binding of albumin, including organic anions, pH, and ionic strength. In the newborn, particularly the premature and the small for gestational age, many factors combine to raise serum bilirubin levels (22). In addition to acidosis, hypoalbuminemia, and hypoxia, which can effect the binding of bilirubin to albumin, there is often an excessive production of bilirubin due to the shorter (90-day) life span of fetal erythrocytes, plethora from delayed clamping of the cord, increased entero-hepatic circulation due to absence of intestinal flora or delayed passage of meconium, hemolysis due to fetal–maternal blood type incompatibility, sepsis, etc. (23–25).

In utero, the bilirubin in the fetal circulation must be excreted trans-placentally; this requires that it be lipid-soluble. After birth, conjugation in the liver (usually with glucuronic acid) is required in order to render the bilirubin sufficiently water-soluble so that it can be excreted into the bile. In some infants, delayed maturation of the uridine disphosphate glucuronyl trans-ferase (UDPGT) enzyme system may contribute to bilirubin accumulation in the circulation by restricting the conjugating capacity of the neonatal liver. When the serum bilirubin concentration reaches about 6 mg/dl the presence of bilirubin in the skin can be observed by the characteristic yellow pigmentation (jaundice) that bilirubin imparts.

In a series of papers, Kapoor and co-workers (26–28) have shown that human (adult) skin and skin epithelium readily take up both free and albumin-bound bilirubin in vitro, with the free bilirubin being absorbed 3.5 times more readily than the bound. Kapoor reported K_m values of 1.8×10^{-3} M for serum-bound bilirubin and 0.3×10^{-3} M for free bilirubin with human skin epithelium. In investigations with purified collagen fibrils obtained from rat tail tendons Kapoor obtained a K_a for the binding of collagen to bilirubin of 5.4×10^3 M^{-1}, with 380 nmol of bilirubin bound per mg of collagen at $37°C$. Salicylate and sulfanilamide, known to displace bilirubin from albumin (29), did not displace bilirubin from collagen, but did displace bilirubin from albumin to collagen. Kapoor also demonstrated that light-irradiated bilirubin in aqueous solution underwent photodecomposition more slowly than when absorbed on human skin segments and that the photodecomposition products were different in the two cases, although they were not identified.

By applying opaque patches to the skin of infants under phototherapy, Vogl (30) concluded that the skin is the principal site for the action of phototherapy in vivo. He observed that, after phototherapy, the patch leaves a sharply defined area of jaundice surrounded by otherwise photobleached skin. The pigment transition region, often as narrow as 1 mm, persists for several hours after the termination of phototherapy. This indicates indirectly that the photoeffect occurs within 1 mm of the surface of the skin. It also demonstrates that the skin binds bilirubin very tightly, since no lateral diffusion was observable.

One possible interpretation of a study (31) of intermittent phototherapy of low-birth-weight infants is that phototherapy has minimal effect on serum bilirubin levels below 6–8 mg/dl, the level at which jaundice becomes clinically evident by virtue of sufficient pigment accumulation in the skin. All these results suggest strongly that the primary site of action of phototherapy is in the skin.

Schmid and Hammaker (32) have shown that in the hyperbilirubinemic rat, an appreciable fraction of the bilirubin pool is in the adipose tissue and in the skin. If the same fraction of the bilirubin pool is present in the skin of infants, this would represent a potent protective mechanism for the infant, since bilirubin is tightly bound to collagen and thus not available for cytotoxic action in the neural tissue. Furthermore, deposition of bilirubin on collagen frees albumin in the serum to bind and transport additional bilirubin. That extravascular sites for bilirubin storage are a significant factor in the newborn is confirmed by the fact that following an exchange transfusion there is a rebound of serum bilirubin concentration that peaks approximately 4–8 hr hours after the exchange (33). This indicates that the release of extravascular bilirubin into the circulation is both slow and of significant quantity.

Photochemistry of Bilirubin

Since the discovery of phototherapy by Cremer et al. (8), considerable effort has gone into the determination of the effects of optical radiation on bilirubin both in vivo and in vitro. These studies have shown that bilirubin in vitro can participate in a large number of photochemical reactions yielding a host of end products that are strongly dependent on the chemical environment of the bilirubin (34). The lability of bilirubin and the large number and short lifetimes of its photochemical intermediates and of many of its end products, complicate precise determinations of pathways and products. For example, Lightner and Quinstad (35, 36) have shown that bilirubin photooxidizes to methylvinylmaleimide, hematinic acid, and propentdyopents. Ostrow et al. (37) have shown that phototautomerism occurs and have also reported the

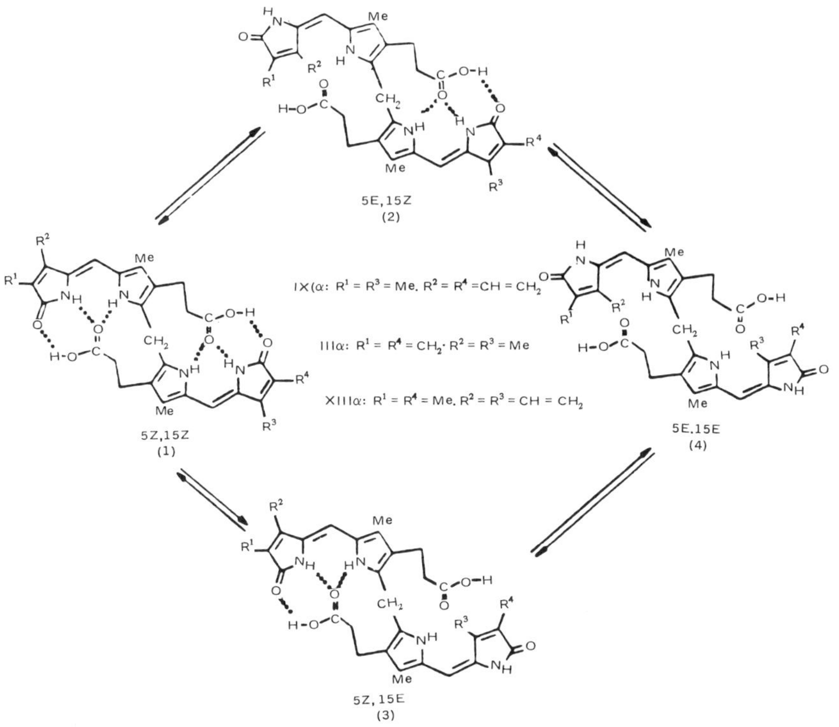

Fig. 16-1. The scheme presented here summarizes the overall photochemical transformations but omits intermediate structures that may be important for the free acid. For example, thermal reversion of (5E,15Z)-BR-IX-α would be expected to lead first to a (5Z,15Z)-conformer (not shown) which is less extensively hydrogen bonded than the more stable (5Z,15Z)-conformer that is finally obtained. [From McDonagh et al. (41).]

formation of mono- and dipyrroles. Garbagnati and Manitto (38) have demonstrated the formation of adducts of bilirubin with substances containing hydroxyl and sulfhydryl groups, such as glutathione and N-acetyl-L-cysteine. McDonagh (39) presented incontrovertible evidence that phototherapy induces the enhanced excretion of a diazo-positve, bilirubin-like substance in the bile of both Gunn rats and infants. This phenomenon at one time led to the speculation that the light may cause the liver to "leak" lipid-soluble substances or to cause the hepatocyte membrane to become permeable to albumin. Ostrow et al. (37) showed this not to be the case. Subsequently it was suggested that in vivo the light acts on the bilirubin so as to form photoproduct(s) and / or adduct(s) that the liver does not recognize as bilirubin, possibly because of increased water solubility, and therefore excretes by an alternative pathway. However, McDonagh (39) and Odell (131) showed that the material isolated after phototherapy increased excretion into the bile duct is IX-α bilirubin. In 1977, Zenone et al. (40) reported the presence

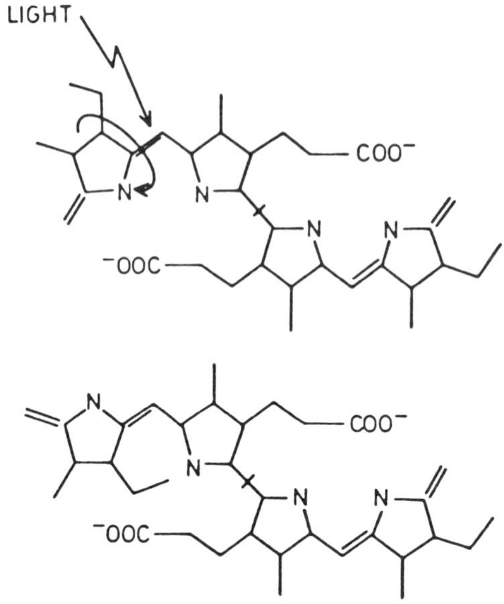

LIGHT

Fig. 16-2. Representation of the photoconversion of bilirubin IX-α. Light converts bilirubin IX-α (Z,Z) to photobilirubin IX-α (E,Z) by a twist of one outer pyrrole ring at the double bond. Photobilirubin does not form an insoluble acid, is rapidly excreted in bile without undergoing conjugation, and is nontoxic to neuronal tissues. [From Broderson (21).]

of bilirubin photoisomers in the bile of Gunn rats, and in 1979 McDonagh et al. (41) showed that bilirubin underwent photoisomerization at the meso double bond to a less lipophylic, less internally hydrogen-bonded form (Fig. 16-1). Under the conditions reported in their paper the main photoproduct of IX-α bilirubin (detected chromatographically) is an unresolved mixture of E,Z and Z,E isomers. This reaction occurs readily in bilirubin solutions exposed to light but is undetectable by silica chromatography and is difficult to detect by simple absorbance measurements. Thus IX-α bilirubin, despite extensive hydrogen bonding, can be photoconverted to more polar configurational isomers that the liver can excrete by a different pathway (Fig. 16-2). The sudden increase in biliary excretion of bilirubin and related bile pigments when jaundiced rats (42, 43) and babies (44) are irradiated with visible light is finally explained.

Dose–Response Relationship of Phototherapy and Time Constant of Bilirubin Diffusion

A series of studies (31, 45–49) have shown that the dose–response relationship of serum bilirubin levels to light exposure is logarithmic (see Fig. 16-3). The curve that describes the intermittent white light phototherapy clearly exhibits unexplained anomalous behavior.

Within broad limits the response of serum bilirubin concentration to phototherapy depends only on the integrated dose, not on whether that dose is delivered intermittently or continuously. Vogl and associates also demon-

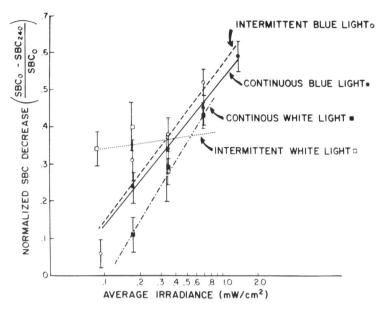

Fig. 16-3. Decrements of serum bilirubin concentration under increasing fluance of white and blue lights, continuous compared to intermittent exposure. [From Vogl et al. (47).]

strated that the decrease in serum bilirubin concentration with time under phototherapy is initially exponential (Fig. 16.4), implying a dominant first-order (passive concentration gradient driven) diffusion process. It is therefore likely that the diffusion time of the bilirubin into or out of the skin is the rate-limiting process. The slowness of the equilibration of serum and skin bilirubin was illustrated by a single series of experiments conducted on a 4-year-old boy with Crigler–Najjar syndrome (132). This child slept prone for

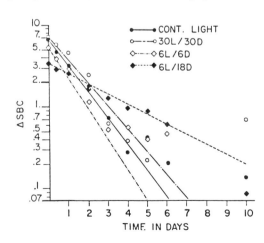

Fig. 16-4. Change in concentration of bilirubin in serum under: constant light exposure; 30 min light/30 min dark; 6 hr light/6 hr dark; and 6 hr light/18 hr dark. [From Vogl et al. (46).]

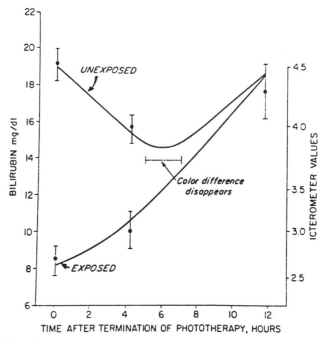

Fig. 16-5. The redistribution of bilirubin bound to skin tissues of a patient with Crigler–Najjar syndrome (congenital deficiency of UDPGT in the liver) after phototherapy. [From Vogl (132).]

12–14 hr per night under Special Blue Lamps (Westinghouse fluorescent lamps F20T12/BB with principal spectral radiance 420–470 nm). During 2 days of observation he had an opaque patch placed over his thoracic vertebrae before going to sleep. In the morning, the unbleached area under the patch was clearly discernible and, by use of a Gossett icterometer (50), his skin color was monitored during the day. As can be seen from Fig. 16-5, the jaundice of the light-bleached skin slowly increased after termination of phototherapy and that of the unexposed area slowly decreased, so that approximately 5 hr after the termination of phototherapy the degree of jaundice in the two areas matched and could no longer be differentiated. From that time on, until the child was again placed under phototherapy for the night, the two areas increased in jaundice together. This clearly indicates that while there is little transverse diffusion of bilirubin in the skin, there is diffusion of untransformed bilirubin from the unpatched area into the circulation when the serum bilirubin concentration is decreased. This experiment indicates a time constant in the range of 3–6 hr, a value in agreement with that found previously in infants (30) and in intact rats (46, 47). The effect of the extravascular compartments on the stabilization of serum bilirubin concentration becomes evident when this time constant is compared to the 5-min response time to phototherapy that is found when bilirubin excretion is measured directly in the bile duct (43).

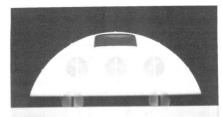
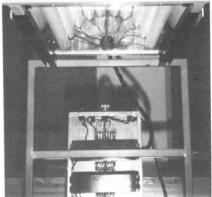

Fig. 16-6. A type of phototherapy unit holding 10 fluorescent lamps in hemicylindrical apposition against a reflecting surface. A Plexiglas shield ½ in. thick at the open side of the unit filters all radiation below 390 nm. The unit rests on a frame which will fit over a bassinet.

Instrumentation and Methods of Measurement

It is not enough merely to bathe an infant in light to correct hyperbilirubinemia. Attention must be paid to the radiant intensity as well as to the spectral distribution incident on the infant. The amount of visible light in the blue range (400–490 nm) and particularly the output around 450 nm, the absorption peak of bilirubin, influences the effectiveness of the therapy. Most phototherapy units under commercial manufacture have 6–8 fluorescent lamps placed side by side in a flat canopy which may be placed over a basinet. A canopy (Fig. 16-6) holding 10 lamps in a hemicylindrical configuration is a more powerful source, and permits more uniform irradiation of an infant.

Regardless of shape, phototherapy hoods or canopies are designed to hold fluorescent lamps, which may be of three types: (1) white or broad-spectrum—so-called "daylight" lamps (F20T12/D); (2) somewhat narrower spectrum standard "blue" lamps (F20T12/B); or (3) narrow-spectrum Special Blue lamps (F20T12/BB) of longer life and much greater output in the critical wavelengths between 420 and 470 nm (Fig. 16-7). This last-mentioned light source is the most efficient (49). In recent years, however, phototherapy units employing quartz–halide lamps with tungsten filaments having a high intensity of broad-spectrum emission have been produced. They are nearly as effective in reducing plasma bilirubin concentration as the Special Blue lamps (51). This effectiveness is the result of the higher intensity of radiation generated by these sources.

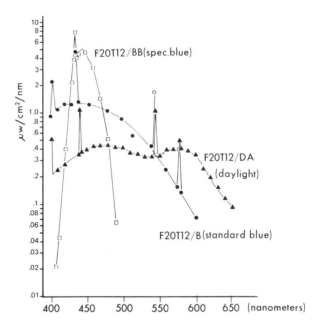

Fig. 16-7. Spectral distribution of various fluorescent lamps commonly used in neonatal phototherapy. The output of energy at 450–460 nm, the absorption peak of bilirubin in sera, is higher in standard blue compared with "daylight" lamps, and much greater in the Special Blue (narrow spectrum) lamps. [From Sisson et al. (49).]

Fluorescent lamp units are generally placed 18–24 in. above the unclothed infant. A Plexiglas shield is used to block UV radiation from fluorescent lamps. The eyes of the irradiated infants must be shielded from the light, lest irreparable damage be done to their retinas.

The amount of radiation to which infants are exposed varies greatly, depending on the energy output of the light sources and the spectral distribution of the lamps used. In general clinical application, constant irradiation in a range of 30–40 $\mu W/cm^2/nm$ (at 420–470 nm) is used (Fig. 16-8), although intermittent exposure (Fig. 16-9) has been employed with more or less success (46, 47, 52). Clinically adequate radiation from the standpoint of rapidity of bilirubin degradation (as measured by daily plasma bilirubin decrement) is about 34 $\mu W/cm^2/nm$ at 420–470 nm (49).

Despite these and other research efforts, much detailed information about the sites and mechanisms of in vivo phototherapy remains unknown. It is remarkable that despite the many man-years of solid scientific effort that have been devoted to the problem, our knowledge of phototherapy and its mechanisms remains so limited. A possible explanatory factor may be the lack of optical and spectrophotometric expertise in the design and execution of both in vitro and in vivo experiments. Commercial instrumentation for determining the absorption spectrum of a bilirubin solution is generally

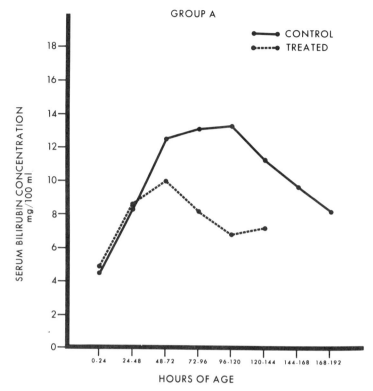

Fig. 16-8. The effect of continuous phototherapy upon the serum bilirubin concentrations of 35 neonates with physiologic hyperbilirubinemia, compared with 37 matched control infants having the same condition but not treated. Mean peak bilirubin concentrations were lower and declined earlier in the treated group. [Modified from Sisson (134).]

available to most investigators. However, experiments in photobiology and photochemistry have often been carried out using white light, or light that has been filtered through relatively wide band-pass filters. Consequently the differences in reaction rates and products have not been studied using spectrally narrow wavelength bands. The execution of these experiments has been hampered to some extent by the unavailability of suitable light sources. It is unfortunate that until very recently the ideally suited tunable dye lasers have been available only in the spectral bands on either side of the bilirubin absorption band, but not in the band of interest. While such equipment is now available, it is relatively expensive, and difficult to set up, and the technologies involved are not familiar to most biomedical researchers.

In vivo the problem is even more difficult. Until 1969, when Sisson et al. (53) and 1972, when Kline (54) pointed out that radiometric, rather than photometric units, were appropriate in the measurement of phototherapy radiance, almost all published papers reported light measurements made with

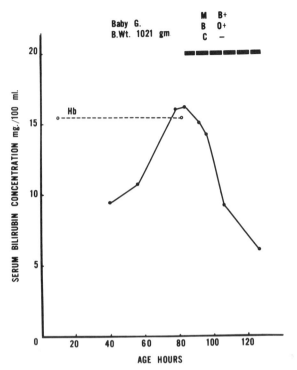

Fig. 16-9. Effectiveness of intermittent phototherapy of a very immature infant in rapid reduction of hyperbilirubinemia. Solid line, serum bilirubin concentration; dashed line, hemoglobin concentration; thick bars, phototherapy, 6 hr on/2 hr off. Light source was standard blue fluorescent lamps F20 T12/B, 40 cm from infant, with an irradiance of 18 μW/cm^2/nm in the 425–475 nm band. (T.R.C. Sisson, unpublished data.)

a photographic light meter. These meters, matched to the spectral sensitivity of photographic film (and the eye), produced values that were misleading to the phototherapeutic situation since the sensitivity of these meters at the far blue end of the visible spectrum is not only very low, but variable and uncontrolled in design.

Since 1972 clinical experiments have increasingly used spectroradiometers for the measurement of incident light intensity. The in vivo action spectrum for phototherapy was finally established by Ballowitz et al. (45) in 1977. Unfortunately, many of the commercially available spectroradiometers likely to be available at moderate cost are not suited to the task, due to a combination of three circumstances: (1) many of these instruments utilize detectors that are more sensitive in the red than in the blue (e.g., silicon photodetectors); (2) the light band to be measured is selected by glass or gelatin filters (most of which permit the passage of between 0.1% and 3% of the incident radiation in the red); and (3) the instrument is calibrated with a tungsten light source that emits several orders of magnitude more energy at the red end of the spectrum than at the blue end. The net result of this combination can be a calibration error of 2 or 3 orders of magnitude when fluorescent sources are measured. Thus a clinical investigator using an instrument whose calibration is reported to be traceable to a National Bureau of Standards calibrated light source (almost all of which are tungsten sources) can be severely misled in his readings when measuring fluorescent light sources with spectral distributions markedly different from tungsten lamps. This unfortunate situation applied to the work of Mims et al. (48), and their careful experiment was marred by a 2 order-of-magnitude error in the calibration supplied with their commercial instrument when it was used to measure the blue light output of fluorescent lamps (55).

For purposes of order-of-magnitude calibration, investigators should be aware that typical clinical phototherapy units (using 6–8 fluorescent tubes) deliver between 0.2 and 1.5 mW/cm^2 in the 425–500-nm band to the infant. Detailed discussions of some of the photometric problems have been published (55, 56). Investigators who are considering approaching this field for the first time are urged to avail themselves of the expertise of competent optical engineers.

NEONATAL JAUNDICE

Neurotoxicity of Bilirubin

A causal relationship between high concentrations of bilirubin in the plasma of the newborn and the more severe form of bilirubin encephalopathy was long suspected. Infants with hemolytic disease of the newborn caused by incompatibility of maternal and fetal blood with respect to the Rh factor usually developed hyperbilirubinemia of marked degree and shortly thereafter developed central nervous system damage. If they lived, these infants often suffered from cerebral palsy, deafness, spasticity, and other crippling neurologic symptoms. In the early 1950s a number of investigators (57–61) recognized the etiologic significance of hyperbilirubinemia in kernicterus. In 1953, Claireaux et al. (62) finally proved that bilirubin appears in kernicteric nerve tissue and that this could be only free bilirubin. Shortly thereafter, Waters et al. (63) isolated bilirubin from chloroform extracts of brain tissue, and Day (64) demonstrated that the respiratory rate of brain cells was diminished 25% by bilirubin, but that oxidation of bilirubin mitigates this effect.

With the knowledge that free unconjugated bilirubin can enter brain tissue and cause irreversible cellular changes or cell death, studies were undertaken to determine those levels that might cause such toxicity. Since hyperbilirubinemia could not be justifiably induced in newborns, retrospective examinations of jaundiced infants of various birth weights and degrees of gestational maturity were made, and those infants who were autopsied were studied for correlations between serum bilirubin concentrations before death and evidence of bilirubin staining of the brain, particularly the basal ganglia. Hsia et al. (59, 60) and Brown and Zuelzer (65) found that kernicterus rarely occurred if serum bilirubin concentrations were below 10 mg/dl, and occurred frequently over 30 mg/dl. Lesser degrees of damage may, however, occur and indeed be so subtle as to be inapparent until school age. For instance, it has been shown (66) that peak concentrations of bilirubin in the serum of full-term newborn infants as low as 15 mg/dl were associated in about 50% of cases studied with some neurologic damage at 4–7 years of age. Such damage is difficult to discern and may, in some instances, appear as visual—motor perception dysfunction. The situation for the small and immature infant is even more uncertain, for incontrovertible histologic proof of kernicterus in such vulnerable infants has been reported when serum bilirubin levels did not exceed 10 mg/dl (67–69).

For many years it was felt that neonatal hyperbilirubinemia did not need treatment when serum levels were below 20 mg/dl because, statistically speaking, kernicterus rarely appeared when only lower concentrations were reached (59). Clinicians are now more sensitive to the fact that kernicterus is an end stage of bilirubin toxicity, and to fail to treat at lower levels than 20 mg/dl may condemn an infant to unnecessary, though perhaps milder, neurologic injury.

We now know that a number of factors significantly influence the availability of free bilirubin in plasma—the villain of the piece. These factors are: (a) the degree of maturity of the infant, (b) the cause of hyperbilirubinemia in the individual patient, (c) the clinical condition of the infant, (d) the available binding sites of bilirubin to albumin and red cells, and (e) interference with bilirubin binding, conjugation, and excretion.

In no sense can these factors be considered as mutually exclusive, for in any given patient at least two will be interrelated. Serum bilirubin concentrations serve only to give a rough approximation of the extent of the accumulation of the pigment in the body. Any level of bilirubin in plasma above 1 or 2 mg/dl indicates that its production exceeds the body's capacity to excrete it at that moment. Serial measurements demonstrating a rapid rise in concentration indicate an excessive production, and help confirm the decision to treat. The clinical manifestations of hyperbilirubinemia in the newborn relate initially to a yellowing of the skin which becomes visible to the practiced eye as plasma concentrations exceed 5–6 mg/dl. Jaundice appears first on the face, then the trunk, and finally the extremities. As jaundice deepens, the skin develops an orange rather than saffron hue, and the plethoric or crying infant takes on an unusual ruddy complexion. This is as easily apparent in the black as the Caucasian infant, although the change is more subtle in the Oriental.

The binding of bilirubin to albumin in plasma ensures its transport to the liver, where it is taken up by acceptor proteins (Ligandin) (70) in the liver cell, conjugated to bilirubin glucuronide by action of UDPGT in the mito-chondria, and then released into the bile. Upon excretion into the gut the bilirubin is in large measure excreted, but a significant amount may be deconjugated, chiefly by β-glucuronidase, an exzyme elaborated in the mucosa, and thence reabsorbed into the circulation. This last process is called the "enterohepatic circulation" of bilirubin and is the physiologic basis of other therapies designed to interrupt its reabsorption. Unfortunately, these therapies are often difficult to administer reproducibly and hence are of uncertain success.

Etiology of Neonatal Hyperbilirubinemia

The causes of noeonatal jaundice are varied. A partial inability to conjugate and excrete this pigment to a degree equal to or greater than its rate of production is common, occurring in nearly half of all infants in the newborn period; it becomes a matter of concern in about 10% of infants. Thus it has been estimated that about 100,000 infants in this country, perhaps more, are annually at risk of bilirubin toxicity and require treatment. Those jaundiced infants not at risk are said to have "physiologic" or, more accu-rately, "developmental" jaundice (L. M. Gartner, personal communication).

The classic cause of pathologic hyperbilirubinemia in infants is hemolytic disease of the newborn (HMD), a rapid destruction of the neonate's red blood cells by autoimmune antibodies from the mother that circulate in the fetus's blood and cause hemagglutination. Originally HMD referred mainly to a maternal–fetal blood group incompatibility of the Rh system, but now also includes the major A–B–O groupings as well as a few minor blood group antibodies. The widespread use of passsive immunization of Rh-negative mothers, who are in danger of sensitization by Rh-positive fetuses, has greatly reduced the incidence of neonatal hemolytic disease due to this blood group system, but there is no preventative in the case of a mother and infant with incompatible A–B–O group blood. Consequently the incidence of the usually milder hemolytic disease from this cause continues unabated.

Increased red blood cell breakdown accompanies other disease states. Studies throughout the world have brought to light variants of glucose-6-phosphate dehydrogenase (G-6-PD) deficiency that cause neonatal hemolysis and severe jaundice among Greeks (71), Bantus (72), and Chinese (73), but such a consequence has not been noted in non-Ashkenazi Jews (74), or in American blacks (75, 76).

Such selective appearance of severe jaundice in some ethnic groups and not in others is due to the large number of variants of this enzyme deficiency with different phenotypic expression.

Several genetically determined disturbances of the glycolytic cycle of erythrocytes have been identified (77). Congenital nonspherocytic hemolytic anemia from any one of these genetic defects may result in hyperbilirubinemia. Jaundice has resulted from such inborn errors of red cell metabolism as pyruvate kinase deficiency, from hereditary spherocytosis, from hereditary absence of glutathione, and, as noted above, in some variants of G-6-PD deficiency. Transient defects of erythrocyte metabolism, infantile pyknocytosis, and glutathione deficiency induced by visible light radiation (78; L. Johnson, personal communication) have also been associated with hemolysis.

If infants deficient in G-6-PD are exposed to certain drugs, hemolysis and hyperbilirubinemia will ensue. This has been reported in relationship to the administration of primaquine, vitamin K, and sulfamethoxypyridazine (79). Drug-induced jaundice has been reported in premature infants who received large amounts of menadione, a vitamin K analog (80).

A common cause of neonatal hemolysis leading to hyperbilirubinemia is infection, either congenital or neonatal. Infection in the newborn often leads rapidly to bacterial or viral sepsis, and a diagnostic sign of this is jaundice.

The newborn infant characteristically is born with relatively high hemoglobin concentration and hematocrit. There is a rapid breakdown of red cells in the first days of life, in part due to the shorter life span of neonatal red cells compared with red cells in the child or adult. This results in an excessive release of heme and production of bilirubin. In the case of the infant who has received a placental transfusion by milking of the cord or other mechanical means, the resulting plethora almost guarantees the appearance of jaundice. The infant of a diabetic mother tends to be plethoric and to develop jaundice to some degree, as does the infant who, for whatever reason, is small for its gestational age, the so-called "low-birth-weight" infant.

Enclosed hemorrhage is a common result of the birth process. Many infants have hemorrhages under the scalp, known as cephalhematoma, or in the skin of those areas excessively squeezed in the birth canal, such as the buttocks in breech delivery. Red blood cells in such hematomata break down, with release of heme and consequent further decomposition to bilirubin, which is absorbed into the circulation. In the full-term infant this is usually innocuous, but in the premature infant the resultant jaundice may be significant.

Interference with the conjugation of bilirubin will also result in hyperbilirubinemia. Hepatic metabolism of bilirubin may be impaired by one of several mechanisms; (1) inadequate production of Ligandin, identified as glutathione transferase B (81), which transfers bilirubin from plasma to the cytoplasm of the liver cell; (2) deficiency of glucuronyl transferase due to immaturity (of liver function or of the whole organism) or a congenital defect—Crigler–Najjar syndrome (82); (3) inhibition of conjugation by hormones (83) or drugs (84), such as maternal steroids or novobiocin; (4) hepatic cell damage from infection, drugs, or hypoxia; or (5) complex metabolic factors, such as maternal diabetes, hypoglycemia, hypothyroidism, or acidosis.

Disturbances of bilirubin excretion may lead to increase in plasma bilirubin levels. Deconjugation of bilirubin in the lumen of the intestine by the action of the enzyme β-glucuronidase allows reabsorption of the now unconjugated pigment into the blood stream. In the neonate with delayed peristalsis or obstruction of the bowel, especially by meconium plug, reabsorption is significant. A few unfortunate infants suffer from congenital biliary obstruction which leads to a regurgitative form of jaundice.

Displacement of bilirubin from its binding site on the albumin molecule has been observed to result when serum free fatty acids exceed four molecules per molecule of albumin, and in the presence of some sulfonamides, parabenes, acetyltryptophan, caprylate, diphenylhydramine (85) stabilizers of antibiotics (84), and benzoate (86).

Since the premature infant tends to be hypoalbuminemic, available binding sites for bilirubin are diminished. The sick infant, especially the immature newborn with respiratory distress and/or sepsis, tends to be acidotic and hypoxic. These two conditions are thought to affect adversely the albumin binding of bilirubin.

Monitoring Hyperbilirubinemia

Serum bilirubin concentrations have been used for over three decades as an indication for exchange transfusion. Nonetheless, no matter how meticulously the determination may be made, there is no firm assurance that the concentration is predictive of the risk of bilirubin toxicity.

It has been determined that the reserve capacity of albumin to bind bilirubin can be measured, though with uncertain accuracy. The more commonly used methods for measuring reserve binding capacity are:

1. Saturation index (87, 88)
2. Phenolsulfonphthalein (PSP) binding (89)
3. HBABA, 2(4'-hydroxybenzeneazo) benzoic acid (66, 90)
4. Sephadex column chromatography (91)
5. Peroxidase (92)
6. Front-face fluorospectroscopy (93)

It is believed that when the reserve binding capacity of albumin is exhausted, excess bilirubin will be present in the plasma not bound to protein and thus able to penetrate cells of the central nervous system. It is believed that if both serum bilirubin concentration and reserve binding capacity of albumin are determined, dangerous bilirubin levels can be anticipated. For a time it was also felt that if one could measure the amount of free bilirubin in plasma, the infant at risk could be identified and treatment instituted. Unfortunately, it is not clear whether unbound bilirubin can actually be measured. It occurs in minute amounts, and the measurements are exquisitely sensitive to minor changes in laboratory conditions.

The correlation of reserve-binding capacity and incidence of bilirubin encephalopathy is not great. This lack of correlation may be due in part to the high margin of error in such determinations (up to 50%). A recently developed instrument employs front-face spectrofluorometry of whole blood. A few drops serve as a sample, yielding total bilirubin level, its conjugated fraction, and the bilirubin-binding capacity of the blood (93). This promising instrument is still under trial and is not commercially available at the time of writing. Few clinical laboratories are equipped to perform any of these reserve binding-capacity tests.

At present the clinician is still forced to rely on serial determinations of the serum concentration of bilirubin, correlating this level at frequent intervals with the clinical condition of the infant, and treating hyperbilirubinemia when experience dictates that the jaundiced infant is at risk of brain damage. No fixed level of safety can be assumed, and clinical interpretation must take its usual course.

There are experimental (94, 95) and clinical (96) observations to support the belief that phototherapy will prevent bilirubin encephalopathy as effectively as exchange transfusion. In these experiments the normal growth and development of congenitally icteric rats was preserved by photoirradiation, kernicterus and nerve damage were prevented (94), and destruction of Purkinje cells did not occur (95). In photo-irradiated low-birth-weight infants no deterioration of neurologic development was observed (96).

As described above, phototransformation of bilirubin in vivo takes place primarily in the skin (30). However, the penetrance of visible light is far deeper than is generally appreciated, and bilirubin in the plasma, especially in the vascular bed of the skin, is also transformed. The transmission of both blue and white light from fluorescent sources through the abdominal wall of the living Gunn rat and infant pig has been shown by Sisson and Wickler (97) to be about 20–23%. Studies by Viggiani et al. (98) demonstrated a significant transmission of white light through the skull and brain tissues of rats. These observations strongly suggest that the action of light on bilirubin is not confined solely to the tissues of skin, but includes at least the peripheral vascular bed and possibly organs and tissues more deeply placed.

REACTIONS AND SIDE REACTIONS

Visible light is a ubiquitous part of our environment. The notion that light can be only beneficial has a seductive and plausible attraction. Nevertheless, we must recognize that light can cause some harm either directly or indirectly. It is a fact that we do not yet know the true extent of the biologic influences of electromagnetic energy on the newborn.

Clinical experience with phototherapy of hyperbilirubinemia has shown no evidence of long-term deleterious effects. Nonetheless, the potential for undesirable consequences of this form of radiation exists, and potentially detrimental effects continue to be discovered in vitro (99).

We do know of certain short-term effects. Rubaltelli et al. (100) have shown that the tryptophan–kynurenine pathway is disturbed in light-irradiated infants because of the photodestruction of the metabolites of tryptophan.

The normal concentration of riboflavin, vitamin B₂, in whole blood is dramatically reduced by phototherapy of the newborn (Fig. 16-10). The in vivo and in vitro reduction of riboflavin has been associated with a deficiency of G-6-PD (101) and with deficiency of glutathione and glutathione reductase (78, 102; T. R. C. Sisson and T. Fiorentino, unpublished observations; L. Johnson, personal communication). These enzyme deficiencies, occurring only under phototherapy, lead to increased hemolysis and consequent light-induced increase in bilirubin concentrations. However, black infants with congenital G-6-PD deficiency do not develop light-induced hemolysis and

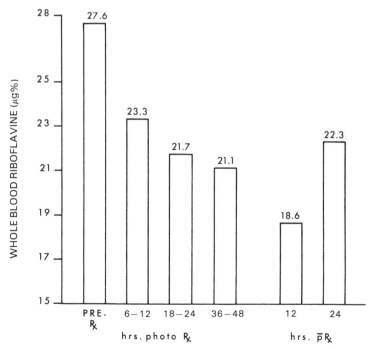

Fig. 16-10. Mean whole-blood riboflavin levels of 21 infants before, during, and after 48 hr of exposure to continuous phototherapy. [From Sisson et al. (101).]

hyperbilirubinemia. Therefore, one may reasonably conclude that the accelerated jaundice under light, a failure of phototherapy, is due to the reduction of erythrocyte riboflavin. Riboflavin is an essential coenzyme for the activity of G-6-PD and glutathione. Therefore, riboflavin is essential for red cell respiration, and its absence will cause red cell hemolysis.

Visible light may induce enzyme production. Yeary et al. (103) have demonstrated increased UDPGT activity in hepatic microsomes of the Gunn rat, and the photoactivation of cytochrome P448 has been demonstrated in liver cell cultures (104). Sisson et al. (105), in preliminary studies on the effect of irradiation of the perfused Gunn rat liver with blue light (420–475 nm), demonstrated that the activity of cytochrome P450, cytochrome b5, p-nitrophenol glucuronidation, benzo(a)pyrene and aniline hydroxylation, and aminopyrine demethylation were all increased an average of 40%. These results have interesting implications for drug kinetics and metabolism in the newborn, whose metabolic activity is notoriously slow (Table 16-1).

Plasma amino acids are affected by phototherapy—minimally in vivo (101) and significantly in vitro in the presence of dye sensitizers (106), when oxidation of histidine residues of albumin will occur. Rubaltelli and Jori (107, 133) have shown that irradiation of bilirubin-bound albumin causes a selective modification of two histidyl residues of albumin that are essential for the binding of bilirubin. Cashore et al. (108) observed that phototherapy does not affect the albumin–bilirubin binding capacity of the newborn.

Of great importance are the findings that visible light has the capacity to inactivate purified DNA and to kill bacteria in cultures (109). Speck and Rossenkranz (110, 111) have shown that when DNA–bilirubin complex in mammalian cell culture is exposed to broad-spectrum light, the bilirubin moiety is photoactivated, causing a cleavage of bonds within DNA. Inter-

Table 16-1. Enzyme Activity of Perfused Gunn Rat Livers (μmol/g)

Enzyme	Dark			Light	
	jj	jj	Jj	jj	jj
Aminopyrene demethylation	3.028	3.77	1.835	5.175	5.089
Aniline dehydroxylation	0.151	0.187	0.147	0.301	0.335
Cytochrome P450	0.435	0.442	0.387	0.608	0.762
Cytochrome b5	0.792	0.551	0.554	0.808	0.794
Benzo(a)pyrene hydroxylation	0.569	0.772	0.351	0.924	1.743
p-Nitrophenol glucuronidation	2.592	1.350	2.082	4.607	4.639
					5.020

mittent phototherapy, far from sparing DNA the disruptive effect of constant irradiation, appears to enhance it instead (112). In light irradiation of newborn infants (whose deep tissues receive significant amounts of photic energy from phototherapy), the potential consequences of cell damage must be considered when weighing the ratio of risk to benefit from the treatment. Permanent cell injury has not been documented (or, for that matter, observed) in the infant, and one must presume that repair mechanisms exist as they do in the case of UV-induced cell damage. Elkind and Han (113) have shown that there are significant differences—at the molecular level—in the effects produced by UV radiation and simulated sunlight (containing near-UV). They further emphasize the need for caution in attempting to extrapolate biologic systems, such as the cell. However, one must not be lulled into complacency by knowledge of related repair mechanisms or lack of observed harmful phenomena. Too little time has passed in the use of phototherapy to dismiss long-range possibilities; the first infants exposed to phototherapy have just entered their childbearing years.

Some short-term effects of phototherapy have modified the management of infants during treatment. A principal side reaction of phototherapy has been frequent loose stools, sometimes actual diarrhea. Several related effects may be involved. An increased gut-transit time has been reported by Rubaltelli and Largajolli (114). This physical effect in the gut (whether direct or indirect) is exacerbated by increased insensible water loss (115, 116) in infants under phototherapy. Any disturbance of fluid and electrolyte balance is poorly compensated by the newborn. Any increase of water loss places an unwanted metabolic demand upon even the healthy infant, and it is a particularly undesirable demand on the jaundiced immature neonate.

The frequent, loose, and usually discolored stools are the result of another effect of phototherapy besides rapid gut-transit time: a dysfunction of carbohydrate digestion. Bakken (117) demonstrated clinically and by histochemical studies of jejunal biopsies that lactase deficiency developed in neonates fed breast milk while under phototherapy. This study contradicted earlier conclusions (118). A prospective, controlled study was made of three groups of infants randomly fed either lactose-free milk or lactose-containing milk: one group of jaundiced infants was treated with blue light; one group of jaundiced infants was not irradiated; and one group of nonjaundiced infants, not irradiated, served as controls (119). It was found that the group of infants receiving a diet containing lactose and exposed to phototherapy developed frequent watery green stools, acidic in character and containing reducing substances (indicating nondigestion of disaccharides). These infants also had abnormal lactose tolerance tests. Matched infants on *lactose-free formula* did not demonstrate these abnormalities. Hyperbilirubinemia itself did not cause these deviations, regardless of diet, nor did control infants have such changes. It was concluded that intestinal lactase deficiency is caused by phototherapy, although the condition is limited to the period of irradiation, and the clinical abnormalities can be avoided by a lactose-free diet during treatment. It is not known whether inhibition of lactase activity is a direct or indirect result of phototherapy.

Direct effects of visible light on cells of the blood have been reported. Erythrocytes maintained in a liquid medium containing bilirubin and irradiated by broad-spectrum light were shown to lose K+, Na+, and ATPase activity and to undergo hemolysis (120). This suggests that red cell damage in an in vitro system is mediated by bilirubin-photosensitized oxidation in the membrane structure. Visible light irradiation of red cells of newborns (normal and jaundiced) causes the cells to swell and to lose glutathione (102; T. R. C. Sisson and T. Fiorentino, unpublished data). Maurer et al. (121) demonstrated in rabbits that exposure to phototherapy lights causes a shortened life span of blood platelets, and also increases the rate of platelet production. No convincing evidence that these events occur in vivo, in clinical phototherapy, has been reported, but the likelihood is disquieting.

The possibility that hyperbilirubinemia may exert an inhibitory effect on cellular immune responses in humans was proposed by Rola-Pleszczynski et al. (122), who demonstrated a significant decrease in cell-mediated immunity as measured by lymphoproliferative response to phytohemagglutin-P (PHA-P) in adult and cord lymphocytes incubated with increasing concentrations of bilirubin in the substrate.

These observations received confirmation from the studies of Rubaltelli et al. (123), who found that lymphoproliferative response to phytohemagglutin-M (PHA-M) in hyperbilirubinemic infants was inhibited in the presence of autologous plasma, contrary to the responses of normal infants and adults. Phototherapy did not overcome the inhibition. Their further investigations of the effect of bilirubin and light-irradiated bilirubin upon the phagocytic activity of granulocytes led them to conclude that bilirubin and phototreated bilirubin both inhibit the phagocytic function of polymorphonuclear cells, and that light exposure, at least in vitro, does not decrease the inhibitory effect of bilirubin (124). In another study this group of investigators showed that the spontaneous motility and chemotactic activity of phagocytes and T-cell function of newborns were decreased when incubated with either bilirubin or light-irradiated bilirubin. On the other hand, light exposure of such cells in the absence of either type of bilirubin had no effect (125, 126).

These studies indicate that phototherapy, though it may not reverse bilirubin's inhibitory effect, does not itself reduce the immunologic capacity of infants so treated. Phototherapy may, however, improve the milieu for resisting or combatting infection by reducing the concentration of bilirubin in an infant's blood and tissues.

Phototherapy in the newborn not only has effects upon molecular and cellular events, but also can exercise a profound influence on intrinsic biologic behavior. As an example, it has been demonstrated that, during the administration of phototherapy, the rapid eye movement (REM) sleep of infants increases not only in frequency but in duration, compared with infants in a normal nursery environment (127). Since it is believed that protein synthesis in cells of the central nervous system occurs mainly, if not entirely, during periods of REM sleep, one might theorize that promotion of this sleep state in the still-developing infant brain is advantageous.

Another important biologic phenomenon that is affected by the light environment of the newborn infant is rhythmicity. Sisson et al. (128–130) selected plasma human growth hormone (HGH, or somatotropin) as a marker for biologic rhythms in the neonate, and in a series of studies determined the pattern of rhythms of HGH in constant nursery light, in cycled light/dark, cycled bright light/dim light, and constant phototherapy (with eyes shielded from light).

They found that under constant nursery illumination normal newborns have ultradian rhythm of HGH of 4–6-hr intervals but no circadian rhythm. However, under cycled light there was not only an ultradian pattern but a circadian rhythm with peak at about midnight, as in the adult. Under phototherapy, constantly administered for 24-hr periods, both ultradian and circadian rhythms of HGH were obliterated (Fig. 16-11).

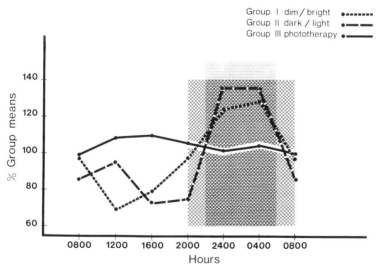

Fig. 16-11. Under cycled light, both dim/bright light and totally dark/light, a circadian rhythm of plasma human growth hormone is noted. Under continuous phototherapy, the circadian rhythm is obliterated. [From Sisson (135).]

Table 16-2. Summary of Side Effects of Phototherapy

Determined in vitro
    1. Albumin denaturation
    2. Diminished riboflavine levels
    3. G-6-PD activity loss
    4. Glutathione reductase activity loss
    5. Mutagenesis in cell cultures
    6. DNA modification
    7. Erythrocyte membrane alteration
    8. Plasma amino acid concentration
Determined in vivo (animals)
    1. Retinal damage
    2. Increased liver glycogen in rats
    3. Retarded gonadal growth (not function) in rats
    4. Inhibition of fertilization and embryonic development in sea urchins
    5. Decrease in circulating platelets
Determined in vivo (human infants)
    1. Excess body heat from thermal output of lamps
    2. Temporary growth retardation (head circumference)
    3. Increased insensible water loss
    4. Decreased G-6-PD and glutathione reductase activity
    5. Loose, discolored stools
    6. Intestinal lactase deficiency
    7. Reduction of whole-blood riboflavin
    8. Alteration of tryptophan–kynurenine metabolism
    9. Alteration of biologic rhythms
    10. Physical hazards from inappropriate phototherapy—unit construction
    11. Increase in gut-transit time
    12. Increase in respiration
    13. Increase in peripheral blood flow
    14. Alteration in plasma amino acids.

These findings suggest that the common practice of maintaining high illumination of nurseries night and day can eliminate the normal circadian rhythms of growth hormone, whereas cycling the nursery lights will permit a normal rhythm.

Phototherapy produces even more profound change by erasing *all* biorhythm of this important developmental hormone. The condition induced by the therapy is surely unphysiologic; its temporary nature may not exert a long-term effect, but certainly delays the establishment of a biologic rhythm normally present in the first day of life. The long-term consequences of this delay are unknown.

Table 16-2 summarizes the various side effects of neonatal phototherapy.

SUMMARY

There are many questions regarding the use of phototherapy in organisms as vulnerable as the newborn infant that remain unanswered. The optimum amount of radiant energy that should be employed to correct hyperbilirubinemia has not been established.

Evidence does not yet exist to indicate that intermittent phototherapy has a clinical advantage or disadvantage over continuous phototherapy. We do know that there are disadvantages to both, either in practical management of infants under treatment or in more subtle biologic effects at the molecular and cellular level.

Proponents of the concept that the wavelengths of light administered should be narrowly tailored to affect only the substance to be degraded (in this instance bilirubin and its absorption band in the blue portion of the spectrum) take the position that using the broad spectrum of visible light will lead to unwarranted photobiologic activity in other molecular or cellular components absorbing light in other spectral regions. Those who do not subscribe to this point of view consider the entire visible spectrum to be more physiologic and beneficial radiation for the human. The latter stand might have more scientific validity if it were not for the fact that light in the near-UV regions, to which we are also exposed naturally, is distinctly harmful. The argument is not easily settled.

The use of visible light as a therapeutic tool in the management of jaundice of the newborn has been uncommonly successful, and has been so easy of application that most physicians have been uncritically accepting of the technique. Some would maintain that investigators have had to go out of their way to find either fault or danger in this treatment. However, it is prudent to retain a certain skepticism about the ultimate effects and safety of phototherapy until medical science and its companion disciplines know more of the biologic impact of nonionizing electromagnetic radiation. It seems quite reasonable to deal with phototherapy as one would with a drug— cautiously.

REFERENCES

1. Shastid, T. H. (1948): The blue glass craze. In: *The Victor Robinson Memorial Volume: Essays on History of Medicine*, edited by S. R. Kagan, pp. 369–373. Froben Press, New York.
2. Pleasanton, A. J. (1876): *Blue and Sun-Lights: Their Influence upon Life, Disease, etc.* Claxton, Remsen & Haffelfinger, Philadelphia.
3. Baldwin, K. W. (1926): The therapeutic value of light and color. *Atlantic Medical Journal* 1926(Oct. 12).
4. Finsen, N. R. (1893): Am lysets indvirkninger paa huden. *Hospitalstidende* 1893(July 5).
5. Finsen, N. R. (1900): Neue Untersuchungen uber die Einwirkung des Lichtes auf die Haut. *Mitteilungen aus Finsens Medizinschem Institut* 1:8–34.
6. Fischer, H., and Herle, K. (1938): Einwirkung von Licht auf Porphyrine. Überführung von Ätio-porphyrin I in bilirubinoid Farbstoffe. *Hoppe Zeylers Z. Physiol. Chem.* 251:85–96.
7. Cremer, R. J., Perryman, P. W., Richards, D. H., et al. (1957): Simultaneous micro-determination of serum bilirubin and serum 'haem-pigments.' *Biochem. J.* 66:600.

8. Cremer, R. J., Perryman, P. W., and Richards, D. H. (1958): Influence of light on the hyperbilirubinemia of infants. *Lancet* **1**:1094–1097.

9. Ferriero, H. C., and Berezia, A. (1960): A super-illuminacio na hiperbilirubinemia da recen nascido. *An. Bras. Ginec.* **49**:147–148.

10. Peluffo, E., and Beltran, J. C. (1962): Luminoterapia en las ictericias neonatorum. *Arch. Pediatr. Uraguay* **33**:98–105.

11. Mininni, G., Violante, N., and Fabiano, M. (1964): La fototerapia nell'ittero dell' immaturo. *Rev. Clin. Pediatr.* **25**:638–647.

12. Broughton, P. M. G., Rossiter, E. J. R., Warner, C. M. B., et al. (1965): Effect of blue light on hyperbilirubinemia. *Arch. Dis. Child.* **40**:666–671.

13. Ballabriga, A., Masclons, R., and Escrin, J. M. (1965): Accion de la luz en la hiperbilirubinemia neonatal: estudio experimental. *Rev. Esp. Pediatr.* **21**:23–31.

14. Sandrucci, M. G., Ansaldi, N., and Colombo, N. L. (1965): Effetto della fototerapia nell'ittero neonatale dell' immaturo. *Minerva Pediatr.* **17**:394–399.

15. Corse, L., Delascio, D., and Guariento, A. (1964); La fototerapia nell'itero neonatale dell' immaturo. *Minerva Pediatr.* **16**:131–134.

16. Alison, F., and Marie, L. (1966): La prevention de l'ictère nucleaire chez le prémature. *Ann. Pediatr.* **13**:115–118.

17. Lucey, J. F., Ferriero, M., and Hewitt, J. (1968): Prevention of hyperbilirubinemia of prematurity by phototherapy. *Pediatrics* **41**:1047–1054.

18. Schmid, R., and McDonagh, A. F. (1975): The enzymatic formation of bilirubin. *Ann. N. Y. Acad. Sci.* **244**:533–552.

19. Jacobsen, J., and Brodersen, R. (1976): The effect of pH on albuminbilirubin binding affinity. *Birth Defects* **12(2)**:175–178.

20. Broderson, R. (1979): Bilirubin solubility, interaction with albumin and phospholipid. *J. Biol. Chem.* **254**:2364–2369.

21. Broderson, R. (1980): Bilirubin transport in the newborn infant, reviewed with relation to kernicterus. *J. Pediatr.* **96**:349–356.

22. Gartner, L. M., Kwang-sun, L., Vaisman, S., et al. (1977): Development of bilirubin transport and metabolism in the newborn rhesus monkey. *J. Pediatr.* **90**:513–531.

23. Maisels, M. J. (1972): Bilirubin. *Pediatr. Clin. North Am.* **19**:447–501.

24. Odell, G. B. (1976): Neonatal jaundice. In: *Progress in Liver Disease,* edited by H. Popper and F. Schaffer, Vol. V, pp. 457–475. Grune & Stratton, New York.

25. Behrman, R. E., Brown, A. K., Currie, M. R., et al. (1974): Preliminary report of the Committee on Phototherapy in the Newborn. *J. Pediatr.* **84**:135–147.

26. Kapoor, C. L., Murti, C., and Bajpai, P. (1973): Interaction of bilirubin with human skin. *N. Engl. J. Med.* **288**:583.

27. Kapoor, C. L. (1974): The physiological significance of the interaction of bilirubin with reconstituted collagen tendrils. *Curr. Sci.* **43**:134–136.

28. Kapoor, C. L. (1975): Interaction of bilirubin with reconstituted collagen fibrils. *Biochem. J.* **147**:199–203.

29. Bratlid, D. (1972): The effects of antimicrobial agents on bilirubin binding by human erythrocytes. *Scand. J. Clin. Lab. Invest.* **30**:331–337.

30. Vogl, T. P. (1974): Phototherapy of neonatal hyperbilirubinemia: bilirubin in unexposed areas of the skin. *J. Pediatr.* **85**:707–710.

31. Vogl, T. P., Hegyi, T., Hiatt, I. M., et al. (1978): Intermittent phototherapy in the treatment of jaundice in the premature infant. *J. Pediatr.* **92**:627–630.

32. Schmid, R., and Hammaker, L. (1963): Metabolism and dispostion of C^{14}-bilirubin in congenital nonhemolytic jaundice. *J. Clin. Invest.* **42**:1720–1734.

33. Brown, A. K., Zuelzer, W. W., and Robinson, A. R. (1957): Studies in hyperbilirubinemia. II. Clearance of bilirubin from plasma and extravascular space in newborn infants during exchange transfusion. *Am. J. Dis. Child.* **93**:274–286.

34. Ostrow, J. D., and Branham, R. V. (1970): Photodecomposition of bilirubin and biliverdin in vitro. *Gastroenterology* **58**:15–25.

35. Lightner, D. A., and Quinstad, G. B. (1972): Hematinic acid and propentdyopents from bilirubin photo-oxydation in vitro. *FEBS Lett.* **25**:94–96.

36. Lightner, D. A. (1974): In vitro photooxidation products of bilirubin. In: *Phototherapy in the Newborn: An Overview,* edited by G. B. Odell, R. Shaffer, and A. P. Simopoulos, pp. 35–55. National Academy of Sciences, Washington, D.C.

37. Ostrow, J. D., Berry, C. S., and Zarembo, J. E. (1974): Studies on the mechanism of phototherapy in the congenitally jaundiced rat, In: *Phototherapy in the Newborn: An overview,* edited by G. B. Odell, R. Shaffer, and A. P. Simopoulos, pp. 74–92. National Academy of Sciences, Washington, D.C.

38. Garbagnati, E., and Manitto, P. (1973): A new class of bilirubin photoderivatives obtained in vitro and their possible formation in jaundiced infants. *J. Pediatr.* **83**:109–115.

39. McDonagh, A. F. (1975): Phototherapy and hyperbilirubinemia. *Lancet* **1**:339.

40. Zenone, E. A., Stoll, M. S., and Ostrow, J. D. (1977): Mechanism of excretion of unconjugated bilirubin during phototherapy. *Gastroenterology* **72**:1180–1181.

41. McDonagh, A. F., Lightner, D. A., and Wooldridge, A. (1979): Geometric isomerization of bilirubin and its dimethyl ester. *J. Chem. Soc. Chem. Commun.* **3**:110–112.

42. Ostrow, J. D. (1971): Photocatabolism of labeled bilirubin in the congenitally jaundiced (Gunn) rat. *J. Clin. Invest.* **50**:707–718.

43. McDonagh, A. F., and Ramonas, L. (1978): Jaundice phototherapy: micro flo-cell photometry reveals rapid biliary response of Gunn rats to light. *Science* **201**:829–831.

44. Lund, H. T., and Jacobsen, J. (1974): Influence of phototherapy on the biliary excretion patterns in newborn infants with hyperbilirubinemia. *J. Pediatr.* **85**:262–267.

45. Ballowitz, L., Gentler, G., Krochman, J., et al. (1977): Phototherapy in Gunn rats. *Biol. Neonate* **31**:229–244.

46. Vogl, T. P., Cheskin, H., Blumenfeld, T. A., et al. (1977): Effect of intermittent phototherapy on bilirubin dynamics in the Gunn rat. *Pediatr. Res.* **11**:1021–1026.

47. Vogl, T. P., Cheskin, H., Blumenfeld, T. A., et al. (1980): Bilirubin dynamics in the Gunn rat: dose response of continuous and intermittent phototherapy. *Biol. Neonate* **38**:106.

48. Mims, L. C., Estrada, M., Gooden, D. S., et al. (1973): Phototherapy for neonatal hyperbilirubinemia—a dose:response relationship. *J. Pediatr.* **83**:658–662.

49. Sisson, T. R. C., Kendall, N., Shaw, A., et al. (1972): Phototherapy of jaundice in the newborn: II. Effect of various light intensities. *J. Pediatr.* **81**:35–38.

50. Gosset, I. H. (1960): A Perspex icterometer for neonates. *Lancet* **1**:87–88.

51. Sisson, T. R. C., Ruiz, M., Wu, K.-T., et al. (1978): Comparison of incandescent and fluorescent light sources in phototherapy (Abstract). *Pediatr. Res.* **12**:535.

52. Maurer, H. M., Shumway, C. N., Draper, D. A., et al. (1973): Controlled trial comparing agar, intermittent phototherapy and continuous phototherapy for reducing neonatal hyperbilirubinemia. *J. Pediatr.* **82**:73–76.

53. Sisson, T. R. C., Kendall, N., Davies, R. E., et al. (1970): Factors influencing the effectiveness of phototherapy in neonatal hyperbilirubinemia. *Birth Defects* **6(2)**:100–105.

54. Kline, R. M. (1972): Shedding light on the use of light. *Pediatrics* **50**:118–126.

55. Behrman, R. E., Brown, A. K., Currie, M. R., et al. (1974): *Final Report of the Committee on Phototherapy in the Newborn,* pp. 24–29. National Academy of Sciences, Washington, D.C.

56. Anderson, R. J., Vogl, T. P., and Schruben, J. H. (1974): The radiometry of phototherapy. In: *Phototherapy in the Newborn: An Overview,* edited by G. B. Odell, R. Schaffer, and A. P. Simopoulos, pp. 1–20. National Academy of Sciences, Washington, D.C.

57. Aidin, R., Corner, B., and Tovey, G. (1950): Kernicterus and prematurity. *Lancet* **1**:1153–1154.

58. Zuelzer, W. W., and Mudgett, R. T. (1950): Kernicterus, etiologic study based on analysis of 55 cases. *Pediatrics* **6**:452–474.
59. Hsia, D. Y.-Y., Allen, F. H., Gellis, S. S., et al. (1952): Erythroblastosis fetalis: studies of serum bilirubin in relation to kernicterus. *N. Engl. J. Med.* **247**:668–671.
60. Hsia, D. Y.-Y., Patterson, P., Allen, F. H., et al. (1952): Prolonged obstructive jaundice in infancy: general survey of 156 cases. *Pediatrics* **10**:243–251.
61. Gowan, A. T. D., and Scott, J. M. (1953): Kernicterus and prematurity. *Lancet* **1**:611–614.
62. Claireaux, A. E., Cole, P. G., and Lathe, G. H. (1953): Icterus of the brain in the newborn. *Lancet* **2**:1226–1230.
63. Waters, W. J., Richert, D. A., and Rawson, H. H. (1954): Bilirubin encephalopathy. *Pediatrics* **13**:319–325.
64. Day, R. L. (1954): Inhibition of brain respiration in vitro by bilirubin. Reversal of inhibition by various means. *Proc. Soc. Exp. Biol. Med.* **85**:261–264.
65. Brown, A. K., and Zuelzer, W. W. (1957): Study of hyperbilirubinemia. *Am. J. Dis. Child.* **93**:263–273.
66. Johnson, L., and Boggs, T. R., Jr. (1974): Bilirubin-dependent brain damage: incidence and indications for treatment. In: *Phototherapy in the Newborn: An Overview,* edited by G. B. Odell, R. Shaffer, and A. P. Simopoulos, pp. 121–149. National Academy of Sciences, Washington, D.C.
67. Gartner, L. M., Synder, R. N., Shabon, R. S., et al. (1970): Kernicterus. High incidence in premature infants with low serum bilirubin concentrations. *Pediatrics* **45**:906–917.
68. Harris, R. C. Lucey, J. F., and MacLean, J. R. (1958): Kernicterus in premature infants associated with low concentrations in plasma. *Pediatrics* **21**:875–884.
69. Stern, L., and Denton, R. L. (1965): Kernicterus in small premature infants. *Pediatrics* **35**:483–485.
70. Litwack, G., Ketterer, B., and Arias, I. (1971): Ligandin: a hepatic protein which binds steroids, bilirubin, carcinogens and a number of exogenous organic anions. *Nature* **234**:466–467.
71. Doxiades, S. A., Fessas, P., and Valaes, T. (1960): Erythrocyte enzyme deficiency in unexplained kernicterus. *Lancet* **2**:44–45.
72. Levin, S. E., Charlton, R. W., and Freiman, I. (1964): Glucose-6-phosphate dehydrogenase deficiency and neonatal jaundice in South African Bantu infants. *J. Pediatr.* **65**:757–764.
73. Lu, T. C., Wei, H. Y., and Blackwell, R. W. (1966): Increased incidence of severe hyperbilirubinemia among newborn Chinese infants with G-6-PD deficiency. *Pediatrics* **37**:994–999.
74. Steinberg, A., Oliver, M., Schmid, R., et al. (1963): Glucose-6-phosphate dyhydrogenase deficiency and hemolytic disease of the newborn in Isreal. *Arch. Dis. Child.* **38**:23–28.
75. O'Flynn, M. E. D., and Hsia, D. Y.-Y. (1963): Serum bilirubin levels and glucose-6-phosphate dehydrogenase deficiency in newborn American Negroes. *J. Pediatr.* **63**:160–161.
76. Wolff, J. A., Grossman, B. H., and Paya, K. (1967): Neonatal serum bilirubin and glucose-6-phosphate dehydrogenase. *Am. J. Dis. Child.* **113**:251–254.
77. Hsia, D. Y.-Y. (1966): *Inborn Errors of Metabolism I: Clinical Aspects,* 2nd ed. Year Book Medical Publishers, Chicago.
78. Blackburn, M. G., Orzalessi, M. M., and Pigram, P. (1972): Effect of light on fetal red cells in vivo. *J. Pediatr.* **80**:640–643.
79. Zinkham, W. H. (1967): The selective hemolytic action of drugs: clinical and mechanistic considerations. *J. Pediatr.* **70**:200–210.
80. Meyer, J. C., and Angus, J. (1956): The effect of large doses of "synkavite" in the newborn. *Arch. Dis. Child.* **31**:212–215.
81. Habig, W., Pabst, M., Fleichner, B., et al. (1974): The identity of glutathione transferase with Ligandin, a major binding protein of liver. *Proc. Natl. Acad. Sci. U.S.A.* **71**:3879–3882.

82. Crigler, J. F., Jr., and Najjar, V. A. (1952): Congenital familial nonhemolytic jaundice with kernicterus. *Pediatrics* **10**:169–180.

83. Hsia, D. Y.-Y., Riabovs, S., and Dowben, R. M. (1963): Inhibition of glucuronosyl transferase by steroid hormones. *Arch. Biochem.* **103**:181–185.

84. Sutherland, J. M., and Keller, W. H. (1961): Novobiocin and neonatal hyperbilirubinemia. *Am. J. Dis. Child.* **101**:447–453.

85. Brodersen, R. (1978): Free bilirubin in blood plasma of the newborn: effects of albumin, fatty acids, pH, displacing drugs, and phototherapy. In: *Intensive Care in the Newborn II,* edited by L. Stern, W. Oh, and B. Friis-Hansen, pp. 331–345. Masson, New York.

86. Nathenson, G., Cohen, M. I., and McNamara, H. (1975): The effect of Na benzoate on serum bilirubin of the Gunn rat. *J. Pediatr.* **86**:799–803.

87. Odell, G. B., Storey, G. N. B., and Rossenberg, L. A. (1970): Studies in kernicterus III. The saturation of serum proteins with bilirubin during neonatal life and its relationship to brain damage at 5 years. *J. Pediatr.* **76**:12–21.

88. Bratlid, D. (1973): Reserve albumin-binding capacity, salicylate index, and red cell binding of bilirubin in neonatal jaundice. *Arch. Dis. Child.* **48**:393–397.

89. Waters, W. J., and Porter, E. G. (1961): Dye-binding capacity of serum albumin in hemolytic disease of the newborn. *Am. J. Dis. Child.* **102**:807–814.

90. Svenningsen, N. W., Lindquist, A., and Dahlquist, A. (1971): HBABA index in neonatal jaundice. In: *Proceedings of the XIII International Congress on Pediatrics,* Vol. 1, pp. 353–355. Visuna Verlog. Wien. Med. Akad.

91. Kapitulnik, J., Valaes, T., Kaufman, N. A., et al. (1974): Clinical evaluation of Sephadex gel filtration in estimation of bilirubin binding in serum in neonatal jaundice. *Arch. Dis. Child.* **49**:886–894.

92. Wennberg, R., Lau, M., and Rasmussen, L. F. (1976): Clinical significance of unbound bilirubin (Abstract). *Pediatr. Res.* **10**:434.

93. Lamola, A. A., Eisinger, J., Blumberg, W. E., et al. (1979): Fluorometric study of the partition of bilirubin among blood components: basis for rapid microassays of bilirubin and bilirubin binding capacity in whole blood. *Anal. Biochem.* **100**:25–42.

94. Sisson, T. R. C., Goldberg, S., and Slaven, B. (1974): Effect of visible light on the Gunn rat: convulsive threshold, bilirubin concentration, and brain color. *Pediatr. Res.* **8**:647–651.

95. Johnson, L., and Schutta, H. S. (1970): Quantitative assessment of the effects of light treatment in infant Gunn rats. *Birth Defects* **6**(2):114–118.

96. Lucey, J. F., Hewitt, J. R., Emery, E. S., et al. (1973): Controlled follow-up study of low-birth-weight infants in 4–6 years of age treated with phototherapy. *Pediatr. Res.* **7**:313.

97. Sisson, T. R. C., and Wickler, M. (1973): Transmission of light through living tissues. *Pediatr. Res.* **7**:316.

98. Viggiani, F., Ciesla, M., and Russo, O. L. (1970): Penetrazione della luce attraverso ed cranio ed il cervello del ratte a diversa eta. Misurazione eseguite separatamente per la cute e per la parte ossea. *Boll. Soc. Ital. Biol. Sper.* **46**:470–473.

99. Speck, W. T., and Rosenkranz, H. (1979): Phototherapy for neonatal hyperbilirubinemia, a potential environmental health hazard: a review. *Environmental Mutagenesis* **1**:321.

100. Rubaltelli, F. F., Allegri, G., Costa, C., et al. (1974): Urinary excretion of tryptophane metabolites during phototherapy. *J. Pediatr.* **85**:865–867.

101. Sisson, T. R. C., Slaven, B., and Hamilton, P. B. (1976): The effect of broad and narrow spectrum fluorescent light on blood consitituents. *Birth Defects* **12**(2): 122–133.

102. Blackburn, M. G., Orzalesi, M. M., and Pigram, P. (1971): Effect of light and bilirubin on fetal red cells in vitro. In: *Proceedings of the XIII International Congress on Pediatrics,* Vol. 1, p. 381. Visuna Verlog. Wien. Med. Akad.

103. Yeary, R. F., Wise, K. J., and Davis, O. R. (1976): Activation of hepatic microsomal glucuronyl transferase from Gunn rats by exposure to light. *Life Sci.* **17**:1887–1890.

104. Paine, A. J., and McLean, A. E. (1974): Induction of aryl hydrocarbon hydroxylase by light-driven superoxide generating system in liver cell culture. *Biochem. Biophys. Res. Commun.* **58**:482–486.

105. Sisson, T. R. C., Granati, B., Sonawane, R., et al. (1978): Effect of light on the perfused Gunn rat liver. *Pediatr. Res.* **12**:399.

106. Odell, G. B., Ralph, S., and Brown, A. B. (1970): Dye-sensitized photooxidation of albumin associated with a decreased capacity for protein-binding of bilirubin. In:Bilirubin Metabolism in the Newborn, edited by D. Bergsma. *Birth Defects* **6**(2):31–36.

107. Rubaltelli, F. F., and Jori, G. (1979): Visible light irradiation of human and bovine serum albumin–bilirubin complex. *Photochem. Photobiol.* **29**:991–1000.

108. Cashore, W. J., Karotkin, E. H., Stern, L., et al. (1975): The lack of effect of phototherapy on serum bilirubin-binding capacity in newborn infants. *J. Pediatr.* **87**:977–980.

109. Webb, R. B., and Malina, M. M. (1970): Mutagenic effects of near UV and visible radiant energy on continuous cultures of *E. coli*. *Photochem. Photobiol.* **12**:457–468.

110. Speck, W. T., and Rosenkranz, H. (1975): Bilirubin induced photodegradation of deoxyribonucleic acid. *Pediatr. Res.* **9**:703–705.

111. Speck, W. T., and Rosenkranz, H. (1976): Intracellular DNA-modifying activity of phototherapy lights. *Pediatr. Res.* **10**:533–555.

112. Santella, R. M., Rosenkranz, H. A., and Speck, W. T. (1978): Intracellular DNA-modifying activity of intermittent phototherapy. *J. Pediatr.* **93**:106–109.

113. Elkind, M. M., and Han, A. (1978): DNA single strand lesions due to "sunlight" and UV light: a comparison of their induction in Chinese hamster and human cells of their fate in Chinese hamster cells. *Photochem. Photobiol.* **27**:717–724.

114. Rubaltelli, F. F., and Largajolli, G. (1973): Effect of light exposure on gut transit time in jaundiced newborn infants. *Acta. Paediatr. Scand.* **62**:146–148.

115. Oh, W., Williams, P., Yao, A. C., et al. (1976): Insensible water loss and peripheral blood flow in infants receiving phototherapy. *Birth Defects* **12**(2): 114–121.

116. Wu, P. Y. K., and Hodgman, J. E. (1974): Insensible water loss in pre-term infants: changes with postnatal development and non-ionizing radiation. *Pediatrics* **54**:704–712.

117. Bakken, A. R. (1977): Temporary intestinal lactase deficiency in light-treated jaundiced infants. *Acta Paediatr. Scand.* **66**:91–96.

118. Chung, C. M., and Fong, Y. F. (1976): No evidence of lactase deficiency related to phototherapy of jaundiced infants. *N. Engl. J. Med.* **295**:1483.

119. Sisson, T. R. C. (1979): Advantages of a lactose-free formula for jaundiced infants undergoing phototherapy. In: *Transactions of the Ross Clinical Research Conference, Sarasota, Florida, January 1979*, pp. 101–107.

120. Odell, G. B., Brown, R. S., and Kopelman, A. E. (1972): The photodynamic action of bilirubin on erythrocytes. *J. Pediatr.* **81**:473–483.

121. Maurer, H. M., Fratkin, M. J., Haggins, J. C., et al. (1975): Effect of phototherapy on thrombopoiesis (Abstract). *Pediatr. Res.* **9**:368.

122. Rola-Pleszczynski, M., Hensen, S. A., Vincent, M. M., et al. (1975): Inhibitory effects of bilirubin on cellular immune response in man. *J. Pediatr.* **86**:690–696.

123. Rubaltelli, F. F., Piovesan, A. L., Semenzato, G., et al. (1977): Immune competence assessment in hyperbilirubinemic newborns before and after phototherapy. *Helv. Paediatr. Acta* **32**:129–133.

124. Rubaltelli, F. F., Piovesan, A. L., Granati, B., et al. (1980): The effects of bilirubin and phototreated bilirubin on the phagocytic activity of granulocytes (Abstract). *Pediatr. Res.* **14**:170.

125. Granati, B., Colleselli, P., Felice, M., et al. (1981): The effects of bilirubin, phototreated bilirubin and light on spontaneous motility and chemotaxis of leucocytes. *Pediatr. Res.* (in press).

126. Rubaltelli, F. F., Piovesan, A. L., Granati, B., et al. (1981): The effect of phototherapy on T-cell function. *Pediatr. Res.* (in press).

127. Sisson, T. R. C., Ruiz, M., Wu, K.-T., (1977): Sleep patterns of newborn infants under phototherapy (Abstract). *Pediatr. Res.* 11:411.

128. Sisson, T. R. C., Root, A. W., Kechavarz-Oliai, L., et al. (1974): Biologic rhythm of plasma human growth hormone in newborns of low birth weight. In: *Chronobiology,* edited by L. Scheving, F. Halberg, and J. Pauly, pp. 348–352. Igaku Shoin, Tokyo.

129. Sisson, T. R. C., Katzman, G., Shahrivar, F., et al. (1975): Effect of uncycled light on plasma human grown hormone in neonates (Abstract). *Pediatr. Res.* 9:280.

130. Park, T. S., Sisson, T. R. C., Padgett, S., et al. (1976): Effect of phototherapy and nursery light on neonatal biorhythms (Abstract). *Pediatr. Res.* 10:429.

131. Odell, G. B. (1976): Roundtable on Jaundice Phototherapy, presented at the 4th Annual Meeting of the American Society of Photobiology, Denver, Colorado, February 18, 1976.

132. Vogl, T. P. (1976): Bilirubin redistribution in the skin of a Crigler–Najjar child under phototherapy. Paper presented at the VII International Congress on Photobiology, Rome, Italy, September 2, 1976.

133. Jori, G., Rossi, E., and Rubaltelli, F. F. (1976): Evidence for visible light-induced covalent binding between bilirubin and serum albumin "in vitro" and "in vivo." Discussion at Roundtable on Jaundice Phototherapy, presented at the 4th Annual Meeting of the American Society of Photobiology, Denver, Colorado, February 18, 1976.

134. Sisson, T. R. C. (1973): Phototherapie der Neugeborenen-Hyperbilirubinämie, *Fortschr. Med.* 91:563–566.

135. Sisson, T. R. C. (1982): Advances in phototherapy of neonatal hyperbilirubinemia. In: *Trends in Photobiology,* edited by C. Hélène, M. Charlier, T. Montenay-Garestier, and G. Laustriat pp. 339–348. Plenum Press, New York.

17

Phototherapy of Psoriasis and Other Skin Diseases

J. A. Parrish

One specific aspect of photomedicine is the use of nonionizing electromagnetic radiation to treat disease. Heliotherapy has been prescribed since ancient times for a wide variety of illnesses. The Nobel Prize for medicine was awarded to Niels Finsen in 1903 for demonstrating the usefulness of ultraviolet (UV) radiation in the treatment of a form of cutaneous tuberculosis. Erysipelas and other infections, both cutaneous and internal, have been treated with UV radiation and sunlight and artificial UV sources were used in the prevention and treatment of rickets. For most of these disorders, specific chemotherapy has replaced phototherapy. However, some forms of phototherapy are still quite useful. Visible light phototherapy is an effective treatment for hyperbilirubinemia of infants. This therapy is discussed in Chapter 16. UV radiation is used to treat skin diseases and to relieve certain forms of itching and, in both cases, offers advantages over other available forms of treatment. This UV phototherapy is the topic of the present chapter.

In many of the disorders treated with phototherapy the clinical improvement is not impressive or consistent. Some of the diseases are self-limiting, and controlled studies using bilateral comparison techniques are seldom done. These factors make it difficult to evaluate the effectiveness of phototherapy. It does appear that eczema, pityriasis rosea, parapsoriasis, and other diseases are occasionally improved by repeated exposures to sun or to artificial sources. Certain photodermatoses can be improved by controlled exposures to UV or visible radiation. Even though polymorphous light

J. A. Parrish • Department of Dermatology, Harvard Medical School, Massachusetts General Hospital, Boston, Massachusetts 02114.

eruption, solar urticaria, and light-sensitive eczema are abnormal reactions initiated by photons and although phototherapy itself causes clinical symptoms in these light-sensitive disorders, eventually with repeated phototherapy treatments the threshold to solar radiation is raised so that patients can better tolerate sun exposures. Phototherapy may deplete mediators, induce melanogenesis, thicken stratum corneum, alter membranes, injure cells involved in the pathogenesis of photosensitivity, or act by other unknown mechanisms.

Acne is often treated with UV radiation from sun or artificial sources. There is debate whether UV radiation diminishes the disease process or simply masks lesions by inducing redness and subsequent tan. Some dermatologists find that phototherapy of acne has no effect. Many acne patients do seem to be improved during summer months or during prolonged visits to sunny climates. Such an observation is difficult to interpret. Acne is made worse by prolonged emotional stress. For adolescents and young adults, summertime, vacation trips, and sunbathing often reflect a time of leisure and diminished stress. UV radiation-induced vasodilitation may also hasten resolution of some types of inflammatory lesions in acne.

Certain forms of itching are reported to be improved by phototherapy. Persons with chronic renal failure are often bothered by severe generalized itching. The exact cause is not known but it is hypothesized that toxic metabolites normally cleared by the kidneys can accumulate in the skin, where they affect superficial nerve endings, resulting in itching. Dryness of the skin increases the itching. Poor health, malaise, depression, and fatigue magnify subjective aspects of cutaneous sensations so that pruritus becomes a significant problem. In 1975, Saltzer (1) reported that seven of eight uremic patients were less pruritic within a month of beginning UV phototherapy. More recent studies (2) confirmed this observation, showing that repeated total-body erythemogenic exposures to UVB led to relief of itching in persons with renal failure maintained with hemodialysis therapy. Black patients have also been effectively treated with UVB (3). Studies by Gilchrest et al. (2, 4) suggest that the effect of UV radiation is more than subjective. They treated patients with equal exposure times in UVB and UVA chambers and only the UVB-treated patients improved. Erythomogenic UVB exposure doses were given. Because the minimal erythema dose (MED) to UVA is 1000 times greater than that for UVB and the UVA intensity was only 10 times that of UVB, the UVA exposure doses were therefore markedly suberythemogenic and were considered placebo therapy. Therapeutic benefit seems to be related to total number of treatments and therefore response occurs sooner in patients treated more frequently. In patients treated with one to three treatments per week, improvement usually follows four to six UVB exposures. Phototherapy may inactivate a circulating substance or substances responsible for the pruritus experienced by many patients with chronic renal failure. This mechanism is supported by the observation that treatment to one half of the body leads to bilateral improvement (4). It has been claimed that observed therapeutic response is only subjective or is caused by a counterirritant effect of sunburn. Pruritus is difficult to evaluate and quantify and some patients are not benefitted. However, if chronically ill uremic patients believe they have less itching and feel more comfortable, the treatment is rewarding for both the patient and the therapist.

A host of chemical, metabolic, and structural changes occur when living cells absorb UV radiation (see Chapter 8). Many of these changes can be considered harmless or reversible, but other changes are injurious to the cell. It is likely that phototoxicity or cell injury is a mechanism which is central to most forms of phototherapy of skin disease. For example, UV radiation may decrease abnormal hyperproliferation, interfere with function of abnormal cells, or kill cells intricately involved in the pathophysiologic expression of disease. It is assumed that the variety of radiation-induced cellular alterations and cascades of tissue reactors known to occur in normal skin also occur in diseased skin and that qualitative and quantitative differences in response to radiation may lead to improvement of diseased skin without irreversible or unacceptable damage to normal skin. In some forms of phototherapy, therapeutic effect may result because abnormal cells are more sensitive to radiation than are normal cells.

In considering potential beneficial effects of nonionizing electromagnetic radiation, several perspectives must be considered simultaneously: the effect of photons on specific biomolecules, the effect on cell function and viability, the inflammatory response and repair of the organ as a whole, and the differential effect on normal and abnormal cells and tissue. There are many chromophores and multiple photobiologic responses with separate action spectra and there are complex interactions among these responses. Quantification of these effects makes it possible to select exposure conditions that maximize beneficial effects and minimize the undesirable side effects.

Acute and chronic phototoxic effects on normal skin and blood are the limiting factors in phototherapy. While most attention has been placed on delayed erythema of normal skin, it is important to remember that this is only one manifestation of ultraviolet effects. Absence of erythema does not mean that no effects have occurred. DNA damage, dyskeratotic cells, and melano-genesis can occur after suberythemogenic exposure doses of UV radiation and other effects are also likely to occur.

PHOTOTHERAPY OF PSORIASIS

The skin disease most often treated by phototherapy is psoriasis. Because the therapeutic effect in this disorder is often quite striking, phototherapy of psoriasis has been the object of many studies and will be discussed in more detail. The kinds of advances made in the therapy of this disorder may improve phototherapy of other skin diseases. Psoriasis is a disease of unknown etiology characterized by increased epidermal cell proliferation. It is a common chronic skin disease that affects from 1% to 3% of people to a variable extent. The tendency to have psoriasis is inherited. Onset is often prior to adult life, but psoriasis may begin at any age, from birth to old age. Once the disease becomes manifest, its course is unpredictable.

The individual lesions of psoriasis are raised, red, circumscribed scaling plaques which tend to occur symmetrically over the body, with a predilection for bony prominences, such as elbows and knees. Lesions may, however, occur at any site. Microscopically there is a marked thickening of the epidermis, with a regular elongation of rete ridges and consequent elongation of dermal papillae, which contain dilated capillaries. There is an increased number of dividing cells in the lower layers of the epidermis, a general acceleration of the epidermal cell cycle, and alterations of cell differentiation. This results in the formation of scales as the outer layers of the epidermis are manufactured rapidly and abnormally.

It has been known for decades that many patients with psoriasis improve in the summer. Dermatologists feel that sunlight is moderately good therapy for many persons with psoriasis and several clinical studies have supported this observation. As early as 1923 Alderson got good results by treating psoriasis with a quartz-jacketed mercury discharge lamp (5). He used erythemogenic exposure and stated, "I am guided by the reaction, and my purpose is to produce a slight hyperemia and eventual pigmentation. I believe this is of great importance . . ." Subsequent observers confirmed that repeated erythemogenic UV exposures improved psoriasis. For example, Bowers et al. (6) found in 1966 that seven of nine patients treated with UV radiation from a mercury-vapor lamp were moderately to much improved. They also selected exposure doses that caused transient erythema and mild desquamation of normal skin. Young (7) found that repeated exposure to artificial UV sources was ineffective, but he treated for as few as 14 days, does not mention whether erythema of normal skin was achieved, and gives insufficient radiometric and dosimetry data.

The effect of erythemogenic UV radiation has been studied using bilateral comparison trials and compared to oral psoralen photochemotherapy (see Chapter 22). Parrish et al. (8) documented that 80% of patients treated with repeated erythemogenic sun exposure improved considerably and that daily treatment was not significantly better than alternate-day therapy. However, complete clearing of all lesions in sun-exposed sites occurred in only two of 34 patients. In the same study, 14 of 17 patients treated with 0.6 mg/kg methoxsalen and sunlight cleared completely. Patients were permitted to use lubricants, but the frequency of use and number of patients using topical lubricants are not recorded. Using a paired comparison technique, Parrish et al. (9) and Wolff et al. (10) compared repeated erythemogenic exposures to artificial UV sources with less frequent treatments using oral psoralen photochemotherapy (PUVA, see Chapter 22). Using their treatment protocols, it was found that PUVA was more quickly effective in clearing psoriasis than was UV radiation alone. In both studies, however, UV radiation led to improvement in most patients. On the other hand, van Weelden et al. (11) found that when using topical 1% salicylic acid in petrolatum in addition to doses of UVB greater than those previously used, phototherapy was equally as effective as oral psoralen photochemotherapy. This study utilized a bilateral comparison technique evaluated after 10 biweekly treatments. In another study, 30 patients were treated either with PUVA or with placebo capsules followed by erythemogenic doses of UV radiation (primarily UVB), and both treatments were equally successful (11). In these studies in which UVB phototherapy was as effective as PUVA, erythemogenic exposure doses were used and all patients applied petrolatum to the skin (see below, "Adjunctive Agents").

The mechanism of the therapeutic effect of UV radiation on psoriasis is not known. Repeated episodes of phototoxicity induced by a variety of wavebands lead to improvement of psoriasis. The precise mechanisms of beneficial effect may vary with the waveband used. All or some of the cellular and organ responses of normal skin to UV radiation may occur in psoriatic skin and repeated occurrence of one or more of these events eventually (usually after 10–35 treatments) leads to the return of skin that appears clinically and histologically normal. The disease process may stay in remission for days to years, but almost always eventually recurs.

Ultraviolet exposure of skin of animals (12–14) and humans (15) causes a biphasic alteration of macromolecular synthesis. A transient decrease in DNA, RNA, and protein synthesis is followed by a rebound increase in synthesis of these biomolecules, and often by a proliferative state. Most hypotheses about the mechanism of phototherapy and photochemotherapy of psoriasis have focused on the assumption that UV radiation of psoriasis tissue also causes a decrease in DNA synthesis which influences the return of more normal cell kinetics. Medications known to be effective in treating psoriasis are those that suppress mitoses, DNA synthesis, or cell proliferation. It is not known whether psoriatic cells are more sensitive to UV damage because they are more metabolically active or are replicating more rapidly or because they differ in other ways. It is not known whether the therapeutic effect results because UV radiation decreases macromolecular synthesis in all psoriatic cells or whether there is selective inhibition or killing of a smaller population of highly proliferative cells. When normal skin is exposed to erythemogenic UV radiation, the rebound hyperproliferative state can lead to thickening of the epidermis or to desquamation. This proliferogenic stimulus, most marked by shorter UV wavelengths, may also occur in psoriatic tissue; it may act to normalize differentiation or it may be an undesirable antitherapeutic influence to be overcome by other, more therapeutic UV effects.

There is a variety of other mechanisms by which UV radiation may benefit psoriasis. Phototherapy may compromise specific cells, such as lymphocytes or polymorphonuclear leukocytes, which are necessary for the pathophysiology of the disease. Metabolites or mediators which are necessary to maintain the hyperproliferative state may be photochemically altered. In the epidermis, UV radiation may alter the recruitment of cells from a resting phase to a proliferative phase, alter differentiation, or act as gene regulator or deregulator. More than one mechanism may be involved. The gradual continuous decrease in the thickness and scaling of a plaque and the complete remission of disease after cessation of treatment may not necessarily result from the same molecular mechanism. The net effect of multiple episodes of phototoxicity may be to gradually decrease total macromolecular synthesis in abnormal keratinocytes. The remission may result from a UV-radiation effect on blood vessels, white blood cells, or on keratinocyte gene regulation. All of the treatments, by some cumulative effect, act in concert to reestablish normal kinetics and differentiation and normal clinical and histologic appearance of the skin.

ACTION SPECTRUM

Several observations define the general shape of the action spectrum for the therapeutic effects of UV radiation (Fig. 17-1). Broadband exposure devices which, when considering the spectral sensitivity of normal skin, are essentially UVB sources, improve psoriasis when erythemogenic doses are used. High-pressure mercury lamps, mercury-xenon sources, fluorescent "sunlamps," and sun are all moderately effective if repeated erythemogenic exposure doses are used. With all of the broadband sources, however, total clearing of psoriasis without the use of adjunctive therapeutic agents is not regularly achieved.

Within the range of 254–313 nm the action spectrum for clearing of psoriasis with repeated doses of UV radiation has been determined and compared to the erythema action spectrum of adjacent unaffected skin (16) (see Fig. 17-1). These observations were made in patients who were also treated with topically applied lubricating agents such as hydrated petrolatum (see "Adjunctive Agents" below). For all wavelengths shorter than 295 nm, no improvement occurred at any site at any exposure dose. At the shorter wavelengths the action spectrum for induction of delayed erythema in normal skin was therefore different from the action spectrum for phototherapy of psoriasis. For instance, at 254 and 280 nm repeated daily exposures to 20 and 50 times MED caused no change in psoriasis. The shorter wavelength UV

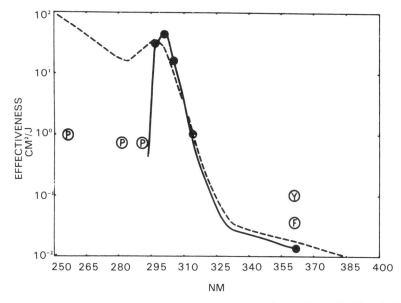

Fig. 17-1. The proposed action spectrum for phototherapy of psoriasis obtained by plotting effectiveness (reciprocal of threshold dose) on a log scale vs. wavelength in nanometers. The dashed line is the human erythema action spectrum. The solid line is the action spectrum for phototherapy of psoriasis based on several studies. The closed circles represent reciprocal of lowest daily dose that clears psoriasis [295, 300, 305, 313 nm from Parrish (16); 365 nm from Parrish (20)]. Open circles are placed at the reciprocal of the highest daily exposure doses tried and found not to be effective [P from Parrish (16); F from Fisher (19); Y from Young and van der Leun (18)]. The action spectrum for phototherapy must fall below these points.

radiation was far more erythemogenic than therapeutic. Other observations using shorter wavelength UV radiation to treat psoriasis are limited. Stern and Kihiczak (17) saw no histologic or morphologic improvement in a psoriatic plaque after a single exposure to a dose of UVC (primarily 254 nm) which caused marked histologic alterations of uninvolved skin. Van Weelden et al. found that UVC did not augment UVB phototherapy (11).

The marked and relatively abrupt decrease in effectiveness of wavelengths shorter than 295 nm may be explained by anatomic differences between psoriatic and normal skin. In psoriasis, the proliferative compartment at the bottom of the epidermis is thicker than in normal skin and its average depth is deeper within the tissue. There is also an increased thickness of the abnormal stratum corneum. Epidermal proteins absorb wavelengths shorter than approximately 290 nm and, in general, transmission decreases exponentially with increased thickness of an optical barrier. Also, optical scattering is inversely related exponentially to wavelength, so that the shorter wavelengths have longer pathlengths, which further increases their chance of being absorbed before reaching the proliferative compartment. Transmission of wavelengths shorter than 290 nm to the proliferating epidermal cells or to blood vessels in psoriasis may therefore be markedly reduced when compared with normal skin.

Within the UVB region the threshold dose for induction of delayed erythema of normal skin and the minimal daily dose required for therapeutic response are quite similar. Studies with monochromatic radiation showed that MED doses of 295 nm improved most patients. At 300 and 305 nm, sites repeatedly exposed to doses less than 1 MED may clear completely. Sites treated with 313-nm radiation also may heal psoriasis at less than MED doses, but exposure of 1.5 MEDs and greater may cause edema and an increase in induration and scaling (16).

The action spectra for delayed erythema of normal skin and for phototherapy of psoriasis may also be closely aligned in the UVA region. UVA is markedly less erythemogenic than is UVB, requiring as much as 1000 times more energy to cause redness in normal skin. At these longer wavelengths it appears that therapeutic effects also require 1000 times greater doses. The evidence for this comes from several studies (see Fig 17-1). Young and van der Leun (18) found that 14 daily exposures to 7–14 J/cm^2 of UVA had no effect on psoriasis. They used a high-pressure mercury arc filtered through its own glass envelope plus an additional 3 mm of window glass to essentially eliminate UVB radiation. No erythema was reported to occur on normal skin. Fischer (19) investigated the therapeutic effects of defined narrow wavebands at longer UV wavelengths by irradiating circular areas within plaques of psoriasis vulgaris. Areas 22 mm in diameter were exposed once daily, five times per week for 3 weeks to a 500-W mercury lamp. Using appropriate filters, spectral lines were isolated and different experimental sites were exposed to 313-nm band (0.5, 1, and 2 times predetermined MED of adjacent normal skin), 334-nm plus 365-nm band (30 J/cm^2), 365-nm bank (30 J/cm^2), and 405-nm band (30 J/cm^2). At these exposure doses the 313-nm band was the most effective and the degree of improvement correlated with increasing exposure dose. Other wavelengths were less effective at the doses used. The MED to these longer wavelengths was not measured; it is estimated that, with the mercury source at 334 or 365 nm, 30 J/cm^2 is near or below the MED for most light-skinned Caucasians. No significant improvement was seen in any site treated with 405-nm radiation. Parrish (20), using larger exposure doses (50–300 J/cm^2), found UVA (320–440 nm but primarily 365 nm) to be effective in clearing psoriasis from small exposure sites. Comparative studies showed these doses of UVA to be as effective as doses of UVB 1000 times smaller. MED to UVA with the same exposure sources was 20–100 J/cm^2.

These observations are of interest because they do suggest that within portions of the UVA band the action spectrum for therapeutic effect is similar to the action spectrum for delayed erythema of normal skin, but the use of such large exposure doses with conventional sources is impractical and possibly unsafe for whole-body treatments. The addition of UVA to UVB phototherapy in an exposure dose ratio of 20:1 does not noticeably improve UVB phototherapy (11). This is not surprising if the therapeutic exposure dose for UVA is 1000 times greater than for UVB. A 20:1 ratio of UVA to UVB would be expected to increase effectiveness of UVB by only 2%.

The marked decrease in effectiveness at wavelengths shorter than 290 nm may have important and practical therapeutic implications. UVC is highly erythemogenic to normal skin and its presence in broad-spectrum photo-therapy exposure sources may therefore limit exposure doses to the more therapeutic longer wavelengths. In a small study with six psoriasis patients (19) 1 MED (about 400 mJ/cm^2) and 2 MEDs of the 313-nm band of a mercury source were compared to 1 MED (20–40 mJ/cm^2) and 2 MEDs of 313-nm band plus the shorter wavelength component (down to 280 nm) of the same source. The therapeutic effect of the 313-nm band alone was "somewhat superior" to that obtained when the wavelengths down to 280 nm were included. Exact dosimetry and detailed evaluation of this small group are not given, but the observations suggest that when the shorter wavelength UV radiation is included the MED of normal skin is lower (sensitivity for induction of delayed erythema is greater), but the therapeutic effect of equally erythemogenic doses (equal multiples of MED) is less. In paired comparison studies the addition of UVC has been shown to decrease the effect of UVB phototherapy (11). In these studies the addition of the markedly erythemo-genic UVC limited the tolerance of normal skin to the more therapeutic UVB. It is also possible that the shorter wavelength UV wavebands have a net proliferogenic influence on the abnormal cells within psoriatic plaques. Parrish (16) observed that psoriasis initially cleared by 305-nm radiation relapsed when subsequently exposed to broad-spectrum UVB (FS40 West-inghouse fluorescent bulbs). Phototherapy with broadband sources may therefore be a complex phenomenon with additive therapeutic effects from photons of different energies, but also with competing and nontherapeutic effects from some wavebands. Further study of waveband interactions is required.

In the past the exposure sources used for phototherapy were selected largely on the assumption that the action spectrum for phototherapy was the same as that for erythema. The type of lamps and exposure doses used were gradually modified by trial and error. More recently, selection of the most appropriate exposure source is based on the action spectrum of acute phototoxicity of normal skin, possible mechanisms of phototherapy, optical properties of skin, and the spectral and geometric properties of available exposure sources. The goal has been to achieve total-body exposure in reasonable time periods in a safe and practical manner. Considerations include the observations that UV wavelengths shorter than 290 nm are more erythemogenic than therapeutic (16), that longer wavelengths (>313 nm) are therapeutic at or slightly below erythema-producing doses but require massive exposure doses (20), and that longer wavelengths penetrate more deeply into tissue and may be more likely to affect abnormal blood vessels and cellular infiltrates possibly important to the pathophysiology of psoriasis. Compared to wavelengths longer than 310 nm, UV radiation of 290–310 nm requires lower exposure doses to be both erythemogenic and therapeutic. It must also be remembered that excessive irradiation with wavebands which are neither therapeutic nor erythemogenic causes a heat load on the skin and results in patient discomfort. Absorbed UVA or visible radiation can raise skin temperature and body temperature during prolonged exposure. The region between 300 and 320 nm may therefore represent an important "compromise region" (20) for phototherapy of psoriasis.

Polychromatic radiation with maximum output between 300 and 325 nm has been claimed as a practical and effective treatment. This treatment has been referred to as "selective ultraviolet phototherapy" (SUP) because it decreases the more erythemogenic, shorter wavelength UV component present in many artificial UV sources, is therefore more like solar radiation (21), and may utilize radiation which is transmitted deeper into the psoriatic tissue (22). In patients treated with erythemogenic exposure doses, results with SUP have been reported to be good (23), better than more conventional broad-spectrum UV treatment (24, 25), and in selected cases as effective as PUVA (22). Other studies have found PUVA to be a better treatment for more difficult cases of psoriasis (26). Because PUVA is activated primarily by UVA, its better results in some cases may be partially explained by optical arguments related to a greater portion of photochemistry occurring deeper within the tissue (22).

A natural spectral shift toward longer wavelengths may partly explain why heliotherapy at the Dead Sea appears to be more effective than solar phototherapy at other locations (27–30). Because the Dead Sea is 1200 feet below sea level, solar radiation must travel a longer column of atmosphere before it reaches the earth. Due to the increased pathlength through air, shorter wavelengths are preferably scattered and absorbed. This results in a net spectral shift to longer wavelength at ground level. This path length effect is small and one might suppose that other mechanisms, such as higher aerosol content near the Dead Sea, account for some of any biologically significant shifts in the terrestial solar spectral power distribution. It is also probable that soaking in the sea water alters optical properties of psoriasis in a way that increases the effectiveness of phototherapy. The water may remove UV-absorbing substances from the skin.

It is probable that the refinement of exposure sources will continue as more information about the action spectrum of phototherapy becomes available and advances in technology create more options for manipulations of the properties of total-body exposure sources. Further spectral narrowing of the wavebands used for phototherapy may result in increase in safety and effectiveness. Preliminary studies with monochromators show that complete clearing of small areas of psoriasis may be achieved with repeated exposure doses slightly less than the MED of normal skin (16). In order to clear psoriasis with broadband sources it is usually necessary to increase the exposure dose as the UV radiation tolerance of normal skin increases; doses of 5–20 times the original MED are often used toward the end of a course of therapy. The total number of treatments required with monochromatic radiation is also reduced (31). This may be further evidence that broadband radiation often includes antitherapeutic effects that are responsbile for the fact that more than 20 phototoxic events are often required before all evidence of disease is absent.

ADJUNCTIVE AGENTS

Standard hospital phototherapy and many clinical studies of UV radiation therapy of psoriasis include the use of tar or related derivatives or other substances applied to the skin. Goeckerman first reported the beneficial effects of application of tar and exposure of the skin to UV radiation in 1925 (32). After evaluating other potential photosensitizing agents, he settled on crude coal tar, which he believed would enhance the therapeutic effects of UV radiation (33). For more than 50 years this combination has been the customary treatment for generalized psoriasis and its effectiveness is without question (34–36). The mess, stain, and offensive odor of tar often make it necessary to hospitalize patients for this treatment. The current trend is to use ambulatory care facilities or day care units to provide tar and UV therapy. Home therapy with tar remains impractical in many instances. Tar is usually applied to the skin at a 1–6% concentration in an ointment or lubricant base, 1 hr to many hours prior to UV radiation.

The therapeutic mechanism of tar plus UV phototherapy of psoriasis and the exact role played by each therapeutic component are the subjects of debate. Tar has been used since ancient times to treat skin diseases. Coal tar is a by-product of the destructive distillation of coal (37). Its distillation products, derivatives, and related chemicals are the only tars now in common medical use (38). Wood tar and bituminous tars, once used by dermatologists, are no longer widely prescribed. Over 10,000 different components are present in crude coal tar and most of these have not been identified. Tar alone has some definite but modest therapeutic effects on psoriasis (6, 7, 37). Most studies find the beneficial effects of tar to be less than that of UV radiation alone (6, 39, 40). UV radiation and tar used in combination appear to be more effective than either used alone (39–41).

For decades after Goeckerman's publications, it was assumed that chemical photosensitization was an important aspect of the widely used tar plus UV radiation therapy. This mechanism is now in question. Topical crude coal tar (42), tar pitch (43), and several commercially available tars (44) are phototoxic, i.e., these compounds reduce the amount of UV radiation necessary to induce injury of normal skin as manifest by delayed erythema. The action spectrum for this photosensitization effect appears to be most easily demonstrated within the UVA spectrum. The treatment sources commonly used with topical tar include both UVA and UVB. However, when considering the spectral power distribution of the sources and the spectral sensitivity of tar-treated normal skin, it is seen that phototoxicity, as manifested by delayed erythema (see Chapter 8), occurs primarily from the UVB component of the sources. Considering this effect on normal skin, exposure is limited by UVB acute phototoxicity long before the sources have delivered enough UVA to induce tar photosensitization. It appears, then, that the erythemogenic effects of tar plus UV therapy as commonly practiced result from the well-known UVB-induced inflammation of skin.

The therapeutic waveband of tar and UV phototherapy as commonly used may also be the UVB component of the exposure sources. Two studies compared the effectiveness of UVA plus tar with that of UVB plus tar in psoriasis therapy and found the UVB–tar combination therapy to be more effective (6, 45). The exposure doses of UVA in both these studies were insufficient to elicit tar photosensitization. However, when using exposure doses adequate to cause cutaneous phototoxicity (manifest by delayed erythema), Parrish et al. (46) found UVA and UVB to be equally therapeutic to tar-treated psoriatic lesions. It was felt that the UVB therapeutic effect was independent of tar photosensitization because the exposure dose of UVB required to cause delayed erythema of normal skin was the same with or without the tar. Special sources, filters, and long exposure time were necessary in order to obtain photosensitizing doses of UVA without inducing phototoxicity from the much more erythemogenic UVB present in most UV treatment sources. Tar–UVA phototoxicity was shown by the fact that less UVA was required to elicit delayed erythema in the presence of tar than when skin was irradiated without tar application. Therefore tar–UVA photosensitization phototherapy is therapeutic, but the dose of UVA required to benefit tar-treated skin is large enough to be impractical with currently available sources.

Tar–UVA photosensitization therapy of psoriasis has additional problems. After application of crude coal tar or tar products to the skin, subsequent exposure to UVA may lead to an unpleasant, burning, or painful sensation that has been referred to as the "smarting reaction" (43, 44, 46). Smarting begins relatively abruptly at some point during UVA exposure, is relieved simply by discontinuing the exposure, and may return when exposure is resumed. Smarting usually occurs at doses of UVA slightly less than those needed to produce delayed erythema in tar-treated skin, but considerable individual variation exists. The action spectrum appears to include UVA, but may extend into visible wavelengths. The mechanism of this uncomfortable reaction is not known. Cutaneous nerve endings may be directly affected by some photochemical event, or they may be indirectly affected via damage of other cells or components in the skin.

The vehicle or ointment used to dilute and apply crude coal tar may enhance the therapeutic effect of UV radiation. LeVine et al. (40) found that when used in conjunction with repeated daily erythemogenic exposures to UVB, the lubricant vehicle without the tar was as effective as the combination of tar and UVB. In a series of reports Petrozzi et al. (39) used bilateral comparison techniques to confirm that crude coal tar combined with UV radiation was equally effective as the same UV source used in combination with the hydrophilic ointment vehicle. They used erythemogenic exposure doses of UV radiation in all cases and compared topical adjunctive agents. In one study they showed topical methoxsalen to be somewhat superior to hydrophilic ointment (47). The second study showed methoxsalen to be superior to crude coal tar and to hydrophilic ointment (48). In both studies observations were discontinued when the methoxsalen side was cleared or markedly improved (an average of 17 and 18 treatments). At that time less than half the patients treated with hydrophilic ointment or crude coal tar were clear, but improvement was about the same with the two agents. In a subsequent study (49), a direct bilateral comparison of crude coal tar and hydrophilic ointment was continued longer (an average of 23 treatments). The two topical compounds proved to be equally effective as adjunctive agents to UV phototherapy. Here again, however, although 83% of patients in each group were markedly improved, only one-half (hydrophilic ointment) to two-thirds (crude coal tar) of them were completely clear of disease. In no case was the ointment alone or the radiation alone as effective as the combination of the two. The exact radiometry and dosimetry in these studies is not clear. Outpatient studies, possibly using more aggressive UVB doses, have further documented that topical application in the petrolatum and subsequent exposure to erythemogenic doses of UVB two times per week (11), three times per week (50), or five times per week (51) leads to clearing of psoriasis vulgaris. The results in these studies were somewhat more impressive, with 80–95% of patients clearing.

It has been shown that hydrated petrolatum and other hydrophilic, nonvolatile substances alter the surface of psoriasis lesions so that less UV radiation is backscattered from the surface of scales (52) (see Fig. 17-2). This reduced remittance is immediate, broad-spectrum, and not due to UV absorption by the topically applied substance. It appears to be caused by an immediate alteration of the optical properties of psoriatic plaques caused by matching of refractive index between the applied material and the numerous

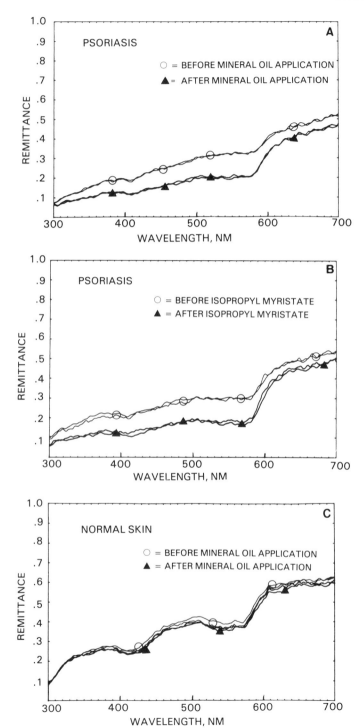

superficial flakes of stratum corneum (see Fig. 17-3). The optical effects may be cosmetic as well as therapeutic; less visible light is backscattered and the lesions appear to be less silvery or white and more the color of normal skin. These optical effects probably account for a portion of the increased effectiveness of UV radiation when used in combination with topical tars; the vehicle used to apply the tar enhances the effect of UV radiation by increasing transmission to the proliferating cells of the epidermis. Because the same effect does not occur in normal skin (52, 53), selective increased UV penetration into psoriasis occurs. Thick applications of tar actually absorb enough UV radiation to decrease effectiveness of phototherapy, but if thin layers and low concentrations are used, this effect will be small and may be offset by the therapeutic effects of tar alone and the optical effects of the vehicle. Lubricants or tar vehicles may also facilitate the removal of scale.

Therefore, considering clinical studies outlined above, the spectral power distribution of treatment sources most often used, and the erythema and photosensitization action spectra of tar-treated skin, it appears that the major therapeutic component of the popularly used tar and UV-radiation treatment is probably UVB. Other factors add to the effectiveness of the treatment program. Tar, hospitalization, and patient–physician and patient–nurse interactions play important roles. The vehicles used to apply the tar and the ointments used to treat scaling, dryness, and itching are also therapeutic in varying degrees. Optical changes induced by certain of these agents improve the effectiveness of phototherapy and it is not necessary to use tar to obtain this enhancement. When suboptimal UV exposure doses are used, the beneficial effects of tar itself may be a recognizable component of the therapy, but with adequate UV doses the messiness and odor may outweigh any therapeutic advantage.

When using broad-spectrum UVB it appears that erythemogenic doses are required Some investigators have claimed to achieve clearing with suberythemogenic exposures (54) to broadband sources, but the studies need confirmation with careful dosimetry and larger numbers of patients. In our experience it is occasionally possible to completely clear psoriasis with

Fig. 17-2. Remittance spectra of 12 psoriatic plaques from four patients were measured using an integrating sphere spectrophotometer before and immediately after application of mineral oil (A) (refractive index, n_D = 1.48), isopropyl myristate (B) (n_D = 1.44), or water (n_D = 1.33). The same was done for normal skin in vivo (C). A marked, broad-spectrum decrease in remittance of psoriatic plaques occurs within seconds after application of mineral oil or isopropyl palmite. Water requires approximately 5 min application time to produce an effect of equivalent magnitude. In contrast, none of the above substances when applied to normal skin produces any discernible change in spectral remittance. Application of lipophilic compounds to psoriatic skin immediately reduces remittance in a manner consistent with a refractive index-matching mechanism. Application of water to psoriatic skin produces a similar effect, but a longer application time is necessary. No such effects were noted for normal skin, which is consistent with the fact than an index-matching mechanism requires multiple air–skin interfaces.

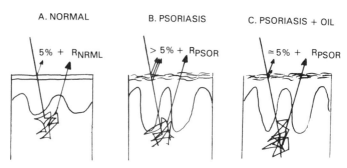

A. NORMAL   B. PSORIASIS   C. PSORIASIS + OIL

5% + R_{NRML} > 5% + R_{PSOR} ≈ 5% + R_{PSOR}

Fig. 17-3. The mechanism by which lipophilic lubricants such as mineral oil affect the optics of psoriatic plaques can be deduced from spectral remittance measurements. To a first approximation, the remittance of skin can be modeled as a summation of the reflectance caused by the step change in refractive index between air ($n_D = 1.0$) and stratum corneum ($n_D = 1.55$), plus the backscattered radiation from within the tissue (A). In psoriasis, incident radiation encounters multiple air–skin interfaces due to scales of dry corneocytes at the skin surface. Hence, psoriatic plaques should have a greater surface reflectance component than that of normal skin (B). The fraction of incident radiation absorbed by skin is simply 1.00 minus the remittance. If remittance is decreased by some treatment of the surface with an optically nonabsorbing substance, by definition a greater fraction of the incident radiation must be transmitted into and absorbed by the skin. Application of lipophilic substances, which readily spread on the surface of the skin, should fill air spaces between psoriatic flakes, providing a better match of refractive index at these optical interfaces, and consequently reduce the remittance of psoriatic plaques (C). Because this mechanism involves index matching, the reduction in remittance should occur over a very wide spectrum. Because only the surface of skin is involved, the effect should occur rapidly, and because normal skin has but one air–skin interface, oils should have little effect on remittance of normal skin. Relatively polar compounds such as water, which do not spread readily on skin, should either require a longer time to reduce remittance of plaques, or have lesser effect than oils, or both.

broadband UVB phototherapy without achieving any erythema, but this requires great attention to detail and some luck, and the doses used are very close to those which would be expected to produce erythema. In any case absence of delayed erythema of normal skin does not necessarily mean absence of phototoxic insult to cells. Dyskeratotic cells (55), DNA damage (56), melanogenesis (57), and decrease in threshold (58) to subsequent exposure have all been documented at suberythemogenic UV exposure doses.

Ultraviolet phototherapy has also been used in combination with other topical agents such as liquor carbonic detergens (42, 59, 60) and with dithranol (61, 62). The relative effectiveness of UV radiation reported in these studies is variable and seems to depend in part on the UV doses and the frequency and number of treatments. The therapeutic effects of dithranol appear least affected by UV radiation. The combination of UV phototherapy with orally administered retinoic acid derivatives appears to offer the short-term advantages of inducing remission with a lesser number of phototherapy treatments and with fewer side effects than seen with the oral agent alone (63,

64). Information about duration of remissions and long-term risks requires further study. Combination of phototherapy with other forms of treatment may decrease the total amount of UV radiation necessary to achieve and maintain clearing. This is important because the long-term risks of therapy include skin cancer and chronic actinic degeneration and are most likely related to both number of treatments and total cumulative exposure dose.

UVB therapy has been combined with PUVA (see Chapter 22) (65). Compared to the use of either modality alone, it was found that less than half the number of treatments were required. The total cumulative UVA dose required was less than half the dose that would be required using PUVA alone with the combination treatment. The cumulative UVB dose was 20% that required using UVB phototherapy. Also, the final dose of UVA or UVB at the time of clearing is considerably smaller than if either treatment is used alone. Because both PUVA and UVB are known carcinogens and may lead to chronic actinic damage, it is hoped that the smaller doses required in this approach will result in less cumulative phototoxic insult to skin. Long-term effects and maintenance requirements require further study.

SUMMARY

To date, all successful forms of phototherapy and photochemotherapy including tar and UV combinations (66–69) are known to induce damage to DNA. Because of the nature of psoriasis, a hyperproliferative disorder, DNA effects may be essential therapeutic mechanisms. The long-term effects of aggressive erythemogenic phototherapy are not certain. Long-term tar and UV phototherapy may increase the incidence of skin cancer in psoriatics (70); both agents are well-known carcinogens (see Chapter 9). More studies are needed.

There are several means by which phototherapy of psoriasis could be made safer and more effective. Methods of selectively increasing UV transmission into psoriatic tissue include refractive index matching, alteration of the optical properties of the surface of psoriasis, mechanical removal of scale, and selective elution of UV-absorbing substances from the abnormal tissue. Waveband selection may further improve effectiveness and reduce risks. Possibilities include the use of monochromatic radiation, collimated radiation, or sources with spectral power distribution matching phototherapy action spectrum. It may prove beneficial to alter the spectral power distribution of the source as therapy progresses, because the optical properties of normal and abnormal skin change after repeated UV exposures. Intelligent use of waveband interactions requires more study. The effectiveness of long-term hazards of maintenance therapy are uncertain. Much more study is needed to find the safest and most convenient way to treat psoriasis, a chronic disease which is often present intermittently throughout the life of an affected individual. Home phototherapy should receive thoughtful consideration.

Therapy of psoriasis with in vivo photochemistry is an effective treatment. Aggressive therapy and individualization of treatment should result in very satisfactory short-term management of over 90% of patients. The short-term side effects of phototherapy and photochemotherapy are avoidable by careful dosimetry. Long-term effects are most likely related to degree of phototoxicity during treatment and to total cumulative exposure dose. Because psoriasis is a life-long disease, it is important to explore ways to utilize photons for therapy but to minimize phototoxicity and total exposure doses. Combination treatments may be very useful in this regard and should be fully studied.* Psoriasis seldom causes death, but its discomfort and psychosocial trauma may in some measure spoil life.

ACKNOWLEDGMENTS. This work was supported by NIH Grant AM 25395-02 and by funds from the Arthur O. and Gullan M. Wellman Foundation.

REFERENCES

1. Saltzer, E. I. (1975): Relief from uremic pruritus: A therapeutic approach. *Cutis* **16**:298–299.
2. Gilchrest, B. A., Rowe, J. W., Brown, R. S., et al. (1977): Relief of uremic pruritus with ultraviolet phototherapy. *N. Engl. J. Med.* **297**:136–138.
3. Schultz, B. C., and Roenigk, H. H., Jr. (1980): Uremic pruritus treated with ultraviolet light. *J. AMA* **243**:1836–1837.
4. Gilchrest, B. A., Rowe, J. W., Brown, R. S., et al. (1979): Ultraviolet phototherapy of uremic pruritus. *Ann. Intern. Med.* **91**:17–21.
5. Alderson, H. E. (1923): Heliotherapy in psoriasis. *Arch. Dermatol. Syphilol.* **8**:78–80.
6. Bowers, R. E., Dalton, D., Fursdon, D., et al. (1966): The treatment of psoriasis with U.V.R., dithranol paste and tar baths. *Br. J. Dermatol.* **78**:273–281.
7. Young, E. (1972): Ultraviolet therapy of psoriasis: A critical study. *Br. J. Dermatol.* **87**:379–382.
8. Parrish, J. A., White, H. A. D., Kingsbury, T., et al. (1977): Photochemotherapy of psoriasis using methoxsalen and sunlight: A controlled study. *Arch. Dermatol.* **113**:1529–1532.
9. Parrish, J. A., Fitzpatrick, T. B., Tanenbaum, L., et al. (1974): Photochemotherapy of psoriasis with oral methoxsalen and longwave ultraviolet light. *N. Engl. J. Med.* **291**:1207–1212.
10. van Weelden, H., Young, E., and van der Leun, J. C. (1980): Therapy of psoriasis: comparison of photochemotherapy and several variants of phototherapy. *Br. J. Dermatol.* **103**:1–9.
11. Wolff, K., Fitzpatrick, T. B., Parrish, J. A., et al. (1976): Photochemistry for psoriasis with orally administered methoxsalen. *Arch. Dermatol.* **112**:943–950.

*Treatments can be "cycled." Patients may depend on one treatment for 1–3 years and then be switched to a second treatment. After several treatments have been used, patients might be recycled through the treatments once again. Physicians presently change treatments when patients begin to respond poorly or when long-term toxicity begins to be evident. It may be a better plan to institute premedicated, planned cycling of therapies from the beginning.

12. Pullmann, H., Galosi, A., Jakobeit, C., et al. (1980): Effects of selective ultraviolet phototherapy (SUP) and local PUVA treatment on DNA synthesis in guinea pig skin. *Arch. Dermatol. Res.* **267**:37–45.

13. Epstein, J. H., Fukuyama, K., and Epstein, W. L. (1968): UVL-induced stimulation of DNA synthesis in hairless mouse epidermis. *J. Invest. Dermatol.* **51**:445–453.

14. Krämer, D. M., Pathak, M. A., Kornhauser, A., et al. (1974): Effect of ultraviolet irradiation on biosynthesis of DNA in guinea pig skin. *J. Invest. Dermatol.* **62**:388–393.

15. Epstein, W. L., Fukuyama, K., and Epstein, J. H. (1969): Early effects of ultraviolet light on DNA synthesis in human skin in vivo. *Arch. Dermatol.* **100**:84–89.

16. Parrish, J. A. (1980): Action spectrum of phototherapy of psoriasis. *J. Invest. Dermatol.* **74**:251.

17. Stern, W. K., and Kihiczak, G. (1974): Photobiology of psoriasis. *Arch. Dermatol.* **109**:502–505.

18. Young, E., and van der Leun, J. C. (1975): Treatment of psoriasis with longwave ultraviolet light. *Dermatoligica* **150**:352–354.

19. Fischer, T. (1976): UV-light treatment of psoriasis. *Acta Derm. Venereol. (Stockh.)* **56**:473–479.

20. Parrish, J. A. (1977): The treatment of psoriasis with longwave ultraviolet light (UV-A). *Arch. Dermatol.* **113**:1525–1528.

21. Tronnier, H., and Heidbüchel, H. (1976): Zur Therapie der Psoriasis vulgaris mit ultravioletten Strahlen. *Z. Hautkr.* **51**:405–424.

22. Tronnier, H. (1977): Derzeitiger stand der Photochemotherapie für die Dermatologisch. *Praxis Dtsch. Dermatol.* **25**:265–276.

23. Mischer, P. (1977): Erste Erfahrungen mit der "selektivan ultravioletten Phototherapie" (SUP) der Psoriasis vulgaris. *Österreichische Dermatologische Gessellschaft, Jahressitzung* **18**:6.

24. Pullman, H., Wichmann, A. C., and Steigleder, G. K. (1978): Praktische Erfahrungen mit verschiedenen Phototherapieformen der Psoriasis—PUVA, SUP-, Teer-UV-Therapie. *Z. Hautkr.* **53**:641–647.

25. Schröpl, F. (1977): Zum heutigen Stand der technischen Entwicklung der selektiven Fototherapie. *Proxis Dtsch. Dermatol.* **25**:499–504.

26. Hönigsmann, H., Fritsch, P., and Jaschke, E. (1977): UV-Therapie der Psoriasis Halbseitenvergleich zwischen oraler Photochemotherapie (PUVA) und selektiver UV-Phototherapie (SUP). *Z. Hautkr.* **21**:1078–1982.

27. Sapeika, N. (1976): Treatment of psoriasis at the Dead Sea. *S. Afr. Med. J.* **50**:2021.

28. Schamberg, I. L. (1978): Treatment of psoriasis at the Dead Sea. *Int. J. Dermatol.* **17**:524–525.

29. Avrach, W. W. (1977): Climatotherapy at the Dead Sea. In: *Psoriasis*, edited by E. M. Farber and A. J. Cox, pp. 258–261. Yorke Medical Books, New York.

30. Goldberg, L. H., and Kushelevsky, A. (1977): Ultraviolet light measurements at the Dead Sea. In: *Psoriasis*, edited by E. M. Farber and A. J. Cox, pp. 461–463. Yorke Medical Books, New York.

31. Parrish, J. A., and Jaenicke, K. F. (1980): Action spectrum for phototherapy of psoriasis. *J. Invest. Dermatol.* **76**:359–362.

32. Goeckerman, W. H. (1925): The treatment of psoriasis. *Northwest Med.* **24**:229–231.

33. Goeckerman, W. H. (1931): Treatment of psoriasis: continued observations on the use of crude coal tar and ultraviolet light. *Arch. Dermatol. Syphilol.* **24**:446–450.

34. Muller, S. A., and Kierland, R. R. (1964): Crude coal tar in dermatologic therapy. *Mayo Clin. Proc.* **39**:275–280.

35. Perry, H. O., Soderstrom, C. W., and Schulze, R. W. (1968): The Goeckerman treatment of psoriasis. *Arch. Dermatol.* **98**:178–182.

36. Sams, W. M., Jr. (1974): Phototherapy of psoriasis. In: *Sunlight and Man: Normal and*

Abnormal Photobiologic Responses, edited by M. A. Pathak, L. C. Harber, M. Seiji, et al., pp. 143–147. Univ. of Tokyo Press, Tokyo.

37. Rasmussen, J. E. (1978): The crudeness of coal tar. *Prog. Dermatol.* **12**:23–29.

38. Grupper, C. (1971): The chemistry, pharmacology and use of tar in the treatment of psoriasis. In: *Psoriasis: Proceedings of the International Symposium, Stanford University*, edited by E. M. Farber and A. J. Cox, pp. 347–356. University Press, Stanford, California.

39. Petrozzi, J. W., Barton, J. O., Kaidbey, K., et al. (1978): Updating the Goeckerman regimen for psoriasis. *Br. J. Dermatol.* **98**:437–444.

40. LeVine, M. J., White, H. A. D., and Parrish, J. A. (1979): Components of the Goeckerman regimen. *J. Invest. Dermatol.* **73**:170–173.

41. Marsico, A. R., Eaglstein, W. H., and Weinstein, G. D. (1976): Ultraviolet light and tar in the Goeckerman treatment of psoriasis. *Arch. Dermatol.* **112**:1249–1250.

42. Everett, M. A., and Miller, J. V. (1961): Coal tar and ultraviolet light. II. Cumulative effects. *Arch. Dermatol.* **84**:937–940.

43. Crow, K. D., Alexander, E., Buck, W. H. L., et al. (1961): Photosensitivity due to pitch. *Br. J. Dermatol.* **73**:220–232.

44. Tanenbaum, L., Parrish, J. A., Pathak, M. A., et al. (1975): Tar phototoxicity and phototherapy for psoriasis. *Arch. Dermatol.* **111**:467–470.

45. Marsico, A. R., and Eaglstein, W. H. (1973): Role of longwave ultraviolet light in Goeckerman treatment. *Arch. Dermatol.* **108**:48–49.

46. Parrish, J. A., Morison, W. L., Gonzalez, E., et al. (1978): Therapy of psoriasis by tar photosensitization. *J. Invest. Dermatol.* **70**:111–112.

47. Petrozzi, J. W., Barton, J. O., Kligman, A., et al. (1979): Topical methoxsalen and sunlamp fluorescent irradiation in psoriasis. *Arch. Dermatol.* **115**:436–439.

48. Petrozzi, J. W., and Barton, J. O. (1979): Comparison of crude coal tar and topical methoxsalen in treatment of psoriasis. *Arch. Dermatol.* **115**:1061–1063.

49. Petrozzi, J. W., and de los Reyes, O. (1980): Ultraviolet phototherapy in psoriasis. *Arch. Dermatol. Res.*, in press.

50. Adrian, R. M., LeVine, M. J., and Parrish, J. A. (1980): Treatment frequency for outpatient phototherapy of psoriasis. A comparative study. *J. Invest. Dermatol.* **74**:251.

51. LeVine, M. J., and Parrish, J. A. (1980): Outpatient phototherapy of psoriasis. *Arch. Dermatol.* **116**:552–554.

52. LeVine, M. J., Hu, J., Anderson, R. R., et al. (1979): Reflectance of psoriatic plaques. Abstract presented at the 7th Annual Meeting of the American Society for Photobiology, June 24–28, Pacific Grove, California. *Programs and Abstracts*, p. 175.

53. Schleider, N. R., Moskowitz, R. S., Cort, D. H., et al. (1979): Effects of emollients on ultraviolet-radiation-induced erythema of the skin. *Arch. Dermatol.* **115**:1188–1191.

54. Frost, P., Horwitz, S. N., Caputo, R. V., et al. (1979): Tar gel-phototherapy for psoriasis. *Arch. Dermatol.* **115**:840–846.

55. Kaidbey, K. H., Grove, G. L., and Kligman, A. M. (1979): The influence of longwave ultraviolet radiation on sunburn cell production by UVB. *J. Invest. Dermatol.* **73**:243–245.

56. Gschnait, F., Brenner, W., and Wolff, K. (1978): Photoprotective effect of a psoralen-UVA-induced tan. *Arch. Dermatol. Res.* **268**:181–188.

57. Kaidbey, K. H., and Kligman, A. M. (1979): The acute effects of longwave ultraviolet radiation on human skin. *J. Invest. Dermatol.* **72**:253–256.

58. Parrish, J. A., Zaynoun, S., and Anderson, R. R. (1981): Cumulative effects of repeated subthreshold doses of ultraviolet radiation. *J. Invest. Dermatol.* **76**:352–355.

59. Everett, M. A., Daffer, E., and Coffey, C. M. (1961): Coal tar and ultraviolet light. *Arch. Dermatol.* **84**:473–476.

60. Ellis, C. C. (1948): The treatment of psoriasis with liquor carbonis detergens. *J. Invest. Dermatol.* **10**:455.

61. Ingram, J. T. (1953): The approach to psoriasis. *Br. Med. J.* **2**:591–594.

62. Comaish, S. (1965): Ingram method of treating psoriasis. *Arch. Dermatol.* **92**:56–58.

63. Beierdorffer, H., and Wiskemann, A. (1978): Kombinierte Therapie der Psoriasis mit einem aromatischen Retinoid (RO 10-9359) und UVB-Bestrahlungen. *Aktuel. Dermatol.* **4**:183–187.

64. Steigleder, G. K., Orfanos, C. E., and Pullmann, H. (1978): Retinoid-SUP-Therapie der Psoriasis. *Z. Hautkr.* **54**:19–23.

65. Momtaz-T., K., and Parrish, J. A. (1981): Combination UVB and PUVA in the treatment of psoriasis. *J. Invest. Dermatol.* **76**:303.

66. Walter, J. F., Stoughton, R. B., and DeQuoy, P. R. (1978): Suppression of epidermal and proliferation by ultraviolet light, coal tar and anthralin. *Br. J. Dermatol.* **99**:89–96.

67. Stoughton, R. B., DeQuoy, P., and Walter, J. F. (1978): Crude coal tar plus near ultraviolet light suppresses DNA synthesis in epidermis. *Arch. Dermatol.* **114**:43–45.

68. Cecht, T., Pathak, M. A., and Biswas, R. K. (1979): An electronmicroscopic study of the photochemical cross-linking of DNA in guinea pig epidermis by psoralen derivatives. *Biochim. Biophys. Acta* **562**:342–360.

69. Pathak, M. A., and Biswas, R. K. (1977): Skin photosensitization and DNA cross-linking ability of photochemotherapeutic agents (Abstract). *J. Invest. Dermatol.* **68**:236.

70. Stern, R. S., Zierler, S., and Parrish, J. A. (1980): Skin carcinoma in patients with psoriasis treated with topical tar and artificial radiation. *Lancet* **1**:732–735.

18

Laser Applications in Medicine

D. E. Rounds

Like conventional light sources, lasers emit photons which can interact with biologic molecules to produce photochemical reactions. However, lasers have unique properties that are not found in conventional light sources. These properties include monochromaticity, coherence, and high intensity.

MONOCHROMATIC CHARACTERISTICS

The earliest laser, such as the helium–neon and ruby lasers, emitted single wavelengths. As laser instrumentation developed, the new devices, such as argon and krypton lasers, offered multiple wavelengths, but monochromatic lines could be easily selected by passing the beam through narrow-band filters. More recently, tunable dye lasers have offered a wide variety of wavelengths, spanning the spectrum from ultraviolet (UV) throughout the visible region.

Although the broad absorption characteristics of most chromophores respond to (1–3), but do not require, monochromatic light activation, this property of laser light can be useful in probing certain biochemical events in living cells. For example, irradiation with a green (5300 Å) laser wavelength selectively prevented cytochrome c from serving as an electron and hydrogen ion acceptor without apparently affecting the functional capacity of cytochrome b (4). These two cytochromes are thought to be located adjacent to each other in mitochondrial membranes and the absorption characteristic of cytochrome b overlaps with that of cytochrome c (5). Similarly, the electron transport activity of cytochromes a and a_3 was found to be selectively inhibited by laser wavelengths of 6013 and 6096 Å, which were not absorbed by cytochromes b and c (4).

D. E. Rounds • Pasadena Foundation for Medical Research, Pasadena, California 99101.

COHERENCE

The coherence property of a laser, with its associated collimated beam, facilitates the directing of light through optical paths that are difficult, at best, with conventional sources. The collimated beam (plus the monochromatic characteristic, which reduces chromatic aberration) permits the focusing of the laser light with significantly less photon dispersion than is common for conventional sources. For example, the argon laser beam has been reported to demonstrate a biologically effective beam diameter of 0.6–0.7 μm (6), promoting the effective use of lasers to perform "cell surgery" by selectively destroying organelles (or parts of such organelles) of cells growing in tissue culture. The collimated property of the beam has also offered easy access to various body cavities through endoscopes (to be discussed later).

INTENSITY

The limited intensity of conventional light sources in the visible and near-UV regions of the spectrum often requires that photosensitizing chromophores be applied to target molecules before a photochemical event will occur. This is not necessarily true with laser sources, where a large number of photons can be made to impinge on a molecule within a 1-msec pulse width or less. This means that even moderate absorption by a target molecule can give a sufficient amount of energy to show a marked response. Moreover, in addition to the absorption of the primary wavelength emitted by the laser, the high photon density of the focused laser beam can also promote a two-photon absorption. This occurs when two photons strike a molecule simultaneously. The total energy of the two-longer wavelength photons absorbed by the target molecule is equivalent to that of a single photon having the energy of the doubled frequency of the primary wavelength. This phenomenon has been demonstrated with the use of organic solutions and crystals (7–9) as well as biochemically active constituents (10). Reduced nicotinamide adenine dinucleotide (NADH) has an absorption characteristic which transmits the primary wavelength from a ruby laser (6943 Å), but absorbs efficiently the doubled-frequency range of 3471.5 Å. When a ruby laser beam was focused in an NADH solution the two-photon absorption phenomenon produced a fluorescence excitation that was proportional to the square of the number of input ruby laser photons. This phenomenon also seems to be operational in laser-irradiated living biologic tissue (11). Therefore, in order to predict the effect of laser energy on biologic material, one must consider not only the degree of absorption of the primary wavelength of the laser beam, but also its doubled-frequency equivalent.

The intensity of laser energy often results in thermal effects in addition to possible photochemical events. In the case of laser emissions with pulse widths of a few milliseconds or less, the absorbed energy can produce a heat rise of up to several hundred degrees. If the temperature exceeds the vaporization point, the water content of the tissue will be converted to steam with a concomitant explosive expansion of the tissue. The heated tissue components will be released as a plume of incandescent particles and gases. A milder reaction, typically produced by continuous-wave lasers, simply results in charring and cratering of tissues. Thermal damage will proceed as long as the laser beam is applied to tissue. Using an appropriate wavelength, photon density, and duration of exposure, one can separate the tissue in the form of a bloodless incision, with blood vessels being coagulated as the beam passes through them.

Although the photons from low-power laser sources do not show any appreciable advantage over comparable conventional sources, the thermal response to high-power lasers has been used to good advantage in a number of medical applications. The remainder of this chapter will be devoted to a survey of some of the historical developments and current applications of lasers in medicine.

APPLICATIONS OF THE LASER TO OPHTHALMOLOGY

Photocoagulation of ocular tissues, using intense xenon-arc sources, was standard practice from the early 1950s as therapy for the repair of retinal detachments or retinal tears (retinoschisis). The light energy, absorbed principally by the pigmented retinal epithelium and the choroid, was converted to heat, which produced thermal coagulation of protein. Later, a scar formed in the site of injury, which strengthened the attachment between the neuronal layer and the choroid. It was a natural transition for ophthalmologists to substitute the ruby laser when this monochromatic coherent light source became available. The red (6943 Å) wavelength from a ruby laser was absorbed efficiently by melanin granules (12–14) and the laser beam was observed to produce smaller diameter retinal lesions than could be produced by the noncoherent light sources (15, 16). As compared with the broad-spectrum emission of the xenon-arc lamp, the longer wavelength of the ruby laser resulted in less transient absorption of the energy through the ocular media (the cornea, the aqueous humor, lens, vitreous humor, and the neuronal layers of the retina) before its absorption by the pigmented epithelium. As a result, less damage was produced in the peripheral tissues surrounding the target area.

Historically, patients were treated with the ruby laser to alleviate three of the more common types of retinopathies. As indicated above, the first type was detachment of the retina, derived from trauma, inflammation, or degeneration. Vitreous humor can enter holes or tears that develop in the retina to force the neuroepithelium away from the pigmented layer of the retina. The ruby laser has been used to seal off these holes, to effectively prevent this type of retinal degeneration (17, 18). Retinoschisis, the longitudinal splitting of the retinal layers, can often extend through the center of the retina (macula), the site of central vision. The laser has also been used effectively to wall off the progress of such a tear, which preserves the acute vision of patients with this pathology (15, 19).

The second major area in which the laser has shown promise is the reduction of macular edema. Photographs of fluorescein dye distribution, following injection of the antecubital vein, serve to outline the retinal vessels and more importantly, demonstrate vascular leaks of the dye. Such photographs also indicate the site and extent of leakage of serum into the vitreous humor (20, 21). This type of leakage interferes with the normal function of the cells in the macula, resulting in reduced acuity of central vision. The leaking retinal vessels can be effectively occluded to restore normal vision in many cases. However, in cases of senile macular degeneration and macular edema following cataract extraction, the laser treatment was effective only when the leakage was from discrete sites, but not when leakage was diffuse (22).

A third kind of retinopathy relates to microaneurysms and neovascular tufts formed in the retinal vessels of diabetics (23). These sites of weakened vascular walls often lead to the formation of intraretinal and vitreal exudates and hemorrhages. As the resulting blood clot contracts, it can produce intractable retinal detachment. Laser destruction of the vascular defects before they become hemorrhagic helps to preserve the patient's vision.

Hemoglobin contained within the retinal vessels transmits the 6943 Å wavelength of the ruby laser energy. Therefore, those laser wavelengths that match the absorption characteristic of hemoglobin were considered for application in ophthalmology. The two most intense wavelengths from the argon laser (4880 and 5145 Å) are absorbed by both hemoglobin and fluorescein (24). When this laser became available for clinical use, preliminary studies suggested that greater success could be achieved by treating diabetic retinopathies with the argon laser (25–28) than with the ruby laser. More recently it has been shown that even this form of therapy is not completely successful (29), but varying the techniques of applying the laser treatment (30) has suggested that methods are being developed to improve its effectiveness.

Early explorations of peripheral iridectomy with lasers seemed promising as a means of relieving the interocular pressure associated with glaucoma (31). Heydenreich (32) has employed this technique to enlarge the pupil, obliterate neovascularization in the area of the iris and lens, and treat iris prolapse. This type of interocular surgery could be performed without the requirement for surgical incision through the cornea. However, Worthen (33) questioned whether this form of therapy was sufficiently safe or effective to replace existing therapeutic techniques.

APPLICATIONS OF THE LASER TO TUMOR THERAPY

Of all the medical applications of lasers, the greatest expenditure of funds, time, and effort has been made in the pursuit of an effective treatment for cancer. From the time the earliest, low-powered devices became available, laser instrumentation has excited the interest of oncologists, who were often frustrated by the limitations of more conventional therapeutic procedures.

The pigmented melanoma was one of the first tumors to be irradiated with the laser. The melanin granules within the tumor cells absorbed energy from both the early ruby and neodymium lasers. Klein et al. (34) observed that laser treatment of the Harding–Passey melanoma in mice showed a variable response, ranging from complete regression to accelerated deterioration of the tumor-bearing host. McGuff et al. (35) reported that human tumors implanted in hamster cheek pouches responded well to the ruby laser in the 100–200 J/cm^2 range. Moreover, fibrosarcomas implanted in hamster flanks responded well to repeated treatments with a 10-mW HeNe laser. Minton et al. (36) demonstrated that irradiation of the S-91 Cloudman melanoma with either the ruby or neodymium laser at energy levels in excess of 1000 $J/pulse/cm^2$ caused tumor regression.

The types of human tumors that seemed to be most responsive to pulsed laser treatment included melanomas, angiosarcomas, basal cell epitheliomas, squamous cell epitheliomas, lymphomas, vascular tumors, metastases of bronchogenic carcinomas, and glioblastoma multiforme (37, 38). By 1968, a total of 27 laser-treated patients had been rendered symptom-free from basal cell epitheliomas for a period of 5 years (39). Regardless of this successful account, most laser investigators have concluded that the more conventional means of treating these tumors still seem better than treatment with pulsed lasers.

The response of tumors appeared to depend upon the wavelength of the laser used. After treating the Cloudman S-91 melanoma and the Lewis T-241 sarcoma with either the ruby or neodymium laser, Minton (40) observed that the energy absorbed by individual tumors (as based on their optical density to the imposed wavelength) must be considered in order to produce the optimized effect.

Another important consideration was the power density imposed upon the tumor. Minton et al. (36) developed probability contours for tumor destruction of both ruby and neodymium lasers. These contours appeared to show a linear relationship between tumor diameters and the imposed laser energy in joules. Energy densities producing a 99% probability of lethality for a tumor 2 cm in diameter would show only a 50% lethality for tumors 5 cm in diameter. Although hundreds of mice with transplantable tumors have been "cured" following treatment with large energy densities from pulsed ruby or neodymium lasers, this approach is impractical for the large tumor masses found in human patients.

Moreoever, it was further observed (41) that when transplantable tumors were irradiated with high-energy neodymium lasers, a plume was formed which contained viable airborne cells. When the contents of the plume were collected and reimplanted into another host animal, the dislodged viable cells were able to form new tumors. If a tumor is not completely encompassed within the area of impact, Hoye et al. (41) speculated that laser pressure could produce regrowth of tumor tissue within adjacent muscle bundles and tissue planes. It was later shown by Mullins et al. (42) that this dissemination could produce tumor emboli in the lungs and distribute viable tumor cells into adjacent liver parenchyma.

The problems of tumor cell dissemination and excessive tumor mass appear to have been circumvented when pulsed lasers were replaced with high-energy continuous-wave argon (3) or carbon dioxide (43) lasers. Instead of relying on selected energy absorption by tumor tissue, surgeons used the laser beam as a "light knife." Due to their water content, all tissues constitute a black body for the 10.6-μm wavelength of the carbon dioxide laser. Hemoglobin within well-vascularized tissues, such as the liver, absorbs the 4880- and 5145-Å wavelengths of the argon-ion laser. As a result, it was found that these continuous-wave lasers could excise tumors with relatively bloodless surgical incisions.

Engineers quickly provided surgeons with experimental CO_2 laser devices (43, 44) which seemed to offer some advantages over electrocautery and scalpels for relative ease of operation and healing rates in experimental animals (45, 46). These devices contained an articulating arm to deliver the focused laser beam through a sterilizable end piece held in the gloved hand of the surgeon. Built-in controls permitted the surgeon to regulate both the laser power and the exposure time.

Initial studies, using tumor-bearing animals, indicated that tumors could be either surgically removed (47) or vaporized (48). Blood vessels of 0.5 mm or less could be sealed during normal flow, while vessels up to 2.0 mm could be sealed if blood flow was prevented during laser treatment (49). Although the CO_2 laser produced a thin zone of thermal necrosis on the margins of the incision, which reduced the healing rate (50), Kaplan and Ger (51) observed that this necrotic tissue could be removed, prior to suturing the wound, by abrading the incision edges lightly with a sterile moist gauze. This procedure resulted in healing rates that were comparable to scalpel wounds. The latter authors concluded, after treating 85 cases of benign and malignant tumors in human subjects, that the CO_2 laser could (a) reduce the operating time by eliminating the need to ligate bleeding points, (b) reduce the amount of necrotic tissue and hematoma formation in the wound, which would lead to a diminished infection rate, (c) sterilize the wound in the case of existing sepsis, and (d) reduce the spread of malignant cells during extirpative surgery, as a by-product of sealing off the blood vessels and lymphatics around the tumor mass.

As previously indicated, the collimated beam of the CO_2 laser could conveniently be directed through endoscopes to reach pathologic tissue within body cavities, e.g., the larynx (52), the cervix (51), and the colon (51). Less accessible regions, e.g., the stomach lining, have been reached by passing a high-powered argon laser beam through a flexible fiber optics bundle. This latter method has been used primarily to quench the flow of blood from experimentally induced ulcers in dogs (53) and subsequently in naturally occurring bleeding ulcers in humans (54). With minor technical improvements, this technique may prove useful in treating stomach cancer as well.

APPLICATION OF THE LASER TO MEDICAL DIAGNOSTICS

Laser instrumentation has been used in a variety of ways to evaluate solutions, suspensions, aberrant cells, immunologic reactions, bacterial cell growth rates, and a variety of other parameters that would offer insight into medical problems. However, most of these systems could function equally well with noncoherent light sources, so are not dependent upon the special properties of the laser. In consideration of the application of lasers to the field of diagnostics, therefore, the discussion will be restricted to two subjects: holography and laser flow microphotometry.

The advent of lasers has made the development of holograms, or three-dimensional pictures, a practical reality. This procedure not only can overcome the depth of focus limitations in conventional photography, but also can detect changes in position of the image as small as one-tenth the wavelength of light being used to record the hologram (55, 56). As a clinical tool, holography of the internal structure of the eye appears valuable (57). Such a preparation will permit a careful study of the intraocular structure without inconveniencing the subject and will also permanently record subtle changes in a pathologic condition over a period of time.

Holbrook et al. (58) have also described a holographic system which offers an "x-ray view" of parts of the human body, but with better resolution of soft tissues than is provided by x-rays. The system uses acoustic waves in the frequency range 1–10 MHz to generate a holographic image of an object immersed in a tank of water. The interference pattern is formed on the surface of the water and is reconstructed into a 12-cm-diameter real-time image by reflecting a low-intensity argon laser beam from that surface into a television monitor or a photographic camera. Cartilage, tendons, and blood vessels can be resolved in addition to bone structure. The system has also demonstrated fibrotic intrauterine tumors, the calyces within a human kidney, and the ventricles of the brain. Structural modifications are being made in this promising system in an attempt to eliminate the need for immersing the patient in a water bath, to enlarge the image size, and to improve the resolution of the image. With these improvements, acoustical holography should be a valuable tool for the diagnostician.

Another laser system that has already proven its usefulness to cell biologists and is expanding into the area of diagnostics is flow micro-photometry (59). In this system, mammalian cells are made to flow in single file through a continuous-wave laser beam at a rate of about 5×10^4 cells/min. Although the HeNe laser can efficiently and reliably score the percentage of viable cells in a trypan blue-stained population (60), an argon-ion laser is more frequently used to excite fluorescence in fixed and stained cell suspensions. By measuring the degree of fluorescence excitation at specific emission frequencies, it is possible to conveniently measure the DNA distribution (and therefore the cell cycle phases) of different cell populations, detect the presence of viruses or other antigens with fluorescent antibody techniques, record the presence of parasites in red blood cells, and dif-ferentially count the major classes of white blood cells in the circulation, all with a high statistical precision (59). By plotting the relative amount of RNA vs. the DNA content in acridine orange-stained cell populations (as based on their red and green fluorescence excitation, respectively), it appears to be possible to discriminate among normal, dysplastic, and malignant cervical cells or other similar exfoliated cell populations (G. C. Salzman, personal communication). The cells showing high red fluorescence values, which are suspected of being abnormal, are automatically given an electrostatic charge. As they fall through a dc field, they are deflected into a sample collection container. These selectively sorted cells, identified as abnormal by machine scoring, can be prepared for microscopic confirmation by a pathologist. When this procedure is packaged for clinical use, it will greatly facilitate the processing of Pap tests and blood cell suspensions.

SUMMARY

Laser biologists have reached a level of experience that premits them to understand the basic principles of laser interaction with biologic tissues. Although diagnostic methods still rely on the ability of cells and tissues to block and scatter laser photons or show fluorescence excitation, most clinical applications involve controlled tissue destruction by producing a thermal event. Although clinicians must become experienced with laser instrumenta-tion to apply the therapy effectively, it is evident that the laser is well established as playing a useful role in the areas of ophthalmology and surgery. Continued development of novel laser instrumentation and expanded explora-tion into other areas of medical applications will no doubt lead to improved solutions to existing medical problems.

REFERENCES

1. Rounds, D. E. (1965): Effects of laser radiation on cell cultures. *Fed. Proc. Suppl.* **13**:S116–S121.
2. Rounds, D. E., Olson, R. S., and Johnson, F. M. (1965): The laser as a potential tool for cell research. *J. Cell. Biol.* **27**:191–197.
3. Brown, T. E., and Rockwell, R. J., Jr. (1967): The argon laser: its effects in vascular and neural tissue. In: *Record of the IEEE 9th Annual Symposium on Electron, Ion and Laser Beam Technology*, edited by R. F. W. Pease, pp. 407–411. San Francisco Press, San Francisco.
4. Rounds, D. E., Olson, R. S., and Johnson, F. M. (1968): The effect of the laser on cellular respiration. *Z. Zellforsch.* **87**:193–198.
5. Chance, B. (1959): Electron transfer in biological systems. *Proc. IRE* **47**:1821–1840.
6. Berns, M. W., and Rounds, D. E. (1970): Laser microbeam studies on tissue culture cells. *Ann. N.Y. Acad. Sci.* **168**:550–563.
7. Peticolas, W., Goldsborough, J., and Rieckhoff, K. E. (1963): Double photon excitation in organic crystals. *Phys. Rev. Lett.* **10**:43–45.
8. Singh, S., and Stoicheff, B. P. (1963): Double-photon excitation of fluorescence in anthracene single crystals. *J. Chem. Phys.* **38**:2032–2033.
9. Hall, J. L., Jennings, D. A., and McClintock, R. (1963): Study of anthracene fluorescence excited by the ruby giant-pulse laser, *Phys. Rev. Lett.* **11**:364–366.
10. Rounds, D. E., Olson, R. S., and Johnson, F. M. (1966): Two-photon absorption in reduced nicotinamide adenine dinucleotide (NADH), *NEREM Record* **8**:158–159.
11. Rounds, D. E., and Olson, R. S. (1967): Photoactivation of smooth muscle with the ruby laser. *USAF School of Aerospace Medicine Technical Report 67-66*, pp. 1–6.
12. Zweng, H. C., Flock, M., and Peabody, R. (1966): Histology of human ocular laser coagulation, *Arch. Ophthalmol.* **76**:11–15.
13. L'Esperance, F. A. (1966): Effects of laser radiation on retinal macular anomalies. *Int. Ophthalmol. Clin.* **6**:351–358.
14. Berler, D. K. (1967): A study of 150 eyes treated with ruby laser. *Am. J. Ophthalmol.* **64**:114–116.
15. Campbell, C. J., Rittler, M. C., and Koester, C. J. (1966): Photocoagulation of the retina. *Int. Ophthalmol. Clin.* **6**:293–318.
16. Vallotton, W. W., and Antine, B. E. (1967): Laser versus xenon photocoagulation. *South. Med. J.* **60**:819–822.
17. Zweng, H. C. (1966): Clinical ocular laser coagulation. *Int. Ophthalmol. Clin.* **6**:319–334.
18. Olivella-Casals, A. (1965): Possibilities of laser in ophthalmology. *Ann. Med.* (*Paris*) **51**:331–339.
19. Little, H. L., Zweng, H. C., and Peabody, R. R. (1970): Argon laser slit-lamp retinal photocoagulation. *Trans. Am. Acad. Ophthalmol. Otolaryngol.* **74**:85–97.
20. Peabody, R. (1967): Treatment of macular disease. In: *Record of the IEEE 9th Annual Symposium on Electron, Ion and Laser Beam Technology*, edited by R. F. W. Pease, pp. 397–401. San Francisco Press, San Francisco.
21. Spalter, H. F. (1968): Photocoagulation of central serous retinopathy. *Arch. Ophthalmol.* **79**:247–253.
22. Zweng, H. C. (1971): Lasers in opthalmology. In: *Laser Applications in Medicine and Biology*, Vol. 1, edited by M. L. Wolbarsht, pp. 239–253. Plenum Press, New York.
23. Cogan, D. G., Toussaint, D., and Kuwabara, T. (1961): Retinal vascular patterns. IV. Diabetic retinopathy. *Arch. Ophthalmol.* **66**:366–378.
24. Rounds, D. E., Olson, R. S., and Johnson, F. M. (1967): Wavelength specificity of laser-induced biological damage. In: *Record of IEEE 9th Annual Symposium on Electron, Ion and*

Laser Beam Technology, edited by R. F. W. Pease, pp. 363–370. San Francisco Press, San Francisco.

25. L'Esperance, F. A. (1969): The retina and the optic nerve. *Arch. Ophthalmol.* **82**:112–136.

26. Zweng, H. C., Little, H. L., and Peabody, R. R. (1971): Argon laser photocoagulation of diabetic retinopathy. *Arch. Ophthalmol.* **86**:345–400.

27. Gitter, K. A., and Robinson, T. R. (1973): Techniques of argon laser photocoagulation. *Ann. Ophthalmol.* **5**:703–714.

28. Bowbyes, J. A., Hamilton, A. M., Bird, A. C., et al. (1973): The argon laser—the effect on retinal tissues and its clinical applications. *Trans. Ophthalmol. Soc. U.K.* **93**:437–453.

29. Francois, J., and Cambie, E. (1976): Further vision deterioration after argon laser photocoagulation in diabetic retinopathy. *Ophthalmologica* **173**:28–39.

30. Little, H. L., Zweng, H. C., Jack, R. L., et al. (1976): Techniques of argon laser photocoagulation of diabetic disk new vessels. *Am. J. Ophthalmol.* **82**:675–683.

31. Hallman, V. L., Perkins, E. S., Watts, G. K., et al. (1968): Laser irradiation of the anterior segment of the eye. *Exp. Eye. Res.* **7**:481–486.

32. Heydenreich, A. (1969): Lichtkoagulation im Bereich des Iris-Linson-Diaphragmas. *Klin. Monatabl. Augenheilkd.* **155**:153–161.

33. Worthen, D. M. (1974): Laser treatment for glaucoma. *Invest. Ophthalmol.* **13**:3–6.

34. Klein, E., Fine, S., Laor, Y., et al. (1965): Interaction of laser radiation with biological systems. II. Experimental tumors. *Fed. Proc. Suppl.* **14**:S143–S149.

35. McGuff, P. E., Deterling, R. A., Jr., Gottlieb, L. S. et al. (1965): Effects of laser radiation on tumor transplants. *Fed. Proc. Suppl.* **14**:S150–S154.

36. Minton, J. P., Zelen, M., and Ketcham, A. S. (1965): Some factors affecting tumor response after laser radiation. *Fed. Proc. Suppl.* **14**:S155–S158.

37. Goldman, L. (1966): Applications of the laser beam in cancer biology (a review). *Int. J. Cancer* **1**:309–318.

38. Goldman, L. (1967): Laser treatment of cancer. *Prog. Clin. Cancer* **3**:205–220.

39. Goldman, L., Rockwell, J., Meyer, R., et al. (1968): Investigative studies with the laser in the treatment of basal cell epitheliomas. *South. Med. J.* **61**:735–742.

40. Minton, J. P. (1966): A correlation of the laser wavelength absorption capability of experimental and human tumor relationship to the quantitation of human tumor destruction by pulsed laser radiation. *Cancer* **19**:266–272.

41. Hoye, R. C., Ketcham, A. S., and Riggle, G. C. (1967): The air-borne dissemination of viable tumor by high energy neodymium laser. *Life Sci.* **6**:119–125.

42. Mullins, F., Hoye, R., Ketcham, A. S. et al. (1967): Studies in laser destruction of chemically induced primate hepatomas. *Am. Surg.* **33**:298–303.

43. Stellar, S., Polanyi, T., and Bredemeier, H. (1970): Experimental studies with the carbon dioxide laser as a neurosurgical instrument. *Med. Biol. Eng.* **8**:549–558.

44. Kaplan, I., Ger, R., and Sharon, U. (1973): The carbon dioxide laser in plastic surgery. *Br. J. Plast. Surg.* **26**:359–362.

45. Hishimoto, K., Rockwell, R. J., Jr., Epstein, R. A., et al. (1974): Laser wound healing compared with other surgical modalities. *Burns* **1**:13–21.

46. Fidler, J. P., Law, E., MacMillan, B. G., et al. (1976): Comparison of carbon dioxide laser excision of burns with other thermal knives. *Ann. N.Y. Acad. Sci.* **267**:254–262.

47. Kaplan, I., and Sharon, Y. (1976): current laser surgery. *Ann. N.Y. Acad. Sci.* **267**:247–253.

48. Hall, R. R. (1971): A carbon dioxide surgical laser. *Ann. R. Coll. surg. Engl.* **48**:181–188.

49. Hall, R. R. (1971): Haemostatic incision of the liver: carbon dioxide laser compared with surgical diathermy. *Br. J. Surg.* **58**:538–540.

50. Hall, R. R. (1971): The healing of tissues incised by a carbon dioxide laser. *Br. J. Surg.* **58**:222–228.

51. Kaplan, I., and Ger, R. (1973): The carbon dioxide laser in clinical surgery. A preliminary report. *Isr. J. Med. Sci.* **9**:79–83.

52. Strong, M. S., and Jako, G. J. (1972): Laser energy in the larynx. Early clinical experience with continuous CO_2 laser. *Ann. Otol. Rhinol. Laryngol.* **81**:791–796.

53. Dwyer, R. M., Haverback, B. J., Bass, M., et al. (1975): Laser-induced hemostasis in the canine stomach: Use of a flexible fiberoptic delivery system. *J. AMA* **231**:486–489.

54. Fruehmorgen, P., Bodem, F., Reidenbach, H. D., et al. (1975): The first endoscopic laser coagulation in the human gastrointestinal tract. *Endoscopy* **7**:156–157.

55. Ansley, D. A., and Seibert, L. D. (1970): Pulsed laser holography. *Ann. N. Y. Acad. Sci.* **168**:475–491.

56. Wuerker, R. F. (1970): Holography and holographic interferometry: Industrial applications. *Ann. N . Y. Acad. Sci.* **168**:492–505.

57. Vaughan, K. D., Laing, R. A., and Wiggins, R. L. (1974): Holography of the eye: A critical review. In: *Laser Applications in Medicine and Biology*, Vol. 2, edited by M. L. Wolbarsht, pp. 77–132. Plenum Press, New York.

58. Holbrook, D. R., Richards, V., and Pitt, W. L. (1976): Medical acoustical holography. *Ann. N. Y. Acad. Sci.* **267**:295–311.

59. Mullaney, P. F., Steinkamp, J. A., Crissman, H. A., et al. (1976): Laser flow microphotometry for rapid analysis and sorting of mammalian cells. *Ann. N. Y. Acad. Sci.* **267**:176–190.

60. Malamed, M. R., Kamentsky, L. A., and Boyse, E. A. (1969): Cytotoxic test automation: a live-dead cell differential counter. *Science* **163**:285–286.

19

Photodynamic Inactivation of Herpesvirus

J. L. Melnick and C. Wallis

Photodynamic inactivation has been known since Raab, at the beginning of the 20th century, observed that acridine was harmless to paramecia in the dark but was lethal when the organisms were exposed to visible light (1). Three decades later viruses were shown to be photosensitive (2, 3). However, assay methods in the 1930s were crude, and no quantitative results were reported. In 1958, Yamamoto (4) reported the first quantitative studies on photodynamic inactivation of bacterial virus; in 1960, Hiatt et al. (5) extended this work to a number of DNA-containing animal viruses, but found that RNA-containing enteroviruses were resistant to photosensitization. We have since learned that naturally photoresistant viruses can be made photosensitive if the virus is grown in cells maintained with medium containing proflavine, neutral red, or acridine orange. During replication of the virus, the photoreactive dye becomes incorporated within the virus structure (6–10). If one looks through the literature, one can see that in most laboratories virus titers could be reduced markedly by "dye–light" treatment, but usually some virus persisted. The point is that, *as usually practiced,* photoinactivation may not be complete. Transformation by such preparations in which some infectious virus is still present (11) cannot be said to be caused by photoinactivated virus. However, if the procedures described in the papers from our laboratory are carefully followed, photoinactivation can be made total (12–17).

J. L. Melnick and C. Wallis • Department of Virology and Epidemiology, Baylor College of Medicine, Houston, Texas 77030.

BACKGROUND STUDIES

Over the past two decades our laboratory has been engaged in photodynamic studies of a number of viruses, and it was from this background of experience (6, 12–16, 18) that our colleagues were led to apply the technique in the clinic. The parameters for the system were worked out with some of the enteroviruses, which are actually resistant to photodynamic inactivation if the dye is added to the virus in a test tube. However, if the dye is added to the cell cultures in which the virus grows, the progeny virus particles can be photosensitized. In the experiment shown in Table 19-1, the virus was allowed to remain in the cell for 24 hr, harvested, kept in the dark, and then titrated in the presence of light of such low intensity as to be barely visible. Aliquots of each harvest were also exposed to white light of high intensity for 15 min. Dilutions of dye up to 1:80,000 produced fully photosensitive virus. Even a concentration of 1:160,000 produced photosensitive virus with over 99.9% of the virus inactivated.

Using a concentration of neutral red of 1:40,000, we were interested in determining how long we had to treat the cells with dye before photosensitive virus developed. As shown in Table 19-2, it took 1 hr for dye to penetrate the cell and be at the location of viral replication, where it could be incorporated into the virus particle, making it photosensitive.

The next experiments were set up to answer the question as to how long cells that were exposed to dye (the dye was then removed and the cells washed) would retain the ability to produce photosensitized virus. At periods of 24–120 hr after exposure to dye, virus was added to the cell cultures and the cultures were harvested 24 hr later and examined for photosensitized virus. The results in Table 19-3 indicate that the cellsd retained the ability to produce photosensitized virus for as long as 72 hr after they were exposed to the neutral red.

We then answered the question of whether the mechanism of inactivation was on the virus coat protein or on the virus genome. Photoinactivated viruses

Table 19-1. Effect of Neutral Red Concentration on Development of Photosensitive Echovirus 7[a]

Concentration of dye	Log PFU/ml	
	Dark	Light (15 min)
None	7.5	7.6
1:10,000	5.2	0.0
1:20,000	7.3	0.0
1:40,000	7.5	0.0
1:80,000	7.4	0.0
1:160,000	7.7	3.2

[a] From Melnick and Wallis (19).

Table 19-2. Effect of Duration of Pretreatment of Cells with Neutral Red on Development of Photosensitive Echovirus 7[a]

Duration of treatment with neutral red[b] prior to virus inoculation (hr)	Log PFU/ml	
	Dark	Light
0	7.7	7.6
0.5	7.5	4.7
1.0	7.3	0.0
2.0	7.6	0.0
4.0	7.3	0.0

[a] From Melnick and Wallis (19).
[b] Concentration 1:40,000.

were prepared from enterovirus, influenza virus, poxvirus, and herpesvirus stocks. In all instances the antigenic potency of the photoinactivated viruses was equal to that of the live virus. This was true even when in vitro antibody-combining tests were carried out. Thus, the possibility of misinterpretation as a result of multiplication of any trace residual virus in the treated preparations was excluded. The results of such a test with herpesvirus are shown in Table 19-4. The results with viruses of all four groups showed that photodynamic inactivation does not alter the immunogenic antigen on the surface of the virus, and thus it must be affecting the nucleoprotein core of the virion.

ASSESSING THE RISK OF PHOTOINACTIVATION

The heterotricyclic acridine and phenazine dyes are photoactive compounds capable of absorbing light energy and participating in photooxidation

Table 19-3. Production of Photosensitive Echovirus 7 from Cells Inoculated with Virus at Various Intervals after 2-hr Pretreatment with Neutral Red[a]

Time interval between dye treatment of cells and virus inoculation,[b] hr	Log PFU/ml	
	Dark	Light
None (inoculated immediately)	7.5	0.0
24	7.3	0.0
48	7.7	0.0
72	7.2	0.0
96	7.5	2.5
120	7.1	4.1

[a] From Melnick and Wallis (19).
[b] Virus harvested 24 hr after inoculation.

Table 19-4. Neutralizing Antibody-Combining Test with Herpesvirus[a]

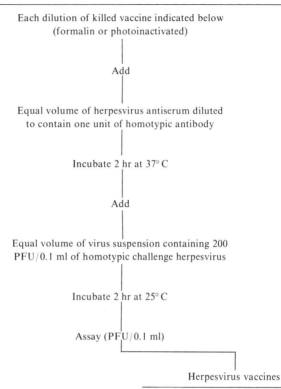

Each dilution of killed vaccine indicated below
(formalin or photoinactivated)

Add

Equal volume of herpesvirus antiserum diluted
to contain one unit of homotypic antibody

Incubate 2 hr at 37° C

Add

Equal volume of virus suspension containing 200
PFU/0.1 ml of homotypic challenge herpesvirus

Incubate 2 hr at 25° C

Assay (PFU/0.1 ml)

| | Herpesvirus vaccines | |
Dilution of vaccine used	Formalinized	Photodynamically inactivated
Undiluted	59	99
1:2	14	102
1:4	2	84
1:8	2	60
1:16	0	20
1:32	0	3
Vaccine potency	1:1	1:8
Controls		
Undiluted vaccine		
+ normal serum	0	0
+ normal serum and live virus	116	120
Control fluids		
+ normal serum and live virus	118	114
+ herpesvirus antiserum and live virus	0	1

[a] Herpesvirus inactivated by photodynamic treatment proved to be eight times more potent antigenically than
virus inactivated by formalin.

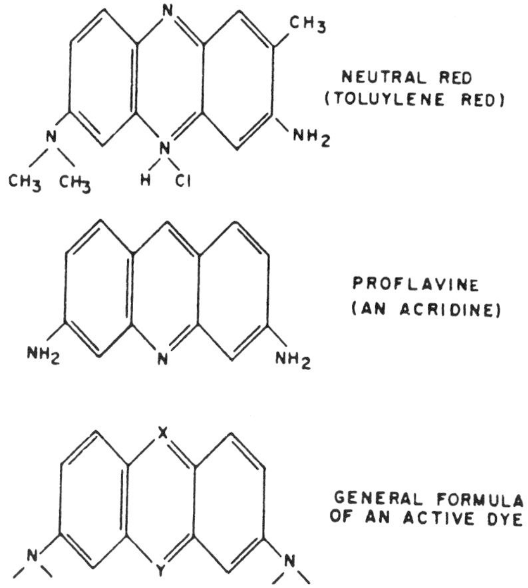

NEUTRAL RED
(TOLUYLENE RED)

PROFLAVINE
(AN ACRIDINE)

GENERAL FORMULA
OF AN ACTIVE DYE

Fig. 19-1. Structural formulas of photodynamically active dyes.

reactions. The acridine family includes familiar names like proflavine, acridine orange, and the antimalarials quinacrine and chloroquine. Neutral red, a phenazine compound (Fig. 19-1), was the first dye used in photodynamic inactivation of herpes simplex skin infections in humans (20). However, since neutral red is a potential contact allergen (21), and since proflavine has proven to be more effective photosensitizer of viruses in vitro (18), proflavine is the dye which has been used for clinical studies.

Proflavine sulfate (Fig. 19-1), a bright yellow, water-soluble acridine dye, was used extensively in the battlefields of World Wars I and II as a topically applied wound antiseptic (22). Laboratory experiments demonstrated bactericidal activity against a wide array of organisms, including *Staphylococcus aureus, Streptococus pyogenes, Bacillus anthracis, Clostridium welchii, Escherichia coli, Salmonella, Pseudomonas, Candida albicans*, and others (23–25).

Herpes simplex virus (HSV) can be irreversibly and permanently made photosensitive by heterocyclic dyes so that brief exposure to visible light renders the virus noninfectious (13). Photodynamic inactivation is dependent upon the dye concentration, temperature, and pH. When grown in cells pretreated with dye, the progeny virus becomes sensitive to light (16).

We have found that purified proflavine is at least 35 times more effective than neutral red in photoinactivating HSV (Fig. 19-2). Furthermore, commercially available proflavine is much easier to purify than the available but highly impure neutral red. Proflavine is a fluorescent dye which in aqueous solution at pH 7 maximally absorbs light at 444 nm (26). Light sources for the photoactivation of proflavine are readily available. Ordinary

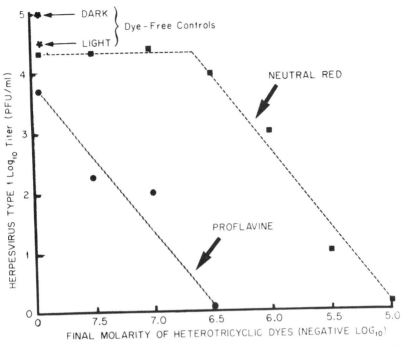

Fig. 19-2. Comparison of neutral red and proflavine for the photoinactivation of herpesvirus. Herpesvirus was diluted 100-fold in glycine buffer to contain 10^5 plaque-forming units per ml. Representative samples, all at pH 9, were treated with dye to attain the final concentration indicated in the figure. After 2 hr of sensitization at $37°C$ in the dark, aliquots were exposed to 5000 $\mu W/cm^2$ 450-nm light for 15 sec.

white fluorescent tube lamps emit only a small part of their total energy output at 450 nm (Fig. 19-3), and therefore are relatively poor sources for the photoactivation of proflavine.

The action spectrum for the photodynamic effect of proflavine corresponds precisely to the absorption spectrum of a mixture of dye and nucleic acid, but not exactly to that of the free dye. Thus, the dye molecules appear to be incorporated into HSV, where they are inserted or intercalated between the stacked bases of the DNA of the virus (27) (Fig. 19-4). The virus is inactivation when the dye-DNA complex absorbs a photon of appropriate energy to produce an oxidation reaction. This leads to a loss of guanine, gaps in the base sequence, and subsequent strand breaks in the DNA of the virus (29).

The question has been raised, based on a single experimental report, as to the cancer hazard of such disrupted DNA (30). HSV treated with neutral red and light was reported to retain transforming ability even though infectivity was destroyed; another report (11) in which 90% inactivated virus was used cannot be properly evaluated because of effects subsequent to the treatment may have been due to the residual live virus. Later (31), the transformed cells

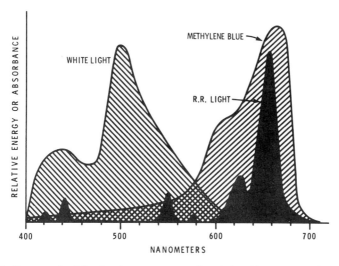

Fig. 19-3. Nomograph of the absorbance spectrum of methylene blue and the emission spectra of Westinghouse 40-W RR Special SHO tubes and of incandescent and fluorescent white lights. For proflavine a special Westinghouse fluorescent tube that emits light chiefly between 440 and 450 nm is also available.

were shown to produce tumors in hamsters, but the serologic response of the hamsters was qualitatively different from the response of hamsters bearing tumors known to be produced by HSV; the reason for this has not been explained.

Our laboratory (32) and others (33; M. Nachtigal, personal communication) have had no difficulty in reproducing HSV transformation induced by ultraviolet (UV)-inactivated virus. However, in spite of several trials, we have yet to induce transformation of hamster cells by photoinactivated virus. In our experiments we used strains with proved transforming ability (19). Similarly, another strain with relatively high transforming capacity was tested in Europe, in both newborn hamster kidney and lung cells, and again the transforming as well as the infecting capacity was destroyed by photodynamic inactivation (M. Nachtigal, personal communication).

More recently, studies have been carried out in our laboratory with viral

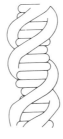 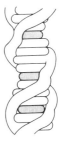

Fig. 19-4. The double-helical structure of DNA (left) and DNA-containing intercalated aminoacridine molecules (right) as proposed by Lerman (27). The base pairs (open disks) and acridine molecules (black disks) are viewed edgewise and the sugar–phosphate backbone is depicted as a smooth tube.

DNA (34). DNA isolated from HSV or HSV-infected cells was infectious when used as a transfecting agent. The specific infectivity of viral DNA isolated from purified HSV type 1 was 1500 plaque-forming units/μg. The DNA isolated from infected cells has much higher infectivity—5400 plaque-forming units/μg. When photodynamically inactivated, all the above DNA preparations rapidly and completely lost not only their infectivity, but also their transforming capacity. Khan et al. (35) also followed the fate of DNA present in photoinactivated virus after it was absorbed to cells. The DNA of the absorbed virus—in untreated or photoinactivated virus—rapidly entered the cell. However, within a few hours most of the DNA molecules from untreated virus went on to replicate; in contrast, in the same short period of time, DNA from photoinactivated virus underwent disintegration and after 6 hr could no longer be detected.

It has also been said that the photoactive dyes, because they are mutagenic, are probably carcinogenic as well. However, recent tests on proflavine by the National Cancer Institute carried out over a period of 2 years in Fisher rats and in hybrid mice that are highly susceptible to carcinogenic chemicals have been negative for tumor induction. Furthermore, Albert (26) in his authoritative monograph states that "no cancer-producing acridines are known." (Proflavine is 3,6-diaminoacridine.) Also, proflavine has long been used, particularly in Great Britain, as an antibacterial agent in the treatment of suppurative wounds, burns, otitis media, mastoid infections, and infections of the mouth and vagina.

In going through the literature, we noticed that some have reported an antitumor effect with some of the acridines, so we tested proflavine in this regard (19). We studied two tumor cell lines—HeLa and a transformed SV40 line—and compared their sensitivity in monolayer cultures with BSC-1, a continuous monkey line, primary monkey kidney cells, and primary rabbit kidney cells. Interestingly, the tumor cells were highly susceptible to proflavine and light, whereas the normal cells were relatively resistant.

As shown in Table 19-5, with no dye or with dye diluted to one in 16 million, no changes in quality were observed in any of the cultures nor in their passages (five for HeLa, SV40-transformed, and BSC-1 cells; and two for the primary cultures). However, the cancer cells and transformed cells were more sensitive to the dye–light treatment. The HeLa and the SV40-transformed cultures lost the ability to be passed after dye treatment at one in eight million concentration; in these two lines the effects increased markedly with increasing dye concentrations, which at one in one million produced the maximum effect scored—immediate rounding of the cells after irradiation. No effect was observed in the normal cell cultures or in their passages after the dye treatment at any concentration from one in 16 million to one in one million. Only after treatment using the highest dye concentration tested, 1:500,000, was there an observable effect on normal cells: after this treatment, the BSC-1 cells and the primary monkey kidney cells could not be passed, and

Table 19-5. Effect of Proflavine and Light on Transformed and Normal Cells[a]

	Effect on cultured cells[b,c]				
Dye concentration	HeLa	SV40 Tr	BSC-1	Primary monkey kidney	Primary rabbit kidney
1:500,000	++++	++++	+	+	++
1:1,000,000	++++	++++	0	0	0
1:2,000,000	++++	++	0	0	0
1:4,000,000	+	++	0	0	0
1:8,000,000	+	+	0	0	0
1:16,000,000	0	0	0	0	0
None	0	0	0	0	0

[a] From Melnick and Wallis (19).
[b] Exposed to light for 15 sec at a wavelength of 450 nm.
[c] Scores:
0: No deleterious effects observed in five serial transfers for HeLa, BSC-1, and SV40 Tr cells; in two transfers for primary monkey kidney and primary rabbit kidney cells.
+: No immediate visible effect, but cells could not be passed.
++: During 5 days of observation, cells showed rounding, ballooning, and syncytium formation.
++++: Immediate rounding of cells after irradiation.

the rabbit kidney cells in addition showed rounding, ballooning, and syncytium formation during the 5-day observation period. It may be that, because these cells have a higher rate of metabolism or DNA turnover, they become more sensitive to the effects of proflavine.

In the above connection, we would like to call attention to two recent papers on photodynamic treatment of experimental tumors (36, 37) (see Chapter 23 for details). In the long run, rather than inducing tumors, photodynamic inactivation may become a method of cancer treatment.

Since the issue continues to be raised, we would like to comment on the significance of in vitro transformation of hamster cells by viruses. Unfortunately, there are no data that allow us to transfer hamster findings to humans. Adenoviruses are highly oncogenic for the immunologically incompetent hamster. Not only do adenoviruses produce transformation in hamster cells, which after transformation can be passed and produce tumors in the hamster, but also the viruses themselves produce tumors in the hamster. Even in this potent system, despite intensive efforts, no evidence has been obtained for oncogenicity of adenoviruses in humans (28).

As regards the alleged production of greater transforming ability in the virus by photodynamic inactivation, this is open to question. We cannot as yet measure quantitatively the transforming capacity of herpesviruses in the absence of the proper cells for assay. The cells that are used are permissive for herpesvirus, so the infective component of the virus must first be inactivated before we can determine whether the virus can transform. In a situation such as that with SV40, where transformation can be measured accurately, UV radiation enhances transformation (38); dye–light treatment works differently and actually decreases its transforming ability (39). In any case, transformation by photoinactivated HSV has been difficult to confirm, so its seems to be a rare phenomenon at best.

IS PHOTODYNAMIC THERAPY EFFECTIVE?

We have dealt with the potential risks of phototherapy. Obviously, they should be considered worth taking only if the treatment is effective. Here, too, there is a controversy, and investigators must proceed with caution.

We first tested photodynamic inactivation as an experimental therapeutic procedure for HSV-induced keratitis in rabbits (40). The experimentally induced herpesvirus keratitis was resolved by the treatment. More recently, Stanley and Pinnolis (41) reported that "when incubation temperature, dye pH, and duration of the intervals between light exposure remain constant, blue fluorescent light (450 nm) caused more effective photodynamic inactivation of proflavine-sensitive HSV in rabbit corneas than did white fluorescent light. Blue light (450 nm) is closest to the light peak for optimum inactivation of the herpesvirus. Incandescent light, as used in our study, appeared to be no more effective than no treatment at all for this virulent herpetic lesion. Rapp's observations should not deter investigations of photodynamic inactivation as an alternate treatment of surface herpetic infections, particularly those caused by a virus resistant to topical chemotherapy."

The favorable in vitro and in vivo studies led our colleagues to test the procedure in the clinic. The therapy consisted of rupturing *early* vesicular lesions with a sterile needle, application of 0.1% aqueous solution of a photodynamically active dye to the base of the ruptured vesicles, and exposure for 30 min to a light source of sufficient intensity and of proper wavelength (450 nm for proflavine). Reexposure to the light was done at 6, 12, 24, and 48 hr. If new lesions developed, the procedure was repeated. The encouraging results obtained in a double-blind study (20) with patients having recurrent herpes simplex led to further trials in patients with herpes lesions of the vulva (42–44), penis (44), eye (45), and oral cavity (46), as well as the lip and skin (47, 48). Some of the results have been favorable, others have not. Additional trials at Baylor College of Medicine conducted as double-blind studies are discussed in Chapter 20 and by Kaufman et al. (49).

Perhaps the most striking example of the effectiveness of photodynamic therapy is provided by Chang and Weinstein (47), who treated the right side of the face and forehead of a 4-month-old child (Fig. 19-5) with diffuse vesiculopustular lesions (eczema herpeticum or Kaposi varicelliform erup-

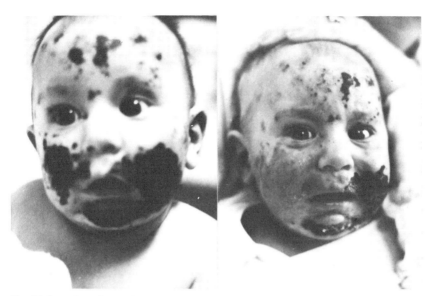

Fig. 19-5. Left, patient before treatment. Right, patient on fifth day of treatment. Lesions on treated side of the face (right side) are healed, whereas untreated ones (left side) are covered by eschar. [From Chang and Weinstein (47).]

tion). The case fatality rate for this serious disease is about 10%. Therapy with topical application of dye, in this case methylene blue (tetramethylthionine, a phenothiazine derivative chemically similar to the phenozine dye, neutral red) and light was started on the third day of illness and repeated the following day. The area was dry on the second day after treatment, whereas oozing was still present in the untreated area. Virus could no longer be recovered from the treated area 24 hr after the initial treatment, in contrast to its recovery for 5 days from the untreated area (Fig. 19-6). Four days after

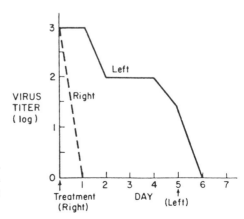

Fig. 19-6. Rapid disappearance of herpesvirus following treatment with methylene blue and light. [From Chang and Weinstein (47).]

therapy was begun, the treated side was completely healed, in contrast to the untreated side (Fig. 19-5). Photodynamic therapy was then applied to the left side of the face and healing was complete 3 days later. This is a fine example of what can be learned from a properly controlled trial, even from a single patient.

Another favorable report comes from London (50) in a study of herpetic keratitis photodynamically treated with proflavine. In such a study of an active disease of the corneal epithelium, the virus-infected cells are readily accessible to the dye and the light, and both the dye uptake and response to phototherapy can be serially observed with a slit-lamp microscope. The British investigators selected 0.1% proflavine for their trial because of its extensive ocular usage in the preantibiotic era; their more recent experience in treating infections did not reveal any toxicity at this concentration. Two stages were observed in the healing process after photodynamic treatment of herpetic corneal ulcers. In the hours immediately after treatment, there occurred debridement or shedding of virus-infected cells that took up the stain; this was transient or lasted for 24 hr. Reepithelialization followed soon thereafter; it was sometimes detectable at 24 hr, but usually became apparent within 48 hr after treatment. In summary, there was a "dramatic response in patients suffering from acute dendritic or ameloid ulcers that had failed to respond to IDU therapy. Such resistant ulcerative cases have the worst prognoses and many pose some of the most difficult problems encountered in patients with ocular herpes infections. The results of photoinactivation therapy were remarkable."

The British investigators, while enthusiastic about the results of photo-dynamic inactivation of herpesvirus in the eye, had serious reservations about the safety of applying proflavine to ulcerated human eyes. When they made small scratches in the corneal epithelium of the rabbit to mimic dendritic ulcers and followed this by proflavine–light treatment, they produced damage to the corneal keratocytes and endothelium with severe uveitis. The observations were similar to those made in certain patients after photodynamic therapy. These complications have led them to discontinue the dye–light treatment for the present, pending elucidation of the problem.

We endorse the conclusions of these investigators: "Before further clinical studies can be undertaken a detailed study must be made of the factors that surround uptake, penetration and persistence of the dye, and the interaction of adsorbed proflavine with light. In view of the apparent effectiveness of photoinactivation in healing certain forms of herpetic keratitis, the question of safety needs to be resolved."

SUMMARY

From the many sufferers of serious herpesvirus illness who still request treatment after being informed about the controversy surrounding photodynamic treatment, there is no doubt that they consider the potential benefit to be far greater then the potential risk. As regards the risk of cancer, it is important to note that in the SV40 system transformation potency was enhanced by UV irradiation (38), but was decreased and even eliminated by photodynamic treatment (39). In our laboratory the situation has been found to be similar for herpesvirus (19). We confirm that UV-inactivated herpesvirus can cause transformation, but we and others have been unable to induce transformation with virus that has been totally inactivated by photodynamic inactivation. Thus, transformation by virus inactivated in this manner does not appear to be a regular event. In some but not all clinical studies, photodynamic treatment of early herpetic lesions was reported to be beneficial. In more recent trials the treatment was of no advantage.

REFERENCES

1. Raab, O. Z. (1900): Ueber die Wirkung fluorescirender Stoffe auf Infusorien. *Z. Biol.* **39**:524–526.
2. Perdrau, J. R., and Todd, C. (1933): Photodynamic action of methylene blue on certain viruses. *Proc. R. Soc. Lond.* [Biol.] **112**:288–298.
3. Shortt, H. E., and Brooks, A. G. (1934): Photodynamic action of methylene blue on fixed rabies virus. *Indian J. Med. Res.* **21**:581.
4. Yamamoto, N. (1958): Photodynamic inactivation of bacteriophage and its inhibition. *J. Bacteriol.* **75**:443–448.
5. Hiatt, C. W., Kaufman, E., Helprin, J. J., et al. (1960): Inactivation of viruses by the photodynamic action of toluidine blue. *J. Immunol.* **84**:480–484.
6. Crowther, D., and Melnick, J. L. (1961): The incorporation of neutral red and acridine orange into developing poliovirus particles making them photosensitive. *Virology* **14**:11–21.
7. Schaffer, F. L. (1962): Binding of proflavine by photoinactivation of poliovirus propagated in the presence of the dye. *Virology* **18**:412–425.
8. Wilson, J. N., and Cooper, P. D. (1962): Photodynamic demonstration of two stages in the growth of poliovirus. *Virology* **17**:195–196.
9. Schaffer, F. L., and Hackett, A. J. (1963): Early events in poliovirus-HeLa cell interaction: acridine orange photosensitization and detergent extraction. *Virology* **21**:124–126.
10. Wilson, J. N., and Cooper, P. D. (1963): Aspects of the growth of poliovirus as revealed by the photodynamic effects of neutral red and acridine orange. *Virology* **21**:135–145.
11. Kucera, L. S., and Gusdon, J. P. (1976): Transformation of human embryonic fibroblasts by photodynamically inactivated herpes simplex virus, type 2 at supra-optimal temperature. *J. Gen. Virol.* **30**:257–261.
12. Wallis, C., and Melnick, J. L. (1963): Photodynamic inactivation of poliovirus. *Virology* **21**:332–341.
13. Wallis, C., and Melnick, J. L. (1964): Irreversible photosensitization of viruses. *Virology* **23**:520–527.
14. Wallis, C., and Melnick, J. L. (1965): Photodynamic inactivation of enteroviruses. *J. Bacteriol.* **89**:41–46.
15. Wallis, C., Sakurada, N., and Melnick, J. L. (1963): Influenza vaccine prepared by photodynamic inactivation of virus. *J. Immunol.* **91**:677–682.
16. Wallis, C., Scheiris, C., and Melnick, J. L. (1967): Photodynamically inactivated vaccines prepared by growing viruses in cells containing neutral red. *J. Immunol.* **99**:1134–1139.

17. Wallis, C., Trulock, S., and Melnick, J. L. (1969): Inherent photosensitivity of herpes virus and other enveloped viruses. *J. Gen. Virol.* **5**:53–61.

18. Wallis, C., and Melnick, J. L. (1965): Photodynamic inactivation of animal viruses: a review. *Photochem. Photobiol.* **4**:159–170.

19. Melnick, J. L., and Wallis, C. (1975): Photodynamic inactivation of herpesvirus. *Perspect. Virol.* **9**:297–314.

20. Felber, T. D., Smith, E. B., Knox, J. M., et al. (1973): Photodynamic inactivation of herpes simplex. *J. AMA* **223**:289–292.

21. Mitchell, J. C., and Stewart, W. B. (1973): Allergic contact dermatitis from neutral red applied for herpes simplex. *Arch. Dermatol.* **108**:689.

22. Mitchell, G. A. G., and Buttle, G. A. H. (1943): Proflavine in closed wounds. *Lancet* **2**:749.

23. Browning, C. H., and Gilmour, W. (1913): Bacterial action and chemical constitution with special reference to basic benzol derivatives. *J. Pathol. Bacteriol.* **18**:144–146.

24. McIntosh, J., and Selbie, F. R. (1944): Sulphathiazole—proflavine powder in wounds. *Lancet* **1**:591–594.

25. Wallis, C., Melnick, J. L., and Phillips, C. A. (1965): Bacterial and fungal decontamination of virus specimens by differential photosensitization. *Am. J. Epidemiol.* **81**:222–229.

26. Albert, A. (1966): *The Acridines*, 2nd ed., p. 193. St. Martins Press, New York.

27. Lerman, L. S. (1964): Acridine mutagens and DNA structure. *J. Cell. Comp. Physiol.* **64**(Suppl. 1):1–18.

28. Gilden, R. V., Kern, J., Lee, Y. K., et al. (1970): Serologic surveys of human cancer patients for antibody to adenovirus T antigens. *Am. J. Epidemiol* **91**:500–509.

29. Simon, M. I., and Vunakis, V. (1962): The photodynamic reaction of methylene blue with deoxyribonucleic acid. *J. Mol. Biol.* **4**:488–499.

30. Rapp, F., Li, J. H., and Jerkofsky, M. (1973): Transformation of mammalian cells by DNA-containing viruses following photodynamic inactivation. *Virology* **55**:339–346.

31. Li, J. H., Jerkosky, M., and Rapp, F. (1975): Demonstration of oncogenic potential of mammalian cells transformed by DNA-containing viruses following photodynamic inactivation. *Int. J. Cancer* **15**:190–202.

32. Melnick, J. L., Courtney, R. J., Powell, K. L., et al. (1976): Studies on herpes simplex virus and cancer. *Cancer Res.* **36**:845–856.

33. De Thé, G., Epstein, M. A., and zur Hausen, H. (1975): *Oncogenesis and Herpesviruses II: Proceedings of a Symposium Held in Nuremberg, Federal Republic of Germany, 14–16 October 1974.* IARC Publications No. 11.

34. Melnick, J. L., Khan, N. C., and Biswal, N. (1977): Photodynamic inactivation of herpes simplex virus and its DNA. *Photochem. Photobiol.* **25**:341–342.

35. Khan, N. C., Melnick, J. L., and Biswal, N. (1977): Photodynamic treatment of herpes simplex virus during its replicative cycle. *J. Virol.* **21**:16–23.

36. Dougherty, T. J. (1974): Activated dyes as antitumor agents. *J. Natl. Cancer Inst.* **52**:1333–1336.

37. Tomson, S. H., Emmett, E. A., and Fox, S. H. (1974): Photodestruction of mouse epithelial tumors after oral acridine orange and argon laser. *Cancer Res.* **34**:3124–3127.

38. Seemayer, N. H., and Defendi, V. (1973): Analysis of minimal functions of simian virus 40. II. Enhancement of oncogenic transformation *in vitro* by UV *J. Virol.* **12**:1265–1271.

39. Seemayer, N. H., Hirai, K., and Defendi, V. (1973): Analysis of minimal functions of simian virus 40. I. Oncogenic transformation of Syrian hamster kidney cells *in vitro* by photodynamically inactivated SV40. *Int. J. Cancer* **12**:524–531.

40. Moore, C., Wallis, C., Melnick, J. L., et al. (1972): Photodynamic treatment of herpes keratitis. *Infect. Immun.* **5**:169–171.

41. Stanley, J. A., and Pinnolis, M. (1976): Light intensity on the photodynamic inactivation of herpes simplex keratitis. *Am. J. Ophthalmol.* **81**:332–336.

42. Friedrich, E. G., Jr. (1973): Relief for herpes vulvitis. *Obstet. Gynecol.* **41**:74–77.

43. Kaufman, R. H., Gardner, H. L., Brown, D., et al. (1973): Herpes genitalis treated by photodynamic inactivation of virus. *Am. J. Obstet. Gynecol.* **117**:1144–1146.
44. Roome, A. P. C. H., Tinkler, A. E., Hilton, A. L., et al. (1975): Neutral red with photoinactivation in the treatment of herpes genitalis. *Br. J. Vener. Dis.* **51**:130–133.
45. Stanley, J. A. (1973): In: *Research to Prevent Blindness*. International Science Writers Seminar, pp. 29–30.
46. Editorial (1974): *Clinical Dentistry* **2**:7.
47. Chang, T. -W., and Weinstein, L. (1975): Eczema herpeticum treatment with methylene blue and light. *Arch. Dermatol.* **111**:1174–1175.
48. Myers, M. G., Oxman, M. N., Clark, J. E., et al. (1975): Failure of neutral-red photodynamic inactivation in recurrent herpes simplex virus infections. *N. Engl. J. Med.* **293**:945–949.
49. Kaufman, R. H., Adam, E., Mirkovic, R. M., et al. (1978): Treatment of genital herpes simplex virus infection with photodynamic inactivation. *Am. J. Obstet. Gynecol.* **132**:861–869.
50. O'Day, D. M., Jones, B. R., Poirier, R., et al. (1975): Proflavine photodynamic viral inactivation in herpes simplex keratitis. *Am. J. Ophthalmol.* **79**:941–948.

20

Dye-Light Phototherapy of Viral, Bacterial, and Fungal Infections

M. Jarratt, W. Hubler, Jr., and W. Panek

In 1899 Oscar Raab (1), a student in Dr. H. von Tappeiner's Munich laboratory, observed that paramecia were killed in the presence of acridine dye and light but were unharmed in the presence of acridine dye in the dark. During the next few years of the early 20th century, von Tappeiner and Jodlbauer (2–4) conducted a long series of experiments with the dye–light reaction and coined the term "photodynamische erscheinung" (photodynamic action). They demonstrated that many dyes photosensitize a wide variety of microorganisms in vitro (Fig. 20-1).

The earliest published attempts to apply photodynamic action therapeutically to skin disease appeared in 1924, when Chavarria and Clark (5) showed that eosin and light enhanced the healing of experimental dermatophyte infections in guinea pigs. Thereafter photodynamic action was investigated in the treatment of cutaneous viral and bacterial infections as well.

PHOTODYNAMIC THERAPY OF CUTANEOUS AND OCULAR VIRAL INFECTIONS

In 1931 Clifton (6) observed photodynamic inactivation of viruses (staphylococcal bacteriophage) with methylene blue and toluidine blue. In

M. Jarratt, W. Hubler, Jr., and W. Panek • Department of Dermatology, Baylor College of Medicine, Houston, Texas 77030.

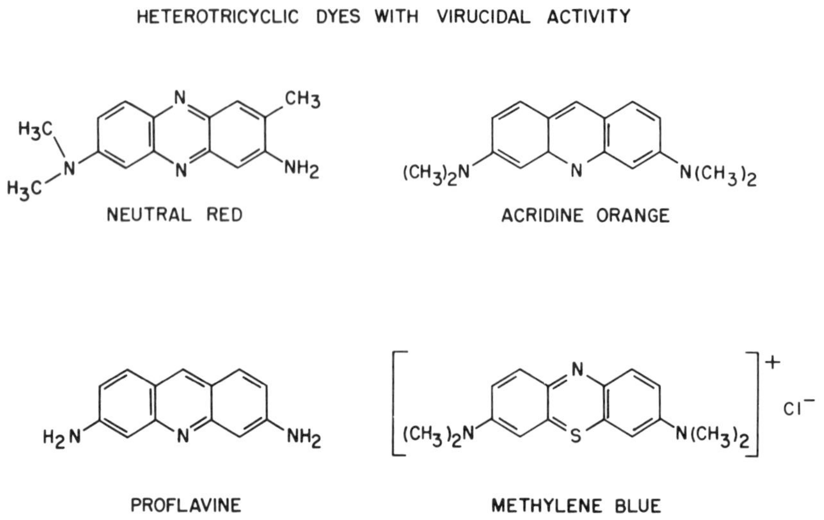

HETEROTRICYCLIC DYES WITH VIRUCIDAL ACTIVITY

NEUTRAL RED

ACRIDINE ORANGE

PROFLAVINE

METHYLENE BLUE

Fig. 20-1. Heterotricyclic dyes that photoinactivate a wide variety of viruses, bacteria, and fungi.

1932, Perdrau and Todd (7) suppressed experimental vaccinia and herpes simplex virus (HSV) infections in the skin and eyes of rabbits with methylene blue and light. In recent years in vitro studies have confirmed the effectiveness of photodynamic action in reducing or eliminating the infectivity of plant viruses (8), bacterial viruses (9), and animal viruses (10, 11).

Interest in the clinical use of photodynamic action in the treatment of cutaneous HSV infection was revived in 1973 by the work of Felber et al. (12). It was reported that the application of neutral red dye and fluorescent light to recurrent herpetic lesions resulted not only in a shortened healing time of recurrent lesions, but also in a reduction in the overall recurrence rate. Kaufman et al. (13), Lefebvre and McNellis (14), and Hinthorn et al. (15) reported similar success in the use of neutral red photoinactivation of cutaneous herpes simplex infection. Rubin and Heaton (16) reported rapid healing and apparent decrease in recurrence rate in patients with herpes labialis and herpes genitalis after treatment with acridine orange and light. Chang and Weinstein (17) reported unilateral healing of facial eczema herpeticum treated initially on one side with methylene blue and light. The untreated control side remained clinically active, with high titers of recoverable HSV for 4 days after the treated side healed. Subsequent methylene blue–light therapy of the control side resulted in rapid healing.

Several publications reported successful dye–light therapy of experimental herpetic keratitis in rabbits (18–20). Although Lahav et al. (21) were not impressed with neutral red–light therapy in shortening the duration of experimental keratitis in rabbits, the therapy dramatically reduced neurogenic spread of the virus from the rabbit eye to the brain, and thus prevented fatal HSV encephalitis in 8 out of 10 dye–light-treated animals. All 10 of the placebo-treated control animals succumbed to HSV encephalitis. Using proflavine–light therapy, O'Day et al. (22) healed 8 out of 10 patients with idoxuridine-resistant herpetic keratitis. Although their human studies indicated efficacy for dye–light therapy of herpetic keratitis, they unfortunately observed instances of phototoxic keratitis and anterior uveitis after exposure of dye-sensitized eyes to excessive amounts of visible light irradiation.

After an initial enthusiastic reception for dye–light therapy of herpes simplex, the tide began to turn as double-blind, placebo controlled studies appeared in the literature. Myers et al. (23) treated 170 episodes of recurrent cutaneous herpes simplex with neutral red and light and found no significant effect either on the duration of herpetic lesions or on the frequency of subsequent recurrences. Taylor and Doherty (24) concluded that proflavine photoinactivation of herpes genitalis was no better than topically applied normal saline. Roome et al. (25) compared neutral red against a nonphotoactive dye, phenol red, and found no difference in response to therapy between the two groups. Kaufman et al. (26) treated 175 women with herpes genitalis in a double-blind, placebo controlled trial with proflavine or with a nonphotoactive yellow vegetable dye, and concluded that there was no difference in the duration of lesions or in the subsequent development of recurrences in the proflavine-treated and the placebo-treated groups.

Soon after the introduction of dye–light therapy for HSV by Felber et al. in 1973, Rapp (27) expressed concern that photoinactivation of HSV might prove to be clinically hazardous. Duff and Rapp (28) previously had shown that hamster cells undergo oncogenic transformation after exposure to HSV type 2. Rapp and his co-workers (29–31) subsequently demonstrated the oncogenic potential of mammalian cells transformed by photodynamically inactivated HSV, and demonstrated enhancement of biochemical transformation of mouse cells by photodynamically treated HSV type 2 over that induced by untreated HSV type 2.

In 1977 it was suggested that Dr. Rapp's fears of the carcinogenic potential of dye–light therapy had been realized. A young man with a history of herpes genitalis treated with dye–light therapy subsequently developed multicentric Bowen disease on the penis (32). The 21-year-old man had a history of recurrent herpes simplex treated with neutral red dye and light on the dorsum of his penis; the lesions of Bowen disease appeared on the ventral aspect of his penis. Since that report, multicentric Bowen disease (Bowenoid papulosis) on the genitalia of young men and women has been reviewed. Most cases of multicentric Bowen disease on the genitalia of young people occur in patients who have no history of genital viral infections or dye–light therapy (33–37). Kopf et al. (38) concluded that "dye–light photochemotherapy is *not* related (to multicentric Bowen disease) in most cases if, indeed, it is in any."

PHOTODYNAMIC THERAPY OF CUTANEOUS
BACTERIAL INFECTIONS

In 1913, Browning and Gilmour (39) demonstrated that acridine yellow and proflavine possessed bactericidal activity in high dilutions against *Staphylococcus aureus, Escherichia coli, Salmonella,* and *Bacillus anthracis.* During World War II acridine dyes first gained widespread use as an antibacterial treatment for wound infections (40); the acridine dye proflavine sulfate was used in treating wound sepsis as an aqueous solution 1 : 1000 and as a powder applied directly into wounds (41, 42). The alkaline pH of proflavine sulfate was found to be the decisive factor in increasing its bactericidal activity over the more acidic acridine derivatives (43, 44). Gordon et al. (45) inoculated mice intradermally with streptococci, treated them with topically applied 1% proflavine, and demonstrated a 50% survival rate in the treated animals as compared to a 10% survival rate in the untreated animals. Rubbo et al. (44) showed that aqueous proflavine 1 : 10,000 killed over 90% of *Streptococcus pyogenes* in 1 hr in serum broth. The minimal bacteristatic concentration of proflavine was shown to be 1 : 160,000 (40). Proflavine is still used as a topical wound antiseptic in Europe. Its clinical use has been characterized by minimal toxicity, a wide spectrum of bactericidal activity, and the rare appearance of resistant bacterial strains.

Investigations of the bactericidal effect of photoactive dyes reviewed above were conducted in ambient light. No attempts were made to demonstrate with dark controls the enhancing effect of photodynamic action. In 1953, Heinmets et al. (46) conducted a sophisticated investigation of the photodynamic bactericidal action of methylene blue on *E. coli* and identified 615 nm as the activating wavelength. In 1964, Wallis et al. (47), with the use of dark and light controls, demonstrated a dramatic accentuation of the bactericidal effect of proflavine on *E. coli* and *Pseudomonas* when cultures

Table 20-1. Photodynamic Inactivation of Bacteria by Proflavine
Sulfate 0.001%

Organism	Bacterial colonies per drop		
	Saline/Light	Proflavine/Dark	Proflavine/Light
Staphylococcus aureus	32	4	0
Staphylococcus epidermidis	102	26	0
Streptococcus pyogenes	84	78	0
Escherichia coli	43	0	0
Clostridium welchii	24	0	0
Pseudomonas	25	0	0
Salmonella	68	0	0
Bacillus anthracis	46	4	0

Table 20-2. Photodynamic Inactivation of Gram-Negative Bacteria by
Proflavine Sulfate 0.0001%

Organism	Bacterial colonies per drop		
	Saline/Light	Proflavine/Dark	Proflavine/Light
Escherichia coli	40	22	0
Clostridium welchii	27	12	0
Pseudomonas	30	17	0
Salmonella	84	28	0
Bacillus anthracis	68	20	0

were exposed to white fluorescent lamps. Cooney and Krinsky (48) demonstrated an identical photodynamic effect of toluidine blue on *Acholeplasma laidlawii.*

Recent in vitro studies in our laboratories confirm that proflavine sulfate photoinactivates a wide variety of gram-positive and gram-negative bacteria (Table 20-1). Gram-negative organisms are more sensitive to proflavine photoinactivation than are gram-positive organisms (Table 20-2).

Gram-positive and gram-negative bacteria were grown in nutrient broth for 12 hr and subsequently diluted with sterile normal saline to a concentration of 1×10^8 colony-forming units per 1 ml of broth. Bacterial suspensions were treated with proflavine sulfate 0.001% or 0.0001% and held in the dark for 1 hr. Bacterial suspensions without proflavine were prepared as controls. One set of bacterial suspensions with proflavine was exposed to two Westinghouse BB 20-W blue fluorescent tubes at a distance of 6 in. for 3 min. Control suspensions of bacteria–proflavine were maintained in the dark. Additional controls of bacteria in normal saline were exposed to light. Subsequently, a cationic resin was added to all bacterial suspensions and agitated for 5 min to remove proflavine. Bacterial suspensions from the three treatment groups (proflavine/light, proflavine/dark, normal saline/light) were transferred to tryptic soy agar plates by the drop plate technique and incubated at 38° C for 48 hr (Fig. 20-2). Average bacterial colonies per drop were recorded. See Tables 20-1 and 20-2 for results.

PHOTODYNAMIC THERAPY OF CUTANEOUS
FUNGAL INFECTIONS

In 1924, Chavarria and Clark (5) produced cutaneous lesions in guinea pigs with *Trichophyton acuminatum* and treated them with eosin and visible light. Control animals treated with eosin in the dark and with light without eosin were compared to animals treated with eosin and light. After 12 days, the guinea pigs maintained in darkness were unchanged. The guinea pigs

PHOTODYNAMIC INACTIVATION

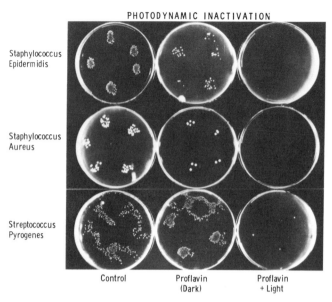

Staphylococcus
Epidermidis

Staphylococcus
Aureus

Streptococcus
Pyrogenes

Control   Proflavin   Proflavin
                         (Dark)   + Light

Fig. 20-2. The antibacterial effect of proflavine is markedly enhanced by visible light.

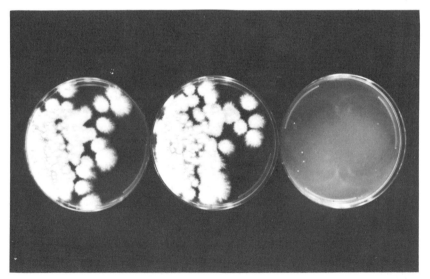

Fig. 20-3. Proflavine and light photoinactivate *Trichophyton mentagrophytes* (shown here) and other dermatophyte fungi. Left, control; center, proflavine–dark; right, proflavine–light.

Table 20-3. Photodynamic Inactivation of Dermatophyte Fungi by
Proflavine Sulfate 0.001%, pH 7

Organism	Fungal colonies per plate		
	Saline/Light	Proflavine/Dark	Proflavine/Light
Trichophyton mentagrophytes	57	60	0
Trichophyton rubrum	56	33	0
Trichophyton tonsurans	50	14	0
Microsporum canis	4	4	0

treated with visible light without eosin showed slight improvement. The
guinea pigs treated with eosin and visible light were cured of cutaneous
dermatophyte infections. In 1962, Dickey (49) demonstrated the photodynamic fungicidal effects of neutral red, methylene blue, and other dyes on
Candida albicans and *Trichophyton mentagrophytes*. Inactivation of *C.
albicans* by proflavine in low concentrations is enhanced by light exposure
(47). Recent in vitro studies in our laboratories show that several dermatophyte fungi are inactivated by proflavine and light but not by the same
concentration of proflavine in the dark (Fig. 20-3) (Table 20-3) and that the
photodynamic fungicidal effect is enhanced at higher pH. (Table 20-4).

Spores obtained from Sabauraud cultures of several dermatophyte fungi
were incubated in aqueous proflavine sulfate 0.01% or 0.001% and irradiated
for 2 hr under two Westinghouse BB 20-W blue fluorescent lamps at a distance
of 4 cm. Control suspensions of dermatophyte spores in proflavine were
maintained in the dark and dermatophyte spore suspensions without
proflavine were exposed to Westinghouse blue fluorescent lamps as described
above. Two identical series of experiments were conducted at pH 4 and pH 10.
After incubation with proflavine, fungal spore suspensions were treated with a
cationic resin to remove proflavine. Samples from each fungal suspension
were streaked onto Mycosel plates and incubated at room temperature for 4
days, after which fungal colonies were counted. See Tables 20-3 and 20-4 for
results.

Table 20-4. Effect of pH on Photodynamic Inactivation of *Trichophyton
mentagraphytes* by Proflavine Sulfate 0.001%

	Fungal colonies per plate		
	Saline/Light	Proflavine/Dark	Proflavine/Light
pH 4	125	120	90
pH 10	110	60	0

SUMMARY

Photodynamic inactivation of viruses, bacteria, and fungi by photoactive dyes and visible light is a well-documented phenomenon. Thus far, however, this potent physicochemical reaction has yet to find its place in modern clinical medicine. Although dye–light inactivation of idoxuridine-resistant herpetic keratitis has been accomplished, the treatment also results in photoinduced keratitis and uveitis (22). Although dye–light inactivation of eczema herpeticum has been observed (17), the treatment does not ameliorate recurrent herpes labialis or herpes genitalis (23–26). And although dye–light therapy has been shown to cure superficial bacterial and fungal infections (5, 45), the treatment has lost out to modern-day nonstaining antibiotics and antifungals. Perhaps the successful application of photodynamic action in clinical photomedicine is yet to come.

REFERENCES

1. Raab, O. (1900): Ueber die Wirkung fluorescierender Stoffe und Infusorien. *Z. Biol.* **39**:524–526.
2. von Tappeiner, H., and Jodlbauer, A. (1904): Ueber die Wirkung der photodynamishen Stoffe auf Protozoen und Enzyme. *Dtsch. Arch. Klin. Med.* **80**:427.
3. von Tappeiner, H., and Jodlbauer, A. (1907): *Die sensibilisierende Wirkung Fluorescierender Substanzen.* Vogel, Leipzig.
4. von Tappeiner, H. (1909): Die photodynamische Erscheinung (Sensibilisierung durch fluoressierende Stoffe). *Ergeb. Physiol.* **8**:698–741.
5. Chavarria, A. P., and Clark, J. H. (1924): The reaction of pathogenic fungi to ultraviolet light. *Am. J. Hygiene* **4**:639–649.
6. Clifton, C. E. (1931): Photodynamic action of certain dyes on the inactivation of Staphylococcus bacteriophage. *Proc. Soc. Exp. Biol. Med.* **28**:745–746.
7. Perdrau, J. R., and Todd, C. (1933): The photodynamic action of methylene blue on certain viruses. *Proc. R. Soc. Lond.* **112**:288–298.
8. Orlob, G. B. (1967): Inactivation of purified plant viruses and their nucleic acids by photosensitizing dyes. *Virology* **31**:402–413.
9. Hessler, A. Y. (1965): Acridine resistance in bacteriophage T2H as a function of dye penetration measured by mutagenesis and photoinactivation. *Genetics* **52**:711–722.
10. Wallis, C., and Melnick, J. L. (1965): Photodynamic inactivation of animal viruses. *Photochem. Photobiol.* **41**:159–170.
11. Wallis, C., and Melnick, J. L. (1965): Photodynamic inactivation of enteroviruses. *J. Bacteriol.* **89**:41–46.
12. Felber, T. D., Smith, E. B., Knox, J. M., et al. (1973): Photodynamic inactivation of herpes simplex. *J. AMA* **223**:289–292.
13. Kaufman, R. H., Gardner, H. L., Brown, D., et al. (1973): Herpes genitalis treated by photodynamic inactivation of virus. *Obstet. Gynecol.* **117**:1144–1146.
14. Lefebvre, E. B., and McNellis, E. E. (1973): Photoinactivation of herpes simplex. *J. AMA* **224**:1039.
15. Hinthorne, D. R., Baker, L. H., Romig, D. A., et al. (1976): Recurrent conjugal neuralgia caused by *Herpesvirus hominis* type 2. *J. AMA* **236**:587–588.

16. Rubin, M. B., and Heaton, C. L. (1972): Phototherapy of recurrent cutaneous *Herpesvirus hominis* infection with acridine orange and ultraviolet light. In: *Proceedings of the 14th International Congress of Dermatology, Padua–Venice, May 22–27*, pp. 162–166.

17. Chang, T., Weinstein, L. (1975): Eczema herpeticum: treatment with methylene blue and light. *Arch. Dermatol.* 111:1174–1175.

18. Moore, C., Wallis, C., Melnick, J. L., et al. (1972): Photodynamic treatment of herpes keratitis. *Infect. Immun.* 5:169–171.

19. Lanjer, J. D., Witcher, J. P., and Dawson, C. R. (1973): Proflavine and light in the treatment of experimental herpetic keratitis (abstract). *Symp. Assoc. Res. Vis. Ophthalmol.*, p. 51.

20. Tara, C. S., Stanley, J. A., Kucera, L. J., et al. (1974): Photodynamic inactivation of herpes simplex keratitis. *Arch. Ophthalmol.* 92:51–53.

21. Lahav, M., Dueker, D., Bhatt, P. N., et al. (1975): Photodynamic inactivation in experimental herpetic keratitis. *Arch. Ophthalmol.* 93:207–214.

22. O'Day, D. M., Jones, B. R., Poirier, R., et al. (1975): Proflavine photodynamic viral inactivation in herpes simplex keratitis. *Am. J. Ophthalmol.* 79:941–948.

23. Myers, M. G., Oxman, M. N., Clark, J. E., et al. (1975): Failure of neutral red photodynamic inactivation in recurrent herpes simplex infections. *N. Engl. J. Med.* 293:945–949.

24. Taylor, P. K., and Doherty, N. R. (1975): Comparison of the treatment of herpes genitalis in men with proflavine photoinactivation, idoxuridine ointment and normal saline. *Br. J. Vener. Dis.* 51:125–129.

25. Roome, A. P., Tinkler, A. E., Hilton, A. L., et al. (1975): Neutral red with photoinactivation in the treatment of herpes genitalis. *Br. J. Vener. Dis.* 51:130–133.

26. Kaufman, R. H., Adam, E., Mirkovic, R. R., et al. (1978): Treatment of genital herpes simplex virus infection with photodynamic inactivation. *Am. J. Obstet. Gynecol.* 132:861–869.

27. Rapp, F. (1973): Medical News: Photoinactivation of herpesvirus may be clinically hazardous. *J. AMA* 255:459–460.

28. Duff, R., and Rapp, F. (1971): Oncogenic transformation of hamster cells after exposure to herpes simplex virus type 2. *Nature [New Biol]* 233:48.

29. Rapp, F., Li, J. H., and Jerkofsky, M. (1973): Transformation of mammalian cells by DNA-containing viruses following photodynamic inactivation. *Virology* 55:339–346.

30. Li, J. L., Jerkofsky, M. A., and Rapp, F. (1975): Demonstration of oncogenic potential of mammalian cells transformed by DNA-containing viruses following photodynamic inactivation. *Int. J. Cancer* 15:190–202.

31. Verwoerd, D. W., and Rapp, F. (1978): Biochemical transformation of mouse cells by herpes simplex virus type 2: enhancement by means of low-level photodynamic treatment. *J. Virol.* 26:200–202.

32. Berger, R. S., and Papa, C. M. (1977): Photodye herpes therapy—Cassandra confirmed? *J. AMA* 238:133–134.

33. Berger, B. W., and Hori, Y. (1978): Multicentric Bowen's disease of the genitalia. *Arch. Dermatol.* 114:1698–1699.

34. Wade, T. R., Kopf, A. W., and Ackerman, A. B. (1979): Bowenoid papulosis of the genitalia. *Arch. Dermatol.* 115:306–308.

35. Wade, T. R., and Ackerman, A. B. (1977): Squamous cell carcinoma in-situ: multiple lesions on the penis in young men. *Arch. Dermatol.* 113:1714.

36. Lupulescu, A., Mehregan, A. H., Rahbari, H., et al. (1977): Venereal warts vs Bowen disease. *J. AMA* 237:2520–2522.

37. Friedrich, E. G. (1972): Reversible vulvar atypia. *Obstet. Gynecol.* 39:173–181.

38. Kopf, A. W., Ackerman, A. B., Wade, T., et al. (1978): Photodye herpes therapy. *J. AMA* 239:615.

39. Browning, C. H., and Gilmore, W. (1913): Bacteriocidal action and chemical constitution with special reference to basic benzol derivatives. *J. Pathol. Bacteriol.* 18:144–146.

40. Albert, A. (1966): *The Acridines*, 2nd ed. Edward Arnold, London.

41. Mitchell, G. A. G., and Buttler, G. A. H. (1943): Proflavine in closed wounds. *Lancet* **2**:749.

42. Rank, B. K. (1944): Use and abuse of local antiseptics on wounds. *Med. J. Aust.* **2**:629–636.

43. Albert, A., Rubbo, S. D., and Maxwell, M. (1942): The influence of chemical constitution on antiseptic activity. I. Study of the mono-amino acridines. *Br. J. Exp. Pathol.* **23**:69–83.

44. Rubbo, S. D., Albert, R. J., Goldacre, M. E., et al. (1945): The influence of chemical constitution on antibacterial activity II: A general survey of the acridine series. *Br. J. Exp. Pathol.* **26**:160–192.

45. Gordon, J., McLeod, J. W., and Mayr-Harting, A. (1947): The value of antiseptics as prophylactic applications to recent wounds. *J. Hyg. (Camb.)* **45**:297–306.

46. Heinmets, F., Vinegar, R., and Taylor, W. W. (1953): Studies on the mechanisms of the photosensitized inactivation of *E. coli* and reactivation phenomenon. *J. Gen. Physiol.* **36**:207–226.

47. Wallis, C., Melnick, J. L., and Phillips, C. A. (1965): Bacterial and fungal decontamination of virus specimens by differential photosensitization. *Am. J. Epidemiol.* **81**:222–229.

48. Cooney, J. J., and Krinsky, N. I. (1972): Photodynamic killing of *Acholeplasma laidlawii*. *Photochem. Photobiol.* **16**:523–526.

49. Dickey, R. F. (1962): Investigative studies in fungicidal powers of photodynamic action. *J. Invest. Dermatol.* **39**:7–19.

21

Transforming Activity of Viruses after Dye-Light Inactivation

F. Rapp and J.-L. H. Li

The phenomenon of photodynamic inactivation was first reported by Raab (1) at the beginning of this century (he observed that paramecia lived while suspended in acridine orange solution and kept in the dark, but were rapidly killed when exposed to normal daylight). More extensive investigations were subsequently carried out with bacteriophages (2-4) and animal viruses (5-11) and the procedure is receiving ever-increasing attention, particularly since it has been applied as a therapeutic measure for the treatment of patients with herpetic infections.

Photodynamic inactivation is a method in which virus is treated with heterotricyclic dyes such as neutral red, proflavine, or methylene blue, and exposed to normal white light in the presence of oxygen; this treatment results in destruction of virus infectivity. The method has been reported to cure herpes keratitis in experimental animals (12-14), and this finding has been applied to patients with primary or recurrent herpes simplex virus (HSV) infections (15, 16). HSV, a widespread human pathogen, is a DNA-containing virus which can be divided into two groups (HSV-1 and HSV-2) distinguishable by biologic, biochemical, and biophysical properties (17). Normally these viruses cause primary or recurrent infections of the skin and mucous membranes in humans, and at present there is no completely effective treatment for these painful infections. Therefore, preliminary results of dye-light therapy which were claimed as promising (9, 10, 15, 16, 18-21) created great enthusiam among clinicians. However, data accumulated from seroe-

F. Rapp • Department of Microbiology, The Milton S. Hershey Medical Center, The Pennsylvania State University College of Medicine, Hershey, Pennsylvania 17033. *J.-L. H. Li* • Department of Microbiology, University of Texas School of Medicine Galveston, Texas 77050.

pidemiologic and biochemical studies have implicated HSV-1 and HSV-2 (22) as possible causative factors in a variety of cancers. HSV-2 was originally found to be associated with cervical carcinoma by epidemiologic methods (23–25) and it has been reported that transformed cells of human cervical origin contain HSV-2 antigen (26) and may occasionally liberate the virus when grown in cell culture (27). A fragment of HSV-2 virus DNA was detected in a human cervical tumor (28), and most investigators share the view that transformation by HSV involves only a small percentage of the virus genome (29). Importantly, transformation by HSV-1 or HSV-2 of hamster embryo cells (30–34), mouse cells (35, 36), rat cells (37), and human cells (34, 38) has been achieved under certain conditions. These studies and the association of herpesviruses with human cancer have been reviewed (29).

Studies employing ultraviolet (UV) irradiation of HSV-1 and HSV-2 have shown that under conditions in which virus infectivity is destroyed, the inactivated virus can morphologically transform mammalian cells in vitro (30–32). The transformants were established as cell lines and subsequently induced tumors when transplanted into a compatible host. Virus-specific proteins were detected in the transformed cells. These results clearly indicate that destruction of the ability of the virus to cause cytopathology does not inactivate the genetic information required for oncogenicity.

Dye–light treatment of HSV also results in inactivation of virus infectivity; however, the studies with virus inactivated by UV irradiation suggested that the dye–light treatment might yield virus particles capable of transforming susceptible cells. Simian virus 40 (SV40), a well-understood model DNA tumor virus, was used as a comparative system for the studies with HSV-1 and HSV-2.

The oncogenic transformation of mammalian cells by photodynamically inactivated HSV and SV40 using neutral red has been reported (39–41). The same results have also been obtained with SV40 following toluidine blue and light photoinactivation (42). This chapter will describe experiments concerning the inactivation of viruses and the transformation of mammalian cells by the inactivated viruses. The properties of the photoinactivated virus-transformed cells and the implications for photodynamic inactivation therapy will also be discussed.

INACTIVATION OF VIRUSES

The information reported on photoinactivation of viruses during the past several decades has suggested that different classes of dyes show widely different effects in a given biologic system. A single dye may have a photodynamic effect on one virus and not another, while a given virus may vary in its photosensitivity to different dyes. Some viruses, such as measles

(43) and parainfluenza viruses (44), are inherently sensitive to large doses of white light even in the absence of photoreactive dyes. Other viruses, such as polio and some enteroviruses, can be photoinactivated by light when they are cultivated in cells pretreated with dye (6, 45–48), but are relatively resistant to light inactivation when the viruses themselves are directly treated with dye (6, 49). Studies on HSV, SV40, and other viruses have revealed that these viruses can be photoinactivated by a wide spectrum of dyes, such as neutral red, proflavine, toluidine blue (6), or methylene blue (50), by growing the viruses in cells containing dye (39) or by treating the viruses with dye directly (6). The mode of action of this dye–light interaction is not well understood, but one possible mechanism that has been suggested by many studies is a photooxidative process (51). DNA has generally been regarded as the target site for this dye–light photoinactivation.

For the inactivation of viruses, the experimental procedures have been described in detail by several investigators (6, 39, 44, 50, 53). We will briefly discuss the two methods that are being used in the transformation studies presented here.

Cultivation of Viruses in Cells Pretreated with Dye

HSV-1, HSV-2, and SV40 can be made photosensitive when the viruses are grown in cells containing neutral red (39). It is hypothesized that during replication of HSV or SV40 in cells pretreated with a dye, the dye molecules are intercalated between the base pairs of the virus DNA. The dye–DNA complex absorbs light energy, which then undergoes a photooxidative reaction that disrupts the structure of the DNA strand. From studies with other viruses (54–56), it is further hypothesized that excision of the guanine moieties in the virus DNA occur, leaving a gap in the base sequences and subsequent single-strand breaks in the virus DNA. This might render the virus particles unable to complete the replication cycle and therefore noninfective. However, the known requirement of only a fragment of HSV or SV40 DNA to achieve transformation makes plausible continued retention of biologic activity of the photoinactivated virus.

Preparation of Photosensitized Viruses. Confluent monolayers of cells grown in bottles were treated for 2 hr with 25 μg/ml neutral red at 37° C. The medium was then removed and the cells were washed four times with Tris buffer (pH 7.4). The drained cultures were subsequently infected with HSV-1, HSV-2, or SV40. After a virus adsorption period of 1 hr, the cultures were washed twice with Tris buffer to remove unadsorbed virus, and were then maintained in Eagle medium free of dye until virus cytopathic effects were observed in 80% of the cells in culture. The subsequent harvest yielded an average titer of 10^6 plaque-forming units per ml (PFU/ml) of photosensitized HSV-1 or HSV-2, and 10^7 PFU/ml of photosensitized SV40.

Inactivation of Photosensitive Virus with Light. Photosensitized virus stocks were exposed to light (Fig. 21-1) for varying time periods with a thermodyne laboratory light (120 V, 0.24 A, and 60 Hz). Viruses were then assayed for surviving infectivity in terms of PFU per ml. It had been shown (39) after 12 min of exposure to light that HSV-1 or HSV-2 infectivity was inactivated and reduced by six logs. No difference was detected in the rate of inactivation between HSV-1 and HSV-2. A seven-log decrease in SV40 infectivity was observed after 45 min of light treatment. In control cultures infected with virus but not treated with neutral red, no loss in infectivity was detected. Likewise, virus–dye samples kept in the dark showed no loss in infectivity.

HSV has been grown in cells pretreated with proflavine (57). In these studies, it was found that proflavine at a concentration of 25 µg/ml was toxic to cells; however, when the concentration of proflavine was lowered to 2 µg/ml, the cells could be maintained without observable toxicity. Virus grown under this condition was not, however, totally photosensitive. These photo-resistant fractions precluded the use of this method for the production of inactivated virus for transformation.

Photodynamic Inactivation by Direct Treatment with Dye

It has been reported that HSV and other viruses can be photoinactivated by directly treating the virus with dye (6, 50). A plausible explanation for this

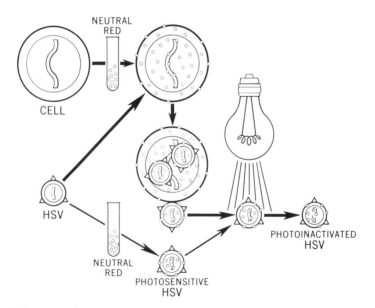

Fig. 21-1. Schematic representation of neutral red and light effect on herpes simplex virus.

effect may be that the reaction of virus and photoreactive dye results in a tightly bound, photosensitive virus—dye complex (44, 49). The dye appears to be able to penetrate the virus coat and combine with the nucleic acid with the result that the virus becomes photosensitive. It has been shown that the effectiveness of a specific dye is frequently a function of its ability to penetrate the virus coat (58). Therefore, HSV has been reported to be exceedingly photosensitive to toluidine blue (6, 29) and less sensitive to proflavine and neutral red (6). Further studies on the effects of these various dyes on HSV in our laboratory (57) have confirmed these observations. The detailed experimental procedures for our studies were orginally described by Wallis and Melnick (6, 44) and employed here with slight modifications. In our studies, we used three different dyes (neutral red, proflavine, and methylene blue) which have been utilized in the clinical treatment of herpes infections. Each dye was dissolved in distilled water to make 1 mg/ml stock solution and sterilized by filtration through a Millipore filter. Dowex cation exchange resin (50 $W-X4-H^+$, 50–100 mesh) was prepared as described by Wallis and Melnick (44).

HSV-1 and HSV-2 stocks were diluted tenfold with Tris buffer (pH 7.4) and mixed with dye to a final concentration of 25 μg/ml. The mixture was then incubated 1 hr at room temperature, with a virus solution free of dye being used as a control. Both virus–dye solutions and control virus samples were then dispensed into plastic Petri dishes and exposed to the laboratory fluorescent light. After exposure to light, virus samples were passed through a Dowex cation exchange resin column to remove the excess dye, and then assayed for surviving infectivity. The results of photosensitization of HSV-1 and HSV-2 to neutral red, proflavine, and methylene blue are shown in Fig. 21-2–21-4. Figure 21-2 shows the photosensitivity of HSV after treatment with neutral red and subsequent exposure to light for varying time periods. A virus infectivity decrease of six logs was noted in HSV-1 and HSV-2 after 10 and 8 min of light exposure, respectively. HSV-2 seems slightly easier to photosensitize. Control samples in dye-free buffer exposed to light (not included in Fig. 21-2) lost no detectable infectivity, thus demonstrating that HSV-1 or HSV-2 grown in cells pretreated with neutral red or directly mixed with the dye in solution have the same photosensitive properties.

The results of experiments concerning the effects of proflavine on virus photoinactivation are shown in Fig. 21-3. A decrease in the infectivity of HSV-1 and HSV-2 was found with prolonged exposure of the virus to light. Within 10–11 min of light treatment, HSV-1 and HSV-2 infectivity were completely inactivated and reduced by greater than six logs. It is interesting to note that in our system, proflavine-treated HSV kept in the dark for 1 hr at room temperature (either passed through the resin column or not) lost only 0.5–1 log of virus infectivity, while other studies (6, 44) have shown that an HSV–proflavine complex kept in the dark resulted in a decrease in virus titer

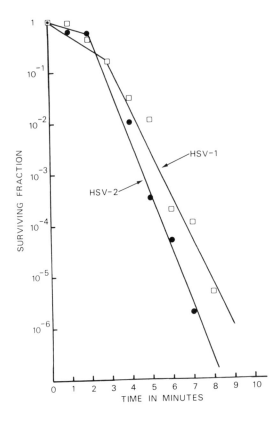

Fig. 21-2. Photoinactivation of HSV-1 and HSV-2 by directly treating virus with neutral red.

of four or five logs. These differences may be due to variations between the different experimental conditions. Both methylene blue and toluidine blue are thiazine dyes, and are very active photosensitizers of coliphage (59). Toluidine blue has been shown to be an extremely photoreactive dye when used with HSV, as mentioned previously. The results of methylene blue photo-inactivation of HSV, presented in Fig. 21-4, suggest that thiazine dyes are also very active photosensitizers of HSV. After 1.5 min of exposure to light, both HSV-1 and HSV-2 samples were totally inactivated. These results indicate that neutral red, proflavine, methylene blue, and toluidine blue are all photosensitizers for HSV. The extent of virus photoinactivation due to these dyes depends on each dye and the experimental conditions employed. Neutral red, proflavine, and methylene blue all have been used in clinical therapy for HSV infections. Indeed, the destruction of the lytic properties of a virus does not necessarily mean that it is inert. Therefore, careful studies on the expression of the oncogenic potential of HSV after dye–light treatment using proflavine and methylene blue have been conducted (57).

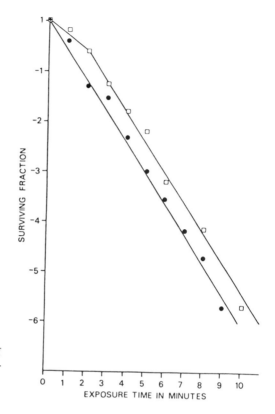

Fig. 21-3. Photoinactivation of HSV-1 and HSV-2 by directly treating virus with proflavine. □, HSV-1; ●, HSV-2.

TRANSFORMATION OF MAMMALIAN CELLS

Photoinactivated HSV-1, HSV-2, and SV40 grown in cells pretreated with neutral red were used in transformation studies (39). Since direct evidence that viruses can transform human cells to malignancy is limited by the availability of susceptible hosts for the transplantation of transformed cells, studies have been conducted with animal cells to prove the involvement of these photoinactivated viruses in the transformation of normal mammalian cells into cells demonstrating a neoplastic phenotype.

The system we used for transformation studies is as follows: primary hamster embryo cells (5×10^5 cells/ml) were mixed with photodynamically inactivated HSV-1, HSV-2, or SV40 in suspension. The mixture was shaken gently for 2.5 hr at 37° C, dispersed into plastic Petri dishes, and maintained in growth medium. Approximately 4 weeks after plating the virus–cell mixture, morphologically transformed foci appeared which had lost contact inhibition with neighboring cells. The transformed foci were picked, and three HSV-1,

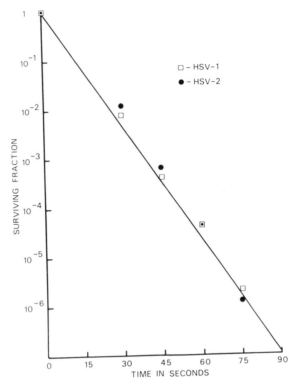

Fig. 21-4. Photoinactivation of HSV-1 and HSV-2 by directly treating virus with methylene blue.

five HSV-2, and two SV40 transformed foci were established into cell lines for further characterization.

PROPERTIES OF VIRUS-TRANSFORMED CELLS

Morphology and Growth Characteristics of the Transformed Cells

The main characteristic of transformed cells that distinguishes them from untransformed cells is their insensitivity to the controls that regulate multiplication. When untransformed cells are cultured in vitro, they will grow until a certain cell density is reached and then stop completely or grow at a much reduced rate. Under the same conditions, transformed cells continue to multiply and reach saturation densities many times higher than those of untransformed cells. It is this sort of differential growth that provides the basis of the transformation assay used with photoinactivated viruses following the establishment of cell lines. The morphologic patterns were examined by conventional staining techniques. Both HSV-1 and HSV-2-transformed cell cultures were found to consist of short fibroblastoid cells mixed with mononucleated and multinucleated cells. Photoinactivated HSV- and SV40-transformed cells grew closely packed together and were easily detached from the glass. They may both be grown in medium with a low percentage of serum. It was particularly interesting that the medium used on cell cultures of one line of HSV-2-transformed cells always became much thicker and more mucoid than the medium on cultures of the other cell lines. This medium was found to contain a high concentration of hyaluronic acid (our unpublished data).

Human cells exposed to neutral red-photoinactivated HSV-2 also demonstrated properties consistent with transformation (60). These included formation of cell aggregates, colony formation in methylcellulose, and retention of synthesis of virus antigens (60).

Alteration of Antigenic Properties in the Transformed Cells

Studies of SV40-transformed cells included four different experiments: (1) rescue of virus from transformed cells; (2) detection of virus DNA sequences by hybridization; (3) detection of virus-specific RNA in transformed cells; and (4) detection of virus-specific proteins in transformed cells. These studies have demonstrated that possibly all or part of the virus nucleic acid persists in transformed cells and is most likely integrated into the cell genome (61, 62). The same phenomenon has also been demonstrated for adenovirus (63, 64). It is unknown whether the entire herpesvirus genome or only part of it is integrated into the transformed cells. In cell lines transformed by HSV, researchers have not been able to detect evidence of the presence of infectious virus or DNA in the transformed cells. Most attempts to induce virus replication by physical and chemical methods have failed, as have attempts to rescue virus from transformed cells by cocultivation with permissive cells or fusion with inactivated Sendai virus. These results suggest that cell transformation by HSV may be due to defective particles, under which condition it would be unlikely that virus could be rescued. Although direct proof of the presence of the HSV DNA genome in HSV-transformed cells has not been produced by hybridization studies, molecular hybridization studies performed with UV-irradiated HSV-2-transformed cells and tumor cells derived from this cell line have revealed the presence of virus-specific messenger RNA equivalent to 10–13% of the HSV-2 genome and cross-reactive with HSV-1 DNA (65). This finding indicates that at least a portion of the virus genome is present and transcribed in the transformed cells. Because it has been impossible to demonstrate the presence of a complete HSV genome capable of undergoing a lytic cycle in the neoplastic virus-transformed cells, and because it has been shown that possibly part of the genome persists in the HSV-transformed cells, the identification of virus-specific proteins whose synthesis could be directed by the virus genome using immunologic methods has become a prerequisite for the determination of virus transformation.

Cells that were transformed by neutral red-photoinactivated HSV or SV40 were tested for the presence of virus-specific antigens by indirect immunofluorescent (IF) techniques (39). Acetone fixed HSV- or SV40-transformed cells were reacted with appropriate antisera. HSV-specific antigens visible as a diffuse fluorescence were found in the cytoplasm of the transformed cells (Fig. 21-5). The amount of fluorescence in the photo-inactivated HSV-1 or HSV-2-transformed cells was about 8–10%. The antigens responsible for the fluorescent reaction were shown to be specific (Table 21-1), since they were not found in cells transformed by SV40 or in

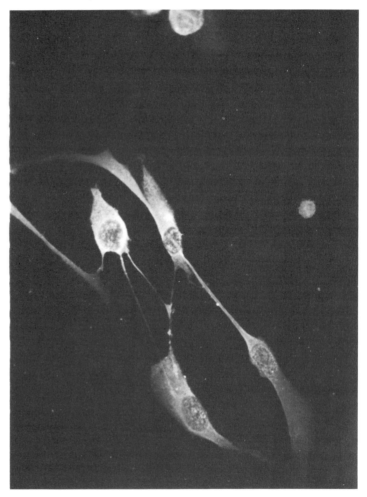

Fig. 21-5. Immunofluorescence photomicrograph of HSV-specific cytoplasmic antigens present in HSV-1-transformed hamster cells (×400).

Table 21-1. Detection of HSV-1 and HSV-2 Antigens in Hamster Embryo Cells Transformed by Photoinactivated Virus

Transforming virus or cell type	Sera			
	Anti-HSV-1[a]	Anti-HSV-2[b]	HSV-2 TB[c]	Anti-SV40 TB[d]
HSV-1	+	+	+	−
HSV-2	+	+	+	−
Normal hamster cells	−	−	−	−
Hamster cells + HSV-1	+	+	+	−
Hamster cells + HSV-2	+	+	+	−
SV40	−	−	−	+
333-8-9[e]	+	+	+	−

[a] Pooled sera from hamsters immunized with HSV-1.
[b] Pooled sera from hamsters immunized with HSV-2.
[c] Sera from hamsters bearing tumors produced by cells transformed by UV-irradiated HSV-2.
[d] Pooled sera from hamsters bearing SV40-induced tumors.
[e] Hamster embryo cells transformed by UV-irradiated HSV-2.

uninfected hamster embryo cells where the same sera were used. When SV40-transformed cells were tested for the presence of virus-specific tumor (T) antigens by the same technique, SV40 T antigens were found in the nucleus of almost all of the transformed cells. Virus (V) antigens were not detected in these transformed cells.

HSV-1- and HSV-2-transformed cells were examined for the presence of the IgG receptor by hemadsorption experiments and binding of [^{125}I]-labeled IgG (66). Following sensitization with rabbit anti–sheep erythrocyte serum, the transformed cells were incubated with sheep erythrocytes, washed free of nonadherent erythrocytes, and then stained with Giemsa for microscopic examination. Three types of results were found with the transformed cells (Table 21-2). One line of HSV-1-transformed cells showed no adsorption of erythrocytes and one line of HSV-2-transformed cells showed adsorption to every cell. The other cell lines of HSV-1- and HSV-2-transformed cells showed adsorption to occasional cells only. These results were confirmed using ^{125}I-labeled IgG (Table 21-2). All the transformed cell lines bound more IgG than either primary hamster embryo cells or the continuous hamster cell line BHK-21. None of the transformed lines bound as much IgG as did primary hamster embryo cells infected with HSV-1.

The results obtained by these two tests correlated well with the results obtained in cells lytically infected with HSV (67–69) and suggest that the phenomenon is due to the appearance on the infected or transformed cells of a receptor for the FC fragment of IgG. These studies favor the view that the receptor is coded by the herpes genome. But it has not yet been proved that the receptors for IgG on lytically infected and transformed cells are identical. However, the results are consistent with the view that herpesvirus functions persist in the transformed cells.

Table 21-2. Antibody-Mediated Binding of Sheep Erythrocytes and Binding
of Radioiodinated IgG to Hamster Embryo Cells Transformed with Neutral
Red-Photoinactivated Herpes Simplex Virus

Virus	Cells	Hemadsorption[a]	IgG bound,[b] counts/min
HSV-1	Infected hamster cells	2	39621
	Transformed hamster cells		
	Clone 1	0	7858
	Clone 2	1	8790
	Clone 3	1	10100
HSV-2	Transformed hamster cells		
	Clone 1	2	19682
	Clone 3	1	8607
	Clone 5	1	9531
	Normal hamster embryo cells	0	3085
	BHK-21 cells[c]	0	4447

[a]0: No hemadsorption.
1: Patchy hemadsorption.
2: Generalized hemadsorption.
[b]Means of three estimations.
[c]Baby hamster kidney cell line.

Oncogenic Properties of Cells Transformed by Photoinactivated Virus

In addition to the morphologic and antigenic changes that occur in the transformed cells, transformed cells form tumors more readily than untransformed cells when transplanted into susceptible animals (70–73). This has become one criterion for determining the malignancy of a cell population. It has been satisfactorily proven that cells transformed in vitro by photoinactivated HSV and SV40 are transplantable (40, 42).

Tumor Formation in Syrian Hamsters. The oncogenic properties of neutral red-photoinactivated HSV- and SV40-transformed hamster cells have been described (40). Approximately 10^6 cells per hamster were subcutaneously inoculated into each newborn hamster during the first 24 hr after birth. The oncogenicity of individual cell lines varied greatly upon initial hamster injection (Table 21–3). One clone of photoinactivated HSV-1-transformed cells produced tumors (Fig. 21-6) in 75% of the injected animals within 6 weeks of incubation. Three clones of photoinactivated HSV-2-transformed cells were injected. They were all malignant, but differed in oncogenic potential. Two clones produced a high percentage of tumors (94% and 90%) within a short latent period of 2 and 4 weeks, respectively. Another clone was less oncogenic, with only 21% of the animals developing tumors within 10 weeks. One clone of the SV40-transformed cells was injected into newborn hamsters and all of the animals produced tumors within 2 weeks. A

Table 21-3. Tumor Formation in Newborn Syrian Hamsters by
Transformed Cells

Virus	Cell Line	Percent of animals with tumors	Latent periods, weeks
HSV-1	HSV-1 clone 1	75	6
HSV-2	HSV-2 clone 1	94	2
	HSV-2 clone 2	90	4
	HSV-2 clone 3	21	10
SV40	SV40 clone 1	100	2

number of tumors were excised and grown in cell culture for further characterization. Most tumor cells were morphologically similar to the original transformed cells. Some cell lines transformed by UV-irradiated HSV were poorly oncogenic in newborn hamsters, but the tumor cells became highly oncogenic upon subsequent passage into additional animals (74). This may be due to the selection within the animal of more oncogenic cells. Tumor cells induced by one clone of photoinactivated HSV-2 primary tumor cells were therefore retransplanted subcutaneously into adult hamsters. Four of five animals developed tumors within 2 weeks.

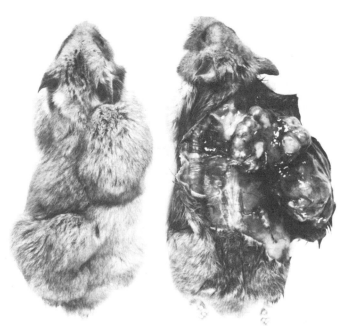

Fig. 21-6. Syrian hamsters with primary tumors 10 weeks after subcutaneous injection of photoinactivated HSV-1 (left) and HSV-2 (right) transformed cells.

The Pathology of Hamster Tumors. The majority of tumors were fibrosarcomas composed of poorly differentiated anaplastic sarcomatous tissue. About 70% of the hamsters bearing primary tumors also showed metastatic lesions in the lung, heart (Fig. 21-7), and lymph nodes, sometimes with the tumor cells also invading the skin or muscles. Metastatic tumors of the lung or heart appeared as small, well-delineated nodules of anaplastic fibroblasts.

Detection of Virus-Specific Antigens in Tumor Cells. Tumor cells

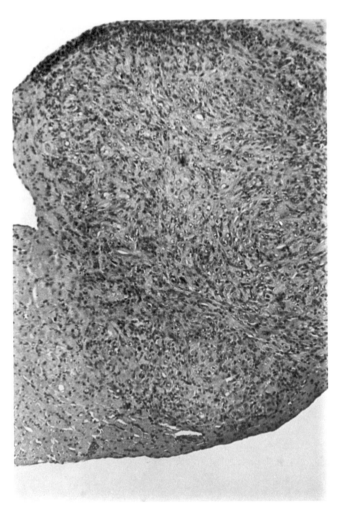

Fig. 21-7. Photomicrograph of a metastatic lesion in the heart of a hamster after subcutaneous injection of photoinactivated HSV-2-transformed cells. (Stained with hematoxylin and eosin; ×100.)

removed from animals and subsequently grown in a cell culture were examined for the presence of virus-specific cytoplasmic antigens using the same methods previously described. All cell lines established from hamster tumors induced by neutral red-photoinactivated HSV or SV40 have been shown to react with appropriate specific sera from tumor-bearing animals (Table 21-4). The sera from tumor-bearing animals carrying different HSV cell lines showed cross-reaction with one another. Tumor cells did not react with anti-HSV-1 and anti-HSV-2 sera. The tumor cells induced by HSV-transformed cells did not react with tumor-bearing serum specific for SV40 and vice versa. HSV tumor cells and their parental transformed cells were also tested for the presence of membrane antigens. Unfixed preparations of either tumor cells or transformed cells were examined by the indirect IF test using sera from hamsters bearing tumors induced by cells transformed with either UV-irradiated or photoinactivated HSV. A membrane fluorescence was seen in 8–10% of the tumor cells or the original transformed cells (Fig. 21-8). This reaction was not found with SV40-transformed cells or with normal hamster embryo cells (Table 21-5).

These antigens detected in the transformed cells or tumor cells by the IF test elicited the synthesis of virus-specific antibodies in hamsters that

Table 21-4. Detection of Virus-Specific Antigens in Fixed Tumor Cells and Virus-Specific Antibodies in Sera from Animals Bearing Tumors

		Specificity of antisera				
Virus	Cells	HSV-1[a]	HSV-2[b]	HSV-1 TB[c]	HSV-2 TB[d]	SV40 TB[e]
HSV-1	HSV-1-infected hamster cells	+	+	+	+	−
	HSV-1 tumor cells	−	−	+	+	−
HSV-2	HSV-2-infected hamster cells	+	+	+	+	−
	Tumor cells, clone 1	−	−	+	+	−
	Tumor cells, clone 2	±	±	+	+	−
	Tumor cells, clone 3	−	−	+	+	−
SV40	Tumor cells, clone 1	−	−	−	−	+
	Normal hamster embryo cells	−	−	−	−	−

[a] Pooled sera from hamsters immunized with HSV-1.
[b] Pooled sera from hamsters immunized with HSV-2.
[c] Sera from hamsters bearing tumors produced by photoinactivated neutral red HSV-1-transformed cells.
[d] Sera from hamsters bearing tumors produced by photoinactivated neutral red HSV-2-transformed cells.
[e] Pooled sera from hamsters bearing SV40-induced tumors produced by photoinactivated SV40 or wild-type SV 40-transformed cells.

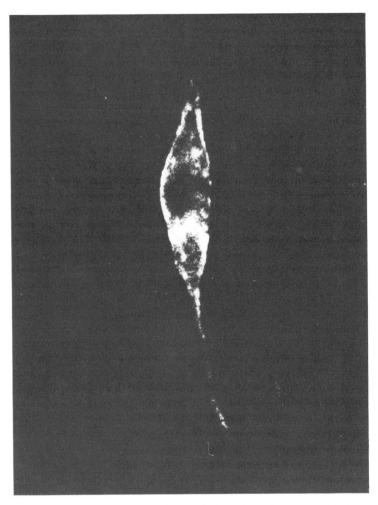

Fig. 21-8. Immunofluorescence photomicrograph of membrane fluorescence detected on HSV-1-transformed hamster cells. (×400)

developed primary tumors and metastases. Although these antibodies had no neutralization activity, they contained the ability to react with the transforming virus and with antigens in the parental transformed cell lines (Table 21-4). This is compatible with the hypothesis that the virus originally transformed the hamster embryo cells. Furthermore, UV-irradiated HSV is capable of transferring the virus gene for synthesis of thymidine kinase more readily to mouse cells exposed to proflavine and light than to untreated cells (75). These observations suggest that low doses of photoinactivation render mammalian cells more susceptible to transformation, possibly by facilitating incorporation of virus DNA during repair of cellular DNA.

Table 21-5. Detection of HSV Membrane Antigens in Unfixed Transformed
Cells and Tumor Cells by Indirect Immunofluorescence Test

Cell	Virus	Specificity of antisera		
		HSV-1[a]	HSV-2[b]	HSV TB[c]
Transformed cells	HSV-1	−	−	+
	HSV-2	−	−	+
	SV40	−	−	−
Tumor cells	HSV-1	−	−	+
	HSV-2	−	−	+
	SV40	−	−	−
Normal hamster embryo cells		−	−	−

[a] Pooled sera from hamsters immunized with HSV-1.
[b] Pooled sera from hamsters immunized with HSV-2.
[c] Sera from hamsters bearing tumors produced by cells transformed by UV-irradiated HSV or neutral red-photoinactivated HSV.

IMPLICATIONS FOR THERAPY

Although photodynamic inactivation has been applied as a technique for treating HSV infection in experimental animals and in human patients, the results of the treatment have been variable in both systems. In animal studies, primarily using a model system involving herpetic keratitis in the rabbit, some workers have reported satisfactory results (12–14), while others have found the treatment to have little if any beneficial effect (76, 77). Reports of treatment of patients with genital herpes infections have been encouraging (9, 10, 15, 16, 18–21) (see Chapters 19 and 20). However, these findings have often depended heavily on self-assessment of progress by patients suffering from recurrent herpes, and there was evidence of a "placebo" effect in some of the reports (18). Studies with controlled systems have demonstrated that the dye–light treatment is of little value for herpes infection. One report (78) demonstrated that proflavine photoinactivation has no greater value than 5'-iodo-2'-deoxyuridine or normal saline in the treatment of genital infection by HSV in the male. Another controlled study (79) of neutral red with photoinactivation in the treatment of herpes genitalis has failed to confirm the favorable reports of treatment by photoinactivation recorded by other workers (9, 10, 15, 16, 21). No benefit was detected from treatment with neutral red when compared with treatment with the placebo dye phenol red. Methylene blue was tested along with proflavine and neutral red for treatment of herpes-infected patients. It was reported that the dye is as effective a vital dye as neutral red or proflavine; however, therapy with three dyes did not prevent or substantially reduce recurrence (80). Therefore, the efficacy of the dye–light photoinactivation as a therapeutic treatment has itself been opened to question.

As early as 1975 (81) it was noted that use of proflavine as a photoactive dye resulted in adverse reactions in patients with herpetic keratitis. Our reports concerning transformation by photoinactivated HSV suggested "caution" to Cusumano and Monif (82) in the use of this modality for the treatment of herpetic lesions. The reported failure of the method to yield significant improvement in a group of patients compared to those receiving a placebo (83, 84) did not deter Melnick and Wallis (10) from continuing to promote the method, dismissing possible adverse effects, and going to great length to criticize the results obtained by the Harvard investigators (83, 84) on the basis that incorrect light was used in the procedure. Finally, Kaufman and his colleagues (85), working in the College of Medicine in which the original favorable results had been obtained, published the results of a double-blind randomized study using proflavine and light that detected no differences in healing time of the lesions, development of recurrences, or virus isolation in the treated vs. the control groups.

Therefore, in the future, such therapeutic maneuvers should be carefully weighed against what is currently known about the biology of DNA tumor viruses. The genetic material of DNA tumor viruses has information for several different virus functions, including lytic function, induction of cellular DNA synthesis, and transformation capacity. It has been shown that virus genetic information for these functions can be differentially inactivated by UV irradiation, x-rays, or photodynamic action (86–88). For several groups of tumor viruses, including viruses of the papova (87–89), adeno (90–92), herpes (30–32, 93), and sarcoma (94) groups, UV irradiation or x-rays can be used to differentially inactivate lytic and oncogenic properties, since these properties have different sensitivities to inactivation. It has also been shown that UV irradiation of certain DNA tumor viruses can enhance their oncogenicity (95–98).

The results of our studies have demonstrated the oncogenic potential of HSV and SV40 following photodynamic inactivation using neutral red and normal white light. These viruses were rendered defective with respect to infectivity, but were able to transform hamster cells in vitro and produce tumors and metastases when implanted into syngeneic hosts. Virus-specific antigenic markers were detected in the cytoplasm or on the surface of the transformed cells and the tumor cells derived from these transformed cells. An analytical study of photodynamic inactivation of SV40 using toluidine blue to determine the minimal function of SV40 (42) has shown that different functions of SV40 were inactivated at different rates. The most sensitive function was the capacity of the virus to replicate, followed in sensitivity by the capacity to induce T antigen and cell DNA synthesis. The transformation capacity was the most resistant function in this dye–light photoreaction. Syrian hamster kidney cells transformed in vitro by toluidine blue light-inactivated SV40 have the same properties as those transformed by non-inactivated SV40. They show an identical morphology, are T antigen positive, contain the same number of SV40 DNA genome equivalents integrated into the host cell DNA, and are oncogenic when inoculated into adult hamsters. These results, together with our studies, suggest that photodynamic inactivation can also differentially inactivate virus lytic function and unmask the oncogenic potential.

Our preliminary results of proflavine photoinactivation have shown that photoinactivated HSV-2 can transform hamster embryo cells. Further studies of these transformed cells are required to verify whether these cells are transformed by proflavine or by dye–light-inactivated HSV-2, since photodynamic action might convert normal cells into malignant cells. Evidence has shown that the dyes used in clinical therapy (proflavine, methylene blue, and toluidine blue) are mutagens in bacterial systems (51, 99). It has also been reported that proflavine can mutagenize RNA viruses, such as measles (100), polio, and tobacco mosaic virus (51). Thus, in terms of potential effects arising from proflavine–light treatment in a cell culture or virus, it is possible that the dye might induce oncogenic potential in individual cells or viruses.

SUMMARY

Data concerning the advantages or disadvantages of photodynamic inactivation as a clinical therapeutic technique accumulated so far are adequate to suggest that physicians should cease to use the method for the treatment of herpetic disease. Most of the results suggest that dye–light therapy is not reliable, since: (1) the efficacy of the treatment is questionable and the results of treatment in patients reported by numerous investigators are inconsistent; (2) careful studies do not support efficacy; and (3) the long-term risks are unknown. Our studies on photodynamic inactivation and transformation in vitro suggest that this method may result in an increased incidence of cancers. Therefore, considering all observations reported thus far, any therapeutic agent suggested for the treatment of clinical herpesvirus infections or any inactivated or attenuated herpesvirus vaccine (52) must be critically evaluated before widespread application to the human population.

ACKNOWLEDGMENTS. This work was supported by Contract No. NO1 CP53516 within the Virus Cancer Program of the National Cancer Institute.

REFERENCES

1. Raab, O. (1900): Ueber die Wirkung fluoresciernder Stoffe auf Infusorien. *Z. Biol.* **39**:524–546.
2. Schultz, E. W., and Krueger, A. P. (1928): Inactivation of staphylococcus bacteriophage by methylene blue. *Proc. Soc. Exp. Biol. Med.* **26**:100–101.

3. Clifton, C. E., and Lawler, T. G. (1930): Inactivation of staphylococcus bacteriophage by toluidine blue. *Proc. Soc. Exp. Biol. Med.* **27**:1041-1042.

4. Clifton, C. E. (1930): Photodynamic action of certain dyes on the inactivation of staphylococcus bacteriophage. *Proc. Soc. Exp. Biol. Med.* **28**:745-746.

5. Perdrau, J. R., and Todd, C. (1933): The photodynamic action of methylene blue on certain viruses. *Proc. R. Soc. Lond.* [*Biol.*] **112**:288-298.

6. Wallis, C., and Melnick, J. L. (1965): Photodynamic inactivation of animal viruses: A review. *Photochem. Photobiol.* **4**:159-170.

7. Hanson, C. V., Riggs, J. L., and Lennette, E. H. (1978): Photochemical inactivation of DNA and RNA viruses by psoralen derivatives. *J. Gen. Virol.* **40**:345-358.

8. Hanson, C. V. (1979): Photochemical inactivation of deoxyribonucleic and ribonucleic acid viruses by chlorpromazine. *Antimicrob. Agents Chemother.* **15**:461-464.

9. Melnick, J., Khan, N. C., and Biswal, N. (1977): Photodynamic inactivation of herpes simplex virus and its DNA. *Photochem. Photobiol.* **25**:341-342.

10. Melnick, J. L., and Wallis, C. (1977): Photodynamic inactivation of herpes simplex virus: A status report. *Ann. N. Y. Acad. Sci.* **284**:171-181.

11. Yen, G. S. L., and Simon, E. H. (1978): Photosensitization of herpes simplex virus type 1 with neutral red. *J. Gen. Virol.* **41**:273-281.

12. Moore, C., Wallis, C., Melnick, J. L., et al. (1972): Photodynamic treatment of herpes keratitis. *Infect. Immun.* **5**:169-171.

13. Lahav, M., Dueker, D., Bhatt, P. N., et al. (1975): Photodynamic inactivation in experimental herpetic keratitis. *Arch. Ophthalmol.* **93**:207-214.

14. Stanley, J. A., and Pinnolis, M. (1976): Light intensity on the photodynamic inactivation of herpes simplex keratitis. *Am. J. Ophthalmol.* **81**:332-336.

15. Felber, T. D., Smith, E. B., Knox, J. M., et al. (1973): Photodynamic inactivation of herpes simplex: Report of a clinical trial. *J. AMA* **223**:289-292.

16. Friedrich, E. G. (1973): Relief for herpes vulvitis. *Obstet. Gynecol.* **41**:74-77.

17. Nahmias, A. J., and Dowdle, W. R. (1968): Antigenic and biologic differences in herpesvirus hominis. *Prog. Med. Virol.* **10**:110-159.

18. Wallis, C., Melnick, J. L., and Kaufman, R. H. (1972): Herpes genitalis management—present and predicted. *Clin. Obstet. Gynecol.* **15**:939-947.

19. Lefebvre, E. B., and McNellis, E. E. (1973): Photoinactivation of herpes simplex. *J. AMA* **224**:1039.

20. Kaufman, R. H., Gardner, H. L., Brown, D., et al. (1973): Herpes genitalis treated by photodynamic inactivation of virus. *Am. J. Obstet. Gynecol.* **117**:1144-1146.

21. Jarratt, M. (1977): Photodynamic inactivation of herpes simplex virus. *Photochem. Photobiol.* **25**:339-340.

22. Randall, J. L., and Plotkin, S. A. (1974): Cytomegalovirus, a model for herpesvirus opportunism. In: *Opportunistic Pathogens*, edited by J. E. Prior and H. Friedman, pp. 261-280. University Park Press, Baltimore.

23. Naib, Z. M., Nahmias, A. J., and Josey, W. E. (1966): Cytology and histopathology of cervical herpes simplex infection. *Cancer* **19**:1026-1031.

24. Naib, Z. M., Nahmias, A. J., Josey, W. E., et al. (1969): Genital herpetic infection association with cervical dysplasia and carcinoma. *Cancer* **23**:940-945.

25. Rawls, W. E., Tompkins, W. A. F., and Melnick, J. L. (1969): The association of herpesvirus type 2 and carcinoma of the uterine cervix. *Am. J. Epidemiol.* **89**:547-554.

26. Royston, I., and Aurelian, L. (1970): Immunofluorescent detection of herpesvirus antigens in exfoliated cells from human cervical carcinoma. *Proc. Natl. Acad. Sci. U.S.A.* **67**:204-212.

27. Aurelian, L., Strandberg, J. D., Meléndez, L. V., et al. (1971): Herpesvirus type 2 isolated from cervical tumor cells grown in tissue culture. *Science* **174**:704-707.

28. Frenkel, N., Roizman, B., Cassai, E., et al. (1972): A DNA fragment of herpes simplex 2 and

its transcription in human cervical cancer tissue. *Proc. Natl. Acad. Sci. U.S.A.* **69**: 3784–3789.

29. Rapp, F. (1974): Herpesviruses and cancer. In: *Advances in Cancer Research*, edited by G. Klein and S. Weinhouse, pp. 265–302. Academic Press, New York.

30. Duff, R., and Rapp, F. (1971): Oncogenic transformation of hamster cells after exposure to herpes simplex virus type 2. *Nature* [*New Biol.*] **233**:48–50.

31. Duff, R., and Rapp, F. (1971): Properties of hamster embryo fibroblasts transformed *in vitro* after exposure to ultraviolet-irradiated herpes simplex virus type 2. *J. Virol.* **8**:469–477.

32. Duff, R., and Rapp, F. (1973): Oncogenic transformation of hamster embryo cells after exposure to inactivated herpes simplex virus type 1. *J. Virol.* **12**:209–217.

33. Kutinova, L., Vonka, V., and Brouček, J. (1973): Increased oncogenicity and synthesis of herpesvirus antigens in hamster cells exposed to herpes simplex type-2 virus. *J. Natl. Cancer Inst.* **50**:759–766.

34. Takahashi, M., and Yamanishi, K. (1974): Transformation of hamster embryo and human embryo cells by temperature sensitive mutants of herpes simplex virus type 2. *Virology* **61**:306–311.

35. Munyon, W., Kraiselburd, E., Davis, D., et al. (1971): Transfer of thymidine kinase to thymidine kinaseless L cells by infection with ultraviolet-irradiated herpes simplex virus. *J. Virol.* **7**:813–820.

36. Duff, R., and Rapp, F. (1975): Quantitative assay for transformation of 3T3 cells by herpes simplex virus type 2. *J. Virol.* **15**:490–496.

37. Macnab, J. C. M. (1974): Transformation of rat embryo cells by temperature sensitive mutants of herpes simplex virus. *J. Gen. Virol.* **24**:143–153.

38. Darai, G., and Munk, K. (1973): Human embryonic lung cells abortively infected with herpes virus hominis type 2 show some properties of cell transformation. *Nature* [*New Biol.*] **241**:268–269.

39. Rapp, F., Li, J. L. H., and Jerkofsky, M. (1973): Transformation of mammalian cells by DNA-containing viruses following photodynamic inactivation. *Virology* **55**:339–346.

40. Li, J. L. H., Jerkofsky, M. A., and Rapp, F. (1975): Demonstration of oncogenic potential of mammalian cells transformed by DNA-containing viruses following photodynamic inactivation. *Int. J. Cancer* **15**:190–202.

41. Rapp, F., and Kemeny, B. (1977): Oncogenic potential of herpes simplex virus in mammalian cells following photodynamic inactivation. *Photochem. Photobiol.* **25**: 335–337.

42. Seemayer, N. H., Hirai, K., and Defendi, V. (1973): Analysis of minimal functions of simian virus 40. I. Oncogenic transformation of Syrian hamster kidney cells *in vitro* by photodynamically inactivated SV40. *Int. J. Cancer* **12**:524–531.

43. Cutchins, E. C., and Dayhuff, T. R. (1962): Photoinactivation of measles virus. *Virology* **17**:420–425.

44. Wallis, C., and Melnick, J. L. (1964): Irreversible photosensitization of viruses. *Virology* **23**:520–527.

45. Crowther, D., and Melnick, J. L. (1961): The incorporation of neutral red and acridine orange into developing poliovirus particles making them photosensitive. *Virology* **14**:11–21.

46. Schaffer, F. L. (1962): Binding of proflavine by and photoinactivation of poliovirus propagated in the presence of the dye. *Virology* **18**:412–425.

47. Wilson, J. N., and Cooper, P. D. (1962): Photodynamic demonstration of two stages in the growth of poliovirus. *Virology* **17**:195–196.

48. Mayor, H. D., and Melnick, J. L. (1962): Intracellular and extracellular reactions of viruses with vital dyes. *Yale J. Biol. Med.* **34**:340–344.

49. Hiatt, C. W., Kaufman, E., Helprin, J. J., et al. (1960): Inactivation of viruses by the photodynamic action of toluidine blue. *J. Immunol.* **84**:480–484.

50. Chang, T. W., and Weinstein, L. (1975): Photodynamic inactivation of *Herpesvirus hominis* by methylene blue *Proc. Soc. Exp. Biol. Med.* **148**:291–293.

51. Spikes, J. D., and Livingston, R. (1969): The molecular biology of photodynamic action: Sensitized photoautoxidations in biological systems. *Adv. Radiat. Biol.* **3**:29–121.

52. Pagano, J. S., and Huang, E. S. (1974): Vaccination against cytomegalovirus? *Lancet* **1**:316–317.

53. Wallis, C., Scheiris, C., and Melnick, J. L. (1967): Photodynamically inactivated vaccines prepared by growing viruses in cells containing neutral red. *J. Immunol.* **99**:1134–1139.

54. Sastry, K. S., and Gordon, M. P. (1966): The photodynamic inactivation of tobacco mosaic virus and its ribonucleic acid by acridine orange. *Biochim. Biophys. Acta* **129**:32–41.

55. Freifelder, D., and Uretz, R. B. (1966): Mechanism of photoinactivation of coliphage T7 sensitized by acridine orange. *Virology* **30**:97–103.

56. Simon, M. I., and Van Vunakis, H. (1962): The photodynamic reaction of methylene blue with deoxyribonucleic acid. *J. Mol. Biol.* **4**:488–499.

57. Li, J. H., and Rapp, F. (1976): Oncogenic transformation of mammalian cells *in vitro* by proflavine-photoinactivated herpes simplex virus type 2. *Cancer Letters* **1**:319–326.

58. Helprin, J. J., and Hiatt, C. W. (1959): Photosensitization of T2 coliphage with toluidine blue. *J. Bacteriol.* **77**:502–505.

59. Yamamoto, N. (1958): Photodynamic inactivation of bacteriophage and its inhibition. *J. Bacteriol.* **75**:443–448.

60. Kucera, L. S., and Gusdon, J. P. (1976): Transformation of human embryonic fibroblasts by photodynamically inactivated herpes simplex virus, type 2 at supra-optimal temperature. *J. Gen. Virol.* **30**:257–261.

61. Butel, J. S., Tevethia, S. S., and Melnick, J. L. (1972): Oncogenicity and cell transformation by papovavirus SV40: The role of the viral genome. *Adv. Cancer Res.* **15**:1–55.

62. Sambrook, J. (1972): Transformation by polyoma virus and simian virus 40. *Adv. Cancer Res.* **16**:141–180.

63. Graham, F. L., van der Eb, A. J., and Heijneker, H. L. (1974): Size and location of the transforming region in human adenovirus type 5 DNA. *Nature* **251**:687–691.

64. Sharp, P. A., Pettersson, U., and Sambrook, J. (1974): Viral DNA in transformed cells. I. A study of the sequences of adenovirus 2 DNA in a line of transformed rat cells using specific fragments of the viral genome. *J. Mol. Biol.* **86**:709–726.

65. Collard, W., Thornton, H., and Green, M. (1973): Cells transformed by human herpesvirus type 2 transcribe virus-specific RNA sequences shared by herpesvirus types 1 and 2. *Nature* [*New Biol.*] **243**:264–266.

66. Westmoreland, D., Watkins, J. F., and Rapp, F. (1974): Demonstration of a receptor for IgG in Syrian hamster cells transformed with herpes simplex virus. *J. Gen. Virol.* **25**:167–170.

67. Watkins, J. F. (1964): Adsorption of sensitized sheep erythrocytes to HeLa cells infected with herpes simplex virus. *Nature* **202**:1364–1365.

68. Watkins, J. F. (1965): The relationship of the herpes simplex haemadsorption phenomenon to the virus growth cycle. *Virology* **26**:746–753.

69. Westmoreland, D., and Watkins, J. F. (1974): The IgG receptor induced by herpes simplex virus: Studies using radioiodinated IgG. *J. Gen. Virol.* **24**:167–178.

70. Aaronson, S. A., and Todaro, G. J. (1968): Basis for the acquisition of malignant potential by mouse cells cultivated *in vitro*. *Science* **162**:1024–1026.

71. Jarrett, O., and MacPherson, I. (1968): The basis of the tumorigenicity of BHK 21 cells. *Int. J. Cancer* **3**:654–662.

72. Pollack, R. E., and Teebor, G. W. (1969): Relationship of contact inhibition to tumor transplantability, morphology and growth rate. *Cancer Res.* **29**:1770–1772.

73. Marin, G., and MacPherson, I. (1969): Reversion in polyoma-transformed cells: Retransformation, induced antigens and tumorigenicity. *J. Virol.* **3**:146–149.

74. Rapp, F., and Duff, R. (1973): Transformation of hamster embryo fibroblasts by herpes simplex viruses type 1 and type 2. *Cancer Res.* **33**:1527–1534.

75. Verwoerd, D., and Rapp, F. (1978): Biochemical transformation of mouse cells by herpes simplex virus type 2: Enhancement by means of low-level photodynamic treatment. *J. Virol.* **26**:200–202.

76. Varnell, E. D., and Kaufman, H. E. (1973): Photodynamic inactivation with proflavine: Quantitative comparison with iodo-deoxyuridine. *Infect. Immun.* **7**:518–519.

77. Thomas, J. V., Dunlap, W. A., and Rich, A. M. (1973): Photodynamic inactivation in the treatment of experimental herpes simplex keratitis. *Br. J. Ophthalmol.* **57**:336–338.

78. Taylor, P. K., and Doherty, N. R. (1975): Comparison of the treatment of herpes genitalis in men with proflavine photoinactivation, idoxuridine ointment, and normal saline. *Br. J. Vener. Dis.* **51**:125–129.

79. Roome, A. P. C. H., Tinkler, A. E., Hilton, A. L., et al. (1975): Neutral red with photoinactivation in the treatment of herpes genitalis. *Br. J. Vener. Dis.* **51**:130–133.

80. Blue dye + light for herpes? *Medical World News.* **1974** (December 20):54–55.

81. O'Day, D. M., Jones, B. R., Poirier, R., et al. (1975): Proflavine photodynamic viral inactivation in herpes simplex keratitis. *Am. J. Ophthalmol.* **79**:941–948.

82. Cusumano, C. L., and Monif, G. R. C. (1975): A word of caution concerning photodynamic inactivation therapy for herpes virus hominis infections. *Obstet. Gynecol.* **45**:335–336.

83. Myers, M. G., Oxman, M. N., Clark, J. E., et al. (1975): Failure of neutral-red photodynamic inactivation in recurrent herpes simplex virus infections. *N. Engl. J. Med.* **293**:945–949.

84. Myers, M. G., Oxman, M. N., Clark, J. E., et al. (1976): Therapy of local herpesviral infections. Photodynamic inactivation in recurrent infections with herpes simplex virus. *J. Infect. Dis.* **133**:A145–A150.

85. Kaufman, R. H., Adam, E., Mirkovic, R., et al. (1978): Treatment of genital herpes simplex virus infection with photodynamic inactivation. *Am. J. Obstet. Gynecol.* **132**:861–869.

86. Cramer, W. A., and Uretz, R. B. (1966): Acridine orange-sensitized photoinactivation of T4 bacteriophage. II. Genetic studies with photoinactivated phage. *Virology* **29**:469–479.

87. Benjamin, T. L. (1965): Relative target sizes for the inactivation of the transforming and reproductive abilities of polyoma virus. *Proc. Natl. Acad. Sci. U.S.A.* **54**:121–124.

88. Latarjet, R., Cramer, R., and Montagnier, L. (1967): Inactivation by UV-, X-, and γ-radiations, of the infecting and transforming capacities of polyoma virus. *Virology* **33**:104–111.

89. Aaronson, S. A. (1970): Effect of ultraviolet irradiation on the survival of simian virus 40 functions in human and mouse cells. *J. Virol.* **6**:393–399.

90. Finklestein, J. Z., and McAllister, R. M. (1969): Ultraviolet inactivation of the cytocidal and transforming activities of human adenovirus type 1. *J. Virol.* **3**:353–354.

91. Jensen, F., and Defendi, V. (1968): Transformation of African green monkey kidney cells by irradiated adenovirus 7–simian virus 40 hybrid. *J. Virol.* **2**:173–177.

92. Casto, B. C. (1968): Effects of ultraviolet irradiation on the transforming and plaque-forming capacities of simian adenovirus SA7. *J. Virol.* **2**:641–642.

93. Albrecht, T., and Rapp, F. (1973): Malignant transformation of hamster embryo fibroblasts following exposure to ultraviolet-irradiated human cytomegalovirus. *Virology* **55**:53–61.

94. Toyoshima, K., Friis, R. R., and Vogt, P. K. (1970): The reproductive and cell-transforming capacities of avian sarcoma virus B77: Inactivation with UV light. *Virology* **42**:163–170.

95. Defendi, V., and Jensen, F. (1967): Oncogenicity by DNA tumor viruses: Enhancement after ultraviolet and cobalt-60 radiations. *Science* **157**:703–705.

96. Schell, K., Maryak, J., Young, J., et al. (1968): Adenovirus transformation of hamster embryo cells. II. Inoculation conditions. *Arch. Gesamte Virusforsch.* **24**:342–351.

97. Duff, R., Knight, P., and Rapp, F. (1972): Variation in oncogenic and transforming potential of PARA (defective SV40)-adenovirus 7. *Virology* **47**:849–853.

98. Seemayer, N. H., and Defendi, V. (1973): Analysis of minimal functions of simian virus 40. II. Enhancement of oncogenic transformation *in vitro* by UV irradiation. *J. Virol.* **12**:1265–1271.

99. Kubitschek, H. E. (1966): Mutation without segregation in bacteria with reduced dark repair ability. *Proc. Natl. Acad. Sci. U.S.A.* **55**:269–274.

100. Haspel, M. V., and Rapp, F. (1975): Measles virus: An unwanted variant causing hydrocephalus. *Science* **187**:450–451.

22

Photochemotherapy of Skin Diseases

J. A. Parrish, R. S. Stern, M. A. Pathak, and T. B. Fitzpatrick

While *phototherapy* is defined as the application of visible or ultraviolet (UV) radiation to the treatment of disease, in photochemotherapy a chemical sensitizer is administered concurrently and the therapeutic effect depends on photochemical interaction of the chemical and radiation. In the doses used, chemical and radiation alone usually have little or no therapeutic effect. Photochemotherapy utilizing psoralen compounds, including 8-methoxypsoralen, and long-wave UV radiation is currently used in the treatment of many common skin diseases. Other forms of photochemotherapy not utilizing psoralens have been used in the treatment of certain tumors (see Chapter 23). Topical forms of photochemotherapy have been proposed for treatment of recurrent herpes simplex (see Chapters 19–21).

PSORALEN PHOTOCHEMOTHERAPY

Definition

Currently, the administration of psoralens (P) and long-wave ultraviolet radiation (UVA) is the most widely used form of photochemotherapy and is commonly referred to as "PUVA." PUVA has been used to treat a variety of diseases, including psoriasis, vitiligo, and mycosis fungoides. Its principal clinical application in the United States and Europe has been in the treatment

J. A. Parrish, M. A. Pathak, and T. B. Fitzpatrick • Department of Dermatology, Harvard Medical School, Massachusetts General Hospital, Boston, Massachusetts 02114. *R. S. Stern* • Department of Dermatology, Harvard Medical School, Beth Israel Hospital, Boston, Massachusetts 02215.

of psoriasis. PUVA therapy usually involves oral administration of psoralens, and that type of therapy will be the main focus of this chapter. Topical psoralen in combination with subsequent exposure to UVA radiation is also used and will be discussed briefly.

Historical Aspects

The use of a specific class of chemicals, the psoralens, to augment the therapeutic effect of sunlight dates back several millennia. Writings dating from 1400 B.C. describe the application of extracts or parts of psoralen-containing plants to the affected skin, which was then exposed to sunlight (1); depigmenting patches of skin, probably vitiligo, were treated in this manner in ancient India and Egypt. Certain photoactive natural or synthetic psoralens continue to be used extensively as the main treatment for vitiligo. It is only in the past few years that the value of this treatment in other skin diseases has been recognized. With the recognition of its therapeutic potential, investigators have attempted to document the dose–response relationship in this therapy and relate its apparent clinical effectiveness to our understanding about basic photobiologic principles.

PSORALENS

While many naturally occurring and synthetic psoralen compounds exist, the most widely used psoralen derivative in dermatologic therapy is 8-methoxypsoralen, also known as 8-MOP or methoxsalen. The bioavailability of 8-methoxypsoralen varies substantially among different commercial compounds (2). In addition, there is substantial variation in serum levels achieved by different individuals after the standard dose (3). The more than 10-fold variation in serum concentrations would appear to be both a result of the differences in pharmacokinetics of different compounds as well as the variation in absorption rates among patients (4, 5). The influence of food intake on absorption (6) causes the additional variation in serum concentration. The quantity of long-wave UV radiation required to elicit a minimal phototoxic dose is lowest between 1–3 hr after the ingestion of psoralens. Cutaneous photosensitization appears to last about 8 hr (7–9). While serum levels are poorly correlated with minimal phototoxic doses, there does appear to be a general reciprocal relationship between serum level and UVA dose required to elicit a phototoxic response, and peak serum levels are associated with the maximal period of sensitization following an oral psoralen dose. Psoralen compounds are metabolized by the liver and primarily excreted by the kidneys (9). Therefore, metabolism and excretion of psoralens are altered in patients with severe impairment of hepatic or renal function.

While 8-MOP is by far the most commonly used agent, a variety of other psoralen derivatives have been used. These include trimethylpsoralen, which has been used both topically and systemically for many years in the treatment of vitiligo. Applied topically, TMP, 8-MOP, and psoralen are potent photosensitizers; a few minutes of sun exposure may result in blistering following application of 0.1 ml/5 cm² skin surface of a 0.1% solution of each of these agents. When given by mouth, methoxsalen is much more erythemogenic and melanogenic to normal skin than is trimethylpsoralen or psoralen. With increased clinical application and the recognition of methoxsalen's side effects, new compounds have been synthesized and used in clinical trials. These include 5-methoxypsoralen, 3-carbethoxypsoralen, and certain alkyl-substituted angelicans (10-12).

Psoralen–DNA Photochemistry

Like a large number of other drugs that interact strongly with nucleic acids (e.g., several antitumor agents such as actinomycin D, adriamycin, and daunomycin, and drugs such as chloroquin, quinacrine, miracil D, and ethidium bromide), the psoralens are known to intercalate between base pairs (13-15). These compounds readily penetrate intact cells or viral particles and intercalate into the DNA. Subsequent exposure with long-wavelength UV radiation (320-400 nm) leads to covalent binding of the psoralen to DNA or RNA (16-19). The photoaddition involves the formation of a cyclobutane bridge between the 5,6 double bond of a pyrimidine base and the 3,4- or 4',5' double bond of the psoralen (13, 16-19). The first step in this photoreaction after intercalation involves the formation of monofunctional adducts of psoralen with pyrimidine bases (thymine, cytosine). This first photochemical reaction is usually a conjugation of the 4',5' double bond of the furan ring of the psoralen molecule with the 5,6 double bond of the pyrimidine base. This results in the formation of a fluorescent adduct that absorbs at 360 nm. Both Cole (14) and Dall'Acqua et al. (15) independently showed in duplex DNA that linear psoralens were able to photoinduce bifunctional adducts by the linkage of one molecule of psoralen to pyrimidine bases of the two complementary strands of DNA.

If two pyrimidines are adjacent at appropriate distances and on opposite strands, subsequent absorption of a second photon by the monoadduct leads to the formation of additional covalent linkages between the 3,4 double bond of the psoralen molecule and the 5,6 double bond of the pyrimidine base of the opposite strand, thus cross-linking the two strands of the double helix (14, 19-22). Thus, reaction of both psoralen double bonds with pyrimidine on opposite strands of a DNA or RNA double helix results in the covalent cross-linkage of the two nucleic acid strands (14-22). Photoconjugation of psoralens to DNA has been established with purified DNA (13-18) in human, mouse, and Drosophilia tissue culture cells (23, 24), and in vivo in bacteria and virus (13, 25), mammalian skin (23, 26, 27), and other biologic systems. The photoreaction with RNA has also been investigated. It appears that this light-dependent conjugation of psoralens with epidermal DNA leads to inhibition of DNA synthesis and cell division (28), and it has been postulated that this effect may account for its therapeutic effect in the treatment of psoriasis (29).

Because of concern about possible mutagenicity and carcinogenicity and alterations in DNA, especially those resulting from bifunctional adducts formed by the photochemical interaction of 8-MOP and DNA, new compounds said to form only monofunctional adducts, including 3-carbethoxy-psoralen, have been developed and used in treating psoriasis. The investigators advocating 3-carbethoxypsoralen claim that with photoactivation this agent damages mitochondrial rather than only nuclear DNA and that the photoadducts may be less mutagenic (11).

While there is some evidence that monofunctional adducts to DNA are repaired by enzymatic mechanisms similar to those that repair photodamage from UV radiation alone, the relationship between type of adduct or site of adduct and mutagenicity is not yet clearly delineated (30). If the therapeutic and deleterious effects of psoralen–DNA damage are in fact separate, the risks of phototherapy could be minimized by utilizing psoralens that preferentially form therapeutic but not toxic photoproducts. In addition to 3-carbethoxy-psoralen, the methylated angelicans, which appear to form monofunctional adducts to DNA, are undergoing study (26). Investigators claim that interstrand cross-links in DNA do not occur as a result of photoactivation of these compounds, possibly making them less mutagenic than 8-methoxy-psoralen (31). Also, it may be possible to preferentially produce mono-functional adducts with existing compounds, including 8-MOP, by using specific wavelengths of UV radiation rather than broadband UV radiation. While there is some evidence that the cross-link (bifunctional) psoralen–DNA photoproduct may be more lethal, it is uncertain which photoproducts cause more mutations per survivor or cause more photocarcinogenesis.

ACUTE EFFECTS OF PUVA ON NORMAL SKIN

Photosensitization occurs when psoralens reach the skin either through diffusion, following topical application, or indirectly, via the bloodstream after ingestion and absorption from the gastrointestinal tract. Since serum levels and skin photosensitivity peak approximately 2 hr after oral administration of psoralens, UVA exposures are given at this time (Fig. 22-1). Following

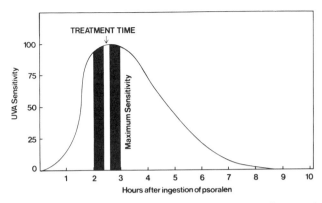

Fig. 22-1. After the ingestion of 8-methoxypsoralen (8-MOP), patients gradually become reactive to UVA. They are maximally reactive 2–3 hr after ingesting 8-MOP and remain reactive to UVA for as long as 6–8 hr.

topical application, however, the skin rapidly becomes photosensitive and may remain photosensitive for a few days, although peak photosensitivity occurs in the first hours.

PUVA causes injury to skin cells and a subsequent inflammatory reaction. The most easily observable acute sign of cutaneous phototoxicity is erythema (redness). Melanogenesis (tanning) is evident several days after a single PUVA exposure. As with sunburn, large doses may cause swelling, blistering, itch, pain, and desquamation. Compared with the UVB-induced sunburn reaction, which appears within 4–6 hr and peaks between 12 and 24 hr after exposure, erythema resulting from PUVA therapy is later in onset, appearing around 24 hr after exposure and peaks 48–72 hr postirradiation. However, a few patients do not show an erythema response until 48 hr and peak as late as 96 hr after exposure. The erythema reaction persists for a longer period than sunburn and may last for many days or even weeks; marked erythema tends to last longer than mild reactions. Unlike the pink to red hue of UVB erythema, the PUVA erythema is a deeper, almost violaceous color, possibly due to dilation of larger, deeper blood vessels. This difference in color may be the result of the release of different mediators by the PUVA reaction or it could be related to the relatively deeper transmission of UVA. The erythema response to UVB is decreased by the topical or intradermal administration of indomethacin, a potent inhibitor of prostaglandin synthesis (see Chapter 8). The erythema response to UVA radiation and to PUVA does not appear to be altered by the administration of indomethacin (32).

Increasing the dose of psoralen or of UVA radiation will increase the erythema response. The PUVA dose–response curve is considerably steeper than that for UVB-induced erythema (Fig. 22-2). A relatively small UVA

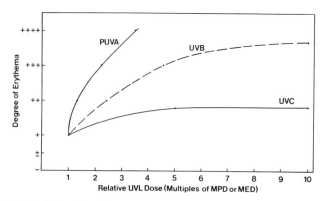

Fig. 22-2. Delayed erythema dose–response curve for PUVA, UVB, UVC.

increment may cause an unexpectedly severe erythema, which, in the case of whole-body exposure, can be akin to a severe burn and life-threatening.

A single PUVA exposure sufficient to cause erythema results in histologic changes in both dermis and epidermis (33). The character and time course of these changes are different than those seen with a comparable erythema response to UVA, UVB, or UVC alone. Epidermal changes seen with PUVA occur later than those seen with UVB and UVC. Fewer dyskeratotic cells are seen. Dermal changes are more marked after PUVA and UVA than after shorter wavelength UV radiation. Endothelial swelling, nuclear dust, and extravasation of red blood cells are seen with PUVA-induced erythema. These findings are still pronounced 7 days after exposure.

In most respects the pigmentation that results from PUVA appears histologically and morphologically similar to normal melanogenesis. Ultrastructural alterations within melanocytes are evident within minutes. A single exposure to PUVA enhances the activity of tyrosinase and there is an increase in the rate of transfer of melanosomes to adjacent keratinocytes (34). Repeated PUVA exposures cause an increase in the number and size of functional melanocytes. In the unstimulated skin of Caucasoids, melanosomes are commonly aggregated in groups of two or more within membrane-limited vesicular bodies commonly referred to as melanosome complexes. Following a single UVA exposure to skin treated with topical psoralens, some melanosomes are found to be singly dispersed, as is characteristic of black skin (35). Grossly, pigmentation appears to maximize about 5–7 days after a PUVA exposure and lasts weeks to months. As with solar or UVB-induced tanning, the individual's ability to tan with PUVA is genetically determined. In some individuals, one or two erythemogenic PUVA exposures may stimulate a greater tanning response than can multiple UVB or sun exposures. PUVA has, in fact, been used for induction to melanization and increased thickening of stratum corneum to increase tolerance to sun (Fig. 22-3).

PUVA FOR PSORIASIS (Fig. 22-4)

Psoriasis is a common cutaneous disease of unknown etiology. It is a disorder that exhibits increased epidermal proliferation which is clinically manifested as red, raised, scaling plaques. The disease varies greatly in extent and response to therapy. A wide variety of agents have been used in the treatment of psoriasis and their mechanism of action is usually considered to be via suppression of DNA synthesis leading to a reduction of epidermal proliferation. Other mechanisms may also be involved.

The earliest studies documenting the effectiveness of PUVA in psoriasis involved the use of topical psoralens (36–38). Topical psoralen photo-chemotherapy is effective but has certain difficulties. The phototoxic response is not entirely predictable, possibly because of variation in percutaneous absorption of psoralen. There is also a tendency to cause irregular hyper-pigmentation around lesions, and the process of applying topical medication to numerous lesions is laborious and time consuming. In Europe, topical application of trimethylpsoralen utilizing a bath followed by exposure to UVA has enjoyed considerable attention in the treatment of psoriasis (39). By using baths for applying psoralens, greater uniformity in psoralen application is possible and uneven pigmentation reduced. Because of substantial photo-sensitization achieved with topical tripsoralen, short exposure times are possible. In the United States, topical PUVA in psoriasis therapy has been used principally for the management of recalcitrant plaques, as a supplement to whole-body oral PUVA (40, 41).

The quantification of oral psoralen photosensitization (42) and the development of a high-output fluorescent UVA treatment system (43) made it possible and practical to treat psoriasis by oral administration of methoxsalen (29). Patients, after taking psoralen by mouth, could receive a therapeutic dose of UVA within a reasonable exposure time. By entering a booth lined with lamps, the entire body could be treated at one time. The striking effectiveness of this therapy in treating psoriasis focused much attention on the concept of photochemotherapy. Many reports have since confirmed the efficacy of oral psoralen photochemotherapy for psoriasis (44–47).

The experience gained in the U.S. cooperative PUVA study (16 centers) demonstrated a high rate of clearing. Of more than 1300 patients initially entering this cooperative trial, 88% cleared completely and 3% failed to improve (45). In general, fair-skinned individuals cleared more rapidly with fewer exposures and smaller UVA exposure doses than did dark-skinned individuals. Patients with a medium complexion cleared with a mean of 23.6

treatments over 11.6 weeks. Two treatments per week cleared the skin with fewer treatments and a smaller total UVA dose than did three treatments per week, but these results were skin-type dependent. Many patients cleared of psoriasis required less frequent treatments (once every 1–3 weeks) to prevent relapse. Short-term side effects included erythema, pruritus, nausea, headache, and dizziness. These symptoms were uncommon and interrupted treatment in only a small number of cases. Cellular and ultrastructural features of psoriasis gradually disappear during therapy (48–50).

Oral PUVA has certain advantages over other treatments for severe psoriasis. Unlike the Goeckerman regimen (tar and UVB radiation), PUVA does not require topical applications, is easily administered, and is suitable for outpatient use. The generalized tanning due to the treatment is usually aesthetically acceptable. PUVA may be effective when other treatments fail. Some patients may be kept free of lesions on a maintenance schedule of relatively infrequent treatments. In one series (44) 85% of patients were kept in remission. Further evidence of PUVA's efficacy comes from a trial (46) which compared treatment response among 224 randomly assigned patients with chronic plaque-type psoriasis. A higher percentage of patients who were treated with PUVA as outpatients cleared compared to patients treated with dithranol as inpatients.

The mechanisms by which PUVA improves psoriasis are not well understood. The effects may or may not be similar to the therapeutic mechanisms of phototherapy (see Chapter 17). It is generally assumed that effect on DNA replication and cellular proliferation is important. Other mechanisms may be operable. For example, PUVA appears to inhibit the chemotactic activity of psoriasis leukotactic factor, and polymorphonuclear leukocytes may be important in the pathogenesis of psoriasis (51). It is possible that PUVA may induce correction of certain immunologic abnormalities noted in patients with active psoriasis. For example, in one study depressed E-rosette formation by peripheral blood T lymphocytes returned to normal after PUVA treatment (52).

The benefit of adjuvant therapy in addition to PUVA in treatment of psoriasis remains controversial. Many investigators have noted more rapid clearing of psoriasis when topical steroids are added to PUVA treatments (53–56). While Schmoll et al. (53) noted no difference in relapse rate between those treated with PUVA alone and those also treated with topical steroids, Morison et al. (55) noted more frequent relapses in the group that also received topical steroids. Morison et al. also failed to note any long-term benefit from the addition of topical tar preparations to PUVA treatment (55).

In Europe, combination therapies for psoriasis using PUVA and oral retinoic acid derivatives have been used. In nonrandomized trails, investigators have noted accelerated response of psoriasis to PUVA following pretreatment with oral retinoic acid derivatives (57). While total number of treatments and UVA dose at clearing is reduced by 30% or more with this combination of photochemotherapy and retinoic acid chemotherapy, the long-term toxicity has not been established.

PUVA therapy of pustular and erythrodermic types of psoriasis has not been uniformly successful. A group in Vienna (58) reported almost 100% success in treating pustular psoriasis of the von Zumbusch type, but this has not been the experience of all investigators. For other groups the management of pustular and erythrodermic psoriasis has been difficult and combination therapy of PUVA and antimetabolites such as methotrexate has been frequently required (59, 60). Utilizing special irradiators that allow delivery of high-energy UVA to local areas, PUVA treatment has been successful in treating a variety of dermatoses of palms and soles, including pustular and plaque-type psoriasis (61, 62). Both topical and oral psoralen have been used successfully in persistent palmoplantar pustulosis (63).

Disadvantages of PUVA include the need to travel to a center where the exposure source is available. Sunlight is a source of UVA radiation and in combination with 8-methoxypsoralen it has been shown to be effective in the treatment of psoriasis (64). There are obvious drawbacks to the use of sunlight; latitudinal variation, climatic variation, and problems of privacy are among them. Without an accurate integrating UVA radiometer, reliable dosimetry is difficult. PUVA is not an effective treatment for psoriasis of the scalp and body folds, because of the difficulty in irradiating the affected areas. Finally, there remain reservations about possible long-term deleterious effects from repeated PUVA treatments; these include accelerated aging of exposed skin, cutaneous carcinogenesis, cataractogenesis, exacerbation of certain photodermatoses and light-sensitive diseases, and alterations in immune function. These potential hazards are discussed more fully later in this chapter.

PUVA FOR OTHER DISORDERS

Vitiligo (Fig. 22-5)

Vitiligo is a disease of unknown cause in which melanin pigment is lost from areas of otherwise normal skin. The histology of vitiliginous skin is normal except that, by light microscopic, histochemical, and electron microscopic ultrastructural criteria, there are no functional dendritic melanocytes present. The absence of pigment in the epidermis results in white patches and makes the affected areas of skin susceptible to sunburn. There are no other symptoms and the condition could be considered a harmless cosmetic problem. However, particularly for dark-skinned people, the disfigurement can be ruinous psychologically, socially, and economically.

Spontaneous repigmentation occurs in less than 5% of patients and is usually limited to minimal perifollicular pigmentation confined to small areas of exposed skin. The skin of most patients does not repigment with exposure to sunlight or to conventional UVB sources. In contrast, PUVA induces some improvement in about 70% of patients with vitiligo. While skin overlying bony prominences responds poorly, other areas, including the face and neck, often respond well. Topical and oral psoralens are used and patients are exposed to either the entire spectrum of sunlight or to artificial sources of UVA radiation.

Several reports document the successful use of PUVA using topically applied psoralens (65–70). There are, however, some disadvantages because penetration of the psoralen through the skin is variable. Also, because topical psoralens are potent photosensitizers, it is often difficult to treat large or multiple sites without occasionally provoking a severe blistering reaction. A dose of UVA close to that which causes erythema is thought to be necessary for treatment, but the minimally effective drug–radiation dose is not known. The fact that in the presence of topical psoralens the dose of UVA required to induce minimal erythema is relatively close to that which causes blistering makes careful dosimetry an essential part of therapy. The unpredictability of the psoralen phototoxic reaction is the major disadvange of topical treatment. Irregular hyperpigmentation of normal skin may be a problem around the margins of a vitiliginous macule that is undergoing topical PUVA therapy. This is due to the striking melanogenic effect of this treatment on normal melanocytes. Finally, patients find it tedious to carefully apply medication to each site, occlude the site to increase penetration of drug, and then expose each site to a measured dose of UV radiation.

Up to 70% of patients with vitiligo improved when treated at least twice weekly for more than 12 months with oral trimethylpsoralen (0.6–0.8 mg/kg) 2 hr before sun exposure (71, 72). Oral methoxsalen, alone or in combination with trimethylpsoralen, was effective in improving the majority of patients with vitiligo who used natural sunlight in a large clinical trial in India (73). Once repigmentation occurs, it appears to be long lasting (74). Oral psoralen photochemotherapy requires larger doses of UVA radiation than does topical therapy. Many of the commercially available artificial sources of UVA are not of adequate intensity to be convenient for oral therapy of vitiligo. However, by using long exposures, fluorescent "black-lights" have been shown to be effective (75, 76). A high-intensity source of UVA has been developed to meet the requirements for indoor oral psoralen therapy of vitiligo (43). Using such a source it appears that trimethylpsoralen (0.5–1.0 mg/kg) is as effective in repigmenting vitiligo as 8-methoxypsoralen (77).

When using 8-methoxypsoralen to treat vitiligo, the doses of drug and UVA radiation are generally the same as those used to treat psoriasis. Repigmentation occurs very slowly and is first noted around the hair follicle. An adequate course of treatment usually requires at least 150 exposures to

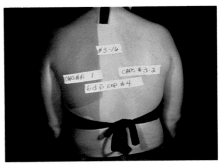

Fig. 22-3. Normal volunteer showing striking melanogenic properties of oral 8-methoxypsoralen. This person exposed the right side of her back to 20 min of noonday sun after ingesting placebo. On a different day the left side of her back was exposed to 20 min of noonday sun 2 hr after she ingested 30 mg of 8-methoxypsoralen. This photograph was obtained 6 days after the PUVA exposure.

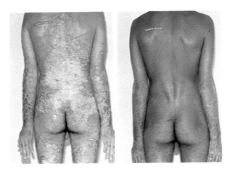

Fig. 22-4. Left: Chronic persistent psoriasis vulgaris which had not responded to conventional topical treatment. Right: Same patient after 20 treatments of oral methoxsalen photochemotherapy. (Photograph courtesy of Klaus Wolff.)

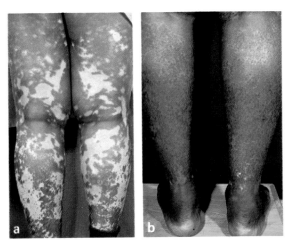

Fig. 22-5. Vitiligo (a) before and (b) after treatment. This patient underwent over 100 treatments with oral trimethylpsoralen.

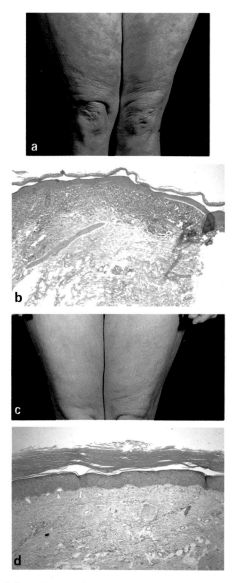

Fig. 22-6. (a) Mycosis fungoides showing plaques and the erythrodermic phase of the disease present continuously for longer than 1 year. (b) Photomicrograph of the same patient before therapy showing dense infiltrate of abnormal cells in the upper dermis. (c) Same patient after 30 treatments with oral methoxsalen photochemotherapy. (d) Photomicrograph of the same patient after more than 30 treatments of photochemotherapy, showing absence of abnormal dermal infiltrate. The thickening of the stratum corneum is the result of repeated PUVA exposures.

PUVA but, in most cases, if a patient is going to respond, signs of improvement are evident after 50 exposures. If patients discontinue therapy, they may lose the recently acquired pigmentation, and new lesions may develop while undergoing treatment. Many patients eventually improve significantly, but total repigmentation is unusual and about 30% of patients do not respond at all despite months of therapy. The face and the exposed areas of hands and feet respond fairly well, but areas involving bony prominences (knuckles, wrists, ankles, etc.) respond poorly.

Mycosis Fungoides (Fig. 22-6)

Mycosis fungoides (MF) is an uncommon cutaneous T-cell lymphoma. It is characterized by a polymorphous cellular infiltrate, with the cell of origin a T (thymus-derived) lymphocyte (78). The disease is mainly confined to the skin early in its course, but usually disseminates to involve visceral organs and may be fatal. The earliest skin lesions frequently lack diagnostic features and may resemble eczema or psoriasis; also, the light microscopic and ultrastructural picture of the skin in early MF is often not diagnostic. Later the skin may become diffusely red, atrophic, or eroded, and plaques or fungating tumors may develop. The histology of these later phases is diagnostic (79).

Conventional treatments of MF include the use of topical steroids, sunburn-spectrum UV radiation, and nitrogen mustard in early phases of the disease. As the disease progresses, modalities including x-irradiation, electron-beam irradiation, and systemic chemotherapy are utilized. However, no therapeutic regimen has clearly been shown to arrest this disease and the long-term benefits of early aggressive treatment remain controversial. Because the morphology and histology are often not diagnostic, the use of potentially toxic agents early in the course of the disease carries the risk of treating patients who do not have MF. For these reasons, in some cases, it appears reasonable to use the least toxic form of therapy (79).

Sunlight has been found to be beneficial to some patients with early stages of the disease (80) and that observation led to an investigation of the effect of PUVA on the disease. Gilchrest et al. (81) demonstrated the efficacy of PUVA in the dermatitic and plaque stages of MF and this has been confirmed by several investigators (82, 83). Early stages of disease appear to respond well. Clinical improvement seen may be due to direct destruction of lymphoid cells in the skin by PUVA. Histologic studies show clearing of the cellular infiltrate in the epidermis and upper dermis (83–85).

While cutaneous lesions are decreased by PUVA, this treatment's effect on survival in MF patients is not known. Histologic evidence of deep cutaneous infiltrates may persist despite clinical evidence of clearing. Some patients treated with PUVA have shown dissemination of their disease (86, 87). Other reports indicate improvement in immune function after PUVA treatment (88). These reports and the lack of long-term follow-up in PUVA-treated MF patients leave the place of PUVA in the treatment of MF still to be determined.

Atopic Eczema

Atopic eczema is a common chronic skin disease which is characterized by severe pruritus. Scratching and rubbing result in red, excoriated, and thickened skin. There is a tendency to secondary bacterial infection. In many cases the skin disease dominates the lives of the patient and family and in some persons it is incapacitating. Treatment is unsatisfactory and centers on avoidance of chemical and physical irritants of all kinds and the use of skin lubricants. Topical corticosteroid preparations are fairly effective in suppressing symptoms, but may have accompanying side effects.

PUVA has been found effective in the treatment of a small group of patients with atopic eczema (89). The principles of treatment are essentially the same as for psoriasis, although there are some important differences. Compared with PUVA treatment of psoriasis patients, about twice the number of treatments is required to clear the skin of patients with atopic dermatitis. Once clear, atopic patients need more frequent maintenance treatments and generally closer supervision and support than do psoriatic patients. When treatments are missed, the eczema rapidly reappears. The need for frequent maintenance therapy and the youth of these patients result in limited enthusiasm for PUVA as a usual treatment in this disease, but it may be useful in cases where no other options exist. The mode of action of PUVA in atopic dermatitis is unknown; a suppression of dermal lymphocytes has been proposed.

Miscellaneous Diseases

Lichen planus is a benign dermatosis, but, as in MF, the skin infiltrate is primarily T lymphocytes. PUVA has been shown to be effective in clearing lichen planus. With PUVA therapy, there was a decrease in clinical symptoms, the infiltrate in the superficial dermis decreased, and in one case immunofluorescent abnormalities returned to normal (90). Urticaria pigmentosa, a disease characterized by an infiltrate of mast cells and monocytes in the upper dermis, has been treated with PUVA. Of 10 patients with adult-onset urticaria pigmentosa treated with PUVA, all improved in exposed areas, but not in covered areas. Only one of three patients followed for at least 6 months without treatment remained symptom free (91). Therapeutic benefit from PUVA in the treatment of polymorphous light eruption (92, 93) has been reported. One presumed mechanism for clinical improvement is PUVA's ability to induce a protective tan in these patients, but depletion of mediators or lymphocytotoxicity may also be involved. PUVA has been used successfully even in cases where patients are sensitive to long-wave (UVA) radiation and it appears to be more successful than treatment with beta-carotene (93). *Alopecia areata*, a disease characterized by local areas of nonscarring hair loss, has been treated with PUVA. No controlled studies have been published, but treatment with oral PUVA has been associated with improvement in patients with chronic disease (94).

DOSIMETRY AND ACUTE SIDE EFFECTS OF PUVA

The erythema response to PUVA increases with increasing cutaneous levels of psoralen and increasing exposure dose of UVA radiation. Depending on dose, the observed clinical response varies from no detectable change to severe erythema and blistering. It is easier to measure and precisely alter the dose of UVA radiation than it is to measure cutaneous levels of psoralen, and therefore therapy aims at keeping the cutaneous drug level constant for a given patient by utilizing a fixed interval from drug administration to radiation exposure and a constant drug dose for that patient. Because nausea often develops at higher doses, the most frequently used starting dose of 8-MOP is 0.6 mg/kg. Since psoralen serum drug levels peak from $1\frac{1}{2}$-3 hr after oral administration, a constant interval of approximately 2 hr has been chosen as the time from drug administration to exposure to UVA radiation. This approach leaves only one variable, namely the dose of UVA radiation.

Features essential to a modern source for UVA radiation have been described in detail (43). Such a source should provide a uniform dose of radiation on the entire exposed surface of a patient. Therefore, the distance from light source to patient must not be critical. The UVA radiation source's output should in ideal circumstances correspond to the action spectrum of the photosensitizer being employed in therapy. Although the relative advantages of monochromatic vs. broadband UV radiation continue to be explored, currently fluorescent lamps enjoy the greatest acceptance because of their relative efficiency and low cost. Currently available fluorescent light sources have outputs in the 6–12 mW/cm^2 range of broadband UV radiation and can deliver sufficient energy to the patient for an average treatment in less than 30 min. In the future, monochromatic or narrowband sources may permit the more rapid delivery of sufficient energy to activate photosensitizers in a shorter time and may permit utilization of possible synergistic benefits resulting from wavelength interaction.

As in the case of UVB phototherapy, with PUVA treatment of psoriasis, repeated inductions of phototoxicity or at least near phototoxic doses appear necessary to improve psoriasis. Phototoxicity is the limiting factor in treating patients. With a constant psoralen dose and a constant time interval between ingestion and exposure, the dose of UVA that can be tolerated can be estimated in two ways: (1) After exposure to graded doses of UVA to 1-cm² areas of normal skin, the lowest dose of UVA that produces a uniform faint pink erythema at 48–72 hr after exposure can be determined. This UVA dose is known as the minimum phototoxic dose (MPD). (2) In a population, MPD, and hence ability to tolerate varying quantities of UVA, appears to be correlated with a patient's previous responses to natural sunlight with respect to burning and tanning. Therefore, these clinical variables have been used to categorize patients with groupings known as "Skin Type." Generally safe initial and incremental exposures of UVA radiation for standard 8-MOP dosage have been established for each skin type and are widely used in clinical practice. Since exposure to PUVA induces pigmentation, which acts as a UVA filter, maintaining erythema requires gradually increasing doses of UVA with subsequent treatments. Because peak erythema response is delayed from 48 to 72 hr, it is common practice in the United States to treat patients at two-to three-day intervals.

POTENTIAL LONG-TERM HAZARDS OF PUVA

As with any new treatment, oral psoralen photochemotherapy utilizing artificial UVA sources causes concern over possible long-term side effects. Some adverse effects may be entirely unpredictable and will be identified only with the passage of time. Others may be anticipated on theoretical grounds by extrapolation from the results of similar treatments or from known in vitro effects and results of animal studies. Long-term hazards for which there is valid theoretically based concern include actinic damage to the skin, cutaneous cancers, ocular damage (keratitis and cataract), and alterations of the immune system.

Actinic Damage

Actinic damage is seen on the sun-exposed areas of fair-skinned individuals whose occupation or recreational activities have resulted in a large cumulative dose of sunlight. The skin is dry, wrinkled, inelastic, and leathery, with irregular pigmentation. In such an individual a comparison of skin of the back of the neck with that of the buttock strikingly confirms the part played by chronic sun exposure. On microscopic examination the collagen of the upper dermis is replaced by masses of amorphous or granular material, which stains slightly basophilic with hematoxylin and eosin (solar elastosis). The epidermis is atrophic. The action spectrum of actinic damage is unknown, although the epidermal change has been attributed to UVB and the dermal changes to more deeply penetrating UVA (95). Approximately 50% of UVA incident on the skin surface can reach the dermis (96) and psoralens located in the dermis may be activated proportionately. Repeated PUVA reactions over a long period may thus injure dermal structures, including blood vessels, fibroblasts, and connective tissue.

Investigators have noted epidermal and dermal changes after both PUVA therapy and UVA irradiation alone. The frequency of these changes with increasing doses of PUVA and their reversibility are not well documented. Increased amounts of amorphous material about dermal blood vessels as well as occasional bizarre connective tissue cells have been noted (97). Histologic changes similar to those seen in chronically sun-damaged skin have been noted in some biopsies from PUVA-treated patients (48, 98). In the dermis, eosinophilic homogenization and a reduction in elastic fibers have been observed (99, 100). Dermal melanophages increase with increasing total exposure to PUVA (101). Freckles induced by PUVA that are histologically indistinguishable from freckles occurring in fair-skinned individuals after sun exposure have been noted (101). Nevus spilus-like hyperpigmentation has also been noted in patients receiving long-term PUVA (102). Increase in number of melanocytes has been noted (99). Since experimental evidence indicates that the frequency and severity of some dermal changes increase with increased number of PUVA treatments, we believe multiple phototoxic insults to skin from PUVA will add to the cumulative morphologic alterations induced by repeated sun exposures.

Carcinogenesis

The association between exposure to UV radiation and the risk of skin cancer has been demonstrated in humans (103). UV radiation is carcinogenic in animals. The carcinogenesis potential of middle-wave (280–320 nm) UV radiation has been most thoroughly documented. The carcinogenic potential of UVA alone has not been well quantified, but appears to be much less than that of shorter wavelengths. In animals, the simultaneous administration of psoralens and UVA is carcinogenic (104). The rate of development of skin tumors was higher in animals given methoxsalen intraperitoneally than when given orally (104–106).

Concern about PUVA's carcinogenic potential is based not only on experimental evidence in animals, but also on the mutagenic potential related to its known DNA photochemistry. The alterations in DNA, if not fully repaired, are likely to increase the risk of cutaneous cancer. In several systems, PUVA is mutagenic and promotes sister chromatid exchanges (107). While there is little doubt that PUVA damages DNA, there is substantial debate about the extent to which this damage is repaired in humans following exposure and the extent to which PUVA-induced alterations in a cell influence its ability to repair other types of damage. Excision repair, a mechanism for repairing UVB damage to DNA, appears to play some role in repairing PUVA-induced DNA damage, but other repair pathways may also be involved (108).

In patients who have received long-term PUVA, cells indistinguishable from those seen in chronically sun-damaged skin have been noted. The frequency of these findings varies substantially among series: one group reported that nearly half of the patients examined exhibited such change, while another group reported that only 3% of patients showed such change (99, 109). Clearly the selection of patients and criteria for grading may account for many of these differences, but irrespective of their frequency, observation of histologic changes similar to those associated with long-term sun exposure suggests that PUVA is adding to the burden of UV-induced cellular damage. It seems logical that the greater the cumulative damage to cells from all types of UV radiation, the greater the clinical actinic change and the higher the risk of nonmelanoma skin cancer.

In 1979, the 16-center cooperative study reported a significant increase in the risk of cutaneous carcinoma among patients treated with PUVA and previously exposed to other carcinogens (110). This increase was not noted in the first year following the initiation of PUVA therapy, but became evident in the second year and has remained elevated for an additional 2 years of observation since that report. Although better ascertainment of cases from careful follow-up was suggested as a reason for this increase in reported incidence compared to both number of tumors expected on the basis of population rates and this population's experience before exposure to PUVA, it is difficult to explain why no such apparent increase in ascertainment of tumors was noted in the first year of treatment, the period during which patients were under closest physician observation. In addition, this study noted that while the incidence of basal cell carcinoma was not substantially different than that experienced by this population pre-PUVA or expected in the general population, the incidence of squamous cell carcinoma was significantly increased. Further, these squamous cell carcinomas appeared in unusual areas, those not normally sun-exposed, and there was a strong association between increased numbers of PUVA treatments and the risk of these tumors. In this study, fair-skinned patients (Skin Types I and II) and patients with previous exposure to ionizing radiation were at highest risk for the development of these tumors. The nature of these risks appeared to be at least additive. The Austrian group reported an increased risk in cutaneous carcinoma among PUVA-treated patients who had previously received arsenic, but failed to detect any overall increase in other patients (111). PUVA's carcinogenic effect in the skin does not appear to be restricted to patients with psoriasis. Patients with mycosis fungoides treated with PUVA and other carcinogens, most notably electron beam and topical nitrogen mustard, have developed multiple squamous cell carcinomas (112). In a large group of East Indians receiving long-term psoralens and sunlight for the treatment of vitiligo, the development of actinic keratoses on vitiliginous areas has been noted (113).

Still, PUVA's role in the development of these cutaneous malignancies remains controversial. Both the European cooperative study (114) and a smaller American cooperative study (115) report a failure to observe any increase in skin cancer risk. These groups do not, however, report on their completeness of follow-up, interval from first dose to reexamination, the risk characteristics, or total doses of PUVA in their populations.

The apparent short latency between exposure and the development of tumors may be an argument against PUVA acting as a primary carcinogen. The rapid development of increased numbers of tumors following substantial PUVA exposure is, however, consistent with its acting as a pseudo-promoter of cutaneous carcinogenesis. PUVA's ability to act as a pseudo-promotor may in part result from its effect on the immune system. PUVA suppresses delayed-hypersensitivity reactions to injected antigens, diminishes allergic contact dermatitis in animals (116, 117), and retards skin graft rejection (118). In vitro and in vivo studies of human peripheral blood lymphocytes have shown dose-dependent decreases in function after PUVA (119–121) (see Chapter 10). The duration and clinical importance of these observed alterations in immune function are not well established, but decreased immunosurveillance either confined to the skin or as a result of changes in systemic immune function could account for the rapid increase in the risk of cutaneous carcinoma that has been observed. Markedly and rapidly increased rates of skin cancer have been noted in nonpsoriatic patients treated with immunosuppressive agents (122).

Alternatively, PUVA may be highly carcinogenic in patients with innate inability to effectively repair PUVA-induced DNA damage. PUVA's ability to rapidly induce skin tumors in patients with grossly defective DNA repair has been demonstrated in one uncontrolled observation (123). Many apparently normal individuals may have subtle decreased ability to repair UV-induced DNA damage, and this decreased ability may increase their risk of developing premalignant or malignant tumors from UV radiation (124). Such patients may also be unable to effectively repair PUVA-induced DNA damage and as a result be at high risk for skin tumors following PUVA.

While observations to date are consistent with PUVA as a pseudo-promotor cocarcinogen of squamous cell carcinoma in the skin of patients who have a genetic predisposition to their development or prior exposure to potent carcinogens, PUVA's potential as a primary carcinogen is not yet determined. It seems quite likely that repeated exposures to PUVA will add to the known carcinogenic risk of repeated exposures to UVB. The magnitude of this effect and its relationship to total dose or patient characteristics remain key questions to be answered in assessing this therapy's long-term risk. At the present time, the physician's and patient's decisions to embark upon PUVA treatment should carefully weigh the patient tumor risk as determined by skin type and previous exposure to carcinogens against the anticipated benefits of this therapy.

PUVA was first used to enhance pigmentation, both in the treatment of vitiligo and in patients desiring increased pigmentation. Clearly, PUVA treatment alters the melanocytes. Following such treatment, increases in the number of melanocytes, individual melanocyte enlargement, and melanocyte clustering, along with increased melanocyte function, have been noted (125, 126). Because of these histologic observations and the data that suggest a higher risk of melanoma associated with a greater exposure to UV radiation, there has been concern that PUVA may increase a patient's risk of melanoma. While malignant melanomas have been seen in PUVA-treated patients, there are no data to suggest that the frequency of such tumors is increased in these patients (127).

Ophthalmologic Risks

Prolonged exposure or high intensities of UVA alone can lead to cataracts. In rabbits and monkeys, permanent lenticular cataracts may be produced by single, high-irradiance or long-duration exposures to UVA. In albino mice, cataracts may be produced by multiple daily UVA exposures that are below the threshold dose of observable corneal damage (128). UV radiation may alter lens crystalline proteins from soluble, lower molecular-weight crystallines to insoluble, higher molecular-weight crystallines, which may alter light scattering within the lens. Tryptophan photochemistry appears to be involved in some forms of UV-induced cataracts (129, 130). Epidemiologic studies suggest that some forms of human cataracts may be related to sun exposure (131, 132).

Photosensitizing drugs may also affect the lens. This is a potentially serious event because the ocular lens is completely encapsulated and never sheds its cells throughout life. Labeling and autoradiographic studies (133–136), bioassays (137, 138), and spectroscopic studies (139, 140) give evidence of the presence of methoxsalen in the eye, specifically in the lens, after parental or oral administration in animals and humans. Free methoxsalen has been demonstrated in human lenses 12 hr after ingestion of a single therapeutic dose (141, 142). Methoxsalen diffuses out of rat and dogfish lenses within 24 hr if they are kept in the dark (140, 142, 143). Up to several hours after methoxsalen administration, photochemistry may take place if the lens is subsequently exposed to UVA (137–141). In the presence of ambient room light as well as UVA there is enhancement of lenticular fluorescence and phosphorescence (140–142). Photoaddition products can be generated with tryptophan as well as with lens proteins (in vitro) in the presence of 8-MOP and oxygen (141, 144). One such photoproduct has been demonstrated in vivo with lenses derived from rats given 8-MOP and exposed to UVA (143, 145). The photoreaction may involve DNA (136), tryptophan (142), or proteins (146).

Cataracts can be induced experimentally by PUVA (147–149) when doses causing striking cutaneous phototoxicity are used. Animal experiments with PUVA doses not adequate to cause cutaneous symptoms (149) or causing only mild chronic phototoxicity (150) did not result in cataracts. When the seeds of the *Ammi majus* were fed to ducklings exposed to the sun for 4–5 hr each day, conjunctivitis was observed within 2–3 days (151). Although no cataracts were observed within 1 month, birds developed mydriasis and severe pigmentary retinopathy (152). The lens of these animals transmits some UVA. if in child- or adulthood the lens of humans is surgically removed because of cataracts, the retina is then at risk for photochemical damage.

Based on all of this evidence, there is concern about the long-term effects of PUVA on the eye. The greatest concern has focused on the development of cataracts. The oral methoxsalen photochemotherapy follow-up study (153) has obtained multiple longitudinal examinations on 1235 patients who had an eye exam at least 1 year after initiating PUVA. There was no evidence to suggest accelerated deterioration in visual acuity for the population as a whole. There have been individual patients who have experienced deterioration of vision over the study period, but the rates and extent of this deterioration of vision or cataract development do not appear to be increased given the age composition of the study population. To date, there appears to be no relationship between PUVA treatment and the risk of developing adverse eye changes.

The absence of ophthalmologic complications of PUVA may be because (1) at the doses used for therapy no risk exists, (2) adequate eye protection has been used for most patients, or (3) it requires many years for long-term eye lesions to occur. Until more is known about this topic, we recommend that UVA-opaque eyewear be worn from the time that methoxsalen is ingested until the end of the treatment day. Transmission of UVA varies substantially among sunglasses. Therefore, sunglasses to be employed for protection should be tested to ensure they do not allow transmission of UVA (154).

Other Potential Long-Term Effects

Acute photosensitivity reactions, including photoallergy, acute onycholysis, and bullae, indistinguishable from those seen in phototoxic and photoallergic reactions to a variety of agents have been noted with PUVA therapy (155–156). Bullous pemphigoid has been seen in patients treated with PUVA. Other nonspecific stimuli, including UVB, have also been associated with the development of this disease (157–158).

Blood cell elements circulating in the dermis are exposed to PUVA. As discussed above, there are some findings that suggest that long-term PUVA may alter immune function. Long-term PUVA therapy leads to suppression of response of peripheral blood lymphocytes to mitogens (121). Effects of PUVA on the immune system are summarized in Chapter 10. If PUVA were to act as an immunosuppressive, the possibility exists that it may increase the risk of systemic as well as cutaneous malignancy. In immunosuppressed individuals, the incidences of lymphoma and leukemia are increased. One case of acute myeloid leukemia developing during PUVA therapy has been reported (159), but no increased incidence has occurred. The PUVA cooperative study has failed to note any increase in the risk of systemic malignancy.

Lupus erythematosus can be precipitated by exposure to UV radiation and a variety of drugs. While a small study indicated there was an increase in ANA titers in patients treated with PUVA, this finding has not been confirmed by subsequent studies (99, 160, 161). In addition, immunoglobulin deposits in the skin such as are seen with lupus erythematosus were not seen in 56 patients after PUVA treatment (99). While scattered reports of lupus occurring in PUVA-treated patients have appeared, there is no evidence to suggest an increased incidence (162, 163). However, PUVA may well be capable of exacerbating latent or asymptomatic lupus erythematosus as does UVB. Therefore, patients should be screened for clinical or laboratory evidence of this disease prior to initiating therapy.

Although hepatotoxic in very large doses in animals, there is no evidence that psoralens are hepatotoxic in doses used in clinical practices (164, 165). There is, however, a reported case of acute allergic hepatitis occurring in a PUVA-treated individual (166). Whether psoralens alone or combined with exposure to UVA are responsible for this acute allergic hepatitis has not been documented. Skin contact allergy to 8-MOP has also been documented (167).

SUMMARY

Psoralen photochemotherapy has been used for the treatment of vitiligo for many centuries. Reports of substantial adverse effects are lacking after long experience with treatment utilizing natural sunlight and psoralens. Introduction of dosimetric parameters and high-intensity artificial UVA sources in 1974 has led to substantial expansion of this therapy, its more frequent utilization for other diseases, especially for the treatment of psoriasis and mycosis fungoides, and has led also to prospective studies of toxicity.

After 5 years' experience, the principal side effect associated with oral methoxsalen photochemotherapy has been an increase in the risk of cutaneous carcinoma among patients with previous exposure to other carcinogens such as ionizing radiation. There is no evidence of accelerated cataract formation nor increased risk of melanoma, two potential toxicities of greater clinical importance. Only long-term scrutiny of the initial cohort of patients treated with PUVA therapy will permit thorough assessment of this therapy's long-term toxicity. For each patient, the potential risks and benefits of this therapy should be shared with the patient and carefully assessed before PUVA treatments are begun. Screening to exclude preexisting photosensitive diseases and exposures, such as ionizing radiation, which increase the risk of side effects should be performed. In addition, patients receiving PUVA therapy should be carefully monitored and attempts to minimize the total dose of therapy should be made.

Phototherapy and oral psoralen photochemotherapy rank with methotrexate as one of several moderately good but not excellent or ideal treatments of psoriasis. The short-term effects of all of these treatments are usually avoidable, controllable, or acceptable with careful dosimetry and attention to detail. The major concern is the long-term toxicity. For example, PUVA and UVB are known to cause actinic degeneration, premalignant mutations in epidermis, and skin cancers in certain susceptible individuals. Long-term use of methrotrexate may lead to liver damage. The character of the long-term hazard and molecular mechanisms involved are not the same for each therapeutic agent. The long-term risks are most likely related to cumulative dose and are probably at least partially reversible over time. Three approaches can therefore be used to attempt to diminish long-term risks:

1. The total amount of therapy can be minimized by raising criteria to enter patients into treatment programs, lowering expectations of patients and physician as far as total absence of any lesions, and undertaking a constant search for protocols which achieve best results at lowest total dose.

2. Two treatments can be combined so that therapeutic effect is achieved at lower cumulative dose of either treatment. Several combinations, such as methrotrexate–PUVA, retinoids–PUVA, retinoids–UVB, and UVB–PUVA, have been successful in this regard.

3. Treatments can be cycled. Patients may depend on one treatment for 1–3 years and then switched to a second treatment. After several treatments have been used, patients might be recycled through the treatments again. Physicians presently change treatments when patients begin to respond poorly or when long-term toxicity begins to be evident. It may be wise to institute premeditated, planned cycling of therapies from the beginning, altering the therapy before obvious difficulties arise.

ACKNOWLEDGMENTS. This work was supported by NIH Contract 1-AM-7-220.

REFERENCES

1. Fitzpatrick, T. B., and Pathak, M. A. (1959): Historical aspects of methoxsalen and furocoumarins. *J. Invest. Dermatol.* **32**:225–228.
2. Andersen, K. E., Menne, T., Gammeltof, T. M., et al. (1980): Pharmakinetic and clinical comparison of two 8-methoxypsoralen brands. *Arch. Dermatol. Res.* **268**:23–29.
3. Ljunggren, B., Bjellerup, M., and Carter, D. M. (1980): Dose-response relations in phototoxicity due to 8-methoxypsoralen and UV-A in man. *J. Invest. Dermatol.*, **76**:73–75.
4. Steiner, I., Prey, T., Gschnait, F., et al. (1978): Serum levels of 8-methoxypsoralen 2 hours after oral administration. *Acta Derm. Venereol.* (*Stockh.*) **58**:185–188.
5. Puglisi, C. V., deSilva, J. A., and Meyer, J. C. (1977): Determination of 8-methoxypsoralen, a photoactive compound, in blood by high pressure liquid chromatography. *Analytical Letters* **10**:39–50.

6. Ehrsson, H., Nilsson, S. O., and Ehrnebo, M. (1979): Effect of food on kinetics of 8-methoxypsoralen. *Clin. Pharmacol. Ther.* **25**:167–171.

7. Parrish, J. A. (1976): Methoxsalen–UV-A therapy of psoriasis. *J. Invest. Dermatol.* **67**:669–671.

8. Wolff, K., Gschnait, F., Hönigsmann, H., et al. (1977): Phototesting and dosimetry for photochemotherapy. *Br. J. Dermatol.* **96**:1–10.

9. Pathak, M. A., Fitzpatrick, T. B., and Parrish, J. A. (1977): Pharmacologic and molecular aspects of psoralen photochemotherapy. In: *Psoriasis, Proceedings of II International Symposium*, edited by E. M. Farber and A. J. Cox, pp. 262–271. Yorke Medical Books, New York.

10. Hönigsmann, H., Jaschke, E., Gschnait, F., et al. (1979): 5-Methoxypsoralen (Bergapten) in photochemotherapy of psoriasis. *Br. J. Dermatol.* **101**:369–376.

11. Dubertret, L., Auerbeck, D., Zajdela, F., et al. (1978): Photochemotherapy (PUVA) of psoriasis using 3-carbethoxypsoralen, a non-carcinogenic compound in mice. *Br. J. Dermatol.* **101**:379–389.

12. Bordin, F., Bacchichetti, F., Carlassare, F., et al. (1980): Methylangelicins as new agents for the photochemotherapy of psoriasis: II) Photobiological properties. Abstract presented at VIII International Congress of Photobiology, July 20–25, Strasbourg, France, Manuscript in press.

13. Cole, R. S. (1970): Light-induced cross-linking of DNA in the presence of furocoumarin (psoralen). Studies with phage lambda, *Escherichia coli*, and mouse leukemia cells. *Biochim. Biophys. Acta* **217**:30–39.

14. Cole, R. S. (1971): Psoralen monoadducts and interstrand cross-links in DNA. *Biochim. Biophys. Acta* **254**:30–39.

15. Dall'Acqua, F., Marciani, S., Ciavatta, L., et al. (1971): Formation of interstrand cross-linking in the photoreactions between furocoumarins and DNA. *Z. Naturforsch.* **265**:561–569.

16. Musajo, L., and Rodighiero, G. (1970): Studies on the photo-C4-cyclo-addition reactions between skin-photosensitizing furocoumarins and nucleic acids. *Photochem. Photobiol.* **11**:27–35.

17. Pathak, M. A., and Kramer, D. M. (1969): Photosensitization of skin *in vivo* by furocoumarins: (psoralens). *Biochim. Biophys. Acta* **195**:197–206.

18. Krauch, C. H., Kramer, D. M., and Wacker, A. (1967): Wirkungsmechanismus photocynamischer Furocoumarine. Photoreaktion von Psoralen (4-14C) mit DNS, RNS, Homopolynucloetiden und Nucleosiden. *Photochem. Photobiol.* **6**:341–354.

19. Musajo, L., Rodighiero, G., Breccia, A., et al. (1966): Skin photosensitizing furocoumarins: photochemical interaction between DNA and $-0^{14}CH_3$ bergapten (5-methoxypsoralen). *Photochem. Photobiol.* **5**:739–745.

20. Dall'Acqua, F., Marciani, S., and Rodighiero, G. (1970): Interstrand cross-linkages occurring in the photoreaction between psoralens and DNA. *FEBS Lett.* **9**:121–123.

21. Johnston, B. H., Johnson, M. A., Moore, C. B., et al. (1977): Psoralen–DNA photoreaction: controlled production of mono- and diadducts with nanosecond ultraviolet laser pulses. *Science* **197**:906–908.

22. Dall'Acqua, F., Marciani-Majno, S., Zambon, F., et al. (1979): Kinetic analysis of the photoreaction (365 nm) between psoralen and DNA. *Photochem. Photobiol.* **29**:489–495.

23. Cech, T. R., and Pardue, M. L. (1976): Electron microscopy of DNA crosslinked with trimethylpsoralen. Test of the secondary structure of eukaryotic inverted repeat sequences. *Proc. Natl. Acad. Sci. U.S.A.* **73**:2644–2648.

24. Wieshahn, G. P., Hyde, J. E., and Hearst, J. E. (1977): The photoaddition of trimethyl-psoralen to *Drosophilia melanogaster* nuclei: a probe for chromatin substructure. *Biochemistry* **16**:925–932.

25. Hallick, L. M., Yokota, H. A., Bartholomew, J. C., et al. (1978): Photochemical addition of

the cross-linking reagent 4,5′,8-trimethylpsoralen (trioxsalen) to intracellular and viral Simian virus 40 DNA–histone complexes. *J. Virol.* **27**:127–135.

26. Dall'Acqua, F., Marciani, S., Vedaldi, D., et al. (1972): Formation of interstrand cross-linkings on DNA of guinea pig skin after application of psoralen and irradiation at 265 nm. *FEBS Lett.* **27**:192–194.

27. Cech, T., Pathak, M. A., and Biswas, R. K. (1960): An electron microscopic study of the photochemical cross-linking of DNA in guinea pig epidermis by psoralen derivatives. *Biochim. Biophys. Acta* **562**:324–360.

28. Epstein, J. H., and Fukuyama, K. (1975) Effects of 8-methoxypsoralen (8-MOP) induced phototoxic effects on mammalian epidermal macromolecular synthesis *in vivo*. *Photochem. Photobiol.* **21**:325–330.

29. Parrish, J. A., Fitzpatrick, T. B., and Tanenbaum, L. (1974): Photochemotherapy of psoriasis with oral methoxsalen and longwave ultraviolet light. *N. Engl. J. Med.* **291**:1207–1211.

30. Gruenert, D. C., and Cleaver, J. E. (1980): Repair of psoralen plus near-UV damage in human cells. Abstract presented at VIII International Congress of Photobiology, July 20–25, Strasbourg, France. Manuscript in press.

31. Dall'Acqua, F., Vedaldi, D., Guiotto, A., et al. (1980): Methylangelicins as new agents for the photochemotherapy of psoriasis: I) Synthesis, dark and photochemical interaction with DNA. Abstract presented at VIII International Congress of Photobiology, July 20–25, Strasbourg, France. Manuscript in press.

32. Morison, W. L., Paul, B. S., and Parrish, J. A. (1977): The effect of indomethacin on long-wave ultraviolet-induced delayed erythema. *J. Invest. Dermatol.* **68**:130–133.

33. Rosario, R., Mark, G. J., Parrish, J. A., et al. (1979): Histological changes produced in skin by equally erythemogenic doses of UV-A, UV-B, UV-C and UV-A with psoralens. *Br. J. Dermatol.* **101**:299–308.

34. Pathak, M. A., Kramer, D. M., and Fitzpatrick, T. B. (1974): Photobiology and Photochemistry of furocoumarins (psoralens). In: *Sunlight and Man: Normal and Abnormal Photobiologic Reactions*, edited by M. A. Pathak, L. C. Harber, M. Seiji, et al. (T. B. Fitzpatrick, consulting editor), pp. 335–368. University of Tokyo Press, Tokyo.

35. Toda, K., Pathak, M. A., Parrish, J. A., et al. (1972): Alteration of racial differences in melanosome distribution in human epidermis after exposure to ultraviolet light. *Nature* [*New Biol.*] **236**:143–145.

36. Allyn, B. (1962): Studies on phototoxicity in man and laboratory animals. 21st Annual Meeting of the American Academy of Dermatology, Dec. 1–6, Chicago, Illinois.

37. Walter, J. F., and Voorhees, J. J. (1973): Psoriasis improved by psoralen plus black light. *Acta Derm. Venereol. (Stockh.)* **53**:469–472.

38. Weber, G. (1974): Combined 8-methoxypsoralen and black light therapy of psoriasis. Technique and results. *Br. J. Dermatol.* **90**:317–323.

39. Fischer, T., and Alsins, J. (1976): Treatment of psoriasis with trioxsalen baths and dysporsium lamps. *Acta Derm. Venereol. (Stockh.)* **56**:383–390.

40. Petrozzi, J. W., and Kligman, A. (1977): Topical psoralen photochemotherapy. In: *Psoriasis: Proceedings of the Second International Symposium*, edited by E. M. Farber and A. J. Cox, pp. 285–290. Yorke Medical Books, New York.

41. Willis, I., and Harris, D. R. (1973): Resistant psoriasis. *Arch. Dermatol.* **107**:358–362.

42. Parrish, J. A., Anderson, R. R., Ying, C. Y., et al. (1976): Cutaneous effects of pulsed nitrogen gas laser irradiation. *J. Invest. Dermatol.* **67**:603–608.

43. Levin, R. E., and Parrish, J. A. (1975): Phototherapy of vitiligo. *Lighting Design and Application.* **5**:35–43.

44. Wolff, K., Fitzpatrick, T. B., Parrish, J. A., et al. (1976): Photochemotherapy with orally administered methoxsalen. *Arch. Dermatol.* **112**:942–950.

45. Melski, J. W., Tanenbaum, L., Parrish, J. A., et al. (1977): Oral methoxsalen photochemotherapy for the treatment of psoriasis: A cooperative clinical trial. *J. Invest. Dermatol.* **68**:328–335.

46. Rogers, S., Marks, J., and Shuster, S. (1979): Comparison of photochemotherapy and dithranol in the treatment of chronic plaque psoriasis. *Lancet* **1**:455–458.

47. Swanbeck, G., Thyresson-Hök, M., Bredberg, A., et al. (1975): Treatment of psoriasis with oral psoralens and long-wave ultraviolet light. Therapeutic results and cytogenetic hazards. *Acta Derm. Venereol. (Stockh.)* **55**:367–376.

48. Hashimoto, K., Kohda, H., Kumakiri, M., et al. (1978): Psoralen-UVA treated psoriatic lesions: Ultrastructural changes. *Arch. Dermatol.* **114**:711–722.

49. Juhlin, L., and Shelley, W. B. (1978): Ultraviolet light inhibition of oriented fibrin formation in psoriasis. *Br. J. Dermatol.* **99**:353–356.

50. Braun-Falco, O., Hofmann, C., and Plewig, G. (1977): Feingene bliche Veranderungen unter Photochemotherapie der Psoriasis. *Arch. Dermatol. Res.* **257**:301–317.

51. Mizuno, N., Enami, H., and Esaki, K. (1979): Effect of 8-methoxypsoralen plus UVA on psoriasis leukotactic factor. *J. Invest. Dermatol.* **72**:64–66.

52. Haftek, M., Glinski, W., Jablonska, S., et al. (1979): T lymphocyte E rosette function during photochemotherapy (PUVA) of psoriasis. *J. Invest. Dermatol.* **72**:214–218.

53. Schmoll, M., Hensler, T., and Christophers, E. (1978): Evaluation of PUVA, topical corticosteroids, and the combination of both in the treatment of psoriasis. *Br. J. Dermatol.* **99**:693–702.

54. Gould, P. W., and Wilson, L. (1978): Psoriasis treated with clobetasol propionate and photochemotherapy. *Br. J. Dermatol.* **98**:133–136.

55. Morison, W. L., Parrish, J. A., and Fitzpatrick, T. B. (1978): Controlled study of PUVA and adjunctive topical therapy in the management of psoriasis. *Br. J. Dermatol.* **98**:125–132.

56. Hanke, C. W., Steck, W. D., and Roenigk, H. H. (1979): Combination therapy for psoriasis. Psoralen plus longwave ultraviolet radiation with betamethasone valerate. *Arch. Dermatol.* **115**:1074–1077.

57. Fritsch, P. O., Honigsmann, H., Jaschke, E., et al. (1978): Augmentation of oral methoxsalen-photochemotherapy with an oral retinoic acid derivative. *J. Invest. Dermatol.* **70**:178–182.

58. Honigsmann, H., Gschnait, F., Konrad, K., et al. (1977): Photochemotherapy for pustular psoriasis (von Zumbusch). *Br. J. Dermatol.* **97**:119–126.

59. Parrish, J. A., LeVine, M. J., and Fitzpatrick, T. B. (1980): Oral methoxsalen photochemotherapy of psoriasis and mycosis fungoides. *Int. J. Dermatol.* **19**:379–386.

60. Vukas, V. (1977): Photochemotherapy in the treatment of psoriatic variants. *Dermatologica* **155**:355–371.

61. Morison, W. L., Parrish, J. A., and Fitzpatrick, T. B. (1978): Oral methoxsalen photochemotherapy of recalcitrant dermatoses of palms and soles. *Br. J. Dermatol.* **99**:297–302.

62. Murray, D., and Warin, A. P. (1979): Phototherapy for persistent palmoplantar pustulosis. *Br. J. Dermatol.* **101**:13–14.

63. Murray, D., Corbett, M. F., and Warin, A. P. (1980): A controlled trial of photochemotherapy for persistent palmoplantar pustulosis. *Br. J. Dermatol.* **102**:659–663.

64. Parrish, J. A., White, H. A. D., Kingsbury, T., et al. (1977): Photochemotherapy of psoriasis using methoxsalen and sunlight. A controlled study. *Arch. Dermatol.* **113**:1529–1532.

65. Lerner, A. B., Denton, C. R., and Fitzpatrick, T. B. (1953): Clinical and experimental studies with 8-methoxypsoralen in vitiligo. *J. Invest. Dermatol.* **20**:299–314.

66. Kanof, N. B. (1955): Melanin formation in vitiliginous skin under the influence of external applications of 8-methoxypsoralen. *J. Invest. Dermatol.* **24**:5–10.

67. Kelly, E. W., and Pinkus, H. (1955): Local application of 8-methoxypsoralen in vitiligo. *J. Invest. Dermatol.* **25**:453–456.

68. Elliot, J. A., Jr. (1959): Methoxsalen in the treatment of vitiligo: an appraisal of the permanency of the repigmentation. *Arch. Dermatol.* **79**:237–243.
69. Fitzpatrick, T. B., Arndt, K. A., and El Mofty, A. M. (1966): Hydroquinone and psoralens in the therapy of hypermelanosis and vitiligo. *Arch. Dermatol.* **93**:589–600.
70. Fulton, J. E., Jr., Leyden, J., and Papa, G. (1969): Treatment of vitiligo with topical methoxsalen and blacklite. *Arch. Dermatol.* **100**:224–229.
71. Farah, F. S., Kurban, A. K., and Chaglassian, H. T. (1967): The treatment of vitiligo with psoralens and triamcinolone by mouth. *Br. J. Dermatol.* **79**:89–91.
72. Fitzpatrick, T. B., Parrish, J. A., and Pathak, M. A. (1974): Phototherapy of vitiligo (idiopathic leukoderma). In: *Sunlight and Man: Normal and Abnormal Photobiologic Responses*, edited by M. A. Pathak, L. C. Harber, M. Seiji, et al. (T. B. Fitzpatrick, consulting editor), pp. 131–141. University of Tokyo Press, Tokyo.
73. Pathak, M. A., Mosher, D. B., Fitzpatrick, T. B., et al. (1980): Relative effectiveness of three psoralens and sunlight in repigmentation of 365 vitiligo patients (Abstract). *J. Invest. Dermatol.* **74**:252.
74. Theodoridis, A., Tsambaos, D., Sivenas, C., et al. (1976): Oral trimethylpsoralen in the treatment of vitiligo. *Acta Derm. Venereol. (Stockh.)* **56**:253–256.
75. Bleehen, S. S. (1972): Treatment of vitiligo with oral, 4,5′,8-trimethylpsoralen (Trisoralen). *Br. J. Dermatol.* **86**:54–60.
76. Kobori, T., and Toda, K. (1973): Treatment of vitiligo with trimethyl-psoralen. *Jpn. J. Clin. Dermatol.* **27**:983.
77. Parrish, J. A., Fitzpatrick, T. B., Shea, C., et al. (1976): Photochemotherapy of vitiligo using orally administered psoralens and high-intensity long-wave ultraviolet light system. *Arch. Dermatol.* **112**:1531–1534.
78. Edelson, R. L. (1975): Cutaneous T-cell lymphomas; perspective. *Ann. Intern. Med.* **83**:548–552.
79. Edelson, R. L. (1979): Cutaneous T-cell lymphoma. In: *Dermatology Update. Reviews for Physicians, 1979 Edition*, edited by S. L. Moschella, T. B. Fitzpatrick, J. J. Herndon, Jr., et al., pp. 195–207, Elsevier, New York.
80. Van Scott, E. J., and Haynes, H. A. (1971): Cutaneous lymphomas. In: *Dermatology in General Medicine*, edited by T. B. Fitzpatrick, K. A. Arndt, W. H. Clark, Jr., et al., pp. 556–573. McGraw-Hill, New York.
81. Gilchrest, B. A., Parrish, J. A., Tanenbaum, L., et al. (1976): Oral methoxsalen photochemotherapy of mycosis fungoides. *Cancer* **38**:683–689.
82. Roenigk, H. H., Jr. (1977): Photochemotherapy for mycosis fungoides. *Arch. Dermatol.* **113**:1047–1051.
83. Bleehen, S. S., Vella, B. D., and Warin, A. P. (1978): Photochemotherapy in mycosis fungoides. *Clin. Exp. Dermatol.* **3**:377–387.
84. Ortonne, J. P., Schmitt, D., Alario, A., et al. (1979): Oral photochemotherapy in lichen planus (LP) and mycosis fungoides (MF): Ultrastructural modifications of the infiltrating cells, *Acta Derm. Venereol. (Stockh.)* **59**:211–218.
85. Lowe, N. J., Cripps, D. J., Dufton, P. A., et al. (1979): Photochemotherapy for mycosis fungoides: A clinical and histological study. *Arch. Dermatol.* **115**:50–53.
86. Fisher T., Van Vloten, W. A., and Volden, G. (1978): Internal dissemination of mycosis fungoides despite successful local therapy. *Acta Derm. Venereol. (Stockh.)* **58**:88–89.
87. Molin, L., Skogh, M., and Volden, G. (1978): Successful PUVA treatment in the tumor stage of mycosis fungoides associated with the appearance of lesions in organs other than the skin. *Acta Derm. Venereol. (Stockh.)* **58**:189–190.
88. Kubba, R., Bailin, P. L., and Roenigk, H. H. (1980): Immunologic evaluation in mycosis fungoides. *Arch. Dermatol.* **116**:178–181.
89. Morison, W. L., Parrish, J. A., and Fitzpatrick, T. B. (1978): Oral psoralen photochemotherapy of atopic eczema. *Br. J. Dermatol.* **98**:25–30.

90. Ortonne, J. P., Thivolet, J., and Sannwald, C. (1978): Oral photochemotherapy in the treatment of lichen planus (LP). *Br. J. Dermatol.* **99**:77–88.

91. Christophers, E., Wolff, K., and Langner, A. (1978): PUVA-treatment of urticaria pigmentosa. *Br. J. Dermatol.* **98**:701–702.

92. Gschnait, F., Hönigsmann, H., Brenner, W., et al. (1978): Induction of UV light tolerance by PUVA in patients with polymorphous light eruption. *Br. J. Dermatol.* **99**:293–295.

93. Parrish, J. A., LeVine, M. J., Morison, W. L., et al. (1979): Comparison of PUVA and beta-carotene in the treatment of polymorphous light eruption. *Br. J. Dermatol.* **100**: 187–191.

94. Claudy, A. L., and Gagnaire, D. (1980): Photochemotherapy for alopecia areata. *Acta Derm. Venereol. (Stockh.)* **60**:171–172.

95. Kligman, A. M. (1974): Solar elastosis in relation to pigmentation. In: *Sunlight and Man: Normal and Abnormal Photobiologic Responses*, edited by M. A. Pathak, L. C. Harber, M. Seiji, et al. (T. B. Fitzpatrick, consulting editor), pp. 157–163. University of Tokyo Press, Tokyo.

96. Anderson, R. R., and Parrish, J. A. (1981): The optics of human skin. *J. Invest. Dermatol.*, **76**:13–19.

97. Kumakiri, M., Hashimoto, K., and Willis, I. (1977): Biologic changes due to long-wave ultraviolet irradiation on human skin. Ultrastructural study. *J. Invest. Dermatol.* **69**: 392–400.

98. Cox, A. J., and Abel, E. A. (1979): Epidermal dystrophy. *Arch. Dermatol.* **115**:567–570.

99. Gschnait, F., Wolff, K., Hönigsmann, H., et al. (1980): Long-term photochemotherapy: histopathologic and immunofluorescent observations in 243 patients. *Br. J. Dermatol.* **103**:11–12.

100. Zelickson, A. S., Mottaz, J. H., Zelickson, B. D., et al. (1980): Elastic tissue changes in skin following PUVA therapy. *J. Am. Acad. Dermatol.* **2**:186–192.

101. Bleehen, S. S. (1978): Freckles induced by PUVA treatment. *Br. J. Dermatol.* **99**:20.

102. Helland, S., and Bang, G. (1980): Nevus spillus-like hyperpigmentation during PUVA therapy. *Acta Derm. Venereol. (Stockh.)* **60**:81–83.

103. Urbach, F. (1969): Geographic pathology of skin cancer. In: *The Biologic Effects of Ultraviolet Radiation (with Special Emphasis on Skin)*, edited by F. Urbach, pp. 635–650. Pergamon Press, New York.

104. Griffin, A. C. (1959): Methoxsalen in ultraviolet carcinogenesis in the mouse. *J. Invest. Dermatol.* **32**:367–372.

105. Langner, A., Wolska, H., Marzulli, F. N., et al. (1977): Dermal toxicity of 8-methoxy-psoralen administered (by gavage) to hairless mice irradiated with longwave ultraviolet light. *J. Invest. Dermatol.* **69**:451–457.

106. Pathak, M. A., Daniels, F., Jr., Hopkins, C. E., et al. (1959): Ultraviolet carcinogenesis in albino and pigmented mice receiving furocoumarins: psoralen and 8-methoxypsoralen. *Nature* **183**:728–730.

107. Wolff-Schreiner, E. C., Carter, D. M., Schwarzacher, H. G., et al. (1977): Sister chromatid exchanges in photochemotherapy. *J. Invest. Dermatol.* **69**:387–391.

108. Hanawalt, P.: Cellular responses to psoralen damage in DNA. In: *Proceedings of the Symposium "Psoralens in Cosmetics and Dermatology," April 13–14, 1981, Paris.* Pergamon Press, Oxford, in press.

109. Cox, A. J., and Abel, E. A. (1979): Epidermal dystrophy. Occurrence after psoriasis therapy with psoralen and long-wave ultraviolet light. *Arch. Dermatol.* **115**:567–570.

110. Stern, R. S., Thibodeau, L. A., Kleinerman, R. A., et al. (1979): Risk of cutaneous carcinoma in patients treated with oral methoxsalen photochemotherapy for psoriasis. *N. Engl. J. Med.* **300**:809–813.

111. Hönigsmann, H., Wolff, K., Gschnait, F., et al. (1980): Keratoses and nonmelanoma skin tumors in long-term photochemotherapy (PUVA). *J. Am. Acad. Dermatol.* **3**:406–414.

112. Verdich, J. (1979): Squamous cell carcinoma: occurrence in mycosis fungoides treated with psoralens plus long-wave ultraviolet radiation. *Arch. Dermatol.* **115**:1338–1339.

113. Mosher, D. B., Pathak, M. A., Harrist, T. J., et al. (1980): Development of cutaneous lesions in vitiligo during long-term PUVA therapy (Abstract). *J. Invest. Dermatol.* **74**:259.

114. Grupper, C., and Berretti, B. (1980): Tar, UV light, PUVA and cancer. *J. Am. Acad. Dermatol.* **3**:643–646.

115. Roenigk, H. H., Jr., and Caro, W. A. (1981): Skin cancer in the PUVA-48 cooperative study. *J. Am. Acad. Dermatol.* **4**:319–324.

116. Morison, W. L., Parrish, J. A., Woehler, M. E., et al. (1981): The influence of ultraviolet radiation on allergic contact dermatitis in the guinea pig. II. Psoralen/UVA radiation. *Br. J. Dermatol.* **104**:165–168.

117. Morison, W. L., Parrish, J. A., Woehler, M. E. et al. (1981): The influence of PUVA and UVB radiation on delayed hypersensitivity in the guinea pig. *J. Invest. Dermatol.*, **76**:484–488.

118. Morison, W. L., Parrish, J. A., Woehler, M. E., et al. (1980): The influence of PUVA and UVB radiation on skin-graft survival in rabbits. *J. Invest. Dermatol.* **75**:331–333.

119. Parrish, J. A. (1981): Photoimmunologic, carcinogenic and ocular effects of *in vivo* psoralen photochemistry in humans. In: *Proceedings of the NATO Advanced Study Institute Program on Molecular Basis of Dermatologic Diseases*, edited by M. A. Pathak. Plenum Press, New York, in press.

120. Morison, W. L. (1981): Photoimmunology. *J. Invest. Dermatol.*, **77**:71–76.

121. Morison, W. L., Parrish, J. A., Moscicki, R., et al. (1981): Abnormal lymphocyte function following long-term PUVA therapy for psoriasis (Abstract). *J. Invest. Dermatol.* **76**:303.

122. Maize, J. C. (1977): Skin cancer in immunosuppressed patients. *J. AMA* **237**:1857–1858.

123. Reed, W. B., Sugarman, G. I., and Mathis, R. A. (1977): DeSanctis-Cacchione syndrome. A case report with autopsy findings. *Arch. Dermatol.* **113**:1561–1563.

124. Lambert, B. O., Ringborg, U., and Swanbeck, G. (1976): Ultraviolet-induced DNA repair synthesis in lymphocytes from patients with actinic keratoses. *J. Invest. Dermatol.* **67**:594–598.

125. Hashimoto, K., Kohda, H., Kumakiri, M., et al. (1978): Psoralen-UVA treated psoriatic lesions: Ultrastructural changes. *Arch. Dermatol.* **114**:711–722.

126. Zaynoun, S., Konrad, K., Gschnait, F., et al. (1977): The pigmentary response to photochemotherapy. *Acta Derm. Venereol. (Stockh.)* **57**:431–440.

127. Durkin, W., Sun, N., Link, J., et al. (1978): Melanoma in a patient treated for psoriasis. *South. Med. J.* **71**:732–733.

128. Zigman, S., and Vaughan, T. (1974): Near-ultraviolet light effects on the lenses and retinas of mice. *Invest. Ophthalmol.* **13**:462–465.

129. Borkman, R. F., Dalrymple, A., and Lerman, S. (1977): Ultraviolet action spectrum for fluorogen production in the ocular lens. *Photochem. Photobiol.* **26**:129–132.

130. Borkman, R. F. (1977): Ultraviolet action spectrum for tryptophan destruction in aqueous solution. *Photochem. Photobiol.* **26**:163–166.

131. Hiller, R., Giacometti, L., and Yuen, K. (1977): Sunlight and cataract: An epidemiological investigation. *Am. J. Epidemiol.* **105**:450–459.

132. Zigman, S., Yulo, T., Paxhia, T., et al. (1977): Comparative studies of human cataracts. Abstracts of the Association for Research in Vision and Ophthalmology, Sarasota, Florida.

133. Goldberg, L. H., Schaefer, H., and Farber, E. M. (1979): PUVA and the eye (Abstract). *J. Invest. Dermatol.* **72**:278.

134. Wulf, H. C., and Hart, J. (1978): Accumulation of 8-methoxypsoralen in the rat retina. *Acta Ophthalmol.* **56**:284–290.

135. Thune, P. (1978): Plasma levels of 8-methoxypsoralen and phototoxicity studies during PUVA treatment of psoriasis with Meladinine tablets. *Acta Derm. Venereol. (Stockh.)* **58**:149–151.

136. Jose, J. G., and Yielding, K. L. (1978): Photosensitive cataractogens, chlorpromazine and methoxypsoralen, cause DNA repair synthesis in lens epithelial cells. *Invest. Ophthalmol. Visual Sci.* **17**:687–691.

137. Glew, W. B. (1979): Determination of 8-methoxypsoralen in serum, aqueous, and lens: relation to long-wave ultraviolet phototoxicity in experimental and clinical photochemotherapy. *Trans. Am. Ophthalmol. Soc.* **77**:464–514.

138. Glew, W. B., Roberts, W. P., Malinin, G. I., et al. (1980): Quantitative determination by bioassay of photoactive 8-methoxypsoralen in serum. *J. Invest. Dermatol.* **75**:230–234.

139. Lerman, S. (1977): A method for detecting 8-methoxypsoralen in the ocular lens. *Science* **197**:1287–1288.

140. Lerman, S., Jocoy, M., and Borkman, R. F. (1977): Photosensitization of the lens by 8-methoxypsoralen. *Invest. Ophthalmol. Visual Sci.* **16**:1065–1068.

141. Lerman, S., Megaw, J., and Willis. I. (1980): The photoreactions of 8-methoxypsoralen with tryptophan and lens proteins. *Photochem. Photobiol.* **31**:235–242.

142. Lerman, S., Megaw, J., and Willis, I. (1980): Potential ocular complications from PUVA therapy and their prevention. *J. Invest. Dermatol.* **74**:197–199.

143. Gardner, K., Lerman, S., Megaw, J., et al. (1980): The prevention of direct and photosensitized UV radiation damage to the ocular lens (Abstract). *Invest. Ophthal. Visual Sci.* **19** (ARVO Suppl.):88.

144. Megaw, J., Lee, J., and Lerman, S. (1980): NMR analyses of tryptophan-8-methoxypsoralen photoreaction products. *Photochem. Photobiol.*, in press.

145. Koch, H. R., Beitzen, R., Dremer, F., et al. (1979): Effect of 8-methoxypsoralen and long UV on the rat lens (Abstract). *Invest. Ophthal. Visual Sci.* **18** (Suppl.):218.

146. Lerman, S. (1979): Photoreaction of 8-methoxypsoralen with tryptophan and lens proteins. Abstract presented at the 7th Annual Meeting of the American Society for Photobiology, June 25–28, 1979, Pacific Grove, California. Book of Abstracts, pp. 92.

147. Griffin, A. C. (1959): Methoxsalen in ultraviolet carcinogenesis in the mouse. *J. Invest. Dermatol.* **32**:367–372.

148. Cloud, T. M., Hakim, R., and Griffin, A. C. (1961): Photosensitization of the eye with methoxsalen. II. Chronic effects. *Arch. Ophthalmol.* **66**:689–694.

149. Freeman, R. G., and Troll, D. (1969): Photosensitization of the eye by 8-methoxypsoralen. *J. Invest. Dermatol.* **53**:449–453.

150. Parrish, J. A., Chylack, L. T., Jr., Woehler, M. E., et al. (1979): Dermatological and ocular examinations in rabbits chronically photosensitized with methoxsalen. *J. Invest. Dermatol.* **73**:250–255.

151. Egyed, M. N., Singer, L., Eilat, A., et al. (1975): Eye lesions in ducklings fed *Ammi majus* seeds. *Zentralbl. Veterinaermed.* [*A*] **22**:764–768.

152. Barishak, Y. R., Beemer, A. M., Egyed, M. N., et al. (1976): Histology of the retina and choroid in ducklings photosensitized by feeding *Ammi majus* seeds. *Ophthalmic. Res.* **8**:169–178.

153. Melski, J., Tanenbaum, L., Parrish, J. A., et al. (1977): Oral methoxsalen photochemotherapy for the treatment of psoriasis: A cooperative clinical trial. *J. Invest. Dermatol.* **68**:328–335.

154. Diffey, B. L., and Miller, J. A. (1980): A comment on routine testing of sunglasses. *Br. J. Dermatol.* **102**:665–668.

155. Plewig, G., Hofmann, C., and Braun-Falco, O. (1978): Photoallergic dermatitis from 8-methoxypsoralen. *Arch. Dermatol. Res.* **261**:201–211.

156. Zala, L., Omar, A., and Krebs, A. (1977): Photo-onycholysis induced by 8-methoxypsoralen. *Dermatologica* **154**:203–215.

157. Robinson, J. K., Baughman, R. D., and Provost, T. T. (1978): Bullous pemphigoid induced by PUVA therapy. *Br. J. Dermatol.* **99**:709–713.

158. Ahmed, A. R., and Winkler, N. W. (1977): Psoriasis and bullous pemphogoid. *Arch. Dermatol.* **113**:845.

159. Hansen, N. E. (1979): Development of acute myeloid leukemia in a patient with psoriasis treated with oral 8-methoxypsoralen and longwave ultraviolet light. *Scand. J. Haematol.* **22**:57–60.

160. Bjellerup, M. (1979): Antinuclear antibodies during PUVA therapy. *Acta Derm. Venereol.* (*Stockh.*) **59**:73–74.

161. Stern, R. S., Morison, W. L., Thibodeau, L. A., et al. (1979): Antinuclear antibodies and oral methoxsalen photochemotherapy (PUVA) for psoriasis. *Arch. Dermatol.* **115**: 1320–1324.

162. Eyanson, S., Greist, M. C., Brandt, K. D., et al. (1979): Systemic lupus erythematosus: Association with psoralen-ultraviolet-A treatment of psoriasis. *Arch. Dermatol.* **115**:54–56.

163. Domke, H. F., Ludwiggen, E., and Thormann, J. (1979): Discoid lupus erythematosus possibly due to photochemotherapy. *Arch. Dermatol.* **115**:642.

164. Hakim, R. E., Freeman, R. G., Griffin, A. C., et al. (1961): Experimental toxicological studies on 8-methoxypsoralen in animals exposed to the long ultraviolet. *J. Pharmacol. Exp. Ther.* **131**:394–399.

165. Melski, J. W., Tanenbaum, L., and Parrish, J. A. (1977): Oral methoxsalen photochemotherapy for the treatment of psoriasis: A cooperative clinical trial. *J. Invest. Dermatol.* **68**:328–335.

166. Bjellerup, M., Bruze, M., Hansson, A., et al. (1979): Liver injury following administration of 8-methoxypsoralen during PUVA therapy. *Acta Derm. Venereol.* (*Stockh.*) **59**:371–372.

167. Weissman, I., Wagner, G., and Plewig, G. (1980): Contact allergy to 8-methoxypsoralen. *Br. J. Dermatol.* **102**:113–115.

23

Photoradiation Therapy of Human Tumors

T. J. Dougherty, D. G. Boyle, and K. R. Weishaupt

Apparently the earliest attempt to use light-activated materials to treat human cancer was in 1903, when Jesionek and Tappenier used topical eosin, activated by white light, on skin tumors (1). Although not well documented, some positive results were indicated. However, no subsequent clinical work, by these workers or others, was reported until the mid-1970s, when Kelly and Snell (2) and Dougherty et al. (3–5) both used a hematoporphyrin derivative— a preparation first introduced by Lipson et al. (6)—as sensitizing dye. Current interest in the use of in vivo light-activated dyes to treat malignant tumors began in the early 1970s in several laboratories. Diamond et al. reported that hematoporphyrin (not the hematoporphyrin derivative of Lipson), administered parenterally and activated in vivo with white light, caused destruction of glioma tumors transplanted subcutaneously in rats (7). About the same time, Dougherty reported that fluorescein (given intraperitoneally) could be activated in vivo by 488-nm light to reduce the growth rate of a mammary tumor transplanted into mice (8). Neither group reported complete tumor control, however, until 1975, when Dougherty showed that hematoporphyrin derivative, given parenterally, could be activated by light in the red region of the spectrum (to increase light penetration into tissue) to cause complete eradication of spontaneous or transplanted mammary tumors in mice and rats (9). Tomson et al. demonstrated that acridine orange fed to mice accumulated in transplanted tumors and caused their destruction following local exposure to blue-green light from an argon laser (10).

T. J. Dougherty, D. G. Boyle, and K. R. Weishaupt • Division of Radiation Biology, Roswell Park Memorial Institute, Buffalo, New York 14263.

The terms photoradiation therapy, photodynamic therapy, and photo-chemotherapy have all been used to describe such processes and have essentially the same meaning, i.e., therapy requiring the use of a photo-sensitizer, applied topically or systemically, which elicits its therapeutic effect only when activated by photons in the visible range of the spectrum (approximately 400–700 nm). Phototherapy is a broader term describing various therapeutic effects of light alone, although even in these cases an endogenous photosensitizer may be acted upon, e.g., treatment of hyper-bilirubinemia (see Chapter 16). We prefer the term photoradiation therapy (although somewhat redundant) to describe the treatment of human tumors by visible light of specific wavelengths following administration of photo-sensitizers showing selectivity for malignant tissue. The term photochemo-therapy, while denoting much the same meaning, puts too much emphasis on chemotherapy, while in fact, the photosensitizers themselves have no therapeutic effect without activation of light. Photodynamic therapy, on the other hand, presumes certain aspects of the mechanism of action, i.e., involvement of oxygen. While this may be likely in many cases, it cannot be taken for granted.

The emphasis on hematoporphyrin derivative (Hpd) as the photoac-tivating dye of choice in photoradiation of tumors is based on two important properties of this material. The first is its ability, as judged by fluorescence, to accumulate and/or be retained to a higher degree in malignant tumors than in surrounding normal tissue or benign tumors. Recent work by Gomer and Dougherty (11), utilizing ^{14}C-Hpd or ^{3}H-Hpd, indicated about twice the concentration of dye in transplanted mouse tumors (7–8 $\mu g/g$ of tissue) compared to skin and 10–15 times compared to muscle 24–48 hr following intraperitoneal injection of 10 mg/kg. Liver, kidney, and spleen, however, accumulated higher concentrations (10–30 $\mu g/g$) than did the tumors. These same workers showed that half-life for clearance of Hpd from serum was 3 hr in mice, 6 hr in rabbits, 10 hr in monkeys, and 24–30 hr in humans with doses of 2.5–10 mg/kg body weight, parenterally administered. The largest single clinical study relating to tumor localization by fluorescence, reported by Gregorie et al. in 1968 (12) with 226 patients, indicated an overall 76% correlation of Hpd fluorescence with positive biopsy for malignancy. Lesions of the skin, cervix, oropharynx, esophagus, lung, larnyx, penis, vulva, urethra, and lymph nodes and adenocarcinomas of the breast, anus, rectum, stomach, and pancreas were included. Lipson et al. have utilized this method for detection of tumors of the esophagus or tracheobronchial tree, as well as the cervix (13). The diagnostic aspects of Hpd fluorescence for early detection of tumors and currently being pursued by Profio and Doiron (14, 15) and Sanderson and co-workers (16).

A second essential property of Hpd, making it useful as a therapeutic tool, is its ability, when properly photoactivated, to cause destruction of cells and tissue in which it resides. While mechanisms of action in vivo are not well understood, evidence exists that in vitro, Hpd and many other photosensitizers require oxygen to be present during the photoactivation in order for an effect to be observed.

In principle, the excited photosensitizer can interact directly with substrate, which subsequently reacts with oxygen to lead to an oxidized form of the substrate, or the photosensitizer can undergo an energy transfer process with oxygen to form singlet oxygen, which subsequently oxidizes the substrate. These processes do not consume the sensitizers. Some sensitizers, on the other hand, may be consumed and may not require oxygen, e.g., the furocoumarins (17). The former two oxygen-requiring processes are termed photodynamic. However, even with furocoumarins, recent evidence indicates that oxygen, in its singlet state, may be involved (18).

There are two pieces of evidence pointing toward singlet oxygen as the most likely cytotoxic agent in porphyrin-sensitized photodynamic processes. Weishaupt and Dougherty (19) showed that a singlet oxygen trapping agent 1,3-diphenylisobenzofuran, when incorporated into cells also containing Hpd, protected the cells from the normally lethal effect of red light. Also, no effect of light in the absence of oxygen was observed. It should be noted, however, that this furan may also trap various free radicals. Also, in 1979, Moan and co-workers (20) demonstrated that D_2O enhanced the photodestruction of cells containing hematoporphyrin (not the derivative). Enhancement of effects in D_2O compared to H_2O is considered to be consistent with singlet oxygen as an intermediate. Thus, the following process is consistent with current evidence

$$S + h_\nu \longrightarrow S^* \text{ (singlet)}$$
$$S^* \text{ (singlet)} \longrightarrow S^* \text{ (triplet)}$$
$$S^* \text{ (triplet)} + O_2 \longrightarrow S + {}^1O_2^* \text{ (singlet)}$$
$${}^1O_2^* + X \longrightarrow X \text{ (oxidized)}$$

where X is a critical cellular constituent. The identity of X in Hpd-photosensitized cellular destruction is not known, although various membrane effects have been noted. For example, Dougherty, Gomer, and Bellnier (unpublished results) demonstrated a 10-fold higher leakage of ^{51}Cr from cells exposed to Hpd plus light than observed in the same cells exposed to sufficient x-irradiation in the absence of Hpd to yield the same survival level. Further, cross-linking of membrane proteins has been observed in cells exposed to mesoporphyrin and light (K. Kohn and D. Kessel, unpublished results). However, single-strand breaks in DNA of cells exposed to Hpd and light have also been observed (C. J. Gomer, unpublished results). Thus, there may be many targets for photosensitized porphyrins in cells and destruction may be a result of attack on several substrates.

An important observation reported by Kelly et al. in 1975 indicated the potentially high therapeutic ratio which might be obtained using Hpd in the treatment of human cancer (21). These workers implanted human bladder carcinoma as well as normal bladder tissue into immunosuppressed mice. Both tissues were then treated by visible light following intravenous injection of Hpd. They found that only the malignant tissue was destroyed. Thus, it appeared possible that tumors might be treated quite specifically utilizing the combination of Hpd and visible light.

Since it was recognized that tissue penetration of visible light required for Hpd activation would likely be the major limitation of this technique, Dougherty et al. investigated the ability of light in the red region of the spectrum to penetrate through large mammary tumors freshly excised from rats (4). The techniques utilized two fiber optics inserted into the tumor, one acting as a detector with the distal end attached to a photometer and the other as a light source with the distal end aligned with a HeNe laser (632.8 nm). The distance between the optics in the tissue was varied and radiation falloff determined (Fig. 23-1).

This method for measuring light transmission does not detect total available radiation, however, since it does not take into account the radiation that is backscattered, which, in tissue, is of significant magnitude. Therefore, a

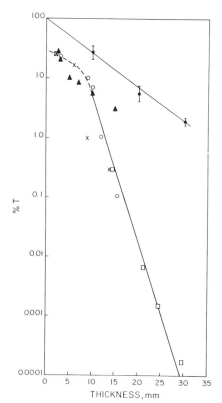

Fig. 23-1. Relative light flux (632.8 nm) at various distances in excised tumor tissue (rhabdomyosarcoma grown in WAG/Rij rats). ○, ×, □, ▲, separate experiments with fiber optics embedded into the tumor; ●, actinometric results with 600–700-nm light. Bars equal standard error.

chemical actinometer was devised for detecting total light flux at various distances from the light source. A light-sensitive mixture (Hpd + 1,3-diphenylisobenzofuran in ethanol) was enclosed in glass capillary tubes placed at various distances from the light source (in this case a xenon-arc lamp emitting 600–700 nm) and periodically analyzed for determination of total received radiation. These data indicated an exponential falloff only $1/10$ to $1/20$ that of the previous method (Fig. 23-1).

In 1976, Kelly and Snell (2) reported a case of necrosis of a portion of a bladder carcinoma treated with white light 24 hr following an intravenous injection of 2 mg/kg Hpd. There have been no further reports on this method by this group.

Since 1976, our group at Roswell Park Memorial Institute has been involved in developing photoradiation therapy as a useful clinical technique for treating various malignant tumors. To date, most patients treated by Hpd plus light have been in terminal stages of their disease. Consequently, only short-term tumor responses are available. In most cases, no other type of therapy was available to these patients or they had failed or recurred on conventional therapies. In some cases, only portions of tumors were treated prior to surgery in order to assess results histologically. Most patients had known or suspected distant metastasis in addition to the cutaneous or subcutaneous disease treated by photoradiation. The initial group of patients was selected with the primary objective of determining whether any type of tumor response could be obtained in a variety of tumor types and to assess toxicity of the treatment.

Drug preparation (Hpd) was essentially as first described by Lipson et al. with modification as previously described (4, 5). Proper drug preparation is essential for obtaining reliable and reproducible results. Drug doses were 2.5 or 5.0 mg/kg body weight, injected intravenously.

Tumor areas (usually 5×5 cm^2 or 7×7 cm^2 fields) were treated using a 5000-w xenon-arc lamp with the following filtration: 6 in. of circulating water, an infrared reflecting mirror, an infrared absorbing filter, and a red cutoff filter (Corning 2418). All filters were immersed in the water filter to prevent breakage. The spectrum emitted by this lamp occurred mainly between 600 and 700 nm, with approximately 25% in the range of Hpd absorption (620–640 nm). The maximum output was 100 mW/cm^2 for a 7-cm-diameter circle. Most exposures were carried out under these conditions. We could see no apparent difference between equivalent exposure doses, e.g., 20 min of exposure at 100 mW/cm^2 and 40 min at 50 mW/cm^2. However, no broader range was investigated. The eyes of patients were protected with dark goggles during the treatment and all patients were warned to remain out of bright sunlight indoors and outdoors for at least 30 days and to then cautiously test their reaction.

More recently, a laser has been used to deliver the activating light. Since light near 630 nm is required, in principle a HeNe laser could be used.

Unfortunately, while this may have limited application, the output of the largest commercially available HeNe laser is nominally rated at 50 mW. Therefore, in order to obtain the necessary power output, we have used a dye laser (rhodamine B dye) pumped by a 4- or 15-W argon laser. The laser is operated without the tuning wedge, which produces a maximum output near 635 nm. For most applications, the dye laser output is coupled to a low-loss quartz fiber (approximately 80% coupling efficiency) which allows the light to be delivered either externally or by insertion directly into the tissue through an 18-gauge or 20-gauge needle.

We determined the action spectrum for this system using response of the feet of albino mice to the combination of Hpd and light at various wavelengths (constant intensity). We found that there appears to be a maximum response at 631 nm, with wavelengths between 625 and 640 nm being nearly as effective. No response was found at 405, 620, or 647 nm, the latter corresponding to the major line in a krypton laser.

Since the spectral output from this system is considerably more narrow than that from the xenon-arc lamp, equivalent results are obtained with a lower radiation dose delivered to the tissue. While not defined exactly, it appears that a factor of one-half to one-third leads to similar effects, i.e., $30–50 \text{ mW}/\text{cm}^2 \times 20$ min for the laser yields similar biologic effects to 100 mW/cm^2 from the lamp for the same time period.

The initial clinical procedure was patterned after our animal experiments (9). Patients were injected intravenously with 5.0 mg/kg Hpd and 24 hr later exposed to the activating light from the 5000-W xenon-arc lamp described above. In the first few patients, the difficulties in extrapolating from animal data directly to humans were apparent. Thus, the skin of patients treated with the same type of lamp, at the same intensity and times, 24 hr following dye injection was found to become extensively necrosed, unlike that of the small animals. As indicated above, the serum clearance of Hpd varies markedly from smaller animals to humans (3 hr in mice vs. 24–30 hr in humans). Thus, in order to improve the resistance of the skin to the combination of Hpd and red light, we increased the time interval between drug injection and exposure to the therapeutic radiation, investigating periods from 1 to 12 days postinjection of 2.5 or 5.0 mg/kg Hpd. At the same time, the exposure times to the lamp were reduced from 60 to 20 min at an intensity of 50 or 100 mW/cm^2 incident on the skin. Since approximately 25% of the emitted spectrum corresponds to the Hpd absorption in the red, the effective intensities were 12.5 or 25 mW/cm^2.

Further, a test of skin reaction prior to treatment was carried out 3 or 4 days post Hpd injection with various exposure times to the lamp. Treatment to the tumor area was then based on the skin reaction judged 24 hr after treatment. An arbitrary scale of skin reaction from zero (no reaction) to 5.0 (complete necrosis) was devised. We found that a skin reaction of moderate erythema or moderate edema subsided within a week without excessive damage. Skin reactions leading to blanching or very heavy edema resulted in skin necrosis with resulting eschars and slow reepithelialization over 1–2 months. The major overall observation, however, was that tumor regression and necrosis could be obtained with acceptable skin reactions in many cases. However, if the skin was extensively involved with tumor, skin necrosis occurred over the area under all conditions that were therapeutically useful. Even in these cases, however, slow reepithelialization occurred over 4–6 weeks without complication. Also, areas of edema, such as in lymphedematous arms, retain Hpd longer than normal areas, resulting in enhanced skin reactions in those areas.

As indicated above, the tumors in this initial study were selected to demonstrate whether a tumor response could be obtained with a reasonable therapeutic ratio. We have studied 12 types of cutaneous and subcutaneous tumors listed in Table 23-1, including sarcomas and carcinomas. These data summarize results of 36 patients comprising over 200 individual treatments, since many patients had very extensive disease (e.g., chest wall recurrence of breast carcinoma) with different areas being treated under different conditions. The main parameters investigated were: time interval between Hpd injection and exposure to the red light, exposure time to the red light, radiation intensity ($D = I_0 t$; were D is the delivered light dose, I_0 is the light intensity incident at the surface of the skin over the tumor, and t is the time exposed to the therapeutic light). A summary of results is given in Table 23-2. In a few cases, single vs. multiple treatments were compared, as well as single vs. fractionated doses (Table 23-3). Drug dose was either 2.5 or 5.0 mg/kg body weight, with the latter generally used for larger tumors (>2 cm).

The major toxicity related to Hpd administration is photosensitivity of

Table 23-1. Tumor Response to Hpd Followed by Red Light

Tumor type	Complete response[a]	Partial response[b]	No response[c]	Total
Basal cell	2	1	—	3
Malignant melanoma	7	1	1	9
Chondrosarcoma	1	—	—	1
Colon adenocarcinoma	2	—	2	4
Prostate	1	1	—	1
Mycosis fungoides	2	1	—	3
Endometrial carcinoma	1	—	—	1
Breast carcinoma	7	2	—	9
Angiosarcoma	—	1	—	1
Squamous cell carcinoma	1	—	—	2
Kaposi sarcoma	—	1	—	1
Fibrosarcoma	—	1	—	1
Total	24	9	3	36

[a] One hundred percent destruction of measurable tumor within a treated field.
[b] Fifty percent or more destruction of tumor in treatment field and/or regrowth.
[c] No apparent reduction in tumor mass during period of observation, which varied from 1 week to 1 month.

Table 23-2. Summary of Photoradiation Conditions and Results[a]

Hpd dose, mg/kg	Interval Hpd treatment, hr	Light intensity, mW/cm²		Time of treatment min	Light dose[b] mW min/cm²	Skin response	Usual tumor response
		Lamp	Laser				
5.0	24	100	—	20	2000	Necrosis	Complete
	48	100	—	20	2000	Necrosis	Complete
	72	100	—	20	2000	Necrosis	Complete
	96	100	—	20	2000	Necrosis	Complete
	120	100	—	20	2000	Extensive reaction	Complete
	144	100	—	10	1000	Moderate to extensive erythema and edema	Complete
	192	100	—	20	2000	Moderate to extensive erythema and edema	Complete
2.5	24	100	—	20	2000	Necrosis	Complete
	48	100	—	20	2000	Necrosis	Complete
	72	100	—	20	2000	Moderate to extensive erythema and edema	Complete
	72	100	—	10	1000	Moderate erythema and edema	Complete
	72	—	60	20	1200	Moderate to extensive erythema and edema	—
	72	—	60	10	600	Moderate erythema and edema	—
	96	100	—	20	2000	Moderate erythema and edema	Complete
	96	—	60	20	1200	Moderate erythema and edema	Complete

96	—	30	20	600	Slight erythema and edema	Partial to complete (depending on depth)
120	100	—	20	2000	Slight to moderate erythema and edema	Partial to complete
120	—	60	20	1200	Slight to moderate erythema and edema	Partial to complete
144 168 192 }	100 or	60	20	1200–2000	Slight erythema and edema	Partial to complete
120–168	—	120	10	1200	Moderate erythema and edema	Partial to complete
120–168	—	120	20	2400	Moderate to extensive erythema and edema	Complete
192–240	—	120	20	2400	Slight to moderate erythema and edema	Partial to complete

[a] In all cases light was applied externally. Results are the usual result based on all patients to date. However, individual variations occur; some patients overrespond and some underrespond to treatment.

[b] Light dose $= I_0 t$, where I_0 is the incident light dose in mW/cm^2 and t is in minutes. In general, I_0 was varied over a range no greater than two.

Table 23-3. Effect of Treatment Fractionation on Tumor and Normal Tissue Response

Tumor	Hpd dose, mg/kg	Time to first fraction, hr	Number of fractions	Exposure time per fraction,[a] min	Time interval between fractions, hr	Skin response	Tumor response
Metastatic breast cancer[b]	2.5	48	6	3	24	Slight erythema	Partial
	2.5	72	3	5, 7, 8	24	Slight erythema	Complete
	2.5	96	2	10	24	Slight erythema	Complete
	2.5	120	1	20	—	Moderate erythema	Complete
	2.5	168	1	10	—	Moderate erythema	Complete
	2.5	96	3	6, 12, 18	24	Moderate erythema	Complete
Endometrial cancer	5.0	96	2	10	72	Moderate erythema	Complete
	5.0	168	1	20	—	Moderate erythema	Complete

[a] Light intensity was 50 or 100 mW/cm^2 full spectrum. Times refer to 100 mW/cm^2 equivalent (i.e., 10 min at 50 mW/cm^2 = 5 min at 100 mW/cm^2).
[b] The first six entries all refer to a single patient.

patients to sunlight for at least 30 days. This has not proven to be a serious problem, since most patients take care to stay out of direct sunlight (indoors and outdoors). Six patients developed moderate to severe edema of exposed areas upon exposure to sunlight within 30 days of Hpd administration. The exact length of photosensitivity is not known at present, although most patients receiving 2.5 mg/kg are no longer photosensitive at 30 days. However, large variations occur. One patient who remained moderately photosensitive for over three months and another who received such a severe reaction within a few days of injection that it could have been life threatening have been reported (D. King, unpublished results).

It should be noted that ulcerating lesions appeared to take up and retain more Hpd than others (judged from fluorescence) and reacted severely to the activating light, resulting in heavy eschars and considerable pain. While, in our hands, this has not led to perforation, the potential clearly exists and, in fact, has been reported by others (see below). We and others have not seen obvious differences in either tumor response or skin reaction in areas previously treated by ionizing radiation. If this result holds with time, this treatment may offer a therapy in many instances where radiotherapy cannot be repeated.

We found highly pigmented melanoma lesions to be particularly refractory to treatment due to absorption of the red light, but this can be overcome to a large extent by using higher intensities from the laser (e.g., 120 mW/cm^2 for 10–20 min) localized just to the lesion to avoid skin exposure.

Currently, we are aware of results from three other clinical centers studying photoradiation therapy whose experience, while similar to ours, adds certain other dimensions to the study and demonstrates the necessity of defining the numerous variables more completely. A group at the Rotterdam Radiotherapy Institute in Rotterdam, Holland, under A. Treurniet-Donker has examined six patients to date with recurrent breast carcinoma on the chest wall (unpublished results). They have used the laser system described above as an external light source in all cases. In general, their cases were rather severe, with most having ulcerating lesions. In one case, a chest wall perforation was caused by the treatment in an area previously very heavily irradiated. In general, these patients have had short-term tumor control, ranging from 3 to 7 months, and have experienced considerable difficulty from apparent over-treatment of the skin.

J. Kennedy, at the Ontario Cancer Foundation in Kingston, Ontario, has treated several very advanced cases of tumors of the head and neck region with very positive results (unpublished results). Using an Hpd preparation similar to that of Dougherty at 2.5 mg/kg and a dye–laser system, he has treated squamous cell tumors inside the skull in excess of 5-cm diameter by repeated exposures to the laser over a period of several weeks. The Hpd was injected several days prior to each laser treatment. Complete clearance of several very large tumors has been achieved.

I. Forbes, at the University of Adelaide in Australia, has treated several breast carcinoma recurrences on the chest wall with much the same results as found by Dougherty. He has used both an arc lamp system delivering 25 mW/cm^2 (620–640 nm) and a dye-laser system as described above. He has had excellent responses (still short observation time) for mycosis fungoides, a tumor type our group has found to be difficult to treat effectively without over-treatment. It is not clear why there is this difference. Forbes has advanced the field considerably by treating a malignant glioma by inserting the light fiber into the mass directly and by treating a peripheral lesion of the lung by inserting the fiber via a needle through the thoracic wall. Results of these cases are not known at present, although there have been no apparent adverse effects.

The potential of photoradiation is further indicated by experimental results using the interstitial implant of the light delivery fiber. In a joint program with R. Thoma, D.V.M., we have treated several primary tumors in pet cats and dogs with excellent results. To date we have treated three osteogenic sarcoma lesions. One of these, a 2.2 × 2.0 cm lesion in the mandible of a cat, was treated 3 days after administration of 5.0 mg/kg of Hpd by placing the fiber, via an 18-gauge needle, directly into the bone lesion. A total emitted intensity of 300 mW was used for 30 min in each of two locations in the tumor. Within 2 months an x-ray indicated essentially complete clearance of tumor with bone remodeling. The most recent x-ray, more than 2 years posttreatment, indicates no tumor. This animal continues to do well.

A second osteogenic sarcoma lesion, in a dog now 3 months post-treatment, appears at this time to be controlled. The third lesion, involving the tibia in a large dog, was more than 6 cm in diameter at the time of treatment, and could not be controlled even with repeated treatments.

Clearly, much needs to be done to adequately develop photoradiation as a conventional therapy for cancer. A great deal more needs to be known about light dosimetry in tissues, optimum drug dose, time interval, and single and fractionated treatment. However, the fact that it offers a therapy where other modalities have failed or are inappropriate should be sufficient to establish it as a new tool in cancer therapy.

Note Added in Proof: Since this article was written clinical reports have appeared for photoradiation treatment of lung cancer (Hayata, Y., Kato, H., Kanaka, C., Ono, J., and Takizawa, N., 1982, Hematoporphyrin derivative and laser photoradiation in the treatment of lung cancer, *Chest.* **81**:269–277); brain cancer (Laws, E. R., Cortese, D. A., Kinsey, J. H., Eagen, R. T., and Anderson, R. E., 1982, Photoradiation therapy in the treatment of malignant brain tumors: A phase I (feasibility) study *Neurosurgery* **9**:(6); 672–678); gynecological cancer (Ward, B. G., Forbes, I. J., Cowled, P. A., McEvoy, M. M., and Cox, L. W., 1982, The treatment of vaginal recurrences of gynecologic malignancy with phototherapy following hematoporphyrin derivative pretreatment, *Am. J. Obstet. Gynecol.* **142**:(3):356–357); and a variety of other tumors (Forbes, I. J., Cowled, P. A., Leong, A. S. Y., Ward, A. D., Block, R. B., Blake, A. J., and Jacka, F. J., 1980, Phototherapy of human tumours using hematoporphyrin derivative, *Med. J. Aust.* **2**:489–493).

REFERENCES

1. Jesionek, A., and Tappenier, V. H. (1903): Zur Behandlung des Hautcarcinomes mit fluoreszierenden Stoffen. *Munch. Med. Wochenschr.* **41**:2042–2044.
2. Kelly, J. F., and Snell, M. E. (1976): Hematoporphyrin derivative. A possible aid in the diagnosis and therapy of carcinoma of the bladder. *J. Urol.* **115**:150–151.
3. Dougherty, T. J. (1977): Phototherapy of human tumors. In: *Research in Photobiology*, edited by A. Castellani, pp. 435–446. Plenum Press, New York.
4. Dougherty, T. J., Kaufman, J., Goldfarb, A., et al. (1978): Photoradiation therapy for the treatment of malignant tumors. *Cancer Res.* **38**:2628–2635.
5. Dougherty, T. J., Lawrence, G., Kautman, J., et al. (1979): Photoradiation in the treatment of recurrent breast carcinoma. *J. Natl. Cancer Inst.* **62**:231–237.
6. Lipson, R., Baldes, E., and Olsen, A. (1961): The use of a derivative of hematoporphyrin in tumor detection. *J. Natl. Cancer Inst.* **26**:1–8.
7. Diamond, I., Granelli, S. G., McDonagh, A. F., et al. (1972): Photodynamic therapy of malignant tumors. *Lancet* **2**:1175–1177.
8. Dougherty, T. J. (1974): Activated dyes as anti-tumor agents. *J. Natl. Cancer Inst.* **52**:1133–1336.
9. Dougherty, T. J., Grindey, G. B., Fiel, R., et al. (1977): Photoradiation therapy II. Cure of animal tumors with hematoporphyrin and light. *J. Natl. Cancer Inst.* **55**:115–121.
10. Tomson, S. H., Emmett, E. A., and Fox, S. H. (1974): Photoradiation of mouse epithelial tumors after oral acridine orange and argon laser. *Cancer Res.* **34**:3124–3127.
11. Gomer, C. J., and Dougherty, T. J. (1979): Determination of [^{3}H]- and [^{14}C] hematoporphyrin derivative distribution in malignant and normal tissue. *Cancer Res.* **39**:146–151.
12. Gregorie, H. B., Horger, E. A., and Ward, J. (1968): Hematoporphyrin derivative fluorescence in malignant neoplasms. *Ann. Surg.* **167**:820–827.
13. Lipson, R. L., Baldes, E. J., and Olsen, A. M. (1964): Further evaluation of the use of hematoporphyrin derivative as a new aid for the endoscopic detection of malignant disease. *Dis. Chest* **46**:676–679.
14. Profio, A. E., and Dioron, D. R. (1977): A feasibility study of the use of fluorescence bronchoscopy for localization of small lung tumors. *Phys. Med. Biol.* **22**:949–957.
15. Dioron, D. R., Profio, A. E., Vincent, R. et al. (1979): Fluorescence bronchoscopy for detection of lung cancer. *Chest* **76**:27–32.
16. Kinsey, J. F., Cortese, D. A., and Sanderson, D. R. (1978). Detection of hematoporphyrin fluorescence during fiberoptic bronchoscopy of localize early bronchogenic carcinoma. *Mayo Clin. Proc.* **53**:594–600.
17. Oginsky, E. L., Green, G. S., Griffith, D. G., et al. (1959): Lethal photosensitization of bacteria with 8-methoxypsoralen to long wave length ultraviolet radiation. *J. Bacteriol.* **78**:821–833.
18. DeMol, N. J., and Beijersbergen Van Henegouwen, G. M. J. (1979): Formation of singlet molecular oxygen by 8-methoxypsoralen. *Photochem. Photobiol.* **30**:331–335.
19. Weishaupt, K. R., and Dougherty, T. J. (1976): Identification of singlet oxygen as the cytotoxic agent in photo-inactivation of a murine tumor. *Cancer Res.* **36**:2326–2329.

20. Moan, J., Pettersen, E. O., and Christensen, T. (1979): The mechanism of photodynamic inactivation of human cells *in-vitro* in the presence of hematoporphyrin. *Br. J. Cancer* **39**:398–409.
21. Kelly, J. F., Snell, M. E., and Berenbaum, M. (1975): Photodynamic destruction of human bladder carcinoma. *Br. J. Cancer* **31**:237–244.

Index